International Symposium on Fluorescein Angiography

Documenta Ophthalmologica
Proceedings Series volume 9

Editor H. E. Henkes

Dr. W. Junk bv Publishers The Hague 1976

International Symposium on Fluorescein Angiography Ghent 28 March-1 April 1976

Edited by J. J. De Laey

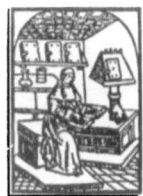

Dr. W. Junk bv Publishers The Hague 1976

ISBN-13: 978-90-6193-149-2   e-ISBN-13: 978-94-010-1573-8
DOI: 10.1007/978-94-010-1573-8

CONTENTS

Session VII – Retina III
Chairman – A. Wessing, Federal Republic of Germany
Moderator – S. Ryan, USA

PREFACE

This volume contains the papers presented at the International Symposium on Fluorescein Angiography held in Ghent, from 28 march to 1 april 1976, under the presidency of Prof. J. François.

The book has been divided in several chapters corresponding to the sessions of the meeting. The same order has been followed as for the presentation of the papers. The discussions, however, immediately follow the papers concerned. During the meeting complications of fluorescein angiography have been discussed; this part will be presented as a separate chapter at the end of the volume.

I wish to express my gratitude to all who contributed to this volume and to all the participants of ISFA-Ghent. I acknowledge also the cooperation of the publishers Dr. W. Junk, B.V.

J.J. De Laey, M.D.

EDITORIAL

We must be respectfully grateful to Her Majesty the Queen, who very kindly extended her high patronage to the International Symposium on Fluorescein Angiography.

Thanks to the chairmen and moderators of the various sessions, thanks to the invited speakers who have kindly presented reports with the conclusions of their research work, thanks also to the participants who brought interesting papers, this symposium on fluorescein angiography has been able to realize its purpose, which should be the aim of every scientific meeting, namely the better understanding and the elucidation of one or other complex and specific problem by the addition of new information to the data already known and by the discussion of recent viewpoints and interpretations, so that we know where we are exactly and from where we can start for further research and wider learning. If we want medicine to progress for the benefit of our patients, whose prophylactic or therapeutic treatment remains our primary concern, we can no longer be satisfied with purely clinical investigations, but we must also devote ourselves to basic and fundamental research. Since the discovery of the ophthalmoscope, fluorescein angiography, more than any other method of examination, has contributed to a better exploration of the eye fundus. This rather new science has known such an important development that ophthalmology is nowadays inconceivable without this technique. But the time has come to move from a pure clinical observation to a more fundamental physio-pathological analysis in order to obtain a more comprehensive pathogenesis of the disease we have to treat. In fact, our symposium which was attended by all the pioneers and experts in the field has revealed new and interesting contributions to stress any more the diagnostic and scientific value of fluorescein angiography.

Moreover, the scientific discussions as well as the human contacts during the meeting have consolidated and enlarged the ties of friendship between scientists of different countries throughout the world for the greatest benefit of science, humanity and peace.

Prof. Jules François

Organizing Committee:
    President: J. François
    Secretary: J.J. De Laey
    Members: P. Amalric, A.C. Bird, A.F. Deutman, E. Norton, J.A. Oosterhuis, K. Shimizu, A. Wessing.

PHOTOGRAPHY WITH CORNEAL CONTACT FUNDUS CAMERAS

LEE ALLEN & OGDEN FRAZIER

(Iowa City, USA)

Conventional fundus cameras, having an air lens between the cornea and front lens of the camera, are usually limited in the area of fundus which can be encompassed to 30 or 35 degrees. Collages are required to show larger areas in single illustrations.

The 100° camera of Pomerantzeff and Govignon eliminates the air lens by applying a special contact lens on the cornea of the subject eye. A capillary film of tears or viscous methylcellulose solution creates optical continuity.

We have one of the early models of the corneal contact camera produced by Govignon and associates and have practiced and developed techniques which we expect to improve upon in the future (Figure 1).

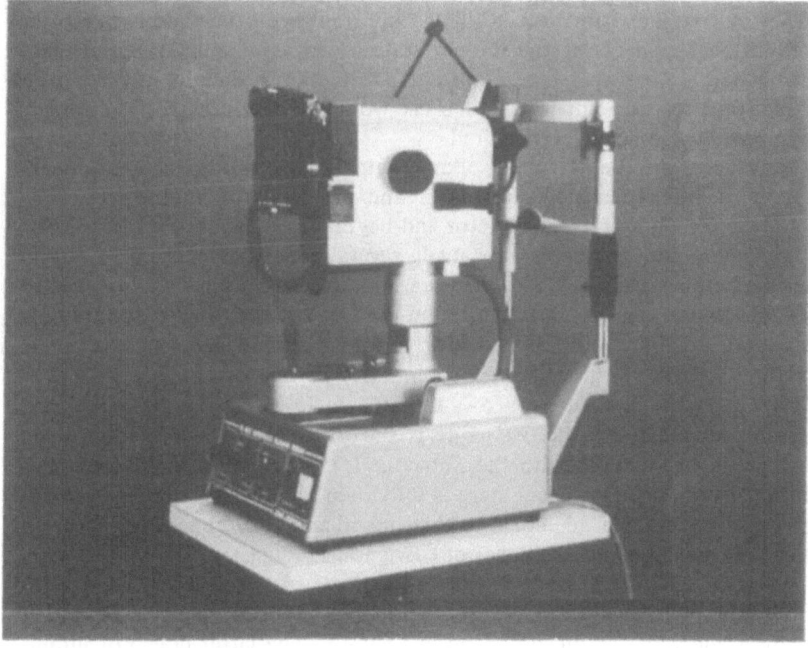

Fig. 1. Photographing ocular fundus of rhesus monkey with corneal contact fundus camera of Govignon and associates.

1

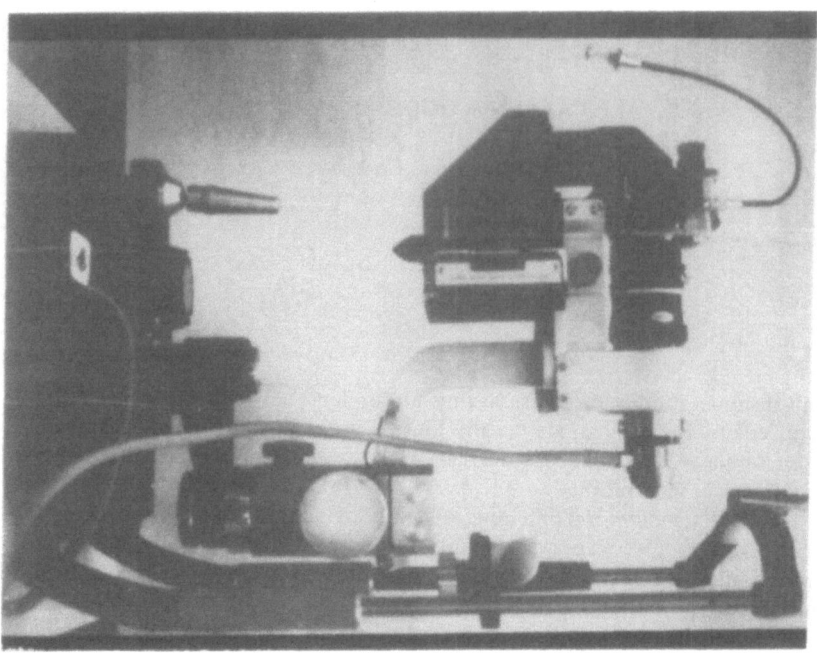

Fig. 2. Pomerantzeff's 'Equator-Plus' camera.

We believe such cameras can fill an important need. They do not displace conventional cameras at the present stage of development but supplement them. Because of this, their present shortcomings should not be over-emphasized to the point where their use would be discouraged and attempts to improve them might be impaired.

Advances are being made. Pomerantzeff has modified the camera (Figure 2) and redesigned the optics and principles of illumination (Figure 3) to photograph to the equator and beyond as shown in Figure 4.

Govignon and associates have made several variations in optics and principles of illumination. These changes are integrated within units referred to as cones which can be interchanged on the front of the camera. We are now using two different 100° cones with different illuminating systems, a 60° and a 30° cone. A photograph taken through one of the 100° cones is shown in Figure 5. Figure 6 shows the area enclosed by the 60° cone, and the area included by the 30° cone is shown in Figure 7. We believe the quality of the pictures with the 30° cone is equivalent to those with con-ventional cameras. However, there is a limit to the distance into the periph-ery possible with the 30° cone, so that the 60 and 100° cones may prove to be the most valuable of the cones of Govignon's design.

Each of the interchangable cones has its own specially-designed fiber optics illuminating system. That for the present 100° cone is shown in Figure 8 and that for the 60° cone in Figure 9. The latter does not illumi-nate as much tissue intervening between the choroid-retina structures and the effective optical exit pupil in the anterior segment of the eye as the

2

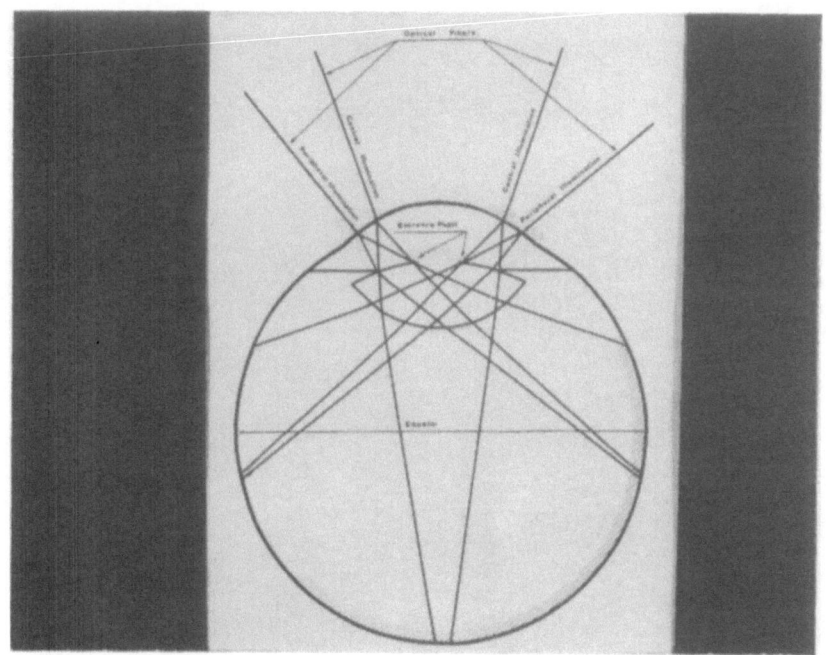

Fig. 3. Illumination principle of 'Equator-Plus' camera.

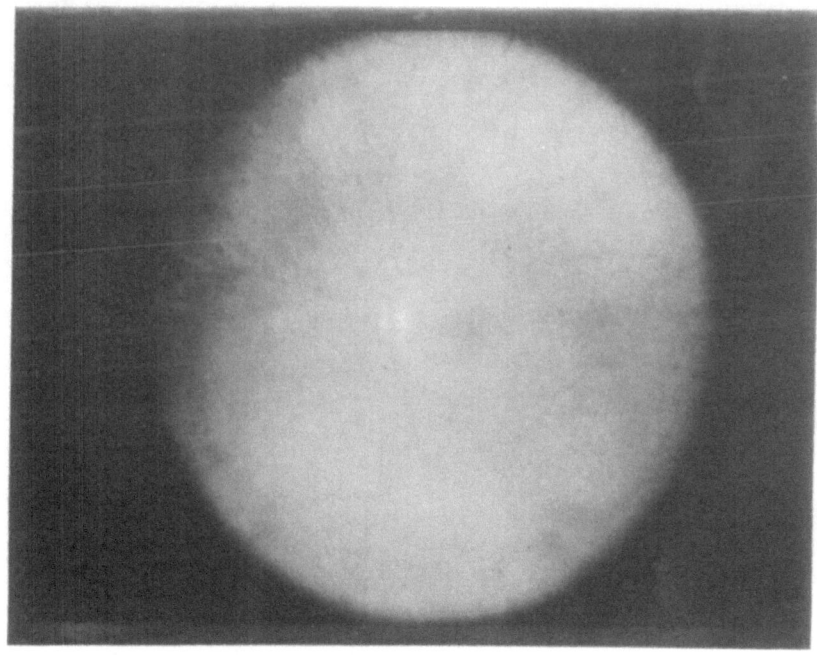

Fig. 4. Black and white copy of 'Equator-Plus' photograph.

3

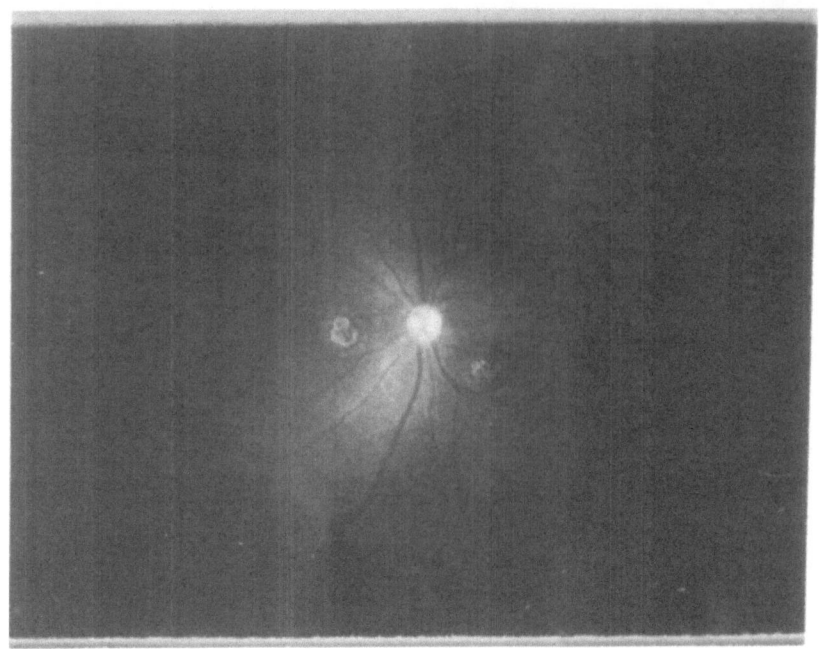

Fig. 5. Copy of a photograph taken with the 100° cone of Govignon.

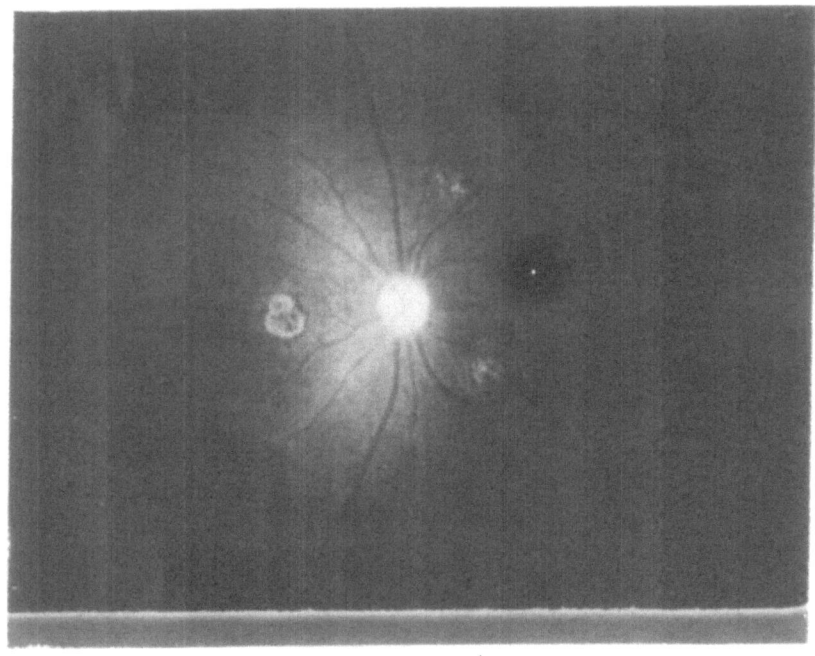

Fig. 6. Copy of a photograph taken with Govignon's 60° cone.

4

former. Thus, less umwanted reflected and dispersed light reaches the camera to 'fog' the film.

We are told a major advance in design of a 100-110° cone is in progress. We can expect continued improvement in quality of photographs with newer designs. Potentially, the large area cameras could quickly and easily map the fundus preliminary to retinal detachment surgery or other procedures. The time needed by the surgeon to draw the map of the fundus could be reduced to a minimum, applied mainly in the far periphery.

In that regard, miniaturation of the image to stay within the 24 mm vertical opening of the 35 mm film format may present a problem in recording small details. Perhaps considerable thought might be given to recording on larger films or paper.

It is not difficult to make good stereograms with the corneal contact cameras. The pupil of the subject eye must be dilated as widely as possible: 8 mm or more. A highly transparent gel-like methylcellulose solution* maintains optical continuity between the surfaces of cornea and cone even when they are tilted away from each other on one side.

The direction of gaze must be established and held with the fixation light before the companion eye. Great care must be taken with present cameras to not abrade the cornea with rapid movement and too much pressure. The feature of interest is framed as desired in the viewfinder and the image sharply focused.

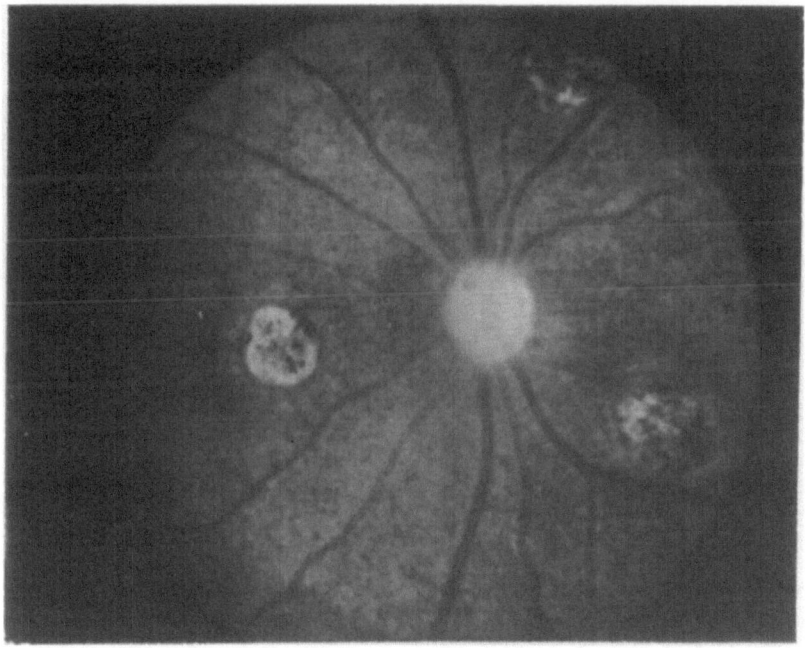

Fig. 7. Copy of a photograph taken with Govignon's 30° cone.

* Gonio-Gel, 2-1/2%, 4000 cps, Muro Pharmacal Laboratories, Inc., Quincy, Massachusetts 02169 U.S.A.

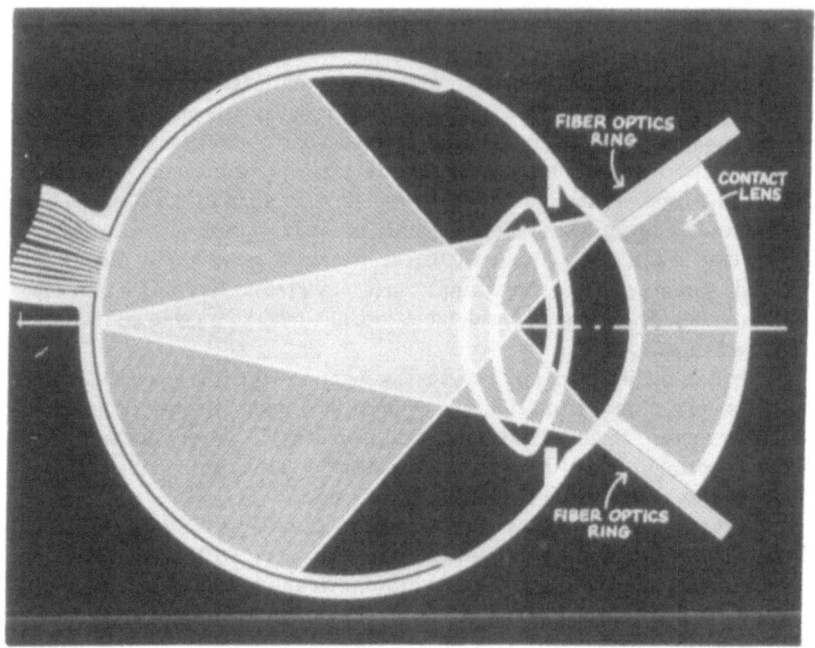

Fig. 8. Diagram of principle of illumination in present 100° cone.

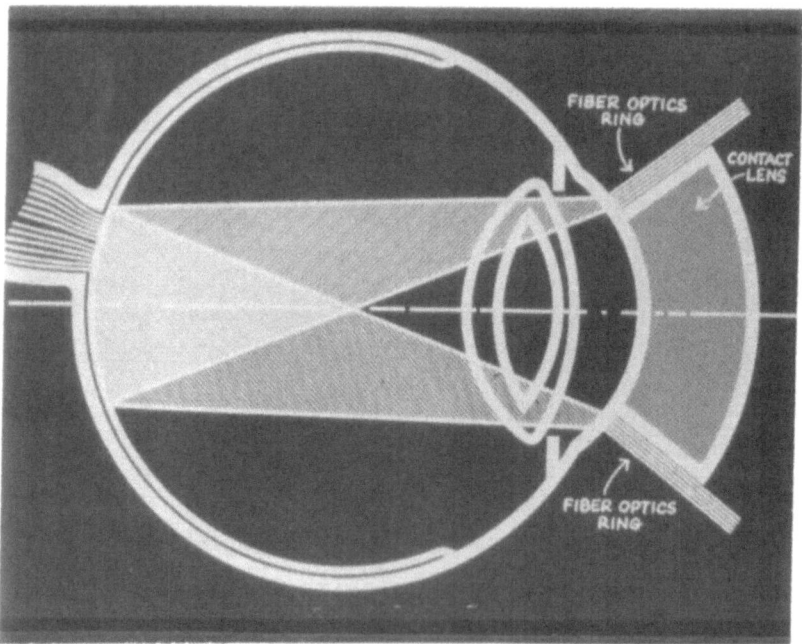

Fig. 9. Diagram of principle of illumination in 60° cone.

To create the stereoscopic effect, two pictures are taken from different vantage points. The camera is shifted by the joy stick approximately 1-1/2 mm to the left maintaining the optical continuity through the gel-like solution. The image is focused and the photographic exposure made for the left frame of the stereo pair. Next, the camera is shifted by the joy stick about 3 mm to the right (1-1/2 mm to the right of the original central corneal position), again maintaining optical continuity. The image is refocused if necessary and the exposure made for the right frame of the stereo pair.

It is not necessary to limit either single frame photography or stereography to the central fundus. The subject eye can be diverted several degrees into eccentric positions if the subject's pupil is large enough. In many cases one edge of the picture may be shadowed, but details can be seen extending gradually into the shadow. The aesthetic loss in more than counterbalanced by the information recorded. If optical continuity is broken on one side of the cornea, it can be reestablished by adding more of the viscous methylcellulose with the camera in place.

Our experiences with one corneal contact fundus camera and different interchangable cones for achieving different amounts of area of view, consideration of their values and estimates of potential value of improved types have been reported. Advantages of large area pictures over collages from conventional cameras have been mentioned. Our best method for making stereograms has been outlined briefly.

REFERENCES

POMERANTZEFF O. & GOVIGNON, J. Design of a wide-angle ophthalmoscope. *Arch. Ophthal.* 86: *420-424* (1971).

POMERANTZEFF, O. Equator-plus camera. *Invest. Ophthalmol.* 14 (5): *401-406* (1975).

GOVIGNON, J. Design of 60° and 30° cones and variations on illuminating systems. (Personal communication)

Authors's address:
Department of Ophthalmology
The University of Iowa
Iowa City, Iowa 52242
USA

CLINICAL TRIALS WITH THE 'EQUATOR-PLUS' CAMERA

OLEG POMERANTZEFF, D. ENG.

(Boston, Mass., USA)

Fig. 1. shows the extent of the field of view provided by the Equator Plus camera. The most valuable information that this camera makes available to the clinician is the overall view of the pathology in the fundus, the localization of large pathological structures in relation to the disk or macula and the comparison of coloration in large areas of the fundus.

Before I begin the main part of this presentation, which is on wide angle angiography, I would like to discuss two of the problem areas we have encountered while working in the general field of wide angle photography. While it is easier to document these problems in relation to wide angle photography, these two problems also affect the techniques in wide angle angiography.

The first and certainly most important of these problems results from the fact that in some patients, particularly diabetics, the pupil is often too small to use direct illumination. Direct illumination means that the light is introduced through fibers in contact with the peripheral cornea.

The second problem stems from the fact that in some patients the media, and particularly the crystalline lens, contain light scattering opacities.

Transillumination, introduced through fibers applied to the sclera at the pars plana, avoids the obstacles posed by both types of problems.

Fig. 2 shows a computer ray plot. Three rays have been traced from several selected points in the retina through the whole system formed by the observed eye, the contact lens, and the system forming field lenses. This system has been calculated so that all the plotted bundles are passing through a 1.8 mm pupil located in the pupillary plane of the observed eye. This diagram shows that the entire fundus can be observed through such a small pupil.

The wide angle photograph in Fig. 1 has been taken through a pupil of 3 mm in diameter.

Transillumination is also a great asset in cases where there are opacities in the crystalline lens. The reason for this is that the light crosses the lens only one time on its way back from the fundus to the camera and consequently there is less stray light in the observation system.

The ocular layers crossed by the transilluminating light constitute a physiological optical filter which substantially changes the spectral content of that light inside the globe. A fundus photograph of a patient taken by direct illumination through a filter extending from 535 nm to 635 nm,

9

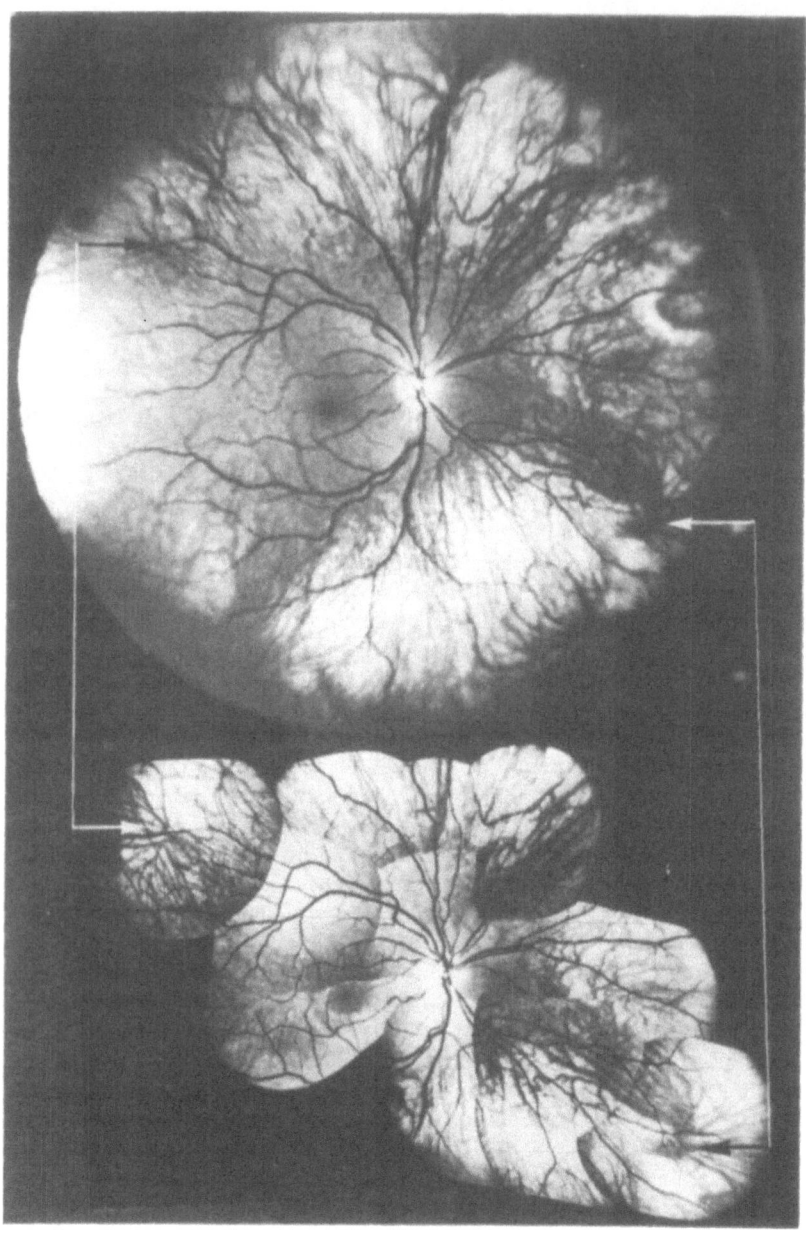

Fig. 1. The composite picture is made of 20 frames taken with the Zeiss fundus camera. The arrows point the corresponding vortex ampulae in both pictures. The field of the composite picture represents approximately one fourth of the field in the wide angle photograph and can hardly be extended beyond these limits.

10

which appears green by transillumination shows a greenish colored fundus. The fundus of the fellow eye of the same patient photographed using the same filter but by transillumination appears red. This change of color in the fundus is due to the spectral filtering by the physiological filter. The spectral characteristics of the physiological filter depend on the peripheral pigmentation of the eye. Using the same filter on two different eyes, one which is lightly pigmented and the other which is rather darkly pigmented, we obtain two distinct pictures. The lightly pigmented eye appears yellowish and shows the retinal vascularization. The darkly pigmented eye appears red and the choroidal vascularization can be seen more clearly than in the lightly pigmented eye. However, this difference in the appearance of the fundus can be controlled by changing the exposure of the film.

Progressive increase of exposure time results in progressive changes from deep red to orange and to yellow.

Fluorescein angiography by direct illumination does not present any special difficulties.

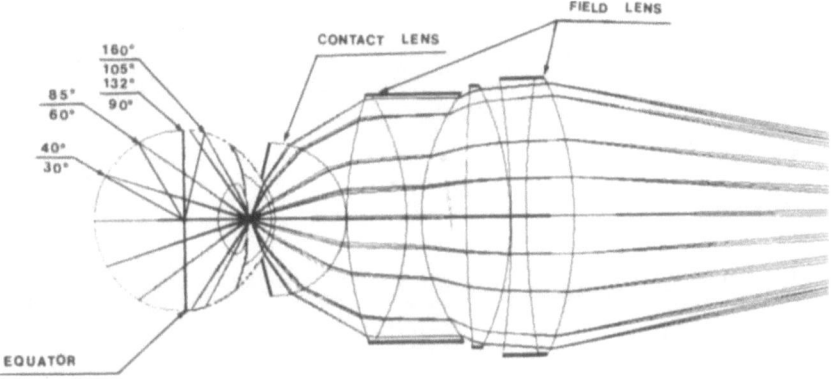

Fig. 2. Computer ray plotting of three ray bundles traced from different points in the fundus. All bundles pass through a 1.8 mm pupil in the pupillary plane.

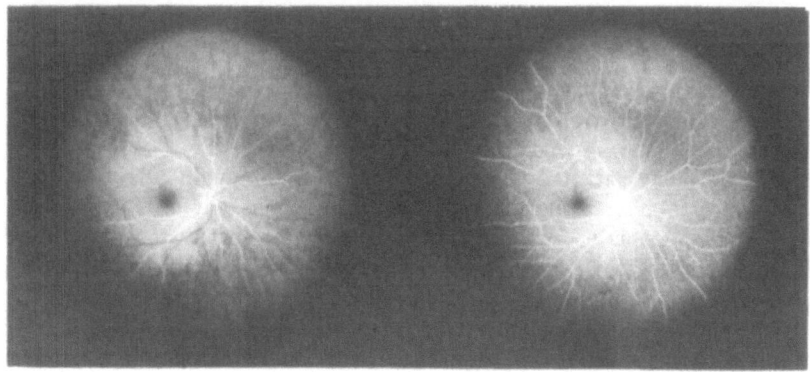

Fig. 3. Fluorescein angiogram by direct illumination. Arterial and venous phases.

11

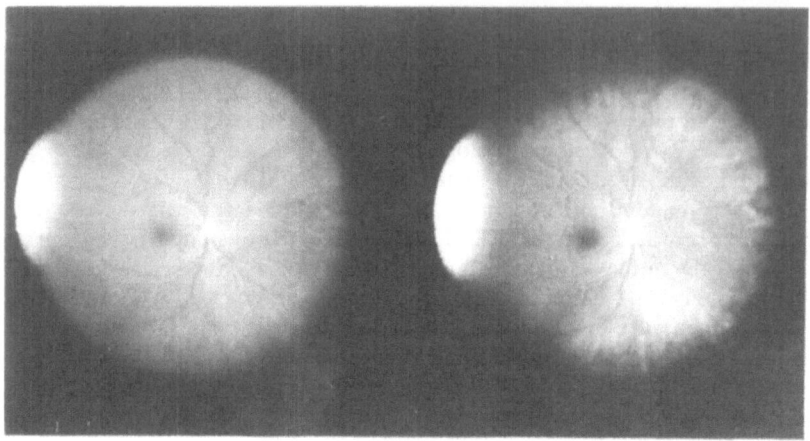

Fig. 4. Fluorescein angiogram by transillumination using SE 40 and SB 50 filters. Arterial and later phase.

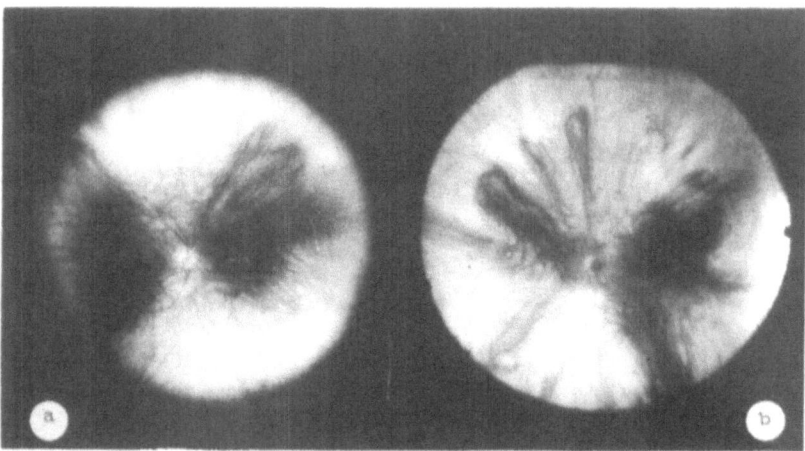

Fig. 5. Cardiogreen (ICG) angiograms; (a) by direct illumination; (b) by transillumination.

Fig. 3 shows two phases (arterial and venous) from a sequence of fluorescein filling using the direct illumination system.

Because many patients have a small pupil, transillumination is also desirable in angiography. Transillumination with the commonly used excitation filter is not possible because too little of these wavelengths are transmitted by the physiological filter. The excitation must be pushed toward the longer wavelengths. By doing so, some efficiency is lost but more light penetrates into the globe.

Fig. 4 shows phases of fluorescein filling using transillumination and using the Delori SE 40 and SB 50 filters. The vessels filled with fluorescein appear to be elevated on the retina. This appearance is due to the fact that

12

the excitation light is incident sideways and fluorescein is emitted laterally. In later phases, the background is seen in more detail but the contrast of the retinal vessels is reduced. This is caused by the fact that the excitation light that is crossing the physiological filter which is partially constituted by blood, strongly excites fluorescence emitted in the direction of the fundus and the latter is illuminated partly in yellow.

Since cardiogreen (ICG) angiography is also a valuable clinical tool, I worked out a technique for wide angle cardiogreen angiography. As you know this angiography can be performed by absorption or by fluorescence. Fig. 5a shows one frame of ICG angiography by absorption using the direct illumination. In this technique the vessels which are filled with the dye appear white on negative and black on positive. Therefore the appearance of the negatives looks more like the conventional fluorescein angiogram, whereas in the prints of Fig. 5 the contrast is reversed.

Fig. 5b shows one frame from a filling sequence of ICG using the transillumination technique. Since the excitation light is red it crosses the physiological filter easily.

ACKNOWLEDGEMENTS

From the Department of Retina Research of the Eye Research Institute of Retina Foundation, Boston, Massachusetts. This work was supported by Public Health Service Research Grant EY-00227 from the National Eye Institute, National Institutes of Health, by United States Army Grant DADA 17-73-c-1344 and by the Massachusetts Lions Eye Research Fund, Inc.

We wish to express our gratitude to Miss Julianne Schneider for her technical assistance and particularly for her volunteering as a patient throughout this study.

Author's address:
Eye Research Institute of Retina Foundation
20 Staniford Street
Boston, Mass. 02114
USA

DISCUSSION

Dr Amalric: Je voudrais revenir sur les présentations qui ont été faites concernant la rétinographie grand angle. Depuis 3 ans j'utilise le rétinographe grand angle. Aussi, ai-je été particulièrement impressionné par les photos de Mr Pomerantzeff. Je pense que la rétinographie grand angle est magnifique pour la choroïde jusqu'à la périphérie, surtout si l'on fait une diaphanoscopie transclérale pour illuminer cette zone. Mais les essais qui ont été faits jusqu'à ce jour au point de vue angiographique sont malgré tout souvent décevants, surtout dans les premiers temps de l'angiographie, parce qu'au temps artériel l'imprégnation est extrêmement réduite et le colorant ne va pas jusqu'à la périphérie. C'est dire que si avec le procédé de Mr Pomerantzeff on utilise en même temps une diaphanoscopie transclérale, j'ai peur que l'angiographie ne puisse donner que des résultats imparfaits. Mais je suis en admiration devant les documents de l'extrême périphérie qu'il nous a présentés.

Mr Pomerantzeff: I think the wide angle angiography gives the same advantages and shows the same drawbacks as the wide angle retinoscopy, that is: it can provide the evidence of a peripheral leak when the conventional angiography shows a normal appearance of the posterior pole. The photographic quality of contrast and resolution is evidently better in the conventional angiogram. It is obvious that for the angiography the best system of illumination is direct illumination and not the transscleral illumination. However, there is the problem of pupil dilatation. The patients very seldom present sufficiently wide pupils, and therefore, the transscleral illumination in angiography is a way of overcoming this and getting something. I have tried cardiogreen angiography with which transillumination is very easy and gives you a very good picture of the choroidal vascularization. By direct illumination you can get some of the retinal vascularization.

HIGH SPEED FLUOROGRAPHY

W.M. HAINING

(Dundee, Scotland)

The essential requirement for rapid sequential fluorography is the ability to record the passage of fluorescein through choroidal and retinal circulations. A method of high speed fluorography has been previously described and the practical advantages of stroboscopic rather than continuous light source illumination have been stressed, HAINING (1974). These advantages are the 'freezing' of micro saccadic ocular movement with consequent absence of any frame blurring in the movie record; and the additional safety factor of preventing retinal overheating, which is of great importance when performing continuous filming of repeated small volume dye injectates. The energy levels employed are from 3.0 to 4.0 joules for pulse rates of up to 80 per second. The electronic circuitry of the first power pack has now been modified to give 200 flashes per second, although at reduced pulse energies. The original optical modification of the standard Zeiss-Littman fundus camera by the insertion of a special prismospherical lens or 'axicon' remains unchanged, making it possible to utilize a rapid re-cycling uncooled short arc flash tube, giving the required improvement of camera efficiency for ultra high speed fluorography. The 'Doiflex' 16 mm cine camera back with electronic synchronization permits filming speeds of up to 40 frames per second, but is unsuitable for the higher filming speeds (200 frames per second). The filter system has been changed to incorporate a 'Barr and Stroud', blue band pass exciter filter type DB1, with a type DB2 barrier filter, also manufactured by Barr and Stroud, Ltd., Glasgow, Scotland.

High speed fluorography is carried out as an out-patient procedure using 5 ml sodium fluorescein (20%) by intravenous injection, or intra-arterial catheter injection of 1.ml of 20% sodium fluorescein, performed in conjunction with concurrent radiological arteriography. Patients have the same tolerance to high frequency flashing as in standard fluorography and premedication of 5 mgm Diazepam is given only where necessary and for repeated runs.

The optimal film characteristics are obtained from 16 mm Kodak Plus-X Reversal film (125 ASA) when processed using Ilford Ilfodata microfilm developer diluted 1 : 3 at 37°, with Ilford Hypam rapid fixer and hardener, give results which cannot be improved upon. The processed film, which is reeled off dry from a modified Cordell 240 Film Processing Machine can be viewed immediately on an 'Analector' variable speed analytical projector. Dry negative film can therefore be evaluated within a few minutes

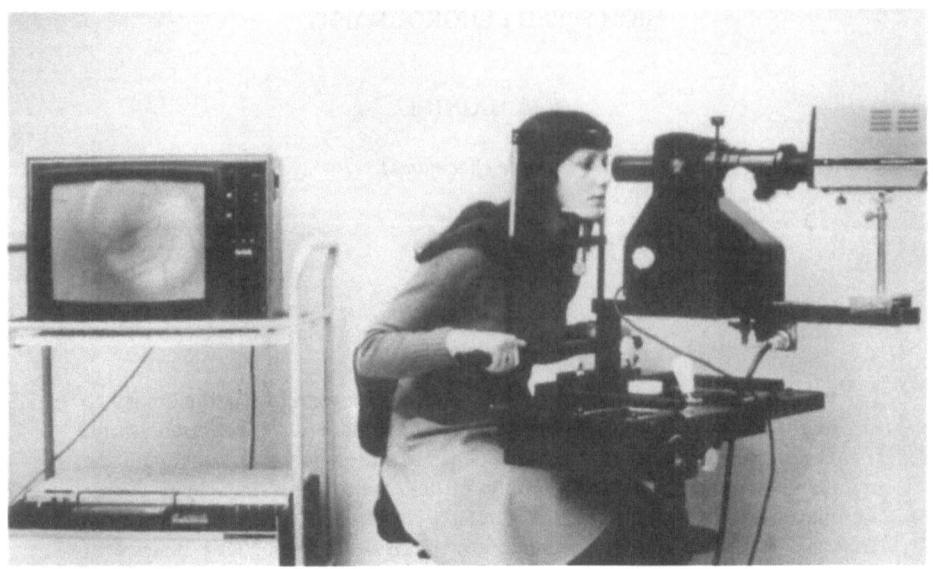

Fig. 1. Colour T.V. System

of completing photography, and a rapid clinical report given to the referring ophthalmologist.

TELEVISION SYSTEMS

Direct visualization of the dye transit on a monochrome video monitor with simultaneous video tape recording of the event provides an alternative approach to cine fluorography. The use of television in fluorescein angiography has been described by LEVERETT et al. (1970) and VAN HEUVEN & SCHAFFER (1973). Existing television camera systems utilize continuous low light level illumination with consequent patient acceptability, but at the same time give recording resolution theoretically equivalent to Kodak TRI-X film (ASA 400), or better depending on the quality of T.V. system. VAN HEUVEN has suggested that a stroboscopic light source would improve the quality of video recording for the same reason as in cinefluorography. We have therefore modified our camera system to introduce the alternative use of a television camera. It seemed logical to use colour rather than monochrome television in order to view and record the fundus in colour immediately prior to carrying out fluorography.

MATERIALS AND METHODS

A simple inexpensive Hitachi Shibadan single gun colour T.V. camera was chosen and the strobe unit electronically synchronized to the vertical retrace frequency. The strobe pulse duration (1/5 ms) was easily recorded without overlap on successive scans (Fig. 1). The vertical scan rate gives an equivalent framing speed of 50 per second, i.e., 10 frames per second faster than in

16

cine fluorography. The camera signal was fed into a Sony colour monitor (Fig. 1) and recorded on $\frac{3}{4}''$ cassette video tape through a Sony U-Matic video recorder with an upper resolution limit of 5 M Hz. It is considerably more economical to record, and easier to retrieve, fluorographic data from cassette video tape than from stored cine film.

The quality of fluorographic recording on colour video tape does not, however, compare favourably with the standard of resolution obtainable from cine fluorography. For this reason, we intend using colour video for standard clinical investigation, whilst reserving cine fluorography for cases of special interest and for clinical research.

ACKNOWLEDGEMENTS

This work was supported by the W.H. Ross Foundation (Scotland) for the Study and Prevention of Blindness. I am indebted to Mr. R. Rimmer, Department Medical Physics, Ninewells Hospital and Medical School, Dundee, for his help in electronic development, and to Mr. F.M. Duncan and Miss Angela Sinclair for their technical assistance.

REFERENCES

HAINING, W.M. Recent advances in the technical aspects of fluorescein angiography. International Clinics Series: *15-29* (1974)

LEVERETT, S.D., JR., BAILEY, P.F., HOLDEN, G.T. & CHEEK, R.J. Fundus cinephotography during gravitational stress. *Arch. Ophthalmol.* 832 (2): *223* (1970).

VAN HEUVEN, W.A.J. & SCHAFFER, C. Advances in televised fluorescein angiography. Presented at the International Symposium of Fluorescein Angiography, Tokyo. In: Fluorescein Angiography, Tokyo: *10-14*. Igaku Shoin (1973).

Author's address:
Ninewells Hospital and Medical School
Dundee DD2 1UB, Scotland

ADVANCES IN TV-FLUORANGIOGRAPHY*

STEPHEN S. FEMAN, M.D., CHARLES SCHAFFER &
WICHARD A.J. VAN HEUVEN, M.D.

(Albany, New York)

For the past seven years, our laboratory has used electronic recording systems with fluorescein angiography. This technique creates a permanent, accurate and immediately available reproduction of the dynamic aspects of retinal vascular flow. The resulting television picture is of value for both the recording of clinical disorders as well as for basic research.

Generally, most angiograms consist of serial photographs. In our studies of blood flow dynamics, serial photography was inadequate to measure the rapid phase of dye transit. For this reason, we were willing to sacrifice the excellence of still photography in order to obtain more data about active physiologic processes.

THE FIRST MODEL (1968)

In theory, this model was quite complex (VAN HEUVEN et al., 1971); it combined an image orthicon television camera, a videotape recording machine, and a Zeiss fundus camera (Fig. 1A). This system emphasized patient safety and reduced cost.

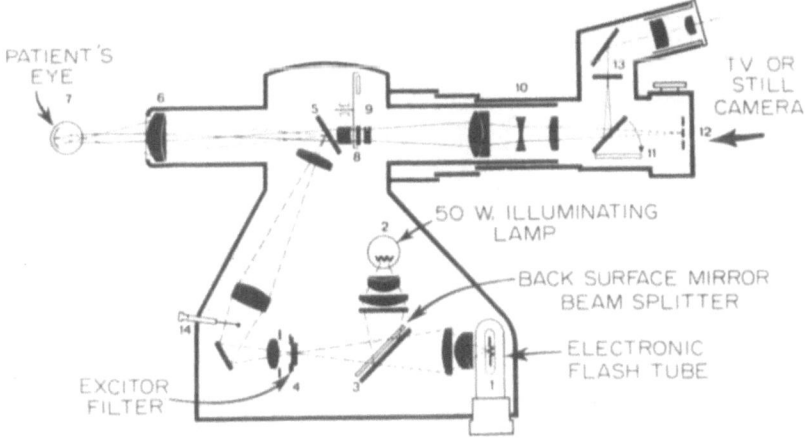

* This work is supported by National Institutes of Health Grant number 2R01 EY00791-05.

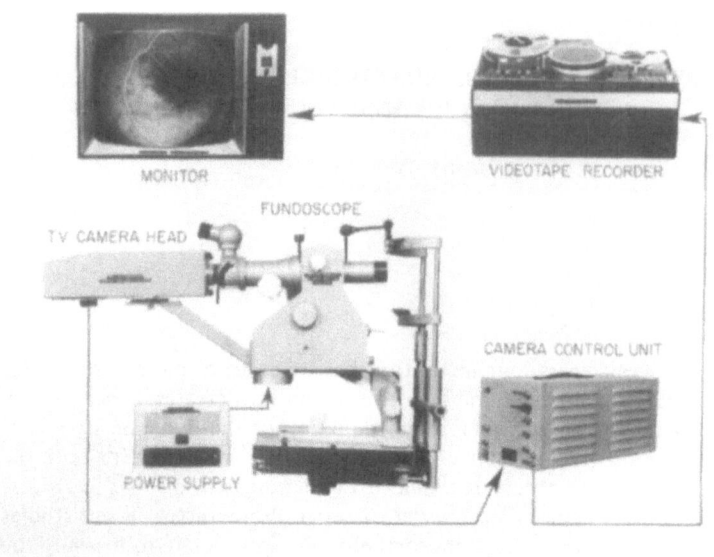

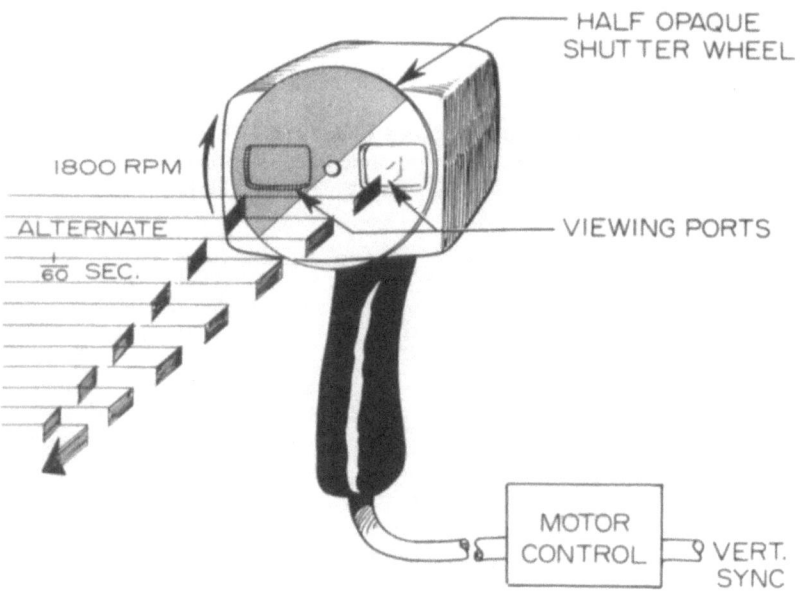

The 50 watt incandescent bulb of the Zeiss camera background illuminating system was its only light source (Fig. 1B). The flash tube was not used; and the beam splitter was replaced by a totally reflecting surface mirror. A special bearing was built on to the fundus camera to counteract the weight of the TV camera.

20

The photocathode of the image orthicon was adjusted to lie in the same plane that had been occupied by the camera film. The picture satisfied American television standards; that is, 60 fields per second, with 525 lines and 30 frames interlaced. The resulting composite signal was recorded on one inch videotape, and could be viewed immediately on a television screen or stored for later study.

EXPERIMENTAL MODIFICATIONS (1969-1972)

In this period various camera tubes were tried — image isocon, secondary electron conduction, silicon matrix, and silicon intensifier target types. Those of adequate sensitivity were too expensive, or too critical in their operation. Others were not sensitive enough, had excessive image retention, or were too noisy.

Stereoscopic television imagery was investigated but suffered from operational complexity (Fig. 2) (VAN HEUVEN & SCHAFFER, 1973; VAN HEUVEN et al., 1974).

By utilizing low-level repetitive flash synchronized to the field frequency we have been able to reduce image blur. This blur was produced by the

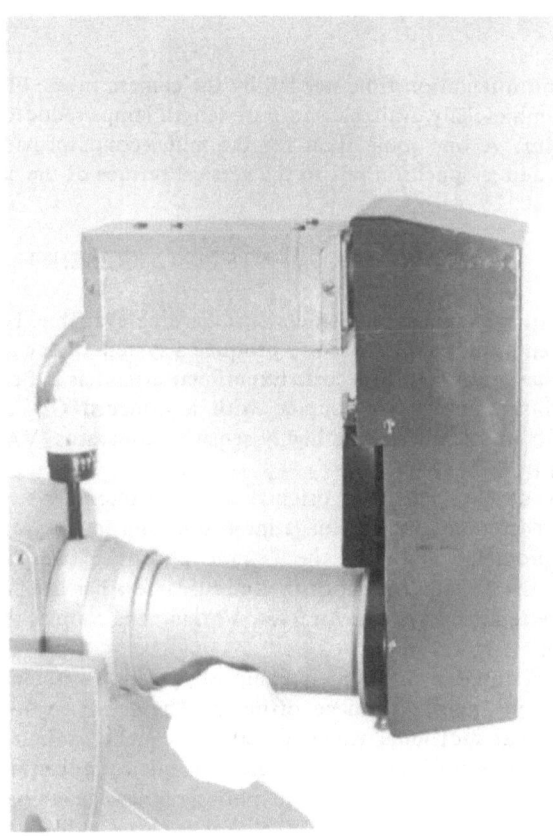

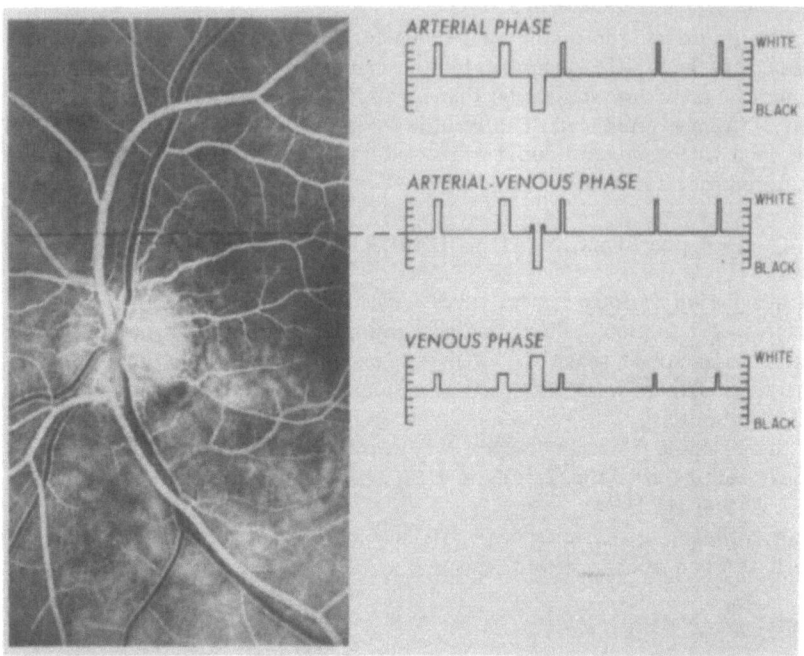

16 millisecond integration time needed by the camera tubes. Flash illumination using commercially available short arc length lamps reduced the integration time blur. A one joule flash for 0.5 milliseconds provides adequate illumination and is synchronized to the vertical retrace of the camera (VAN HEUVEN et al., 1974).

RECENT DEVELOPMENTS (1972-PRESENT)

In 1972, multistage image intensifiers first became available. Now commercial components can be purchased to produce a system of adequate sensitivity, simple operation, and low cost. Experimentation has indicated that the RCA 4550 image intensifier coupled with a Concord CTC 33 television camera results in a low cost, and highly sensitive apparatus (VAN HEUVEN & SCHAFFER, 1974).

With this development, the original image orthicon system has been replaced by a combination of image intensifier and image vidicon camera. The major problem of joining the 18 mm. photosensitive surface of the intensifier to the 35 mm. format of the funduscamera has been overcome by an image size reducing system. An f 1.4, 17 mm. lens couples the intensifier to the vidicon.

This has resulted in a simpler, compact system. It is ten times more sensitive to light than the image orthicon. The signal to noise ratio has improved so that individual videotape frames can be examined. The electronic components no longer need individual critical adjustments and the picture is brought to focus by the photographer-cameraman using the control stick of the standard Zeiss camera.

In 1974 and 1975 the intensifier-vidicon system was mechanically modified to mount above the fundus camera (Fig. 3). This has resulted in a low cost, compact, TV unit that is designed to fit most existing fundus cameras.

The performance of the improved TV system now permits the study of dye dillution curves of the retinal vessels. This is achieved by applying photoelectric sensors to the TV monitor. At present, attempts are being made to quantify regionally localized retinal flow (Fig. 4).

FUTURE DEVELOPMENTS

Solid state imaging devices are now being examined. Integrally coupling the intensifier to a charge coupled device (CCD) or a charge injected device (CID) should permit direct computer processing of image information and a better understanding of retinal vascular dynamics.

REFERENCES

VAN HEUVEN, W.A.J., SCHAFFER, C.A. & MEHU, M. The use of low light level television in fundus imaging. *Mod. Probl. Ophthal.* 9: *9-16* (1971).

VAN HEUVEN, W.A.J. & SCHAFFER, C.A. Advances in televised fluorescein angiography. Fluorescein Angiography. Tokyo: *10-14*. Igaku Shoin (1973).

VAN HEUVEN, W.A.J., SCHAFFER, C.A. & MEHU, M. The evolution of electronic recording systems for fluorescein angiography. Regina Congress. Pruett, R.C. & Regan, C.D.J. (eds.). New York, Appleton-Century-Crofts: *173-180* (1974).

VAN HEUVEN, W.A.J. & SCHAFFER, C.A. Electronic imaging systems for fluorescein angiography. International Ophthalmology Clinics 14: *31-47* (1974).

Authors' address:
Retina Offices
Department of Ophthalmology
Albany Medical College
Albany, New York 12208
USA

Address reprint requests to:
Dr Stephen S. Feman
Retina Offices
Department of Ophthalmology
Albany Medical College
Albany, New York 12208
USA

IMPROVED INTERFERENCE FILTERS FOR
FLUORESCEIN ANGIOGRAPHY

F.C. DELORI & I. BEN-SIRA

(Boston, USA)

The filter combinations presently used for fluorescein angiography of the ocular fundus were selected on the basis of the fluorescence characteristics of sodium fluorescein in aqueous solution (WESSING 1969) or sodium fluorescein diluted in blood (HODGE 1966, HAINING 1968). The excitation filter usually transmits wavelengths below approximatively 500 nm; the barrier filter those above 500 nm. In recent years efforts were directed towards improving the transmission of the filters while consistently keeping a wavelength between 490 and 500 nm as the separation between the spectral ranges of excitation and emission (HODGE 1966, HAINING 1968, ALLEN 1972, ZONDIROS 1974). Recently a filter combination with separation wavelength at 505 nm was proposed and evaluated by WESSING (1974).

The excitation and emission spectra of fluorescein dye during its transit in the human ocular circulation were recently determined (DELORI 1975). Both spectra were found to be markedly shifted towards the longer wavelengths relative to the spectra of fluorescein in aqueous solution. The shift towards a longer wavelength of the excitation and emission spectra is most pronounced in the fovea and decreases for the choroidal background and even more for the retinal vessels.

Maximal fluorescence emission is achieved by matching the transmission bands of the filter combination with the excitation and emission spectra from the fundus. Therefore the filter combinations presently used do not provide the highest attainable efficiency for angiography of the fundus. Calculations based on the *in vivo* measured spectra indicate that a pair of filters with separation wavelength at 525 ± 7 nm would yield the highest overall efficiency.

A new filter combination based on these theoretical predictions was developed and subjected to clinical evaluation. This combination consists of an excitor filter Z6 transmitting between 460 and 530 nm and a matched barrier filter for the spectral range of 530 to 650 nm (Fig. 1).

* This work was supported in part by Public Health Service Research Grant EY-00227 from the National Eye Institute, National Institutes of Health, and by the Research to Prevent Blindness, William Friedkin Award for 1974. This work was presented at the ARVO Atlantic Section Meeting, November 1974, Bethesda, Maryland.

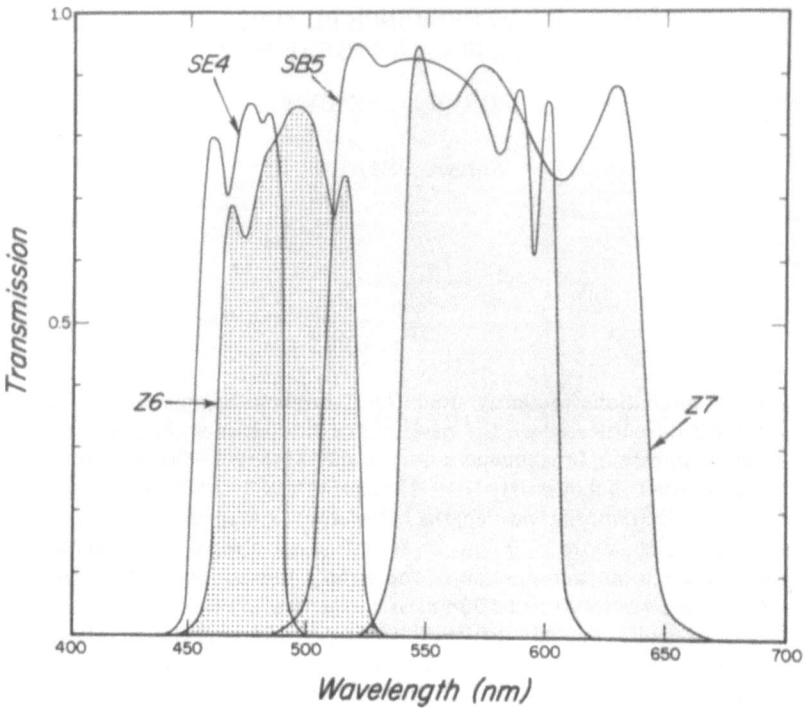

Fig. 1. Transmission characteristics of the new filters Z6-Z7 (shaded areas) and those of the standard SE4-SB5 filters (interrupted lines). The separation wavelengths are 495 nm for the standard pair and 530 nm for the new pair. The bandwidth of filter Z6 is larger than that of filter SE4: the total excitation energy reaching the subject's eye is 1.8 times higher with Z6 than with SE4.

MATERIALS & METHODS

Fluorescein angiography using a Zeiss Fundus camera was performed on 20 subjects using both the new filters and standard filters SE4-SB5 for comparison (Fig. 1). In eleven subjects the filters were compared from angiograms obtained in different angiography sessions. In nine subjects an angiogram was obtained by alternating – by means of special filter wheels – the filter combinations during the same injection. All other parameters were kept constant throughout the experiments: injection of sodium fluorescein dye (500 mg in 5cc) in the antecubital vein; flash energy of 80 Watt sec. per flash; Kodak Tri-X film developed in Kodak D19 (1 : 1 dilution) for 10 minutes at 20° C. The gain in exposure of the negatives provided by the new filters was measured by microdensitometry of various sites of the fundus image for the angiograms of the Z6-Z7 filter and for corresponding sites in the SE4-SB5 angiograms.

Furthermore the new filters have been used routinely since August 1974 at the fluorescein angiography facilities of the Massachusetts Eye and Ear Infirmary.

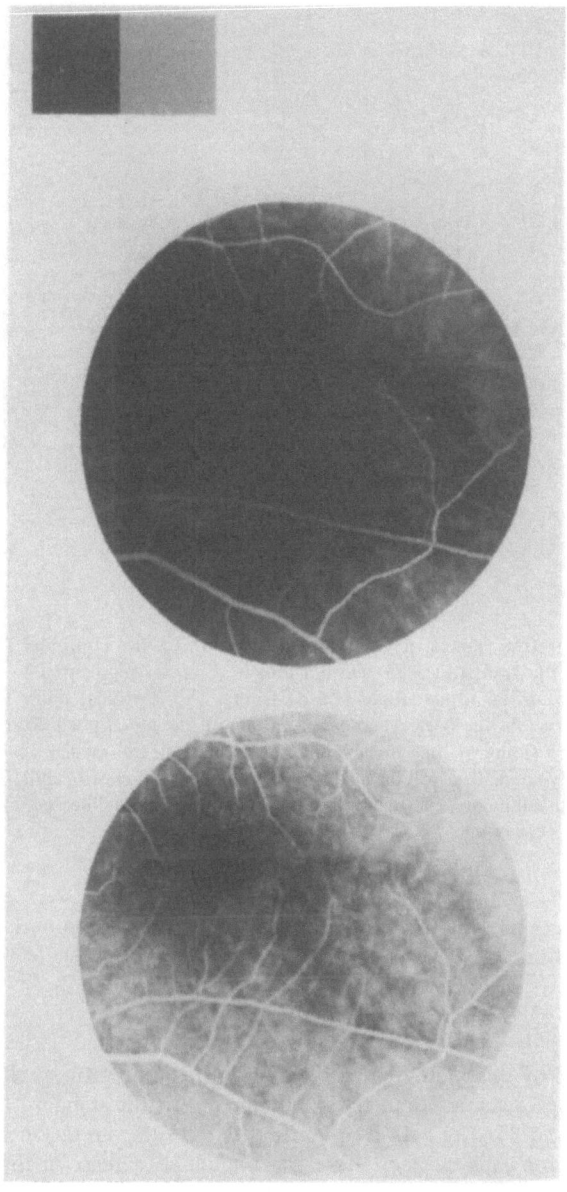

Fig. 2. Successive frames of an angiogram taken with alternating filter combination on a 70-year-old male with choroidal mass temporal to macula. Top: SE4-SB5 filters, 31 sec. after injection. Bottom: Z6-Z7 filters, 33 sec. The choroidal mass is better delineated, the macular dark spot reduced in size. The two negatives were printed simultaneously on Kodak 2 paper.

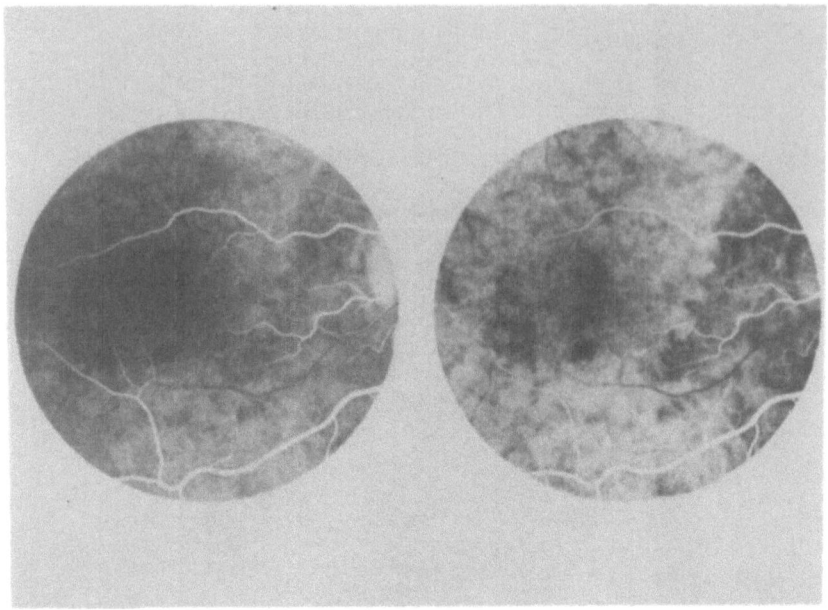

Fig. 3. Comparative frames of two angiograms showing the choroidal filling at the same stage of the transit in a 35-year-old female – darkly pigmented – with normal fundus. Left: SE4-SB5 filters. Right: Z6-Z7 filters. The choroidal filling is more vivid and the demarcation line between the early filling of the lateral posterior ciliary artery and the delayed filling of the choriocapillaris supplied by the medial posterior ciliary artery is clearly seen. The lobular pattern of filling of the choriocapillaris is demonstrated. A small 'filling defect' (just below the fovea) is better delineated.

RESULTS AND DISCUSSION

The new filters present the following characteristics in comparison to routinely used filters.

1. Higher film exposure

The negatives of the angiograms obtained with the new filters showed consistently higher densities than those obtained with the standard filters SE4-SB5 (Fig. 2 and 3). The gain in exposure of the film varied somewhat with subjects but for each subject there was a gradual increase in the exposure gain for retinal veins, arteries, choroidal background and fovea in that order. The average values of the gain for nine subjects were 3.04, 3.34, 3.49 and 4.28 respectively.

2. Better demonstration of the choroidal vasculature

The increased efficiency of the new filters permits improved demonstration of the choroidal vasculature, especially since the gain in exposure for choroidal fluorescence is higher than that for the retina. The contrast of details of the choroid is enhanced since the density of the negative in this area is now significantly higher than the fog level of the film. The enhancement of choroidal fluorescence is most marked in the macular area: the size of the 'macular dark spot' is reduced and demonstration of sub-pigmented epithelium vascularization and site of leakage are much improved.

3. Reduced demonstration of retinal vasculature

The higher choroidal background level reduces somewhat the contrast of retinal vessels outside the macular area. However the use of slower and less granular film or of less flash energy would reduce the density of the choroidal background on the film and therefore improve the image quality for the retinal vasculature.

4. Improved visualization

An important advantage of the new filters is that observations of the subject's fundus with the blue-green illumination of the Z6 excitor filter provides a significant increase in brightness over that obtainable with the blue light of the routinely used excitor filter. This results from an increase in transmission of the media, in reflectance of the fundus and in the sensitivity of the observer's eye. Thus improved visualization and focusing of fundus details, and better recognition of patient's movements during the dye transit are achieved, as well as reduced fatigue for the observer or photographer.

5. Reduced scattering in the media

Angiography with standard filters is often impaired by scattering of light in the ocular media caused by various opacities, especially nuclear sclerosis. Scattering of light veils the visibility of the fundus details, reduces the excitation for the dye in the fundus and impairs the image quality of the angiogram. The new filters improve the situation considerably because both the excitation light and the useful fluorescent light contain longer wavelengths which are less scattered by turbid media.

CONCLUSION

The transmission characteristics of a new filter combination for fluorescein angiography were selected on the basis of *in vivo* measurements of the excitation and emission spectra. This combination is characterized by the separation at 525 nm between the spectral ranges of transmission of the excitation and barrier filters, instead of about 500 nm for the standard filter combination. Compared to the latter filters, the new filters provide an enhancement of the film exposure for all sites of the fundus especially for the choroidal fluorescence. Hence there is an improvement in demonstration of the choroidal vasculature, especially in the macular area, but a slight decrease in the contrast of the retinal vessels. Improved visualization of the fundus for the observer and reduction of scattering in the ocular media of older subjects further improves the overall quality of the angiograms.

REFERENCES

ALLEN, L. & FRAZIER, O. The results of tests on broad band filter combination for fluorescence angiography. Proceedings of the International Symposium on Fluorescence Angiography, Tokyo, 1972. Tokyo, Igaku Shoin (1974).

DELORI F. & BEN-SIRA, I. Excitation and emission spectra of fluorescein dye in the human ocular fundus. *Invest. Ophthalmol.* 14: *487* (1975).

HAINING, W.M. & LANCASTER, R.C. Advanced techniques for fluorescein angiography. *Arch. Ophthalmol.* 79: *10* (1968).

HODGE, J.W. & CLEMENT, R.S. Improved method for fluorescence angiography of the retina. *Am. J. Ophthalmol.* 61: *1400* (1966).

WESSING, A. Fluorescein Angiography of the Retina. St. Louis, The C.V. Mosby Company, 1969, p. *14.*

WESSING A. Erfahrungen mit neuen filtern fur fluoresenz angiographie. *Klin. Monatsbl. Augenheilkd.* 165: *302* (1974).

ZONDIROS, G. Personal Communication 1974: Spectrotech. SE4 and SB5 Interference Filters.

Authors' address:
Eye Research Institute of Retina Foundation
20 Staniford Street
Boston, Mass. 02114
USA

FLUORESCEIN CYCLOSCOPY

K. MIZUNO & M. ASAOKA

(Sendai, Japan)

A good knowledge of the physiology and pathology of the human ciliary process has until now been accumulated only from indirect evidences gained by clinical and experimental studies. In other words, only a little information available has been provided directly from the human ciliary process in situ.

SLEZAK (1971) had examined the posterior chamber with the help of a depression contact lens, but photography of the ciliary process had not been

MAGNIFYING
GONIO - CYCLOSCOPE

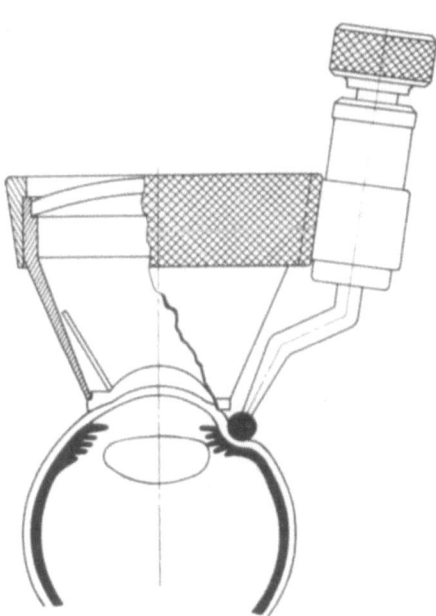

Fig. 1. A schema of 'gonio-cycloscope' which consists of a convex contact lens, an empty funnel, a mirror, an indentor and a cover for the funnel.

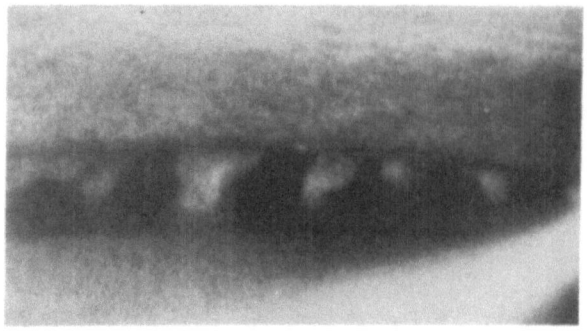

Fig. 2. A fluorescein cyclogram of the normal ciliary process 30 seconds after injection. Continuous flow of the dye from the summit forwards to the lens equatro is clearly visible.

Schema of Fluorescein Cyclogram

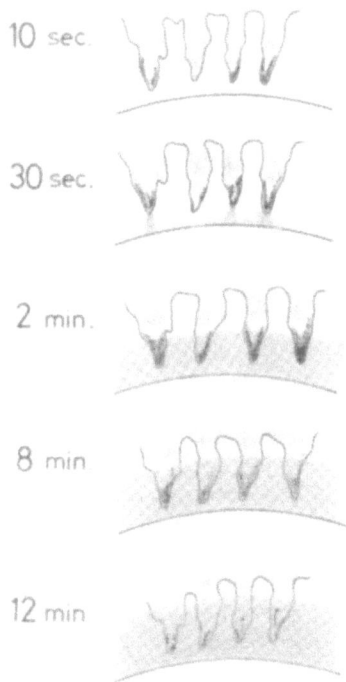

10 sec.

30 sec.

2 min.

8 min

12 min

Fig. 3. A schema of sequence of cyclograms in the normal eye.

accomplished. In our pilot study (MIZUNO & ASAOKA, in press) we placed an indentor on a Hirano gioniolens, and succeeded in taking pictures of the human ciliary body. The present experiment was conducted to obtain clearer stereoscopic images of the ciliary body and to take more precise cyclograms and fluorescein cyclograms.

To visualize the ciliary body in situ, we designed a new contact lens 'magnifying gonio-cycloscope' which consists of a + 5 diopters lens, an empty funnel, a mirror, an indentor and a cover for the funnel (Fig. 1). The convex contact lens, 15 mm in diameter, is able to magnify the object by utilizing a Zeiss photo-slitlamp. A mirror is placed at an angle of 52 degrees to the front surface. The chamber angle and ciliary body are respectively visualized through the mirror by titling the contact lens. A T-shaped depressor is attached to the funnel, depressing the sclera at a point 3 to 6 mm from the limbus by means of several adjusting screws, so that both static and kinetic cycloscopy may be performed.

In the normal adult subject, the ciliary process was found to be such that the 'summit' was steep and the 'valley' was deep. This observation was enabled by depressing the ciliary process about 2.5 mm inwards after mydriasis. The extent to which the ciliary process is accessible with slitlamp examination is greater inferiorly and superiorly than laterally and nasally.

However, it is apparent that scleral indentation is nonphysiological condition to the circulation in the ciliary vessels. Therefore, cases which had an iridolenticular space, aniridia, iris coloboma and iridodialysis were, as a rule, assumed to be a good indication for fluorescein cycloscopy, because their ciliary processes are readily accessible without indentation. The same dosage of sodium fluorescein solution and filters as those in fluorescein fundus angiography were utilized.

The summit of the ciliary process in the normal eye was first stained lineally or spottily with the dye 10-15 seconds after injection, spreading near the summit at 30 seconds. At that time, continuous flow of fluorescein from the summit forwards to the lens equator appeared (Fig. 2). At 5 min, fluorescein remained in the posterior chamber, forming a fluorescent layer around the equator. Subsequently, this fluorescein became diffused in the posterior and anterior chamber, making it impossible to view the ciliary body. It is remarkable that the ciliary process, except the summit and its boundary, was not likely to stain and leak fluorescein in the normal eye. The sequence of cyclograms in the normal eye is schematically illustrated in Fig. 3.

When the intraocular pressure (IOP) was increased artificially with a suction cup or Bailliart ophthalmodynamometer, fluorescein leakage from the summit began to decrease at a calculated IOP of 30 mmHg and stopped completely at 50 mmHg or more. The result obtained well agreed with that of open angle glaucoma, in which only traceable staining occurred from the summit during an observation period at 30 mmHg of the IOP, with no leakage occuring at 50 mmHg or more. When a liter of water was consumed by a normal subject 30 min prior to fluorescein cycloscopy, fluorescein staining already spread to the boundary of the summit several seconds after injection, leaking vigorously during the next 10-20 seconds therefrom into the posterior chamber so that the posterior chamber was brilliantly fluores-

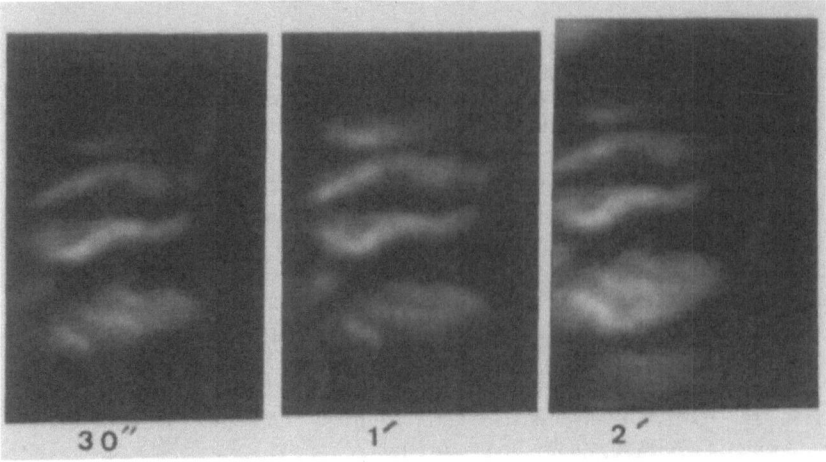

Fig. 4. A fluorescein cyclogram of traumatic aniridia 30-120 seconds after injection. Although, penetrating injury was confined to a place far from these cycliary processes, fluorescein spreaded quickly throughout the whole ciliary process.

cent soon after injection; but it diminished significantly within 5 min after injection. When a normal subject was given 100 ml of glycerol 1 hour prior to fluorescein cycloscopy, the summit was barely stained even 20-30 seconds after injection, with a little leakage from the summit occurring thereafter, resulting in slight accumulation of fluorescein in the posterior chamber. Thus, hemodilution and condensation, produced by water-drinking and an osmotic agent respectively, would result in an increase and decrease respectively in ultrafiltration of fluorescein from the ciliary epithelium.

The features observed by fluorescein cycloscopy presented a significant variety of changes in pathological conditions. Absent or little leakage of fluorescein from the rudimentary ciliary process was of interest in cases of aniridia without buphthalmos. The IOP has been sustained within normal limits in these cases, though their outflow facility was less than 0.1. It is, therefore, probable that a highly reduced production of aqueous humor may be equally balanced with the reduced outflow facility of the humor, resulting in no evidence of glaucoma in spite of the persistent mesodermal tissue in the anterior chamber angle. On the other hand, in a case of traumatic aniridia, although the penetrating injury was confined to a 3 o'clock position, the processes at 9 o'clock revealed very slight atrophy involving partial depigmentation and thinning of the stroma. Fluorescein appeared lineally in the summit at 9 o'clock 5-10 seconds after injection, spreading quickly throughout the whole ciliary process 30 seconds after injection (Fig. 4). It is of particular importance to note that traumatic aniridia, artificial iris coloboma or iridodialysis appears to be an inadequate indication for performing normal fluorescein angiograms, because some sort of traumatic influence upon the ciliary process is assumed to be unavoidable even at a prolonged post traumatic period. In other words, the injured eyes is not preferable to use as indications for performing normal fluorescein cycloscopy, even though they appear to be normal cycloscopically.

Fluorescein cycloscopy reveals diversity in diseases of the uveal tract. In iridocyclitis, fluorescein appeared diffusely or spottily, not only at the summit but also at the 'mountainside' of the ciliary process in accordance with the severity of inflammation. It is of interest to note that fluorescein diffused already out of the ciliary process 5-10 seconds after injection to stain the posterior chamber (Fig. 5). It appeared there so early after injection, that considerable disfunction in the blood-aqueous barrier is conceivable.

Typical of this category was a case of chronic granulomatous cyclitis of sarcoidosis. Coinciding with its cyclogram in which swelling and partial depigmentation of the process were apparent, the whole ciliary process was brilliantly stained already with the dye 10 seconds after injection (Fig. 6).

Finally and further typical of this category was a case of uveal effusion whose ciliary processes were so extremely swollen that they actually touched each other. The most pronounced fluorescence appeared immediately after its injection in whole ciliary process, and leaked vigorously from it into the posterior chamber (Fig. 7).

In these cases, such as severe uveitis and uveal effusion, even intensive indentation was applied on the sclera to increase the IOP up to more than 50 mmHg, fluorescein leakage was so vigorous that the posterior chamber was soon fluorescent, an effect which lasted about one hour. Therefore, fluorescein cycloscopy conclusively demonstrates that uveal effusion manifests itself not only in the choroid but also in the ciliary body.

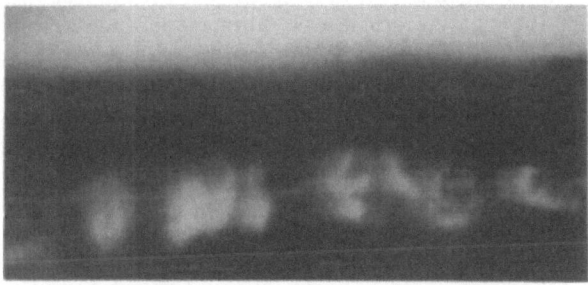

Fig. 5. A fluorescein cyclogram of iridocyclitis 10 seconds after injection. Fluorescein leakage appeared already from the brilliantly stained ciliary process.

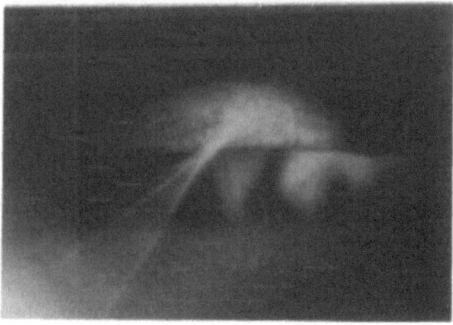

Fig. 6. A fluorescein cyclogram of sarcoid cyclitis 10 seconds after injection. The whole ciliary process was brilliantly stained.

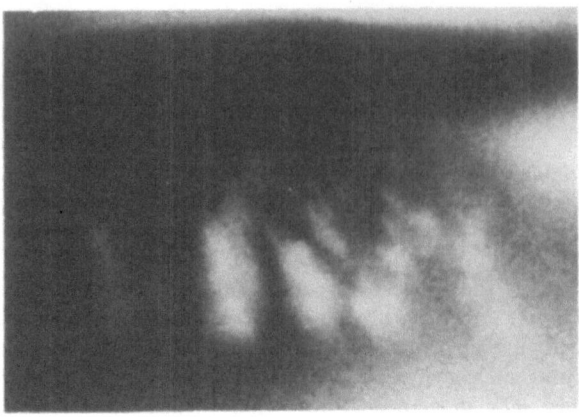

Fig. 7. A fluorescein cyclogram of uveal effusion 15 seconds after injection. The most pronounced leakage appeared immediately after injection.

SUMMARY

A new technique and device for observing the ciliary process in situ was developed, and cycloscopy and fluorescein cycloscopy have been performed as a routine clinical examination. Fluorescein was seen to leak mainly from the summit of the ciliary process in the normal eye. Increased intraocular pressure, hemodilution and -condensation can have a pronounced effect on fluorescein cyclograms. Congenital or acquired abnormalities of the ciliary process also cause fluorescein cyclograms to vary significantly. Accordingly, fluorescein cycloscopy makes available the in vivo study on the physiology and pathology of the ciliary process.

ACKNOWLEDGEMENT

The authors acknowledge Mr S. Iijima, Ricky Contact Lens Co., for his technical assistance.

REFERENCES

MIZUNO, K. & ASAOKA, M. Cycloscopy and fluorescein cycloscopy. *Invest. Opthalm.* in press.
SLEZAK, H. Results of depression biomicroscopy of the posterior chamber. *Amer. J. Opthalm.* 72: *1073-1078* (1971).

Authors' address:
Department of Ophthalmology
Tohoku University School of Medicine
Sendai, Japan 980

A NEW, TV-GUIDED FUNDUS CAMERA

KOICHI SHIMIZU, M.D.

(Maebashi, Japan)

The purpose of this paper is to publish some latest information on a new type of fundus photography using infrared television in alignment and in focusing. A few weeks ago, a well-known photo-equipment manufacturer in Japan developed a new fundus camera which promises to open an entirely new field in fundus photography in general. The most unique feature of the system is that the alignment and focusing are done with infrared light monitored through TV screen.

The whole process of fundus photography is supposed to proceed in complete darkness. By setting the selection button on 'alignment' position, the photographer sees the face of the patient on the TV screen placed beside the fundus camera. The optical axis of the fundus camera and the eye of the patient can be aligned by manipulating the fundus camera so that the patient's eye comes to the center of the TV screen.

The view of the fundus seen by infrared appears on the TV screen by setting the selection button on 'photography' position. The fundus camera and the eye are brought into proper distance by moving the fundus camera to bring the flare to the minimum. Focusing is done not as during ordinary fundus photography but by adjusting two horizontal bars of light projected on the fundus, similar to when we use a refractometer. Instillation of mydriatics is not necessary, as focusing and alignment are conducted by infrared ray and therefore in complete darkness. The optical system is so constructed that high-quality fundus picture can be taken with the pupil diameter of 5.5 mm. Photography can therefore be performed under physiological mydriasis after having kept the patient in darkness for a few minutes.

The actual fundus photography is done by ordinary and visible flash and is recorded on 35 mm color film. The picture covers a fundus area of 45 degrees in diameter. Necessary data, such as the name of the patient and the date of photography, are recorded on the corner of the film. Motor-driven camera body is the standard.

The present camera seems to open a new field in fundus photography because, theoretically and practically speaking, almost anyone can take the fundus picture because of its ease of operation and because it dispenses with forced mydriasis. The operation is so simple that you could train anyone in just half an hour to become a skilled fundus photographer.

The quality of the fundus picture is consistently good and would satisfy the general clinical demands. The focusing by just adjusting two horizontal bars on the TV screen may not satisfy an exacting photographer as he can not do the fine adjustments as, for example, whether to focus on the retinal surface or on the level of the pigment epithelium. This seems to be the major but correctable weak feature of the present system.

Author's address:
Department of Ophthalmology
Gunma University
3-39-15 Showamachi
Maebashi 371
Japan

CIRCULATION PARAMETERS: COMPARISON OF BOTH EYES BY SIMULTANEOUS FLUORESCEIN ANGIOGRAPHY

U.R. LAUX

(Ulm, W. Germany)

Circulation times vary greatly from one investigation to another even in the same patient, due to constantly changing circulation dynamics. In contrast, symmetric parts of the body have almost identical circulation times if determined simultaneously; therefore, side differences are indicative of circulation abnormalities. Of greatest interest to the ophthalmologist are: (1) the arm-retina time, for diagnosis of carotid artery occlusions; (2) the retinal circulation time, as a possible indicator of retinal circulatory disease; and (3) the dye filling pattern of the disc and peripapillary area. In all these problems successive determination of circulation times introduces an error that cannot be calculated. Simultaneous fluorescein angiography of both eyes allows the synchronous measurement of circulation times bilaterally and the synchronous comparison of circulation characteristics in both eyes. The first simultaneously taken fluorescein pictures were published by KOOIJMAN in 1970, then later by HISATOMI & SUZUKI in 1972. We have developed a new method of bilateral angiography that has been presented in detail at the 1975 meeting of the German Ophthalmological Society. I just want to mention that we are using two fully synchronized Zeiss fundus cameras and an automatic injector that has been described recently (LAUX, 1976). Fig. 1 demonstrates the first 12 pictures of the bilateral angiogram of a 24 year old healthy male patient. At the beginning and at the end of the injection an exposure is triggered by the automatic injector, thus permanently marking these important times on the film. Five seconds after the beginning of the injection, the uninterrupted serial angiogram with a picture sequence of 0.6 seconds is started by an electronic timer. It is most important to adjust the sensitivity of the system (flash energy, filter combination, and film speed) so that prior to the dye entrance the fundus is barely visible. Only in this way can we later demonstrate on the film the exact alignment of the cameras and assess with accuracy the time of dye entrance into the fundus.

So far we have used this method primarily for the diagnosis of carotid artery insufficiency, as demonstrated in this 69 year old female patient (Fig. 2). We found that patients with unilateral carotid obstructions showed a prolonged arm-retina time on the involved side. In most of these cases there was also a reduction of ophthalmic artery pressure as measured by ophthalmodynamometry on the same side. In some patients, however, a difference between both sides could only be demonstrated by measurement

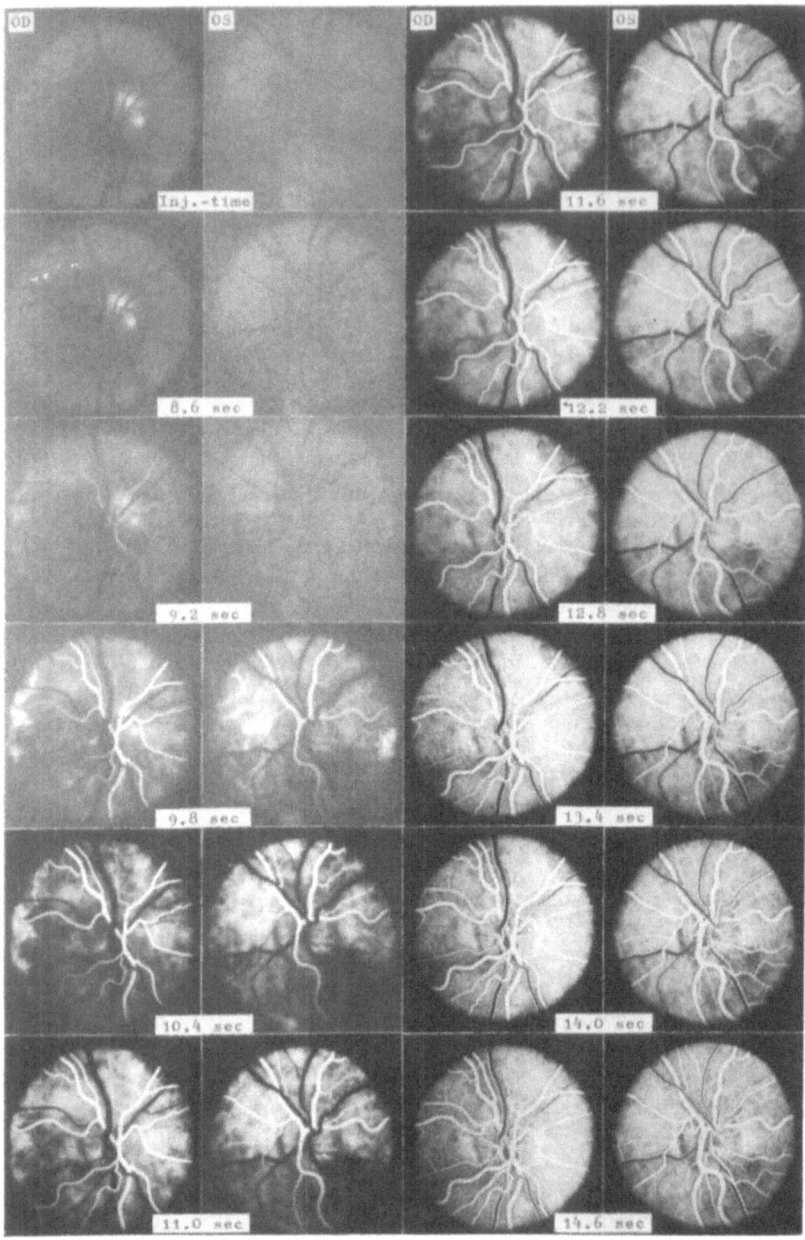

Fig. 1. First 12 pictures of the simultaneous angiogram of a 24 year old healthy male patient. (Note drusen of the optic disc on the right side).

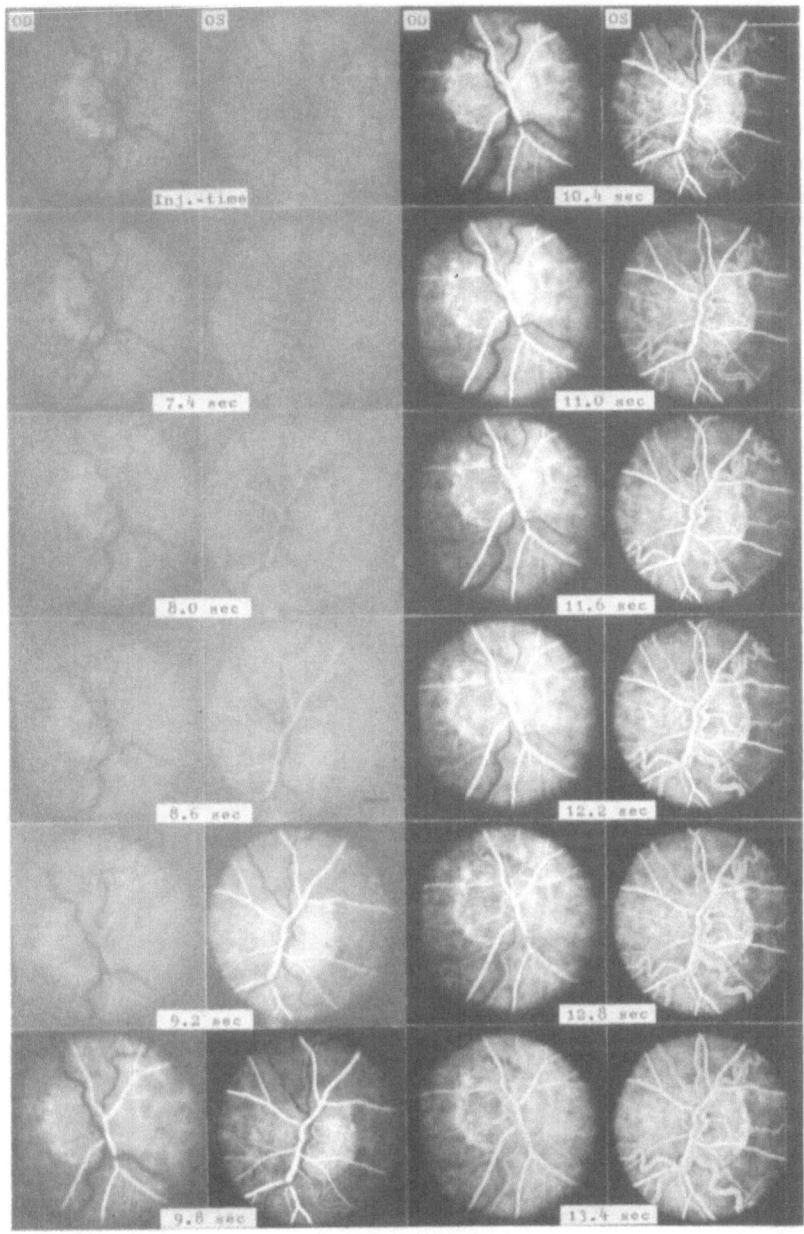

Fig. 2. First 12 pictures of the simultaneous angiogram of a 69 year old female patient with stenosis of the right carotid artery as demonstrated by arteriography.
Arm-retina time delay 1.2 sec on the right. No side difference in ophthalmodynamometry (OD 120/66, OS 115/68).

41

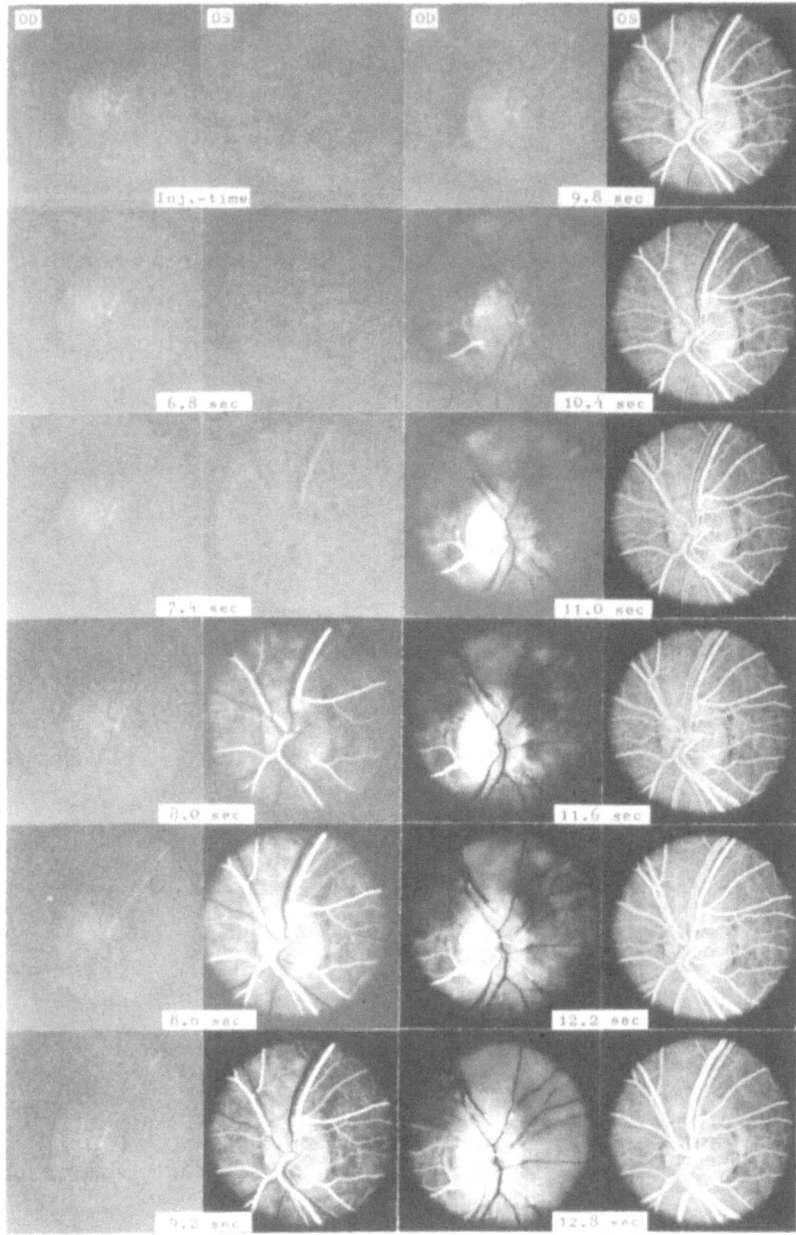

Fig. 3. First 12 pictures of the simultaneous angiogram of a 52 year old female patient with central retinal artery occlusion in the presence of a patent cilioretinal vessel. Arm-retina time delay 3.0 sec on the right.

of the arm-retina time, in others, only by ophthalmodynamometry. Both techniques used together will yield more positive results in cases of carotid artery insufficiency than either method alone. A most interesting case is demonstrated in Fig. 3. This 52 year old lady came to us with a central retinal artery occlusion in the right eye with a patent cilioretinal vessel. The bilateral angiogram showed not only the typical angiographic findings of a central retinal artery occlusion, but also a right arm-retina time delay of 3.0 seconds. An arteriography was immediately done and it showed a complete obstruction of the right internal carotid artery.

REFERENCES

HISATOMI, Ch. & SUZUKI, Y. Simultaneous bilateral angiography. Proc. Int. Symp. Fluorescein Angiography. Tokyo, 1972. Igaku Shoin Ltd., Tokyo. *269-272* (1974).
KOOIJMAN, A.C. Binocular fundus fluorescence angiography. Netherl. Ophthal. Soc. 164th Meeting, 1970. *Ophthalmologica* 164: *398-401* (1972).
LAUX, U.R. Standardisierte Fluoreszein-Injektion zur Serienangiographie. *Albrecht von Graefes Arch. klin. Ophthal.* 198. *57-62* (1976).
LAUX, U.R. Bilaterale Simultanfluoreszenzangiographie. 74. Tagung der Deutschen Ophthalmologischen Gesellschaft 1975. *Ber. Dtsch. Ophthalmol. Ges.* (in press).

Author's address:
Universitäts Augenklinik
Prittwitzstrasse 43
D-79 Ulm, W. Germany

DISCUSSION

Dr. Matsui: Two years ago we reported on our first type of simultaneous stereo fundus angiography camera (TRC-SS-I), with a modification of a Topcon fundus camera TRC-F. The pairs of stereo photographs obtained by the first type gave satisfactory results in pathologically elevated fundus lesions as in choked disc, while the results were unimpressive for normal fundi.

The second type provided satisfactory stereopsia as well in the normal fundus as in pathological cases.

The second slide shows the principle of the system schematically. The inverted image, focused through an aspheric objective lense is separated horizontally into a pair of images by means of a beam-splitter at the conjugate point at the plane of the subject's pupil. The beam-splitter is made of a pair of stereo-pupil and a pair of poro prisms. A pair of stereo-images, made by the beam splitting system is focused on the film through a pair of relay lenses and prisms. The paired stereo-images are documented on a single frame of 35 mm film. The elapsed time after the beginning of the dye injection is also documented on the same frame.

The stereo angiograms obtained by this system provide a satisfactory stereopsia, because of a 3 mm stereo-base at the subject's pupil. With a power supply unit, which enables one exposure a second, serial stereo angiograms can be obtained.

The observation of the stereo angiograms is made through a single-frame stereo-viewer. Each picture of the stereo-angiogram is a little smaller than an usual plane fundus picture. However, this stereo-angiogram can cover the center of the disc and the fovea in one frame.

Dr Haining: A practical point for Dr Laux: since it is of extreme importance to have identical processing of the films, how does he insure that the processing is completely comparable for the two sides?

Dr Laux: Of course this is an important problem. We try to take care of it by processing the two films just identically. We process each pair of films individually in small tanks, so that processing solutions, temperatures and times are all identical for the two films.

Dr Norton: Dr Laux said that usually ophthalmodynamometry showed a comparable impairment. Has he made any attempt to quantitate the degree of occlusion of the carotids with the changes obtained with circulation times? Has he compared this with dynamic scans? Generally we estimate that a carotid has to be occluded somewhere between 60-70% before you pick up much on opthalmodynamometry. Is this a more sensitive test?

Dr Laux: We are in the process of doing this; we are going to use rabbits and compare the arm-retina time with pressure measurements after carotid artery ligation. It is indeed very important to see which method is more sensitive. As I showed you, there were some patients who had a delay in the arm-retina time on one side, but normal ophthalmodynamometric readings. Also the opposite was true, some patients with differences in the ophthalmodynamometric reading showed equal arm-retina times on both sites. I think this has to be evaluated on a quantitative basis.

Dr Norton: Have you compared it with radio-isotope dynamic studies?

Dr Laux: No, we have not.

Dr Stojanovic: Est-ce que vous avez mesuré la vitesse de la circulation périphérique générale dans le cas avec obstruction partielle de l'artère centrale de la rétine?

Dr Laux: If I understand you correctly you were asking if we measured the peripheral circulation in the case with occlusion of the central retinal artery?

One problem with this method is that we need a diaphragm, which excludes large areas of the fundus from exposure. As you could see, so far we can photograph only the papilla and the peripapillary area. Otherwise the stress for the patient is too great and I think unless you exclude the light-sensitive areas from exposure this method is very difficult to perform. So we only photograph the papilla, and the peripapillary area. Therefore, we cannot measure the peripheral circulation time.

FIVE YEARS EXPERIENCE WITH AUTOMATED PROCESSING FOR FLUORESCEIN ANGIOGRAPHY

E.S. ROSEN & E. YOUNG

(Manchester, Gr. Britain)

Very few Ophthalmic Departments have access both to a fundus camera and a photographic service able, on demand, to immediately develop angiographic films and produce prints, thus permitting diagnosis and treatment whilst the patient is still in the unit.

In 1972 E.S. ROSEN presented a paper at Tokyo describing his early efforts (a) to overcome this deficiency, (b) to make the unit self-reliant with the minimal use of skilled photographic personnel, and (c) to still produce angiographic prints of high quality.

This paper represents a four years update of the original paper and details progress since that date.

The film processor selected was an American Cordell 240 Varifilm Rapid Processor, and an Intercop Stabilisation Paper Processing Machine for the processing of the enlargements.

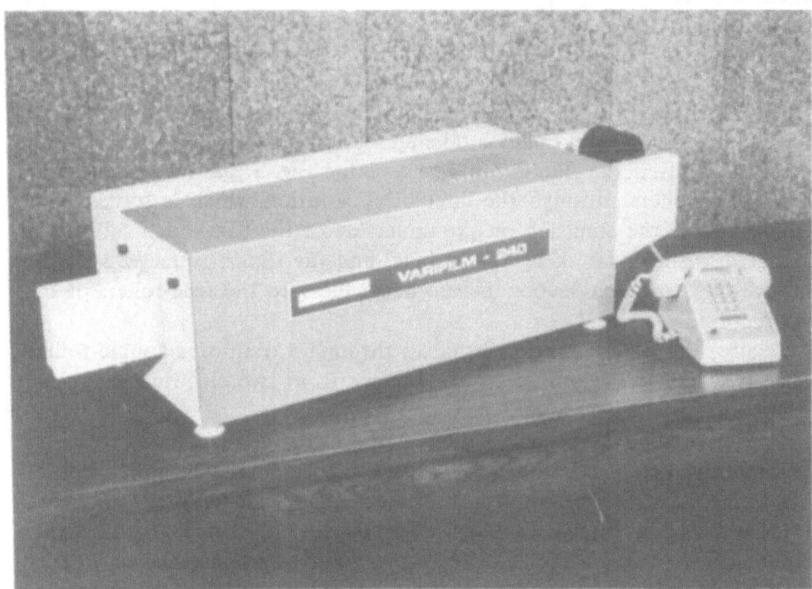

Fig. 1.   Cordell 240 Varifilm Processor.

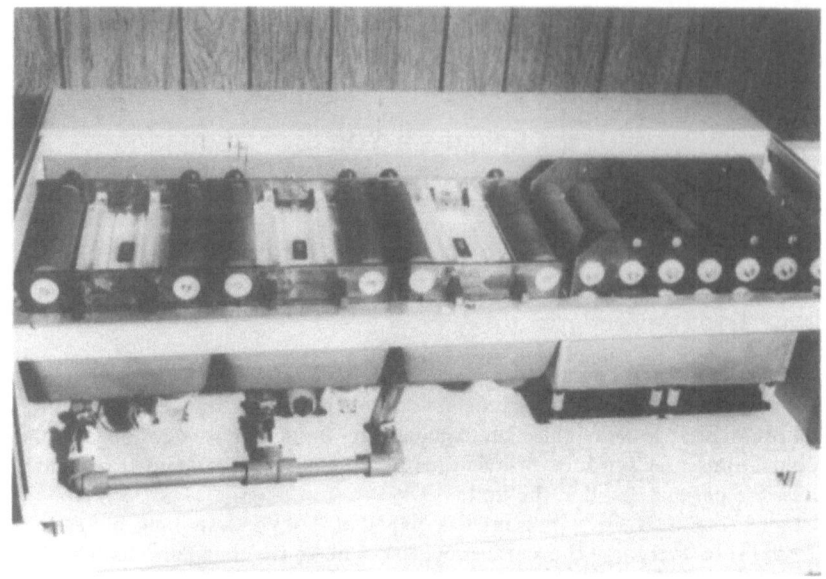

Fig. 2. Cordell 240 Varifilm Processor with light-tight cover removed.

This Cordell machine, though not in its latest form, is demonstrated in a film made of the Retinal Photographic Unit at the Manchester Royal Eye Hospital, being shown elsewhere at this Meeting. This illustrates the production of high quality, enlarged fluorograms in less than five minutes after the patient has been photographed.

Equipment designed for one specific purpose rarely fits the need, without modification, of a different field. This was the case with the 240 Processor and the modifications made are detailed in this paper.

The machine consists of sections for loading film, developing, fixing, washing and drying, and finally a take-up section. (Figs. 1 & 2). At each wet processing section the film is fed into a platen Fig. 3, passing between the driven feed-rollers, through the circulating solution which is forced by a turbine against the emulsion on the underside of the film. Each solution is circulated within its tank by the turbine, and the film is squeegeed by the output-rollers of each section before being fed into the feed-rollers of the next section.

Finally, the film is dried as it passes through a train of 7 double rollers between which it is exposed to the hot air from two electric fans placed behind a heater element and thermostat.

As the machine is normally supplied, the developer and fixing solutions are thermostatically controlled by heaters placed in the feed-pipelines of both baths; a single thermostat – in the developer-pipeline – controls both of the heaters in these two baths. It is important, therefore, that equal volumes of the two solutions, at the same temperature, are loaded initially into their respective tanks. The solutions are then accurately maintained at 38°C.

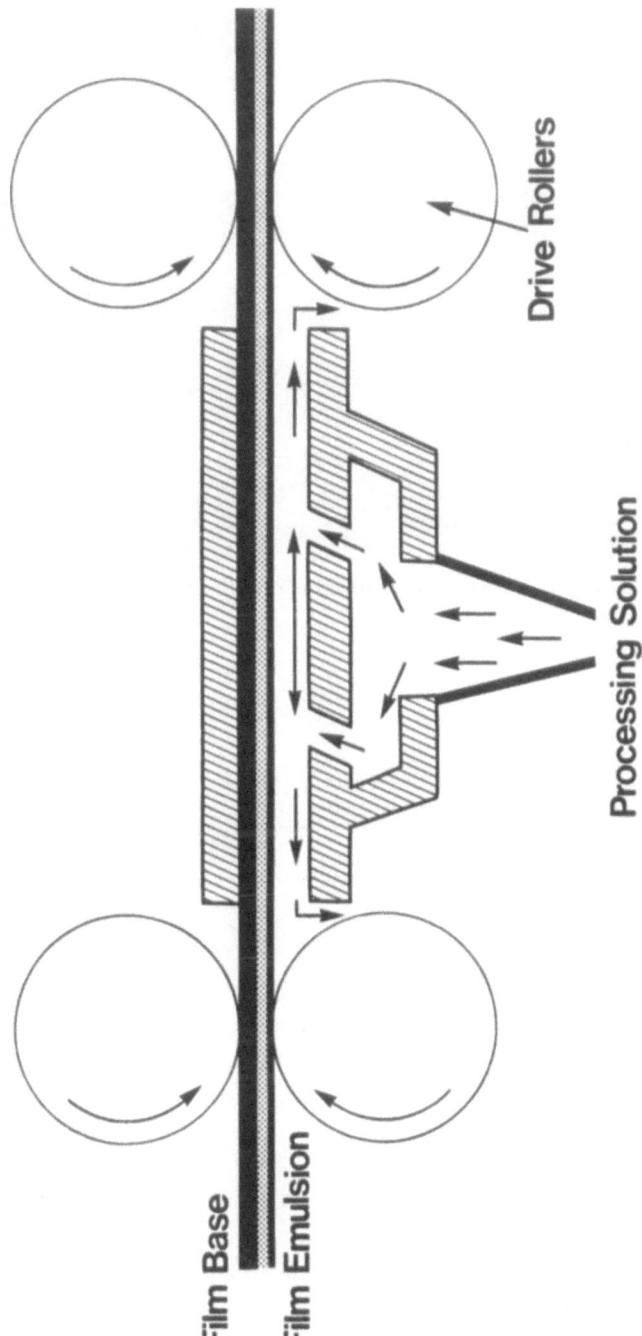

Fig. 3. Section through processing platen showing film path and circulation of solution.

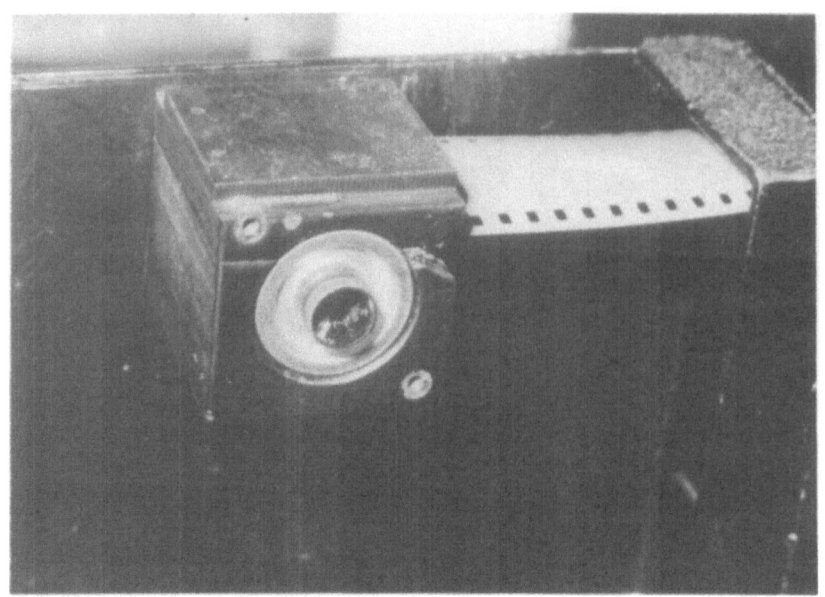

Fig. 4. Cassette holder fitted to Cordell 240 Varifilm Processor.

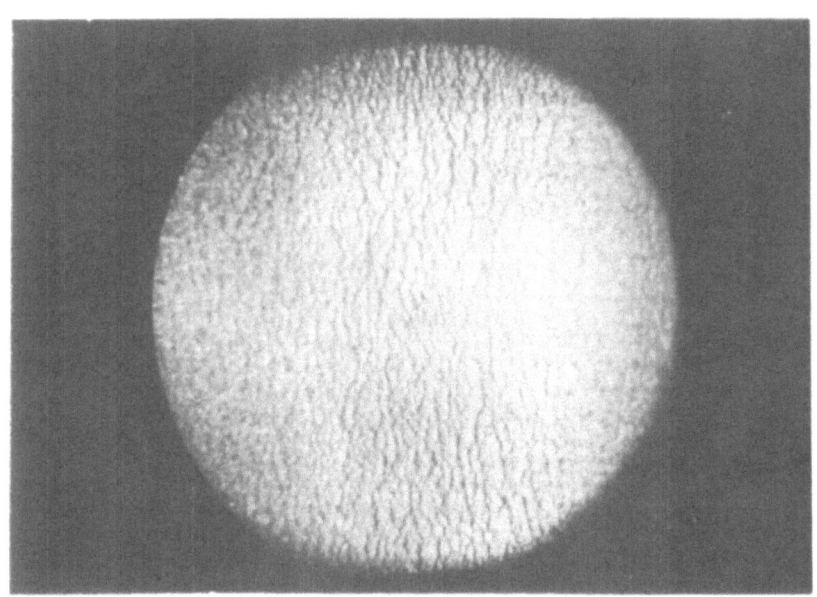

Fig. 5. Rubber drive-roller, showing surface deterioration after several weeks use.

48

Water for the washing of the film is delivered at the rate of 9 litres per minute from an external source. In order to achieve this the machine, as supplied, has to be modified by the removal of a restrainer in the washwater feedline. The wash-water temperature is extremely critical, (± 0.5°C) of the required 38°C. In our system we have provided an external tank of 120 litres of water into which a Griffin & George 'Accurostat', which incorporates a thermostat, heater and a centrifugal pump, is fitted. This supplies water well within the required temperature tolerance and at an adequate volume. The outflow from the wash-tank is returned to the reservoir for re-circulation. It would be preferable to have an in-line thermostatically controlled heater fitted into the cold-water line, the volume being controlled by a needle-valve and flowmeter, this requires, however, a power supply of 60 amps. at 240 volts which is not available to us. In the drying section the heater-thermostat, as fitted, is not sufficiently accurate to maintain the drying air within ± 2°C. of the required 50°C. This has been replaced with a thermostat, fitted by Cordell to their larger Micro-Data Processing Machine, which achieves the necessary temperature tolerance of the drying air. Problems have been encountered with fixation of the film which was not completed in a consistent fashion. This was solved by reducing the speed of film transportation to 1 cm. per sec. by replacing the 24 tooth main-drive sprocket by a 17'tooth drive sprocket, available from the distributors. At the same time it was necessary to remove two links from the main-drive chain.

Parallel scratch lines were apparent on many of our early films. These resulted from abrasion of the film in the feed section of the machine. This problem was eliminated by fitting a cassette holder in direct line with the feed slots of the processing section (Fig. 4).

By far the severest problem encountered was the rapid deterioration of the surface of the rubber rollers. In some instances, this was apparent within weeks and quickly developed into the state shown in Fig. 5.

This pattern always became imprinted onto the softened emulsion of the film, degrading the image. Our first attempt to overcome this problem, was by undercutting the bottom rubber rollers in the area between the sprocket holes, as is shown in our film. This was acceptable providing the film being processed did not track in the wash section. Also, in order to dry the film the final pair of rubber rollers in the wash section had to be left solid in order to squeegee the film before it passed into the drying section, which inevitably caused some impression of the roller texture on the film emulsion. This fault has been overcome by the development of hydrophobic polyurethane rollers. These are fitted in place of the lower rubber rollers in the processing and drying sections and give a mirror like finish to the emulsion surface. We have now used these rollers for almost three years on our machine and, unlike the rubber rollers, they show no sign of deterioration. (Fig. 6).

In collaboration with Messrs. Ilford Ltd., the developer, Ilford Photodata Com., used as a 25% aqueous solution, was devised for use with Ilford FP4 35 mm. film. This developer met the criteria already published by ROSEN & YOUNG in 1974, in that a high contrast image with a low base-fog level was achieved, and co-incidentally increases the apparent film

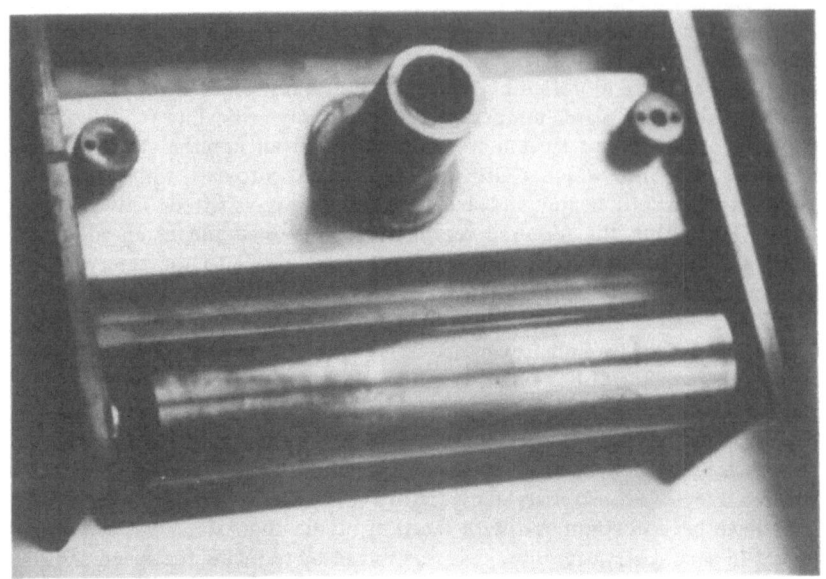

Fig. 6. Underside of platen showing hydrophobic polyurethane roller after 3 years use.

Fig. 7. Unexposed, processed films showing (a) High base-fog level film, (b) a satisfactory film.

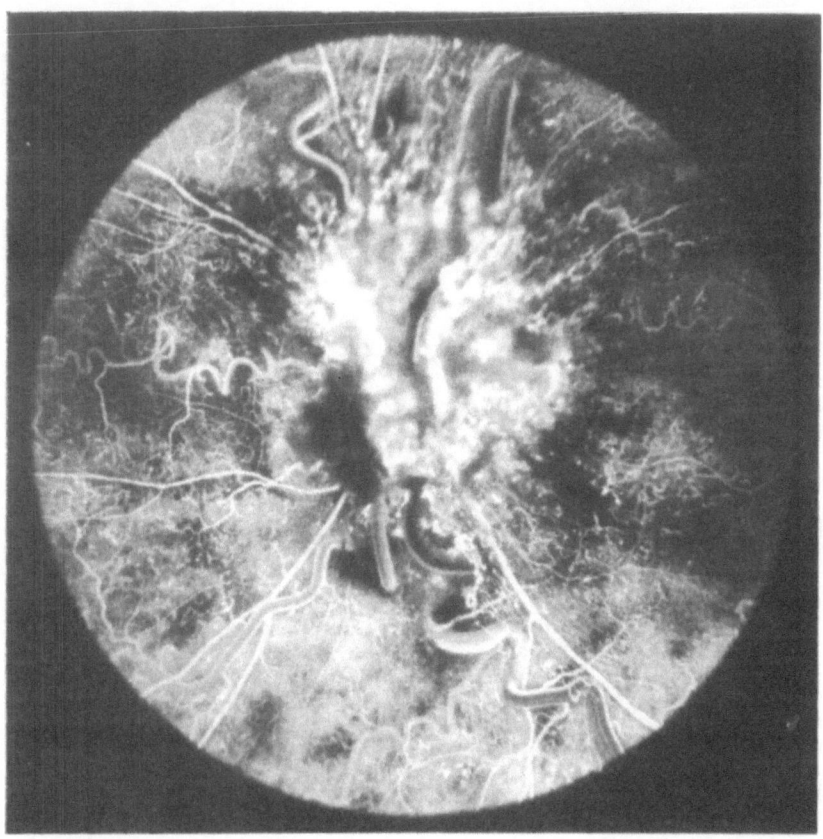

Fig. 8. Prints made from angiographic films processed in the Cordell 240 Varifilm Processor.

speed by a factor of up to about three and a half times. Slight variations in the subsequent formulations of both the film emulsion and the developer, will, with some batches of film, give a base-fog level too high for our requirements. Fig. 7 illustrates the difference between unexposed processed films, the one on the left having a high base-fog level and the other being a satisfactory emulsion.

Co-operation with the local Ilford distributing depot has enabled us to resolve this, we hope, our final problem. Sample films of several different bulk batches held by the depot are forwarded to us and immediately processed. This test ensures the selection of the best emulsion and a bulk order for this particular batch is then placed on the depot. It should be emphasised that bad batches of emulsion are rare and that no other make of film, tested by us, has proved satisfactory under our processing conditions.

In conclusion, we consider angiograms of a very high standard can be achieved if the following precautions are taken:
1. The developer, fixer and wash-water be maintained at 38° centigrade.
2. The heater air be maintained at 50° centigrade.

51

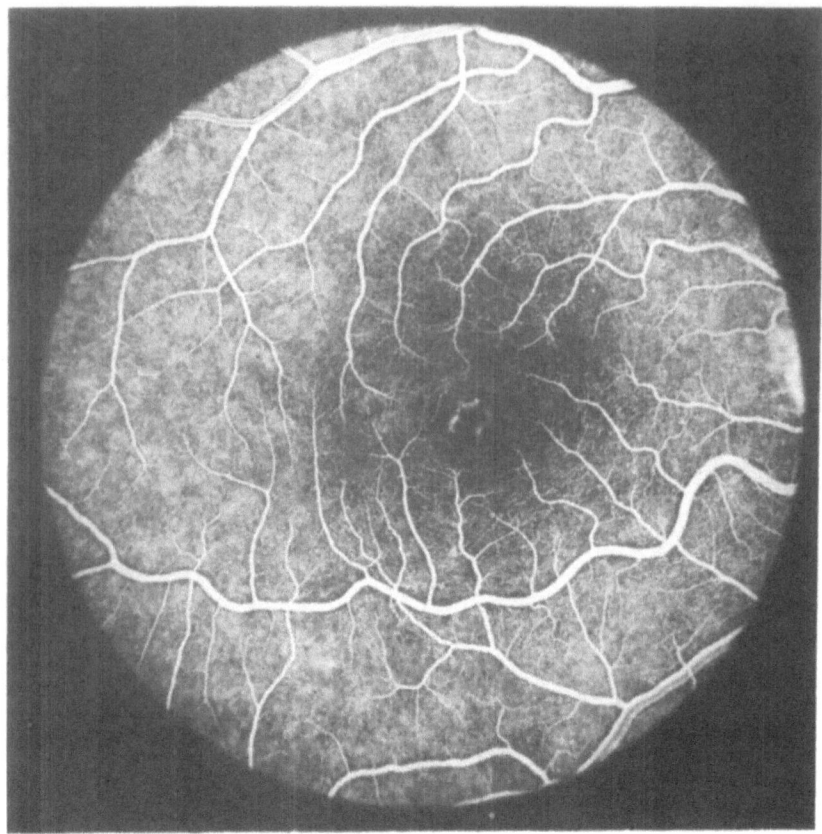

For legend, see p. 51

3. The motor speed be reduced to transport the film at 1 cm. per second.

4. That if hydrophobic polyurethane rollers are used:

a. The lower rollers should make contact with the developer and fixer solutions at all times during processing.

b. The rollers should never be left standing in the machine when not in use.

c. The rollers should be thoroughly washed after each processing session with warm water.

d. The rollers must not be allowed to rest on any rough or gritty surface, nor cleaned with any abrasive materials.

e. A slight positive tension should be maintained, by hand, to the leading end of the film after it emerges from the exit slot.

5. That a semi-stiff leader, 18 cm. long, 3.8 cm. wide and 0.45 mm. thick should be attached to the leading end of each film processed.

6. That the tail end of the film be severed before becoming taught on the inner spool of the cassette.

Fig. 8. illustrates the quality of angiographic films which can be obtained using the Cordell 240 Machine by closely observing the criteria set out.

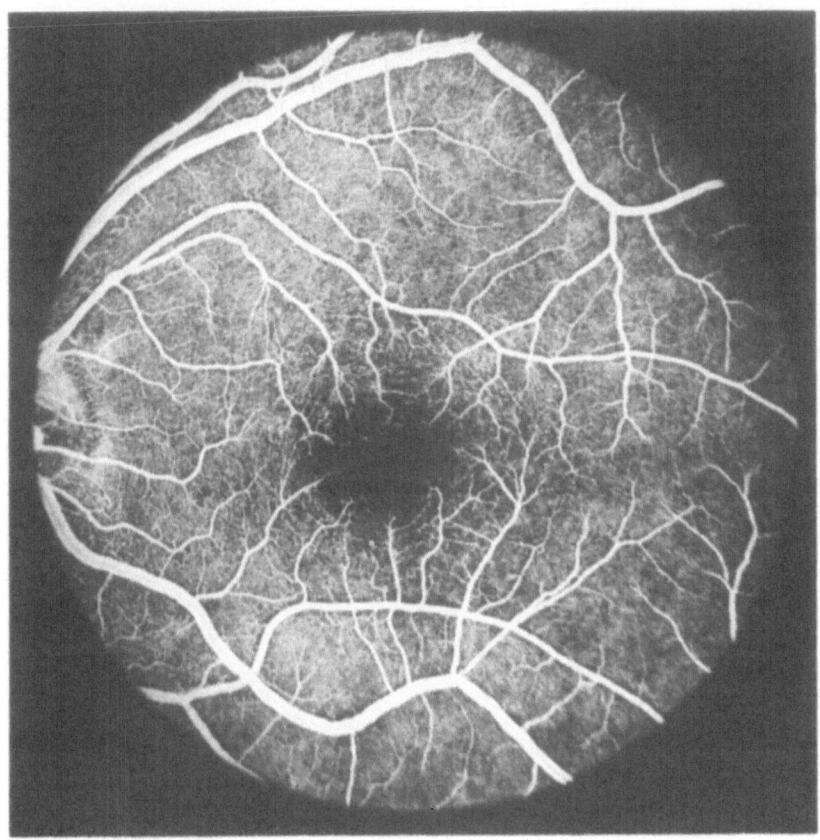

For legend, see p. 51

REFERENCES

ROSEN, E.S. Technical developments in the provision of a retinal angiographic service. Proc. ISFA Tokyo 1972: *41-47*. Igaku Shoin, Tokyo (1974).

ROSEN, E.S. & YOUNG, E. Retinal fluorography: a rapid semi-automatic processing system. *International Ophthalmic Clinics* 14 (3): *63-79*. Publ. by Little, Brown & Co., Boston (1974).

Authors' address:
Manchester Royal Eye Hospital
Nelson Street
Manchester M13 9WH, Great Britain

APPENDIX

Equipment used in the Retinal Photographic Unit,
Manchester Royal Eye Hospital, and sources of supply

1. Cordell 240 Varifilm Processing Machine manufactured by Cordell Engineering, Inc, 210, Broadway, Everett, Massachusetts, U.S.A.

2. Beseler 23C, Series 2 Enlarger fitted with 'Negatrans' film holder. } manufactured by Charles Beseler Co., 219, South, East Orange, New Jersey, 07018, U.S.A.

3. Intercop Stabilisation Paper Processing Machine, Ex. John Blishen & Co. Ltd., 75, Kilburn Lane, London, W. 10.

4. Developer: 25% solution Ilford Photodata Com.

5. Fixer: (20% solution Hypam
       (2.5% Hypam Hardener on Fixer Content.

6. Printing Paper: Ilford Stabilisation Printing Paper. Grade YR.4.1P.

7. Paper Processing Chemicals: Pack of Ilford HD3. Processing solutions.

} Available from Ilford Ltd., Ilford, England., and local depots.

8. Film: Ilford 35 mm. F.P.4 in either 20 or 36 exposure lenghts.

9. Wash-water supply: Accurostat No. S15 − 162, Ex. Griffin & George Ltd., P.O. Box 14, Wembley, Middlesex, England. (alternative in-line supply − Eltron LW Circulation Heater, Ex. Eltron (London) Ltd., Accrington Works, Strathmore Road, Croydon, CR9 2NA, Surrey, England.

10. Hydrophobic Polyurethane Rollers, Ex. Photorollers Ltd., 11, Ollerbarrow Road, Hale, Altrincham, Cheshire, England.

ANGIOSCOPY AND COLOUR ANGIOGRAPHY

P.-A. GROUNAUER, R. FAGGIONI
& VO VAN TOI

(Lausanne, Switzerland)

This paper is chiefly intended for the practitioner, in order to present him with our method and the apparatus involved. However, the F.A.* in colour is not without interest for the university. It is a synthetic method putting the accent on the scopy-graphy association which is a necessary, if not indispensable, diagnostic exercise. It allows time to be gained with an economy of means: one film, no individual processing laboratory. The slides obtained are positive, stereo if necessary.

The F.A. is a complementary examination, among others (GROUNAUER et al., 1975, GROUNAUER & VO VAN TOI, 1976) which is often useful, sometimes decisive. Our means are as follows: Balzers interferential filters mounted on all instruments (Fig. 1), the Olympus GRC-II or the Zeiss camera, the Schultz-Crock ophthalmoscope, an original fluoroscope (Fig. 2), the Rodenstock 2000 slit lamp. With Agfachrome Professional

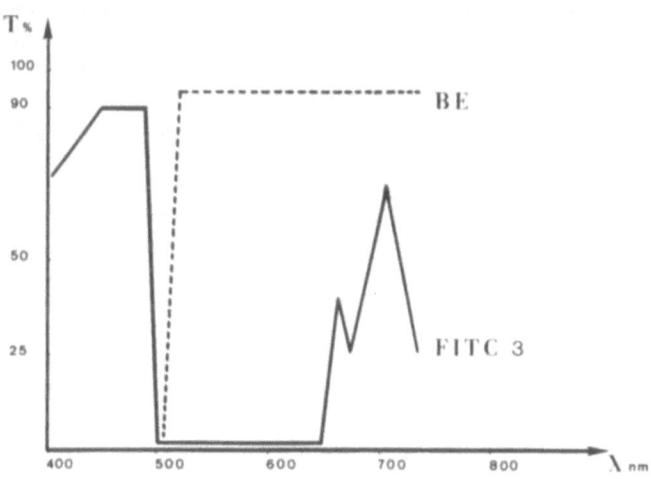

Fig. 1. Interferential filters Balzers, Liechtenstein.

* F.A. = Fluorescence angiography.
This work has been supported by the National Swiss Fund for Scientific Research.

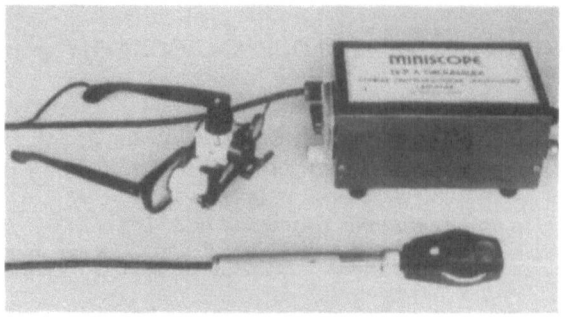

Fig. 2. Instruments used for angioscopy (Heine and Schultz-Crock ophthalmoscope).

50 S 5500° K 18 din overdevelopped to 23 din, we are able to do the retinography and the F.A. on the same film. The Polaroid film No 108 provides an initial document, film No 107 a capillary time in recirculation phase. We inject 5 cc fluoresceine 20% in two shots: first 4 cc then 1 cc for the Polaroid photograph or the slit lamp study.

At the late AV time we interrupt the exam and make a binocular ophthalmoscopy (Fig. 2). The position of the FITC 3 excitative filter may change in relation to the beams: we carry out the ophthalmoscopy in red light at an angle of 45°; at 90° we excite the fluorescence. Passing quickly from one position to another we add or substract fluorescence at will. Once the peripheral lesions are recognized, we resume F.A. Finally, we inject the last cc under biomicroscopic control.

At the end of the F.A. we already have a probable diagnosis which generally confirm the graphic result. Each ocular tissue has its own hue, realising a kind of 'in vivo histology' (Fig. 3 and 4). The origine of the versicoloured effect is described elsewhere (GROUNAUER & FAGGIONI, 1975).

In the discussion only the disadvantages are presented: initially a slight loss of contrast, then the chromatic differences due to individual variations and to the flashes of the retinographs; finally the price of the quadrichromy! Note that Polaroid camera No MP-4 gives, in one minute, a paper copy of a colour F.A.

SUMMARY

Synthetic method, scopy + graphy, giving positive colour dias offering the aspect of an 'in vivo histoangiography'.

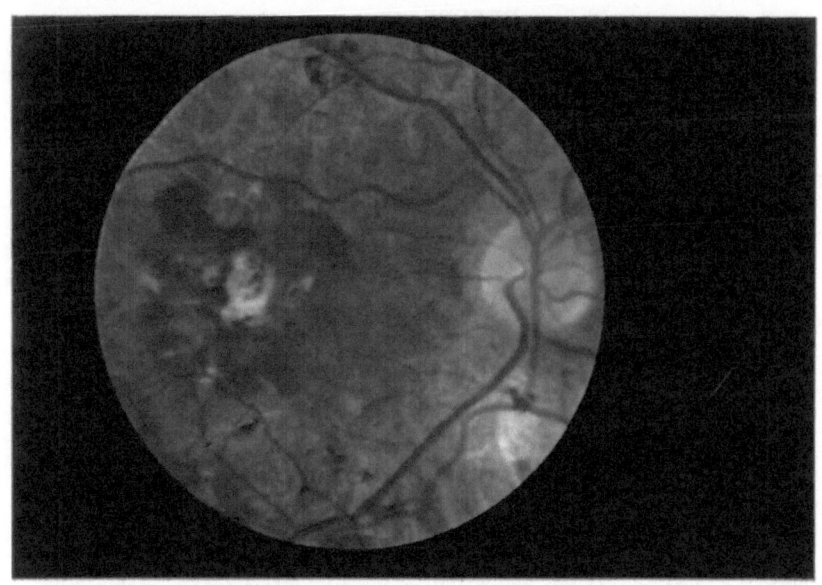

Fig. 3. Retinography (white light).

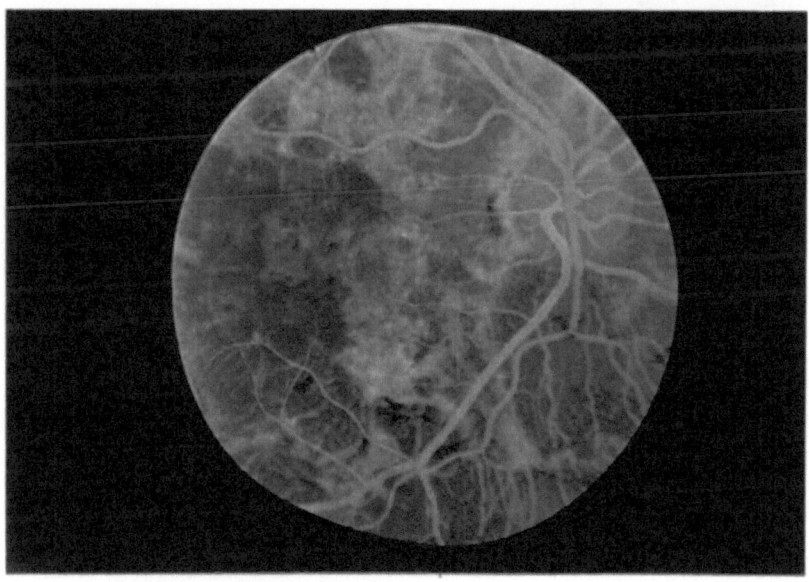

Fig. 4. Angiography in colour. It appears as a 'histoangiography in vivo' in which the colour of the vessels depends on that of the background ('versicoloured effect').

REFERENCES

See also *Ophthalmologica* Basel 170: *426-433* (1975).

BORGIOLI, M. & VOLPI, U. Fluoroscopia a colori. *Annali di ottalmologica* 100: *791-794* (1974).

GROUNAUER, P.-A. & FAGGIONI, R. Colour angiography and angioscopy. *Ophthalmologica*, Basel 170: *426-433* (1975).

GROUNAUER, P.-A., FAGGIONI, R. & HUNGERBÜHLER, P. Angiographie fluorescéinique en couleur – fluoroscopie et équidensitométrie photographique. *Méd. et Hyg.* 33: *523-525* (1975).

GROUNAUER, P.-A. & VO VAN TOI. Fréquence critique de fusion dans le champs visuel central et périphérique. Résultats préliminaires. *Klin. Mbl. Augenheilk.* 168: *90-93* (1976).

IWATA, O. & UI, K. Studies on colour fluorescence fundus angiography. *Acta Soc. Oph. Japon* 78: *524* (1974).

JENSEN, V.A. & OLSEN, W. Colour fluorescein angiography of the fundus. *Acta Ophthalmologica* 52: *501-511* (1974).

LANTZ, J.-M., SHUSTERMAN, M. & RUDNICKI, L. Colour fluorescein angiography of the ocular fundus. *Canad. J. Ophthal.* 9: *29-36* (1974).

PATZ, A. *Highlights of Ophthal.* 14: *31-35* (1972).

WESSING, A. Erfahrungen mit neuen Filtern für die Fluoreszenangiographie. *Klin. Mbl. Augenheilk.* 165: *302-308* (1974).

Authors' addresses:
Clinique ophtalmologique universitaire
15, avenue de France
CH-1004 Lausanne
Switzerland

Institut de Microtechnique EPFL
114, route Cantonale
CH-1025 St. Sulpice
Switzerland

Requests for reprint to Dr P.-A. Grounauer at the Lausanne address

HIGH SPEED HUMAN CHOROIDAL ANGIOGRAPHY
USING INDOCYANINE GREEN DYE AND A
CONTINUOUS LIGHT SOURCE

ROBERT W. FLOWER

(Laurel, Md., USA)

Fluorescein angiography has not proved to be an ideal dye for study of the human choroidal circulation. There are two main reasons for this: First, its unbound molecules readily 'leak' from the fenestrated choriocapillaris; and second, its absorption and fluorescence spectra lie in a region where the ocular tissues do not efficiently transmit light energy – this is particularly true of the macular area. On the other hand, indocyanine green (ICG) dye does not tend to leak from the choroidal vessels and has its absorption and fluorescence spectra in the near-infrared region where light energy is transmitted fairly efficiently by the ocular tissues. An attempt has been made therefore, to develop a clinically feasible and relatively simple method of routinely visualizing the human choroidal circulation using ICG.

During the course of this work, several different clinical angiographic techniques were developed. These include ICG infrared absorption angiography (FLOWER, 1972), ICG fluorescence angiography (FLOWER & HOCHHEIMER, 1973), and a method whereby either or both types of choroidal ICG angiography can be done simultaneously with standard fluorescein angiography of the retinal circulation (FLOWER & HOCH-HEIMER, 1976). This latter method resulted in construction of the so-called multispectral, fundus camera, but it is useless to reiterate details of its operation here since it was constructed primarily to ascertain the strong and weak points of both types of ICG choroidal angiography.

Results of studies performed with this modified fundus camera which involved intravenous injection of a mixture of fluorescein and ICG dyes may, however, be briefly summarized as follows:

1. *ICG infrared absorption angiography* permits visualization primarily of the choroidal veins. In absorption angiography, the fundus is illuminated with light of 8050 Å wavelength – the wavelength maximally absorbed by ICG dye in blood. With no dye present in the choroidal vessels, light from the fundus camera is reflected back from the sclera to the photographic film in the camera, and the entire film area is exposed. Dye-filled vessels absorb some light energy, however, and energy is no longer uniformly reflected back to the entire film area – underexposed areas correspond to dye-filled choroidal vessels. Those blood vessels having the largest diameters (the veins) also have the greatest infrared energy absorptive capacities since the path-length of light through them is greatest, hence, they are most easily seen in the angiograms.

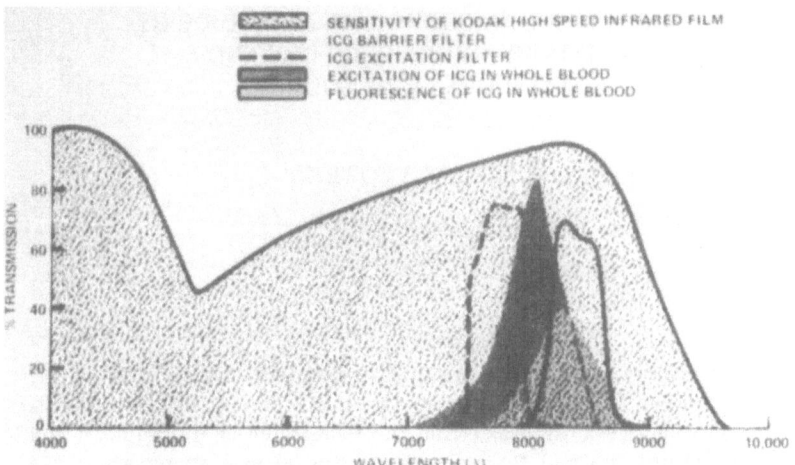

Fig. 1. Spectral characteristics of dye, filters and film used in ICG fluorescence angiography. Although it is not indicated in this figure, the ICG excitation filter has a transmission band which extends from below 4000 Å and up to 7000 Å. Within this band, transmission varies from between 40% to 60%.

2. *ICG fluorescence angiography* permits visualization of both choroidal arteries and veins. In fluorescence angiography, fluorescent light energy which exposes the photographic film arises predominantly from a thin surface layer of the blood-dye mixture. Thus, ability to visualize choroidal blood vessels by this method is not as dependent upon diameter of the vascular lumen as it is in absorption angiography. Unfortunately, in most of the patients studied, it was difficult to distinguish between choroidal arteries and choroidal veins without referring to the other two types of simultaneously made angiograms.

3. *Simultaneous fluorescein angiography*, although it provided little information about dynamics of the choroidal arterial and venous filling phases, did clearly indicate the point in time at which dye-filling of the choriocapillaris took place, marking onset of the choroidal venous filling phase. Noting when this event took place in each sequence of simultaneously made ICG angiograms made it apparent that temporal resolution in choroidal angiography was severely limited by the maximum frequency at which a standard fundus camera xenon flash tube light source could be fired (approximately once every 0.7 seconds).

Specifically, only the first two or three frames in a sequence of angiograms contained information about the choroidal arterial filling phase; the rest related to venous filling. This lack of temporal resolution, of course, largely accounts for the difficulty in differentiating between choroidal arteries and veins in a sequence of ICG fluorescence angiograms.

It was nevertheless clear, in spite of the problem of limited temporal resolution, that of the two types of choroidal angiography developed, ICG fluorescence angiography contains the most information about choroidal blood flow dynamics. It also did not seem likely that ICG choroidal angiography would be widely accepted as either a research or clinical tool if instrumentation as complex as the multispectral fundus camera must be used. It was an important decision, therefore, that further development of choroidal angiography would concentrate only on ICG fluorescence angiography and on improving its temporal resolution. Another important decision was to design simple modifications which could be quickly added to and removed from conventional fundus cameras rather than to attempt construction of an entirely new type of fundus camera.

As indicated in Figure 1, the methodology of ICG fluorescence angiography is straightforward and identical in principle to that of sodium fluorescein angiography, except for the fact that one must work in the near-infrared region of the spectrum instead of with visible light. However, to compensate for the relatively low level of ICG fluorescence intensity and at the same time to correct for chromatic aberration which results from photographing infrared instead of visible light wavelengths, an additional lens must be installed on the standard fundus camera. This lens (see Figure 2A), reduces the image size of the fundus to a diameter of approximately 17 mm in the film plane of a motorized 35 mm camera which fires at a rate of approximately 4 frames per second and has a shutter speed of 1/15 second.

In order to permit making choroidal angiograms at this rapid rate, the usual fundus camera xenon flash tube is replaced with a continuous light source (a General Electric FCS, 150 watt quartz halogen lamp) as shown in Figure 2B. An annealed glass 7000 Å cut-on filter in a special holder is placed on the fundus camera's condenser lens in front of the quartz halogen lamp in order to eliminate nearly all visible light wavelengths from the continuous light source (thus, the patient perceives only a faint, red glow). The ICG fluorescence excitation filter may be placed on the filter wheel or

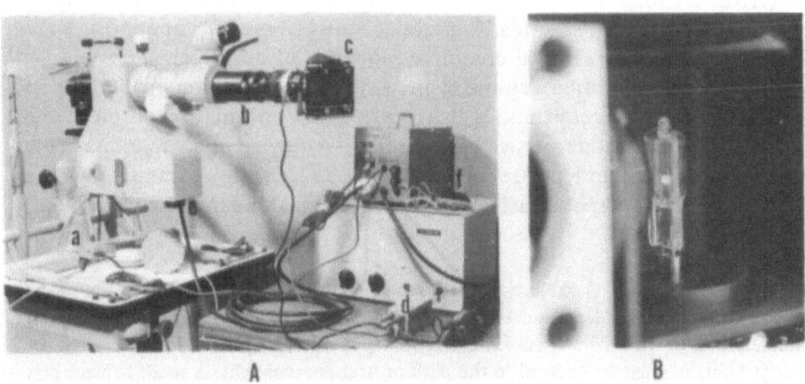

Fig. 2-A. Standard Zeiss fundus camera modified for ICG fluorescence choroidal angiography using a continuous light source. a: control box for automatically turning background light on and off. b: prefocused relay lens. c: 35 mm motorized Nikon camera. d: Nikon battern power supply and control box. e: base of quartz halogen lamp assembly. f: auxiliary power supply with foot switch.
2-B. Quartz halogen lamp in position inside Zeiss fundus camera.

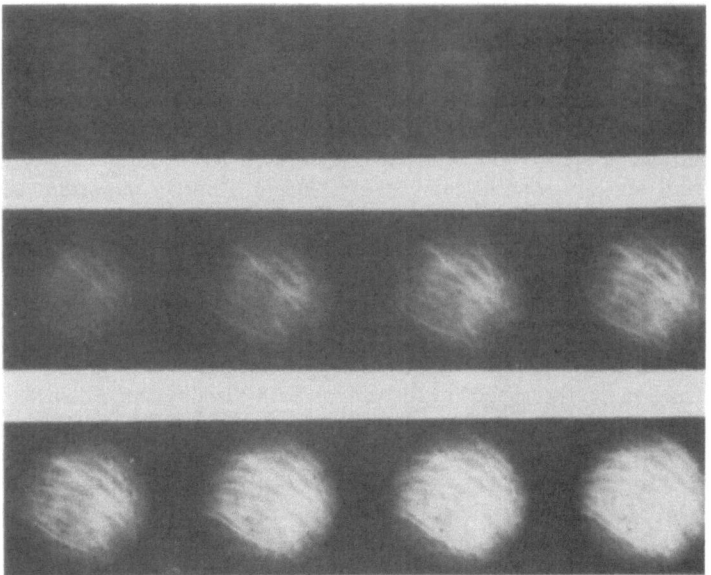

Fig. 3. Sequence of ICG fluorescence angiograms of human peripheral choroidal circulation. The angiograms were made at a rate of 5 per second and progress in time from left to right and from top to bottom in the figure.

in the auxiliary filter holder of the fundus camera*. When operated at maximum recommended voltage and with both filters in position, the continuous light source produces retinal irradiance of 140 milliwatts per square cm. within a bandwidth of 7480 Å to 7950 Å. This is below the maximum permissible level specified by the American National Standards Institutes, Inc. (ANSI Z136. 1-1973) for this region of the spectrum with continuous exposures of up to 24 seconds. In practice, only 12 seconds of exposure are required in order to record a complete sequence of angiograms. Of course, in order for this modified fundus camera system to function properly, perfect alignment of the continuous light source and optimal operation of the motorized 35 mm camera must be assured. A sequence of angiograms made at the rate of 5 frames per second (using a 35 mm movie camera with a 1/15 second shutter speed instead of a motorized standard 35 mm camera) is shown in Figure 3.

* Preferentially, the ICG excitation filter may be permanently mounted in the recess between the condenser lens and the fundus camera beam splitter. Since transmission characteristics of this band-pass, interference type filter depend upon the angle of incident light, it must be located in the path of near-parallel light. A small control box (a, Figure 2A) installed in the fundus camera background lamp power cable turns off the background lamp whenever the quartz halogen lamp is on. Thus, no unfiltered light enters the eye when angiograms are being made, regardless of the location of the ICG excitation filter. Since this filter also transmits virtually all visible light wavelengths below 7000 Å, mounting it permanently in the fundus camera does not significantly limit the camera's use for fluorescein angiography or color photography except for some attenuation of light energy.

In making ICG fluorescence angiograms, it must be born in mind that ICG dye undergoes fluorescence quenching just as sodium fluorescein dye and that ICG dye fluorescence efficiency is not nearly as high as that of sodium fluorescein dye. Thus, injection of ICG dye must be made in such a way that by the time the dye bolus travels from the cubital vein injection site to the ocular blood vessels it is diluted to exactly that concentration producing maximum fluorescence intensity. Excessive dye dilution beyond this ideal concentration results in reduced fluorescence intensity. Injection of a 1 ml bolus of ICG dye having a concentration of 20 mg per ml in aqueous solvent followed immediately by a 5 ml saline flush appears to produce best results (FLOWER, 1973). Development of this regimen was based on the facts that maximum ICG fluorescence in blood occurs at a concentration of approximately 0.03 mg/ml and that, following injection into the cubital vein, a dilution in blood of approximately 600 times takes place by the time the dye bolus reaches the eye.

Figure 4 tabulates the limitations to spatial resolution of choroidal structures attributable to the optics of the eye, optics of the modified fundus camera, and characteristics of the photographic film emulsion used. Based upon these data alone, photographic film seems to be the limiting component in the angiographic process, and it would appear little can be done to improve this situation as better films are not now available (all photographic films work on the same silver halide process, hence, they all have the

Diffraction Limit of the Human Eye Having a **Pupil Diameter of 1 5 mm**	$7 \mu m$ @ 5200Å Wavelength $11 \mu m$ @ 8300Å Wavelength
Equivalent Retinal Resolution Obtained by **Photographing a High Contrast Resolution Chart with the Modified Zeiss Fundus Camera** using	
A. Kodak High Resolution Holographic Film (Ultra high resolution, but very low sensitivity)	$5 \mu m$ @ 5200Å Wavelength
B. Kodak Tri-X Film (Usual film for sodium fluorescein angiography)	$11 \mu m$ @ 5200Å Wavelength
C. Kodak High Speed Infrared Film (Film used for indocyanine green angiography)	$20 \mu m$ @ 8300Å Wavelength

The above data clearly demonstrates that spatial resolution in angiograms of the eye is limited by the photographic film used rather than by the optical system of the fundus camera or the eye.

Fig. 4. Tabulation of factors contributing to limitation of spatial resolution of fundus structures. Note calculations are based on the 1.5 mm effective pupillary diameter used in the Zeiss fundus camera. Use of a larger pupillary diameter would require correcting for the relative large range of variations in spherical aberration which exists in human eyes.

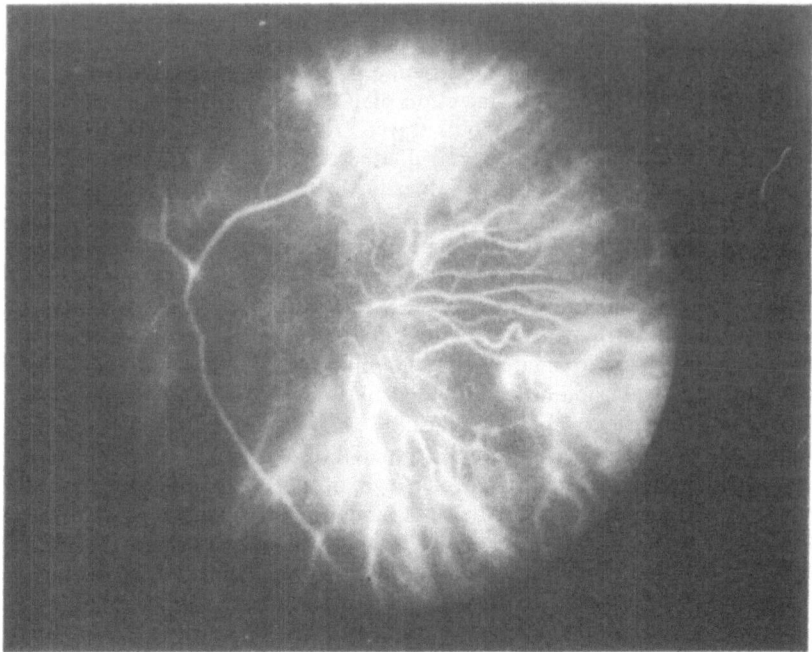

Fig. 5-A. ICG fluorescence angiogram of patient with lesion of unknown origin resulting in loss of pigment epithelium and underlying choriocapillaris.

same quantum efficiency). Yet, there is evidence to suggest that a still more significant limitation to spatial resolution of choroidal structures in the angiograms actually results from characteristics of the eye associated with its anatomy. Specifically, it appears that pigment in the pigment epithelium and in the choroidal interstices causes significant scatter of light emitted by the fluresceing ICG dye. The presence of blood in the two retinal capillary nets and in the choriocapillaris probably also contributes to this scattering. Figure 5A is an ICG angiogram showing a lesion of unknown cause resulting in segmental loss of pigment epithelium and some loss of underlying choriocapillaris. Sharply defined vessels under the lesion may be followed directly to the margin of the lesion at which point they become extremely blurred. Consequently, with respect to spatial resolution attainable in the normal eye where pigment epithelium and choriocapillaris are entirely intact, one would expect to see angiograms resembling the areas surrounding this lesion.

The effect in choroidal angiograms of reduced contrast of smaller choroidal vessels due to fluresceing dye in underlying vascular layers must also be considered. In Figure 5B the angiogram of a diabetic patient with numerous photocoagulations in the nasal fundus shows patchy filling of the choriocapillaris. Areas under coagulation spots are not as well profused with ICG dye as surrounding areas. Note the patch of choriocapillaris in the periphery (between 2 and 3 o'clock) almost surrounded by photocoagulation spots. In this patch, which drains into a single vein (arrow), capillary level vessels are just resolved. Evidence such as this suggests that of all the possibilities

64

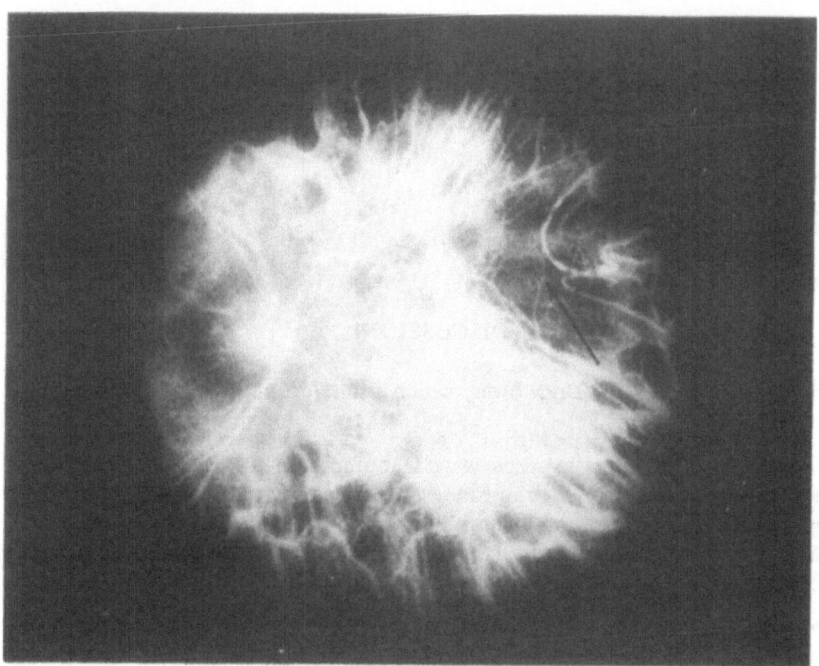

5-B. ICG fluorescence angiogram of nasal fundus of diabetic patient following fairly extensive argon laser photocoagulation. Note drainage of capillary bed into single choroidal vein (arrow).

considered thus far (including photographic films), it is the anatomy of the eye which constitutes the greatest limit to resolution of vascular detail in choroidal angiograms.

The optical components of the modified fundus camera have apparently been refined to the extent that resolution of choroidal vascular structures is limited by properties inherent in the eye itself. Therefore, the technique of choroidal angiography might now be used to first study characteristics of choroidal circulation in normal eyes and then in eyes having known pathology in order to determine the possible extent of clinical application of indocyanine green dye angiography (ORTH, PATZ & FLOWER, 1976).

REFERENCES

FLOWER, R.W. Infrared absorption angiography of the choroid and some observations on the effects of high intraocular pressures. *Am. J. Ophthalmol.* 74: *600-614* (1972).

FLOWER, R.W. Injection technique for indocyanine green and sodium fluorescein dye angiography of the eye. *Invest. Ophthal.* 12: *881-895* (1973).

FLOWER, R.W. & HOCHHEIMER, B.F. A clinical technique and apparatus for simultaneous angiography of the separate retinal and choroidal circulations. *Invest. Ophthal.* 12: *248-261* (1973).

FLOWER, R.W. & HOCHHEIMER, B.F. Indocyanine green dye fluorescence choroidal angiography performed simultaneously with infrared absorption and fluorescein angiography. *Johns Hopkins Med. Journal* 138: *33-42* (1976).

ORTH, D.H., PATZ, A. & FLOWER, R.W. Potential clinical applications of indocyanine green choroidal angiography – Preliminary report. *Eye, Ear, Nose & Throat Monthly* 55: *15-28* (1976).

Author's address.
The Johns Hopkins University
Applied Physics Laboratory
Johns Hopkins Road
Laurel, Maryland 20810, USA

DISCUSSION

Dr Querioz Marinho: Dr Flower, which filters do you use for ICG angiography?

Dr Flower: The filters we used were manufactured for us by Ditric Optics in Massachussets. However, you can get the necessary filters made by almost any manufacturer. I recommend shopping in order to get them made as cheaply as possible. The peak excitation wavelength for ICG fluorescence is about 795 nM; the peak of fluorescence is at 8350 Å.

Dr Tokoro: Using infrared color film we have done infrared absorption angiography with intravenous injection of ICG. We tried to use band pass filters and got better images of choroidal vasculature. Dr Flower, do you have experience with infrared color films?

Dr Flower: The infrared color film was first used by Kogure in Miami some time ago. They tried to do this type of angiography with intra-arterial injection of dye in monkeys. It was a 'false color' technique. We abandoned that immediately, in fact we never even tried it because determination of proper exposure levels and proper control of development of color films is extremely difficult. The variations from patient to patient are too hard to handle so we have never considered even attempting that technique.

Dr Amalric: Je voudrais demander à Mr Flower s'il a utilisé sa méthode à l'indocyanine dans des cas d'albinisme ou de sclérose choroidienne pour mieux préciser les grands axes vasculaires artériels et veineux.

Dr Flower: As a matter of fact we have done two or three albinos. As I mentioned when I gave the paper, this is fairly easy to do since one does not have all the problems with photopic people when attempting to make the angiograms. But in fact interpretation of albino angiograms might be harder than those of normally pigmented eyes. Since the dye enters from the back of the eye, in these lightly pigmented eyes you can possibly see dye fluorescence arising from episcleral blood vessels. I am not certain from where you first see fluorescence, but the speed with which the dye fills vessels is such that it is very difficult to separate fluorescence from the underlying vascular layers which fill first from those which are higher up. I do not know if Dr Patz is going to mention some of this. He has a lot of still slides to show, but we have not seen much in our albino studies that has helped us more than looking at the normal pigmented fundus.

CINE ANGIOGRAPHIC INFLOW MEASUREMENTS USING FLIUORESCEIN AND INDOCYANINE GREEN

D.W. HILL & S. YOUNG

(London, England)

Measurement of the retinal blood flow even with the invasive techniques available in animal studies is difficult. The use of cine angiography reported by BULPITT & DOLLERY (1970) has been widely exploited by that group of workers. The present report concerns the results obtained by two principal modifications of their technique, a faster framing rate using speeds up to 141 p.p.s. and the employment of alternative dyes, fluorescein or indocyanine green (I.C.G.). Additionally this work was carried out on the cat whereas DOLLERY and colleagues used either the pig or the monkey. Details of the methods and background studies have been reported (YOUNG, 1975; HILL & YOUNG, 1976).

ACCURACY

As has already been reported (HILL & YOUNG, 1976) the appearance of the dye bolus varies considerably in different arterioles. To ease the difficulties of measuring linear flow velocity, particularly in unfavourable circumstances, measurements were made by observing the number of frames elapsing whilst the dye bolus travelled between two landmarks whose separation was measured. Using this technique the accuracy varied from site to site; when grouped angiograms were analysed the 95% confidence limits fell within ± 10% of the mean in two thirds, and ± 6% in one third of the sites. Because these variations are unpredictable careful statistical planning of experiments when using this technique is essential.

QUALITATIVE DIFFERENCES OF FLUORESCEIN AND I.C.G.

Angiograms, taken with the two dyes, show by the appearance of the arterio-venous crossings that the blood column is opaque in fluorescein, but translucent in I.C.G., angiograms (HILL & YOUNG, 1976).

The dyes differ photographically, fluorescein being detected by light emission in a different wavelength, and I.C.G. by negative contrast as it reduces the background infra red (I.R.) image by absorbing the illuminating radiation. Despite the lower contrast of I.R. angiograms, the background variance of grouped angiograms, when pulse effects are discounted, is significantly smaller in I.R., as compared to fluorescein, angiograms of the same sites (Table I). The explanation of this phenomenon is not certain, but it may lie with the slight variation of exposure found in rapid stroboscopic flash, which will produce a varying penetration of the blood column in fluorescein angiograms, thereby recording faster or slower flowing laminae of blood.

Table I. Residual variance in pulse grouped angiograms

Dye	Mean Frames Lapse	Variance	D.f.
Fluorescein	7.61	1.44	72
			F 3.00 0.001 > p
I.C.G.	6.26	0.48	54

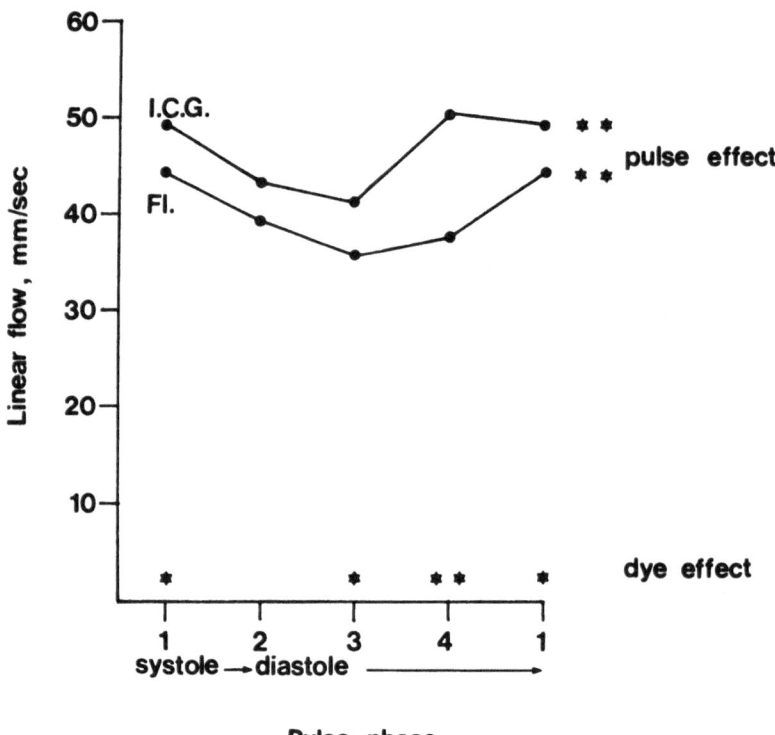

Fig. 1. Graph of the mean linear inflow rates, mm/sec at the retina, prepared from 40 fluorescein and 31 I.C.G. angiograms divided according to the pulse phase of inflow. The statistical significance of variance ratios, F, is indicated: *$0.05 > p > 0.01$, **$0.01 > p > 0.001$. The upper line refers to the pulse effect for each dye separately; the lower line to the dye effect at each pulse phase.

68

PULSE EFFECTS

BULPITT, KOHNER & DOLLERY (1973) reported large fluctuations of inflow in relation to the pulse phase at which the measurement was made; in the present study, of the cat, a less marked fluctuation was found. Fig. 1 shows the plot of the mean inflow velocities from 8 sites studied with both fluorescein and I.C.G. by repeated angiograms within a short interval. The angiograms were grouped according to the pulse phase at which the inflow commenced, 1, systolic, 2-4, early, mid, and late, diastolic. Two features are apparent; the I.C.G. inflow is always faster, and there is a gradual slowing of the inflow rate through diastole. In addition a phase difference is seen, for the flow rate in phase 4, the last third of diastole, has already increased with I.C.G. whilst with fluorescein this is the slowest phase. A three factor variance analysis of the results, by sites, pulse phase, and dye, shows a significant variance for the sites and the interaction of pulse phase with dye, but the pulse phase, and dye, main effects are not significant. When the data is broken down, two factor analyses show significant pulse phase and site effects for each dye individually; whilst similar analyses of dye and site effects by individual pulse phase show significant dye effects in phases 1, 3, and 4 (Fig. 1). The ratio of I.C.G. to fluorescein inflow rates fluctuates widely, but the mean value is 1.19.

CROSS SECTIONAL FLOW VELOCITY PROFILE

The more rapid inflow seen on I.R. angiography coupled with the greater translucency of the blood column to radiation of this wavelength, supports the idea that there is a central core of blood, shown by the I.C.G, moving more rapidly than the peripheral annulus shown by fluorescein. Furthermore there is a phase difference between the central core, which is flowing rapidly in phases 4 and 1, and the peripheral annulus which is only flowing rapidly in phase 1. The most likely explanation of these results is an earlier onset of the systolic phase in the central core, even though phase 4 is nominally diastolic. The results of the phase difference must be a change in velocity profile across the arteriole, but further analysis is inhibited by the irregularity of bolus distribution. BULPITT, KOHNER & DOLLERY (1973) have also described alterations in bolus profile, as well as changes in flow rate in different pulse phases, by measuring changes in the manifest bolus profile using fluorescein angiography. These results are difficult to accept in view of the poor penetration of blood by the fluorescent emission, though this may be partly improved by increasing the illumination (YOUNG, 1975).

CONCLUSION

These results have formed a part of validation studies. Differential flow rates with I.C.G. and fluorescein are of importance not only to rheology, but for the interpretation of future laser doppler studies.

REFERENCES

BULPITT, C.J. & DOLLERY, C.T. Retinal cine angiography. *Brit. Kinematography Sound & Television* 52: *14-16* (1970).

BULPITT, C.J., KOHNER, E.M. & DOLLERY, C.T. Velocity profiles in the retinal microcirculation. *Bibl. Anat. Basle* 11: *448-452* (1973).

HILL, D.W. & YOUNG, S. Arterial inflow studies of the cat retina, using high speed angiography. *Exp. Eye Res.* (1976, in press).

YOUNG, S. High speed cine angiography. *Medical & Biological Illustration* 25: *199-204* (1975).

Authors' address:
Research Department of Ophthalmology
Royal College of Surgeons of England
London, England

DISCUSSION

Dr Kohner: I would like to ask Prof. Hill about his findings with indocyanin green. Like fluorescein indocyanin green is also bound to plasma proteins; therefore, how does he explain the differences he gets? The second question is, how does he explain on physiological grounds that the maximum flow with indocyanin green is in late diastole? It does not seem to make much sense?

Prof. Hill: Thank you very much. I was not sure of the first point you wanted to raise; the answer to the second point is that I said that it is an apparent diastole. It was taken from a crude pulse tracing the femoral blood pressure and there may be a phase difference. I am sure there must be. I agree it is nonsense to expect the fast flow in diastole. We are not getting the beginning of systole with the pulse tracing properly. What was the first point about protein binding?

Dr Kohner: If both substances are protein bound, why should one be apparently flowing at a different rate than the other one?

Prof. Hill: Well, I think it is a question of the degree of penetration of the vessel, which I tried to show in the two simultaneous projected frames of the angiogram and in the diagram I drew of the cross-section of velocity profile. Indocyanin green will give total penetration of the vessel and you will see a more axial stream of dye than you see with fluorescein.

Dr Kohner: But if you get higher intensity of illumination, would you abolish, to some extent at least, differences in the penetration effect?

Prof. Hill: I think there is evidence that if you get more illumination you do reduce that difference. There is a small differential in the apparent flow rates with my apparatus between stroboscopic flash and a continuous illumination system, which gives you a slightly higher level of illumination and slightly faster flow.

70

RIBOFLAVIN FLUORESCENCE ANGIOGRAPHY

M. SHIMOTORI, J. CHIBA & S. AOKI

(Chiba, Japan)

ABSTRACT

Solution of riboflavin shows intense fluorescence. The wavelength of emitted fluorescence is distributed with a peak of 530 nm. Absorption peaks of riboflavin are 266 nm, 373 nm and 445 nm. The Olympus fundus camera which is equipped with exciting and barrier filters for fluorescein angiography was used in this experiment. Albino and pigmented rabbits were injected with riboflavin phosphate through the ear vein. The angiogram was similar to that of sodium fluorescein. Retrobulbar injection of riboflavin revealed a faint background fluorescence.

Fluorescence photography with riboflavin is greatly dependent upon the quantity and concentration of riboflavin phosphate solution.

INTRODUCTION

Since NOVOTNY & ALVIS (1961) first described the method of fluorescence angiography, sodium fluorescein dye was used to perform angio-

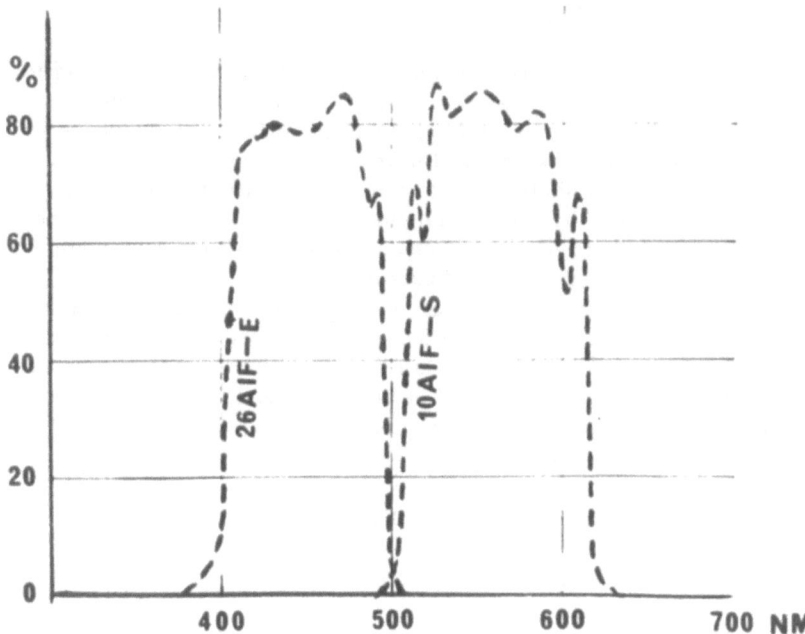

Fig. 1. Transmission characteristics of the filters of the Olympus fundus camera.

71

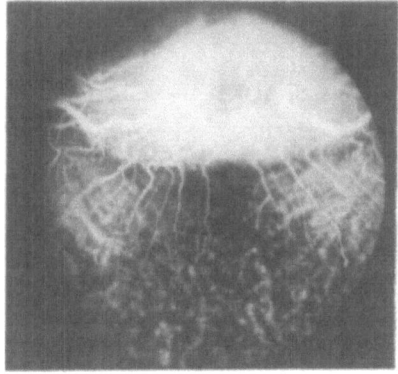 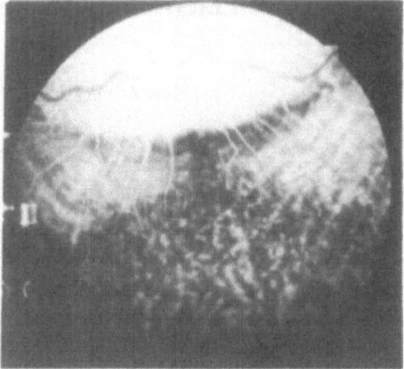

Fig. 2. Riboflavin angiography with a 1% Fig. 3. Fluorescein angiography with a 5%
solution.   solution.

graphy in the human; other dyes including Lissamine Rhodamine B
(MACHEMER, 1970) and acridine orange (KUWAMOTO, 1969) were confined to animal experiment. Indocyanine green dye was used to study the
retinal and choroidal vasculature in animals and the human (KOGURE,
1970; FLOWER et al., 1973). Riboflavin has been used clinically in riboflavin deficiency. Solutions of riboflavin show intense fluorescence, and
fluorescence angiography was performed in rabbit (SHIMOTORI et al., 1975).
    The purpose of this paper is to describe riboflavin fluorescence angio-
graphy comparing it to that of fluorescein sodium.

MATERIALS AND METHODS

Albino and pigmented rabbits weighting 1.5-2.0 kg were used. The animals
were given an intravenous injection of 1 ml/kg of 1% or 4% solution of
riboflavin without anesthesia. After general anesthesia with ketamine, a
retrobulbar injection of 0.5 ml or 1 ml of 4% solution of riboflavin was
given. In some animals photocoagulation was applied to the retina with the
Zeiss photocoagulator. Riboflavin phosphate was used in solution. The absorption peaks of riboflavin are 266 nm, 373 nm and 445 nm, and the fluorescent emission is distributed with a peak of 530 nm.
    The Olympus fundus camera was equipped with an exciter filter of
26 AIF-E and a barrier filter of AIF-S (Fig. 1). This pair of filters is appropriate for riboflavin angiography because of a maximum transmission of the
emitted fluorescence of riboflavin. The flash exposure of the camera was
300 joules. Kodak Tri-X film (ASA 400) was used and developed for
30 minutes.

RESULTS

1. Intravenous injection of riboflavin

When a 1% solution of riboflavin was injected rapidly through the ear vein
of a normal animal, the retinal arteries were clearly demonstrated in a dark

72

fundus because of the faint choroidal pattern. Venous filling of dye and a bright background fluorescence followed. In the late venous phase background fluorescence decreased, leaving a dark fundus.

When a 4% solution was administered, background fluorescence increased in the arterial phase and the retinal vessels became more intensly fluorescent than with a 1% solution. A high quality angiogram was demonstrated, both retinal vessels and background fluorescence were distinct for a long period.

2. Retrobulbar injection of riboflavin

After injection of riboflavin, the optic disc became gradually fluorescence and background fluorescence developed. Retinal veins and arteries were

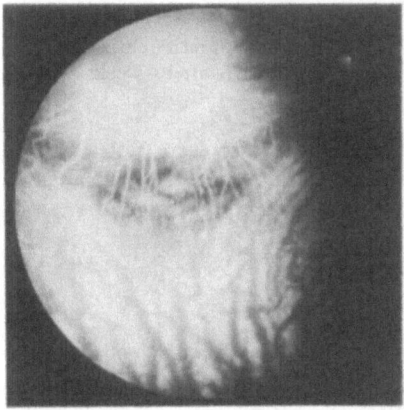

Fig. 4. Riboflavin angiography with a 4% solution by intravenous injection.

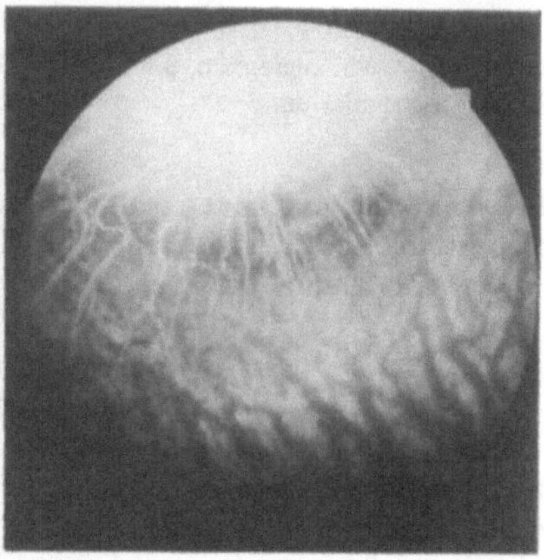

Fig. 5. Riboflavin angiography with a 4% solution by retrobulbar injection.

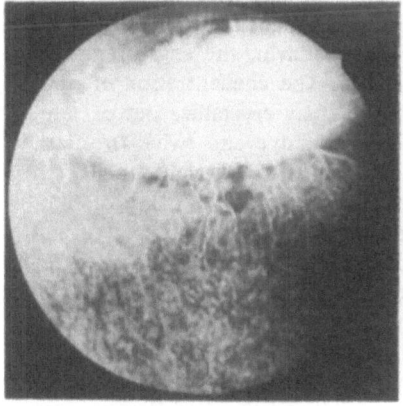
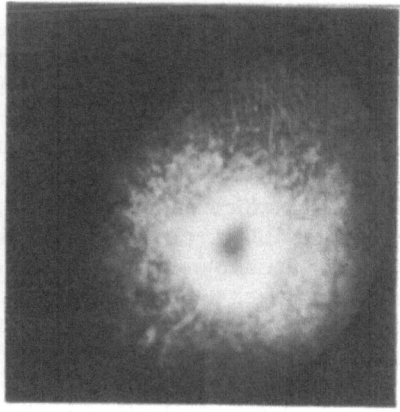

Fig. 6. Riboflavin angiography.

Fig. 7. Diffusion of riboflavin dye after photocoagulation.

73

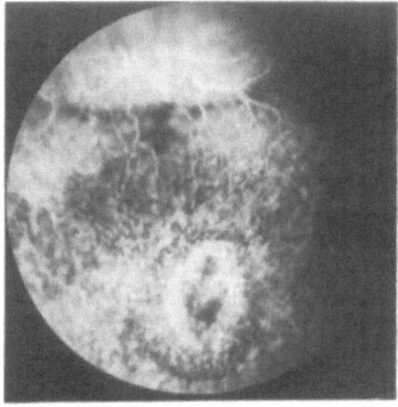

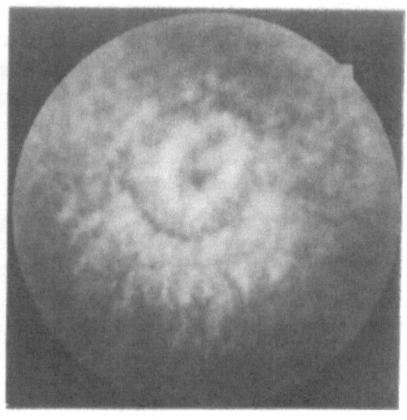

Fig. 8. Riboflavin angiogram, 3 weeks after photocoagulation.

Fig. 9. Angiogram of retrobulbar injection of riboflavin after 4 weeks.

filled with the dye, but small vessels around the disc were not clearly demonstrable in the angiogram. The intensity of fluorescence of the angiogram depended upon the quantity of riboflavin injected.

3. Riboflavin angiogram of the photocoagulated eye

In the photocoagulated eye the lesion looked slightly grey with a white centre; the angiogram revealed an early fluorescent staining of the periphery and delayed fluorescence in the centre. Diffusion of fluorescence continued after the venous phase. Intense fluorescent areas were visible in the dark fundus for 15 minutes after injection.

DISCUSSION

The fluorescence of riboflavin is less intense than that of fluorescein sodium. In normal eyes, after injection of riboflavin, the angiogram corresponded exactly to a fluorescein angiogram. The concentration of riboflavin cannot be raised beyond 4% because it may crystallize out of solution. Theoretically about twice the quantity of dye and twice the flash intensity are necessary to produce an angiogram of equivalent quality to that obtained with sodium fluorescein. After retrobulbar injection of riboflavin in the rabbit, the disc became increasingly fluorescent and retinal vessels near the disc were filled with fluorescent dye. Between the big choroidal vessels which remained dark an increasing fluorescence became visible; but small vessels around the disc were not clearly demonstrable as compared with the appearances of an intravenous angiogram.

Diffusion of riboflavin seemed to occur slowly in photocoagulated areas and remained for 30 minutes after injection; the pattern of fluorescence with riboflavin corresponded to that with fluorescein sodium.

The quality of fluorescent photography with riboflavin is greatly influenced by the quantity of riboflavin and the choice of appropriate filters.

As the intake of riboflavin is increased above the minimal daily requirement, a large proportion is excreted unchanged in the urine. In general high concentration of riboflavin are found in the retina, kidney, liver and heart. The presence of riboflavin in the retina seems to be in some way related to the visual process. The clinical symptoms of riboflavin deficiency in the human are described as dimness of vision, impaired visual acuity and photophobia, accompanied by a cornal lesion. Administration of a high concentration of riboflavin to the retina caused a transient decrease of C-wave amplitude of the ERG, which gradually recovered and increased in 20 minutes.

The action of riboflavin on the retina should be studied before clinical use as a fluorescent dye.

REFERENCES

FLOWER, R.W. & HOCHHEIMER, B.F. A clinical technique and apparatus for simultaneous angiography of the separate retinal and choroidal circulation. *Invest. Ophthalmol.* 12: *248-261* (1973).

HEIMAN, M. Riboflavin significance of its photodynamic action and importance of its properties for the visual act. *Arch. Ophthalmol.* 28: *493-502* (1942).

KOGURE, K., DAVID, N.J., YAMANOUCHI, U., et al. Infrared absorption angiography of the fundus circulation. *Arch. Ophthalmol.* 83: *209-214* (1970).

KUWAMOTO,,K. Fluorescence fundus photography by acridine orange. Proc. Int. Symp. Fluorescein Angiography, Albi 1969, pp. *12-15*. Karger, Basel (1971).

MACHEMER, R. Angiographic-histologic correlation of eye vessel permeability with protein-bound fluorescent dye. *Amer. J. Ophthalmol.* 69: *27-38* (1970).

SHIMOTORI, M. & AOKI, S. Riboflavin fluorescence angiography. *Acta Soc. Ophthalmol. Jap.* 79: *1748-1752* (1975).

YAGI, K. Biochemistry of flavin. Kyoritsu Shupan (1957).

YANO,T. Electroretinographic studies on the influence of vitamins upon the experimental endopthalmitis of the rabbit. *Acta Soc. Ophthalmol. Jap.* 68: *1962-1977* (1964).

Authors' address:
Department of Ophthalmology
School of Medicine
Chiba University
Chiba-shi
Japan

EXPERIMENTAL ANGIOGRAPHY COMBINED WITH ROUTINE BLACK-AND-WHITE ANGIOGRAPHY MADE POSSIBLE BY UTILIZING A DOUBLE-CAMERA 'MADO' HEAD

P. HENDRICKSON & C. KAYABA

(Joban, Japan)

V. DRAGOMIRESCU

(Bonn, W. Germany)

The investigation and refinement of new angiographic techniques, including experimental combinations of exciting and barrier filters, of films and developers, as well as of new tracer materials, has up to now been hampered by the necessity of securing test results in addition to a routine, clinical black-and-white fluorescein angiography, requiring a return visit for the patient to receive a second injection of dye 'only for research'. To perform a second, simultaneous infrared angiography in rabbits, BESSHO et al. (1975) utilized a beam-splitting 'filter mirror' to distribute the fundus image to two motorized cameras which, by means of appropriate barrier filters, differentiated between the fluorescent-yellow and the infrared-sensitive components of the light returning from the retina and choroid which had been illuminated by

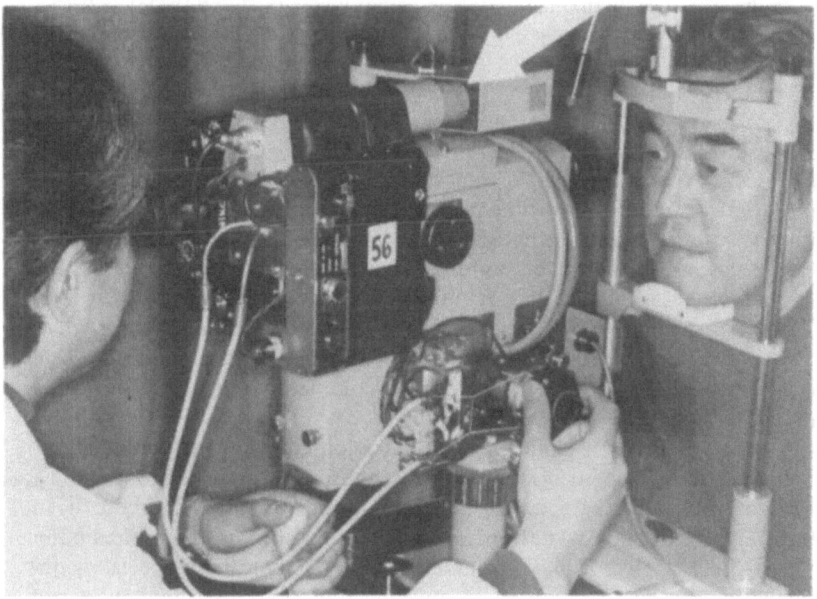

Fig. 1. Utilization of the MADO head mounted on an Olympus GRC fundus camera, permitting normal juxtaposition of photographer and patient. The overhead location of the digital timer and its optical system is indicated by an arrow.

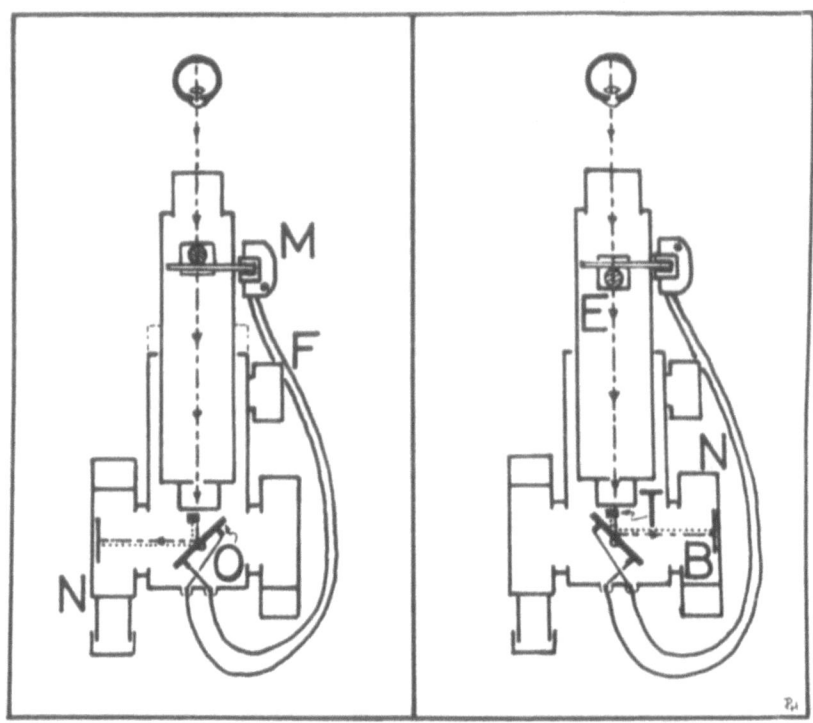

Fig. 2a, b. Sketches of the photographing pathways for the left-side (2a) and right-side (2b) camera bodies. (M = master knob; F = focussing knob; O = optical mirror; N = Nikon F2 camera body; E = exciting filter; B = barrier filter; and T = timing at its point of entrance into the fundus camera optical pathway).

flash through a wide band interference filter, offering a combination of Na = Fluorescein-exciting blue light at 490 nm with 50% transmission, and an appropriate infrared absorption peak for Indocyangreen (ICG) at 805 nm with 65% transmission. Although somewhat handicapped by transmission losses, such a system can be useful in angiographic situations such as that just mentioned, which permit an interdependence of filtration. However, the performance of certain other double-angiographic combinations, such as black-and-white fluorescein angiography combined with color fluorescein angiography, necessitates the usage of two, completely independent exciting and barrier filter sets.

In order to perform clinically such filtration-independent double angiographies with a single injection of contrast substance, we have constructed a so-called 'Multiple Angiographic Documentation' or 'MADO' photo head which replaces the normal automatic mirror reflex housing and camera body of an Olympus GRC fundus camera (Fig. 1). By turning a specially-constructed master knob mounted to an elongated shaft to which the usual Olympus filter-holding plates are affixed, the blue-interference exciting filter for black-and-white fluorescein angiography is brought into its normal location in the fundus camera's light path while a swinging optical mirror in the MADO head is simultaneously turned by means of a cable drive into a position 45° to the optical axis of the fundus camera to direct the retinal image into the motorized Nikon F2 camera body mounted on the left (Fig. 2a). The master knob, when turned slightly further, triggers that left-side camera which is equipped with a Kodak KW15 barrier filter and Tri-X film, thus providing a normal, black-and-white angiogram. For the next exposure, the master knob is turned through 90° in the opposite direction, to a point at which the other exciting filter plate, fitted, for example, with a Kodak KW32 filter for color fluorescein angiography, comes into position in the fundus camera light path. This turning of the master knob also turns the MADO head's mirror through 90° (Fig. 2b), thus directing the retinal image into the right-side motorized Nikon F2 camera body fitted with the necessary Kodak KW56 barrier filter and High Speed Ektachrome film. Further turning of the master knob triggers the right-side camera, while the 90° turning motion of the exciting filter plate is appropriately arrested. The left-side camera is equipped with a Nikon 6X magnifying viewfinder, permitting a normal juxtaposition of photographer and patient, as seen in Figure 1.

Hence, by repeated back-and-forth turning of the master knob, two alternative and completely independent angiographies can be performed (Fig. 3a, b), with the only difference from a routine angiography that the patient must experience being the alternating color of the flash. Mirrored into the frame with each angiogram, digital timing is also photographed to further secure the independence of the two angiographies while allowing their time-wise correlation when desired. The exposure levels of the two films employed can be balanced, when necessary, by using either neutral density filtration, development manipulation, or a combination thereof.

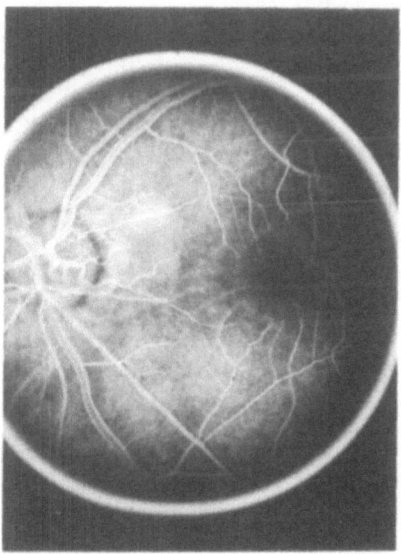 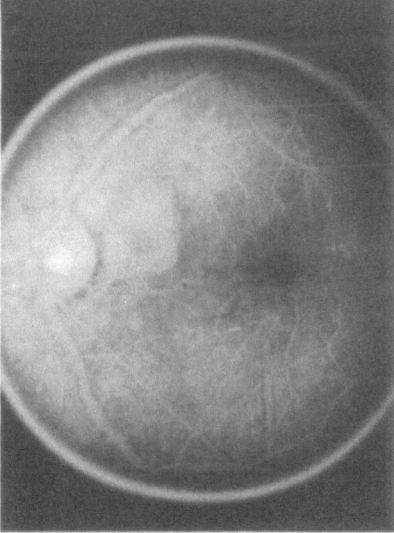

Fig. 3a, b. Sequential photographs from a double angiography. (3a) black-and-white fluorescein angiogram at 9 seconds, and (3b) color fluorescein angiogram at 10 seconds following the injection of 5 cc of 10% Na = Fluorescein in a 49 y.o. man.

The choice of usage of the experimental side of the MADO head is one to be made based upon the interests of the individual researcher. Due to the authors' long-standing interest in the field of color fluorescein angiography (HENDRICKSON et al., 1970), this choice in our case has been, moreover, that of color angiography, a technique suffering from a lack of clinical experience that could provide a reference against which routine clinical results could be interpreted. Such basic experience is now being gained in our clinic utilizing the MADO head equipped with the above-mentioned filter combinations.

ACKNOWLEDGEMENTS

The authors would like to express their deep appreciation to Dr. Masaya Takeuchi, Director of Joban Hospital, for his kind support of this research. Appreciation should also be expressed to Mr. F. Maruyama of the Olympus Optical Co., Tokyo, for his assistance in securing some of the mechanical parts used in the construction of the MADO head.

REFERENCES

BESSHO, T., SUDA, T., NISHIKAWA, N., KOBAYASHI, K. & MANABE, R. Simultaneous Fluorescence and Infrared Fundus Photography. *Jap. J. Clin. Ophthal.* 29: *1177-1181* (1975).

HENDRICKSON, P., ONIKI, S. & ELLIOTT, J. The Matsui Color Fluorescein Angiography Technique: Adaptation to the Zeiss Fundus Camera. *Arch. Ophthal.* 83: *580-583* (1970).

Keywords:
Multiple angiographic documentation
MADO head
Filtration-independent double angiographies
Master knob
Juxtaposition
Digital timing
Time-wise correlation

Authors' address:
Department of Ophthalmology
Joban Hospital
Ueno Dai 2
Joban, Iwaki-shi 972
Japan

ILLUMINATION THRESHOLDS

A. VASSILIADIS

(Palo Alto, Calif., USA)

INTRODUCTION

It is the intent of this paper to examine the limitations imposed by retinal damage on the light requirements for fundus photography and angiography. To this end we briefly review the retinal damage mechanisms and levels and then compare measured light output of fundus cameras with these levels.

The retina is the most vulnerable part of the eye to radiation in the visible and near infrared parts of the spectrum. This is due to the transparency of the ocular media, the high absorption by melanin granules, and the focusing properties of the eye.

Retinal damage from optical radiation has been studied for many years by many investigators (GEERAETS et al., 1965; HAM et al., 1970; VASSILIADIS et al., 1969; VASSILIADIS et al., 1971). The exposure times of the majority of these studies were short, less than one second duration, and the damage that resulted was shown to correspond to an acute lesion caused by thermal effects. The criterion for damage for most of these studies was based on ophthalmoscopic observation of experimental animals. However, other studies using histological, histochemical, and functional damage criteria have given support to these data so that they can be used to establish safe limits of exposure.

Investigations have also been made for the case of prolonged or repeated exposures. The duration of exposure in these investigations have been of the order of many minutes and up to several hours. The first such study was made by NOELL et al. (1966) who demonstrated retinal degeneration in rats exposed to ordinary levels of light when the animals' body temperature was raised above normal. Studies in rhesus monkeys have shown similar results using white light such as provided by an indirect ophthalmoscope (KUWABARA & GORN, 1968; ISO, 1973), and repeated flash lamp exposures (VASSILIADIS et al., 1969). The observed damage occurs at levels of light that are far below those associated with thermal damage – thus, a photochemical mechanism appears to be the basis of long term damage exposures. More recently, using laser light of various wavelenghts, long term damage has been shown to be wavelength dependent (HAM, private communication; LAWWILL, 1973; VASSILIADIS, 1975).

THRESHOLD DAMAGE AND FUNDUS CAMERA

Retinal damage due to optical radiation may be discussed in terms of duration of exposure. Two regions of retinal damage are identified – short exposure (nominally less than 10 sec duration) where damage is thermal in nature, and long exposures (equal to or greater than 10 sec duration) where damage is apparently photochemical and partly thermal. It is important to examine both areas since the fundus camera is operated in both regimes and in the transition between the two.

In the short exposure regime, the damage is due to thermal processes such as the denaturation of proteins and the inactivation of proteins. At very short times, the damage is primarily determined by the incident power density independent of the diameter of the exposed site and the damage is related to a constant energy density. At longer times there is considerable variation in threshold power density as a function of the spot diameter because thermal conduction to tissues surrounding the exposed site plays an important role, and the damage is related to approximately a constant power density.

In the long exposure regime, experimental evidence indicates that the damage mechanism is basically photochemical in origin. Thus, the power density required is again more or less independent of the diameter of the exposure and the damage is associated with a constant energy density.

Experimental data appropriate for exposures similar to fundus camera exposures are not available. Thus, in order to evaluate fundus camera hazard levels it is necessary to use extrapolation from other experimental data. All the data points shown in Figure 1 involve extrapolations or assumptions from the original experimental data. For short times (curve for less than 10 sec exposures) allowance has been made for thermal conduction variation as a function of spot diameter. For the longer exposures, however, it has been assumed that there is no variation in threshold power density as a function of spot diameter.

Power and energy measurements were taken on Zeiss fundus cameras. The data for typical clinical settings were measured as follows:

	Fundus Flash II	Fundus Flash III
Viewing Light		
Standard	4.2 mW	3.5 mW
Fluorescein	0.95 mW	0.6 mW
(Spectrotech Filter)		
Flash		
Photography	54 mJ	73 mJ
Angiography	22 mJ	26 mJ
(Spectrotech Filter)		

Examination of the consequences of a single flash on the retina shows that even for the highest measured value (73 mJ) the energy density at the retina is well below the damage threshold level for white light (GEERAETS et al., 1965). There is a safety factor at approximately 20 in this situation.

We examine next the possible danger from the viewing light over long duration exposures. We find that the retinal power density for the highest value corresponds to about 6.5 mW/cm^2 which, referring to Figure 1, is apparently safe even for exposures of hours in duration.

The most hazardous situation occurs when the fundus camera is flashed for 2 to 3 times per second for several seconds. The average power associated with this condition is shown in Figure 1 for the Zeiss Fundus Flash III. It is apparent that the operation is safe under conditions of exposures lasting for 10-20 seconds (at 2.5 frames per second) for photographic exposures with only a safety factor of approximately 2.5. However, in experimental situations of cinematography, under similar flash exposures, frame rates of 8 or higher would be dangerous.

For fluorescein angiography (at 2.5 frames per sec), there appears to be a safety factor of approximately 8. Again for cinematography application, hazardous levels would be reached at rates of about 16 frames per second. Additionally, there is recent evidence[3] that the damage level in the exposure duration of 1 to 10 second for the shorter wavelengths is appreciably lower than that shown in Figure 1. Thus, the safety factor for fluorecein angiography may be lower than discussed above.

CONCLUDING REMARKS

We have seen that photography and angiography using a standard fundus camera is safe when photographs are taken at low repetition rates. However, when the rates are increased to levels above the standard systems, hazardous retinal levels are approached.

It must be emphasized that the information used for comparison was based on rhesus monkey experimental data, and its extrapolation to humans must necessarily be guarded. At short exposures it has been shown that the human fundus is somewhat less sensitive to damage than the rhesus. However, for long exposures, the threshold levels are probably comparable and

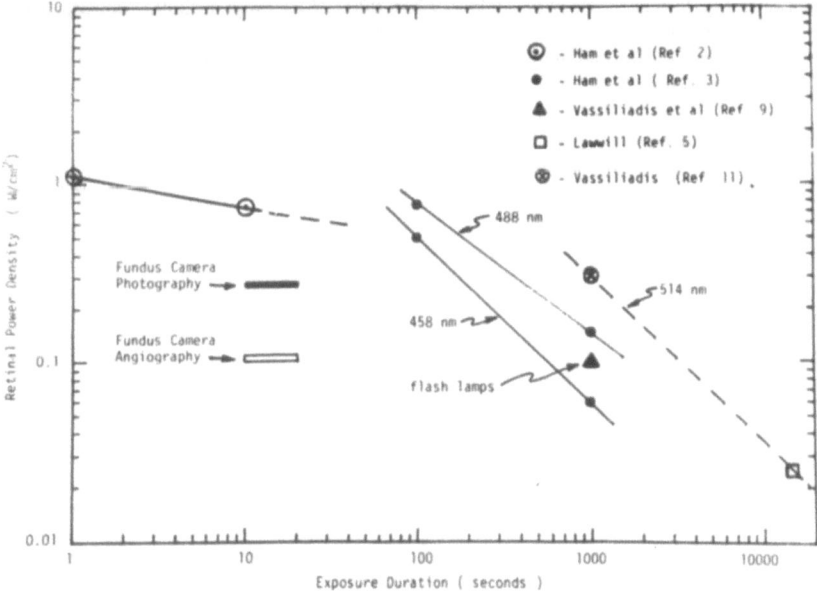

Fig. 1. Threshold retinal power density as a function of time.

possibly lower for humans. Thus, extension of the hazard findings to humans, particularly for longer duration exposures, must be made with great care.

Finally, it is of interest to point out that according to the ANSI Report on the Safe Use of Lasers, the levels in fundus photography and angiography discussed above are higher than the recommended maximum permissible exposure levels.

REFERENCES

GEERAETS, W.J. et al. Laser versus light coagulator: a fundoscopic and histological study of chorioretinal injury as a function of exposure time. *Federation Proc.* 24 (1), Part III, Suppl. 14 (1965).

HAM W.T., Jr. et al. Retinal burn thresholds for the helium-neon laser in the rhesus monkey. *Arch. Ophthal.* 84: *797-809* (1970).

HAM, W.T., Jr. Private communication.

KUWABARA, T. & GORN, R.A. Retinal damage by visible light. *Arch. Ophthal.* 79: *69* (1968).

LAWWILL, T. Effects of prolonged exposure of rabbit retina to low-intensity light. *Invest. Ophthal.* 12: *45* (1973).

NOELL, W.K. et al. Retinal damage by light in rats. *Invest. Ophthal.* 5: *450* (1966).

TSO, M.O.M. Photic maculopathy in rhesus monkey. *Invest. Ophthal.* 12: *17-34* (1973).

VASSILIADIS, A., ROSAN, R.C. & ZWENG, H.C. Research on ocular laser thresholds. Final Report. Contract F41609-68-C-004, SRI Project 7191. Stanford Research Instistute, Menlo Park, California (1969).

VASSILIADIS, A., et al. Investigation of retinal hazard due to pulsed xenon lamp radiation. Final report, Contract Xerox Corp., SRI Project 7112. Stanford Research Institute, Menlo Park. California (1969).

VASSILIADIS, A., ZWENG, H.C. & DEDRICK, K.G. Ocular laser threshold investigations. Final Report, Contract F41609-7-C-0002, SRI Project 8209. Stanford Research Institute, Menlo Park, California (1971).

VASSILIADIS, A. Retinal damage by long exposures to light. Macular Workshop, Bath, England (1975).

Author's address:
Palo Alto Medical Research Foundation
860 Bryant Street
Palo Alto, California 94301
USA

DEMONSTRATION OF AQUEOUS OUTFLOW BY FLUORESCEIN INJECTION INTO THE ANTERIOR CHAMBER AFTER VARIOUS TYPES OF GLAUCOMA OPERATIONS

A. TENNER & W. JAEGER

(Heidelberg, W. Germany)

The demonstration of aqueous outflow after glaucoma operations by means of fluorescein injection into the anterior chamber of the eye was first satisfactorily performed by KLEINERT in 1953. He could observe the outflow of aqueous humor from the filter pleb after Elliot's trepanation through the lymph vessels of the conjunctiva. Consequently, he was basically the first to have successfully performed fluorescein-angiography. This was long before the publications of NOVOTNY & ALVIS appeared in 1961 regarding fluorescein-angiography of the retina. We now find ourselves once again referring back to the examination methods of KLEINERT now that new micro-surgical glaucoma operations in the chamber angle and on Schlemm's canal have developed and interest in the demonstration of newly-formed outflow-pathways has become so acute. At the same time, modern fluorescein-angiography, expecially fluorescein-cineangiography, provides exceptionally good possibilities for analyzing the effectiveness of new types of glaucoma operations.

Our examinations were carried out on eyes with very poor function, under sterile condition in the operation room. For cineangiography we used a Zeiss slitlamp with a xenonbulb type XBO 15o as a light source. A film camera (Bolex H 16) was mounted on a beam-splitter with a barrier filter (Kodak-Wratten 15 Gelatine-Filter) inserted into the diaphragm opening. After careful puncture of the anterior chamber with a discission needle on the limbus at a position across from the filter plebs, a solution of 0.1 to 0.2% Fluorescein sodium was injected from a short canula (10 mm) into the chamber. We attempted to hold the intraocular pressure at a normal or moderately raised level.

The fluorescein injection into the anterior chamber, after Elliot's trephining confirmed the findings of KLEINERT. Should the intraocular pressure climb during the filling of the anterior chamber, for example, to above 20 mm Hg, then the filter pleb is the first to fill with the solution. This effect shows itself in a circumscribed, more plane-like coloration under the conjunctiva in the region above the trephining opening. Gradually, the draining from the filter pleb begins through the lymph-vessel-like structures of the conjunctiva in a somewhat limbus-parallel direction to the inner and outer lid angle. (Fig. 1) Proof that we are dealing here with the lymph-vessels of the conjunctiva has not yet been obtained. There are certain indications, however, that this presumption is justified. Foremostly, BENEDIKT

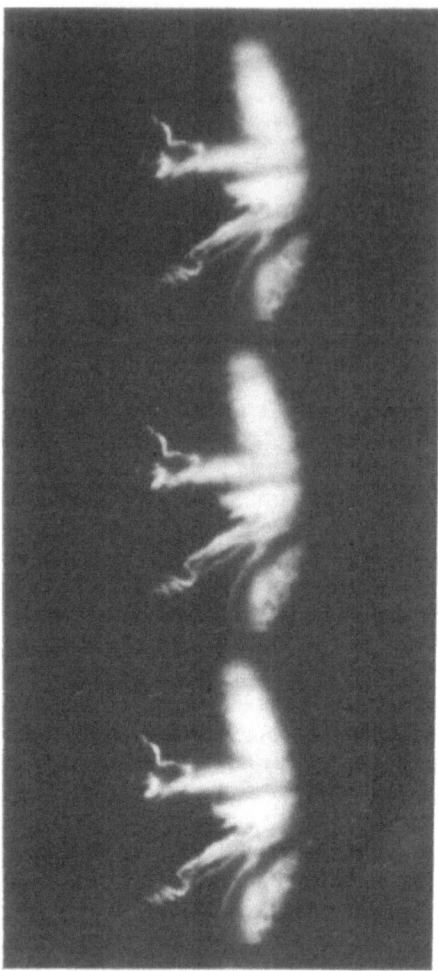

Fig. 1. Aqueous outflow out of a filtering pleb into the lymph-vessel of the conjunctiva after Elliot's trephining, demonstrated by Fluorescein injection into the anterior chamber.

(1975) was also able to observe a drain-off of aqueous humor through these lymph-vessel-like structures of the conjunctiva during examinations on eyes after trabeculectomy.

The trabeculotomy was performed in such a manner that an absolutely water-tight closure of the scleral flap was intended with five sutures of 10-0 nylon. No drainage of aqueous humor through the filter pleb, for example, was revealed, but rather a drainage solely through the aqueous veins, and, interestingly, over those veins which had exposed themselves prior to the operation. Observation of the patient over almost 2 years showed a reliable pressure drop through surgery from pre-operative 40 mm Hg with maximum medication to post-operative 16 mm Hg without medication. Our findings, regarding the outflow of aqueous humor mainly through the aqueous veins, indicated that by re-opening Schlemm's canal to the anterior chamber with opening the trabecular mashwork, the natural drainage pathway was opened once again (Fig. 2). The main drainage resistance in this patient could well have been localised in the trabecular mashwork.

The trabeculectomy was performed by us in the same manner as demonstrated recently by BARRAQUER in 1973: Opening of the conjunctiva at approx. 8 mm away from the limbus with a straight incision and blunt pushing off to the limbus. Preparation of a scleral flap of approximately 4 x 4 mm in 1/2 scleral thickness to the blue-white-border. Excision of the trabecular mashwork in an area of approx. 1.5 x 1.5 mm with opening of the anterior chamber. Removal of the irisprolapse with basal iridectomy; closure of the scleral flap with 2 single sutures of 10-0 nylon, whereby the

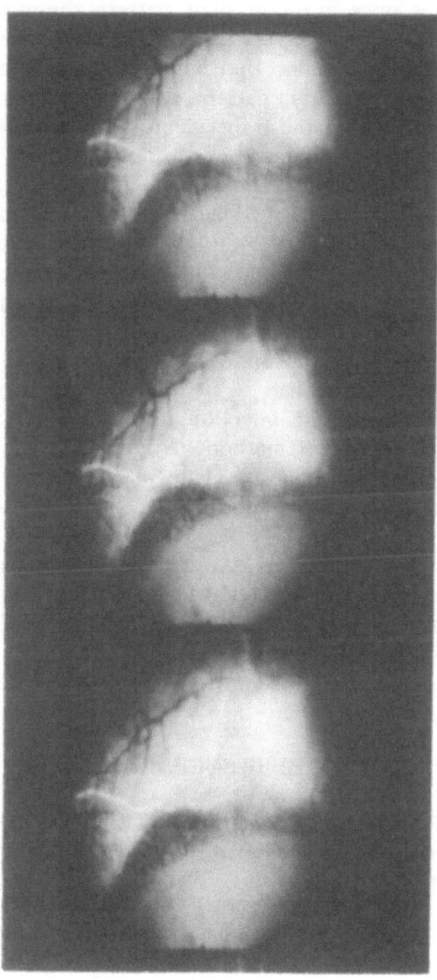

Fig. 2. Aqu ous outflow into aqueous veins after trabeculotomy.

sutures are only relatively loosely tied, in order for the scleral flap only to adapt and to avoid a water tight closure.

The results of the fluorescein injection in the anterior chamber show that, on the basis of a trabeculectomy performed in this manner, we are dealing here with a 'protected' filtering operation.

In the patient approximately 4 months after surgery, clinical examination shows a vascularized and relatively less prominent, but, at the same time, diffuse filter pleb running out to all sides with a intraocular pressure of 17 mm Hg without medication. Immediately after filling the anterior chamber with fluorescein, dye appears in several of the vessels emerging from the depths of the filter pleb. We could be witnessing here intra- or episcleral veins newly opened during the operation. BENEDIKT was also able to demonstrate such veins in his examination regarding the operational function of the trabeculectomy. As secondary drainage, the lymph-vessels presented themselves once again in their pattern running parallel to the limbus toward the outer and inner lid angles. Finally, we note a diffuse distribution of coloration under the conjunctiva. This diffuse drain-off could be described as a third drain pattern. As a result, fluorescein injection in the anterior chamber after the trabeculectomy can demonstrate at least three different pathways of drainage of various swiftness. An outflow of aqueous humor over the newly-opened Schlemm's canal, originally discussed as the main operational function of trabeculectomy, appears, on the basis of our findings and those of BENEDIKT, to play no essential role.

Also the findings of the Tuebingen glaucoma study regarding the pressure patterns after protected filtering procedures point especially to well-opened draining pathways. Our examinations are able to confirm these findings on the basis of the exposure of the draining vessels by Fluorescein injection into the anterior chamber.

Taken together, fluorescein injection into the anterior chamber has shown itself to be an excellent method of demonstrating the outflow of aqueous humor after various types of glaucoma operations. Consequently, the effectivity of the new micro-surgical glaucoma operations can now be better analyzed.

This method appears to be less suitable for routine diagnosis. LINER (1975) cites a more conserving method of introducing fluorescein into the anterior chamber, namely with Iontophorese. On the basis of our experience with this method, unfortunately, however, we have not succeeded in attaining an adequate concentration of fluorescein in the anterior chamber.

REFERENCES

KLEINERT, H. Die Vitalfärbung des Kammerwassers und seiner epibulbären Abfluss-wege nach Fluoresceininjektion in die Vorderkammer. *Klin. Mbl. Augenheilk.* 122: 665 (1953).

KLEINERT, H. Der sichtbare Kammerwasserabfluss glaucomkranker Augen nach Fluorescein-Füllung der Vorderkammer. Ein Beitrag zur Pathologie des intraocularen Flüssigkeitswechsels. *Klin. Mbl. Augenheilk.* 123: 653 (1953).

BENEDIKT, P. Zur Wirkungsweise der Trabekulektomie. Kongress der Österreichische Ophthalmologischen Gesellschaft. Insbruck (1975).

NOVOTNY, H.R. & ALVIS, D.L. A method of photographing fluorescence in circulating blood in the human retina. *Circulation* 24: *82* (1961).

TENNER, A., JAEGER, W. & KOCH, W. Darstellung von Kammerwasservenen durch Fluorescin-Injektion in die Vorderkammer beim Kaninchen. *Klin. Mbl. Augenheilk.* 164: *628-632* (1974).

TENNER, A. & JAEGER, W. Darstellung von Kammerwasservenen durch Fluorescein-Injektion in die Vorderkammer. *Ber. d. DOG* 1972: *479-481* (1974).

TENNER, A. & JAEGER, W. Darstellung des Kammerwasserabflusses nach Glaucom-operationen durch Fluoresceininjektion in die Vorderkammer. Filmdokumentation v. Kongress der Bayrischen Augenärztevereinigung, Oktober 1974.

LINER. Diskussionsbemerkung beim Symposion. Operative Behandlung des Glaucoms mit offenem Kammerwinkel. Tübingen, April 1975 (in press).

Authors' address:
University Eye Clinic
Heidelberg, W. Germany

FUNDAMENTAL ASPECTS OF POSTERIOR OCULAR CIRCULATION

PAUL HENKIND, M.D., Ph.D., F.A.C.S.

(Bronx, N.Y., USA)

Fluorescein angiography can be understood if one appreciates the fundamental aspects; anatomic, physiologic, and pathologic, of the posterior pole circulation. This paper considers some of those basic aspects of the retinal, choroidal, and optic disc head circulation particularly as they relate to fluorescein angiography. The fundus angiogram is simply a series of photographs documenting the passage of a dye through vascular pathways. Fluorescein enters and leaves the posterior pole circulation in a well defined manner and by analysis of the angiogram quantitative and qualitative statements about the circulation can be made. For example, the various circulation times, arm-retina, intraretinal, choroido-retinal, are 'quantitative' measurements, while filling patterns, defects, leaks, etc. are 'qualitative' evaluations.

We will consider three aspects of the posterior circulation: 1) Vascular pathways including angioarchitecture and vessel structure; 2) Some physiologic parameters; and 3) Pathologic responses.

1) VASCULAR PATHWAYS

a) Gross anatomy

The blood vessels of the retina, choroid, and optic disc, all originate from branches of the ophthalmic artery. The inner portion of the retina is nourised by the central retinal artery, generally a separate branch of the opthalmic artery, while the outer half of the retina and the optic nerve head are supplied by branches of the posterior ciliary arteries. Due to the differing path lengths and calibers of these vessels we find different circulation times for the retina and choroid. Usually the choroidal and disc vessels are perfused earlier than the retinal vessels, but the opposite situation may also occur. The sequence of filling, and the various circulation times are determined basically by anatomic and hemodynamic factors.

b) Retinal vasculature

The retinal circulation is an end artery system with only one major afferent and one major efferent vessel, the central retinal artery and central retinal vein respectively, and an interposed capillary bed. The major vessels and their ramifications are basically the plumbing bringing blood to the capillary bed, where the acts of nutrition and purification are carried out. The retinal capillary bed forms several layers at the posterior pole and while these layers are readily obvious on analysis of histological specimens, particularly those prepared by ink injection or retinal digestion, the only easily distinguishable capillaries seen by routine fluorescein angiography are the perifoveal arcade and the most superficial retinal capillaries making up the layer of radial peripapillary capillaries (RPC's). Much has been made about the presence of a capillary-free zone around retinal arteries and a less prominent capillary-free zone around retinal veins. In the embryonic development of the retinal circulation such a zone is absent, and it occurs due to the normal vascular remodeling necessary to ensure a mature bed which will distribute blood evenly through the retina.

The deeper retinal capillary bed is considered more closely related to the venous side of the circulation while the superficial bed(s) is more intimately involved with the arterial side. This has practical application when considering the variety of hemorrhages seen in the fundus. In venous occlusive conditions including diabetes, deeper retinal hemorrhages, of a 'dot and blot' nature are frequently encountered, whereas linear 'flame-shaped' hemorrhages occurring in the superficial retina are a hallmark of arterial disease. The RPC's seem to be particularly involved in a variety of ocular conditions including hypertensive retinopathy, papilledema, posterior inflammatory disorders, and perhaps also in glaucoma. Most 'flame-shaped' hemorrhages and cotton wool spots occur in the region of the RPC's and this territory of distribution is seemingly an anatomic counterpart of the Bjerrum area of field defects.

Recent angiographic studies (YEUNG et al., 1973) have demonstrated the appearance of capillaries crossing the foveal zone of the retina, normally considered to be an area free of vessels. These vessels are simply the remnants of an embryonic capillary bed which has not fully disappeared, and the significance of the persistent vessels in unknown (HENKIND et al., 1975). More important is the predilection of the macular capillaries to be involved in processes distant from the macula. We find cystoid macular edema and macular exudation, a reflection of 'leaking' capillaries in disparate conditions such as anterior uveitis, 'pars planitis', Irvine-Gass syndrome, peripheral angiomatosis, etc. This situation has been termed by WISE (1966) the 'exaggerated macular response'.

The presence of arterio-venous crossings in the retina is certainly significant. Such crossings are most common in the temporal portion of the posterior pole. At such crossing sites the artery and vein (which generally lies beneath the artery) share a common adventitia. Disease of the wall of one vessel significantly affects the adjacent crossing vessel. Thus, in hypertension, there may be arterial alterations which affect the vein and cause a branch retinal vein occlusion. Another site where there is a common adventitial coat is at the lamina cribrosa and this is the favored locale of central retinal vein occlusion. The question of whether a retinal vein occlusion can occur without significant ischemia due to arterial pathology has been raised by HAYREH and others.

Fluorescein angiography has helped to clarify the status of the cilioretinal artery(s). Recently, JUSTICE et al. (in press) demonstrated by angiography, that approximately 50% of humans possess one or more cilio-retinal arteries. Such vessels, generally 'hook' around the disc margin temporally and almost always fill prior to the rest of the retinal arteries, reflecting the fact that they arise from a source other than the central retinal artery. Presumably, they originate from either an independent posterior ciliary artery or a branch of a posterior ciliary artery which also supplies a segment of the choroid. Angiography has demonstrated that the cilio-retinal artery serves a distinct intraretinal territory and that in occlusive episodes a discrete zone is either spared or obliterated without significant overlap from the surrounding retinal circulation. For example, in the case of cilio-retinal artery occlusion, the surrounding retinal capillary bed, fed by a patent central retinal artery, does not protect the infarcted area.

The composition of the retinal vessels is worthy of comment. The central retinal artery and its branches almost to the retinal periphery are muscular arteries. Past the first bifurcation of the central retinal artery there is a lack of an internal elastic lamina. Sympathetic nerve endings are absent from the intraretinal vessels. All retinal vessels are lined by a continuous layer of endothelial cells whose walls are joined by 'tight' junctions. The retinal capillaries are fine, thin-walled vessels lined by endothelial cells and covered by a layer of intramural pericytes (IMP). The function of these latter cells is unknown but they seem to be selectively destroyed in diabetes mellitus.

c) Choroidal vessels

The choroid is supplied by a number of ciliary arteries each of which has its own territory of supply. On the practical level we find this expressed by a variety of segmental choroidal filling patterns which have led to the 'watershed' hypothesis of Hayreh. We also find *spatial* filling 'defects' of the choroidal capillary bed which were, at one time, interpreted, as pathologic defects, but which are now recognized as physiologic variations in filling time without any particular significance. The choriocapillary network, once considered to be a continuous vascular bed, anatomically and physiologically, now has been shown to consist of virtually independent vascular segments each with its own 'end' artery. This information helps us to explain the often patchy pattern of choroidal disease. The capillaries of the choroid are broad channels, more like sinusoids, lined by endothelium which is fenestrated. The majority of these fenestrations occur on the side of the vessel apposed to Bruch's membrane. Presumably, this is important in a functional sense. Federman, who has been studying the choroidal fenestrae, feels that they may be a dynamic phenomena, and that there are significant differences in their number in the various regions of the choroid (personal communication). He has also found alterations in the position of the fenestrae in macular degeneration and in choroidal tumors.

d) Optic nerve head vessels

Anatomic and angiographic data support the view that the optic disc is nourished by the short ciliary rathar than by the central retinal artery circulation. Furthermore, it is obvious that the disc head has its own separate arterial supply which divides into a capillary bed independent of the choriocapillaris. Support for these statements is seen in conditions such as central retinal artery occlusion where the disc circulation is normal on angiography; and ischemic optic neuropathy where the central retinal artery blood flow is normal in spite of absent perfusion of the disc. One question that is often raised concerns the association of pathologic damage in the juxtapapillary choroid with that in the disc. While the capillary beds to the regions are entirely separate it is conceivable that processes affecting the feeding arteries to the contiguous areas could lead to vascular damage affecting both the choroid and disc. Ultrastructurally, the capillaries of the disc head resemble retinal capillaries.

e) Central retinal vein

An anatomic feature of importance is that the central retinal vein is the major efferent channel for both the retinal and the disc head circulations and the vortex veins drain the choroid. Intercommunications of capillaries do exist between the optic disc and the retina, but these tend to be insignificant. On the other hand, the intercommunication of disc and choroidal vessels can lead to the formation of rather substantial collaterals veins – opticociliary veins – in instances of central retinal vein obstruction.

2. PHYSIOLOGY

We will briefly consider the concepts of blood flow and autoregulation, innervation of vessels, and permeability.

a) Blood flow

It is pertinent to consider how blood flows through the vessels at the back of the eye. Are all of these blood vessels freely communicating open conduits or are there intermittently closed pathways? As far as we know the retinal vessels including the capillaries are open all of the time, and they do not show evidence of intermittent closure typical of visceral capillaries. Retinal blood flow seems to follow the path of least resistance, and while sphincters at arterial branchpoints have been conjectured about as a means of routing blood, such structures are lacking in man and other primates.

We should not lose sight of the fact that ophthalmoscopically we *do not* see a retinal blood vessel per se, but rather a column of moving blood. The visible column is comprised basically of the axially flowing red blood cells, the peripheral plasma is invisible. During fluorescein angiography the plasma layer is made visible hence the blood column appears wider in angiogram than in color photograph. If the blood flow becomes sluggish in the vessel then segmentation of the blood column occurs, i.e., 'box car' or sludging effect. Walls of retinal vessels are normally invisible but occasionally can be seen as a congenital sheathing at the disc, or in pathologic situations such as arterio-sclerosis or inflammatory diseases where secondary vascular changes occur.

Though retinal blood vessels appear to remain open all of the time, constriction and dilation of the major vessels can be seen ophthalmoscopically. Since nervous innervation to these vessels is absent, an internal mechanism within the vessel must control the vascular tonus. This has been termed autoregulation. The site of autoregulation is presently unknown. The stimulus for autoregulation seems to be the level of the blood pressure or perhaps some metabolic factor. For example, in systemic hypertension the retinal blood vessels constrict – if their walls are not sclerotic from arteriosclerosis. In conditions leading to stasis the retinal vessels dilate suggesting the presence of a metabolic initiator.

When retinal blood vessels constrict or dilate they must do so in three dimensions. Thus, a narrowed vessel is also a straighter one; and a dilated one is tortuous.

The choroidal vessels are richly innervated and presumably respond to sympathetic stimulation. The choriocapillary bed seems to be continually open and has a high rate of blood flow. The function of this two dimensional network is more than merely nutritional. The choriocapillaris also acts to remove the heat generated during the visual process from the back of the eye. In the monkey choroidal blood flow is approximately 20 times that of the retina. The high rate of blood flow through the choroid leads to a very low oxygen extraction compared to the greater degree of oxygen extracted from blood passing through the retina. It is a high rate of oxygen extraction that gives the color difference between retinal arteries and veins. In situations where there is no interposed capillary bed in which the oxygen extraction takes place then no difference in color can be discerned between the afferent and efferent vascular loop, (i.e. racemose angiomas).

Too little is known about the blood flow within the vessels of the disc head to make any meaningful comment at this time.

b) Permeability

The most important elements at the back of the eye are the neurons. The other components, blood vessels and glia, serve to sustain the nervous cells. Such cells must be nourished from the outside environment and yet must be insulated from it. This is done eminently well at the level of the retina. A dual blood supply assures that nutrition reaches the various retinal layers. The inner retina being supplied by intraretinal vessels and the outer retina receiving its oxygen and other nutriment from the choriocapillaris. The retinal vessels never directly contact the neurons but rather are coated with glial elements, mainly Müller cells, which also surround the neurons. It appears that there is a transfer of nutritive material from the capillaries to the investing glia and thence to the nerves. Not all of the vascular contents are poured out, rather there is a selective outflow of nutrients from the vessels. Here we invoke the concept of *permeability*. The holding back of certain substances including fluorescein, in the vessels of the central nervous system is the so-called bloodbrain barrier. In the eye we have the similar or identical bloodretinal barrier, and a retinal pigment epithelial barrier. The latter is an exquisite nonvascular adaptation necessary to preserve the integrity of the outer retina from being flooded by material from the porous choriocapillaries. It is the intactness of the various barriers that makes fluorescein angiography feasible. For if the dye immediately 'leaked' out of the retinal vessels and permeated the surrounding tissue we would not be able to examine the circulation. One area where there is a lack of a barrier is at the rim of the optic nerve head. Here, fluorescein leaking from the choriocapillaris crosses the marginal disc tissue and stains the periphery of the nerve. This, of course, must be distinguished from the abnormal staining found in papilledema and papillitis. Unknown at present are the exact mechanism(s) responsible for permeability. Is the process mediated simply by a physical barrier at the level of 'tight' junctions, or is there an active metabolic component allowing or preventing egress of material from the vessel? Exactly what blood borne substances pass through retinal vessels is still unclear. Studies using fluorescein labeled dextrans of known molecular weight promise to provide important data about the permeability of ocular vessels (BELLHORN & BELLHORN, personal communication).

Alterations in the permeability of retinal vessels are seen in diabetes, uveitis, vascular occlusive disease, and macular edema of many causes. It is the terminal end of the capillary, the post-capillary venule which seems to be the most susceptible locus for a breakdown of normal permeability.

3. PATHOLOGIC RESPONSES

Here we will concern ourselves simply with the two major developmental pathological responses of retinal blood vessels, namely neovascularization and collaterals. These two entities have tended to be confused with each other but they are non-related. By definition retinal neovascularization is new vessels originating from and contiguous with the pre-existing retinal vascular bed. They are located either within or adjacent to the retina, in areas where vessels are not normally present. Retinal collaterals are vessels which develop within the framework of the existing retinal vascular network. Collaterals originate from the retinal capillary bed, joining obstructed to non-obstructed adjacent vessels, or by-passing obstructions in a single vessel, i.e. veins are linked to veins, arteries linked to arteries, and less frequently arteries are joined to veins. Flow through these channels is generally slow, rarely normal. Fluorescein angiography shows the difference between these vascular responses. Neovascularization leaks fluorescein, indicating an altered permeability of the new vessels, while collaterals rarely leak dye except in their early stage of development.

We have touched upon some of the fundamental 'facts' about the posterior pole circulation. Some of the 'facts' will undoubtedly prove incorrect and other bits and pieces of information will be added to further our knowledge of the posterior ocular circulation.

REFERENCES

Hundreds of articles have appeared in recent years dealing with one or another of the aspects touched upon in this paper. For recent works dealing with gross vascular anatomy, I suggest the various papers of HAYREH, for those dealing with ocular circulatory physiology the works of ANDERS BILL and co-workers are admirable.

The Book 'The Retinal Circulation' by WISE, DOLLERY & HENKIND (Harper and Row, 1971) provides an overview of the subject area.

Specific references

HENKIND, P., BELLHORN, R.W., MURPHY, M.E. & ROA, N. *Brit. J. Ophth.* 59: *703* (1975).
WISE, G.N. & WANGVIVAT, Y. *Amer. Jl Opth.* 61: *1359* (1966).
YEUNG, J., CROCK, G., CAIRNS, J., HEINZE, J., TROSKI, S. & BILLSON, F. *Aust. J. Ophthal.* 1: *17* (1973).

Author's address:
Department of Ophthalmology
Montefiore Hospital & Medical Center
111 East 210 Street
Bronx, New York 10467
USA

QUANTITATIVE ASPECTS OF FLUORESCEIN ANGIOGRAPHY

PETER Y. EVANS, M.D., JOSEPH M. TERRY, M.D.,
SURESH R. LIMAYE, M.D. & ROGER C. LANCASTER

(Washington, D.C., USA)

Generally, the evaluation of clinical angiograms is done on a qualitative basis. Since the normal structures and fluorescence patterns of the fundus are well known, it is usually fairly easy to be certain whether any given angiography feature is normal or abnormal. Given sufficient photographic quality and good magnification, such observation and interpretation lead often directly to diagnosis and treatment without the need for any time consuming measurements and calculations. That, in addition to its purely aesthetic appeal, is probably a major practical reason why this method has found such universal clinical acceptance within a rather short span of time.

On the other hand, Flocks, Miller & Chao's (1959) attempts to document retinal circulation time date back to several years before the birth of modern fundus angiography. Quantitative studies have continued to intrigue some of the fluorescein fans ever since. Time was the first factor to be checked. Retinal transit times (Oberhoff et al., 1965; Evans & Wruck, 1970), arm-to-retina as opposed to arm-to-choroid circulation times, were measured by many, including Shimizu and his group (1974). Densitometry was used by Hickam & Frayser (1965) to estimate a mean retinal circulation time of 5.4 seconds, and cineangiography was finally employed for the direct determination of arteriolar retinal flow velocity by Dollery (1968), who found 20-40 mm/sec. for the superior temporal artery, and Evans et al. (1974). By combining arteriolar caliber measurements with the established flow velocity, the latter two authors were able to arrive at estimates for retinal volume flow. And serial measurements of fluorescein diameters in our lab from consecutive cine frames gave a somewhat surprising magnitude for normally invisible arteriolar pulsation for systole and diastole. All those results have been previously reported. Some of our own published cineangiography data are briefly summarized in Table I.

Other workers used rapid sequence fundus angiography for measurements of vascular reactivity to various vasoactive agents, and infrared photography for determinations of retinal blood oxygen saturation, both based on Hickam's and his co-workers' (1963) original work. Reflectometry and fluorometry were applied to studies of the choroidal and other intraocular circulations. And, finally, another factor and its effect on choroidal and retinal perfusion with fluorescein was studied: the intraocular pressure. Some of the conclusions drawn from the suction cup experiments may have been somewhat hasty but they certainly stimulated discussion.

Table I. Summary of own previous cineangiography data

Arm-to-choroid time	8.4 sec.	(5.0-14.6)
Arm-to-retina time	8.8 sec.	(5.4-14.7)
Macula transit time	1.7 sec.	(1.2-2.5)
Arteriolar peak velocity in 80-108 μm diameters	8-12 mm/sec.	
Volume flow for same diameter macular arterioles	1.2-3.5 μl/min.	
Amplitude of expansile pulsations in same aa.	6.5-9%	

PRESENT STUDY

One aspect of fluorescein angiography has in the past found only scanty attention. Although 5% and 10% sodium fluorescein solutions have been available for many years, the optimal concentration of fluorescein solutions to be administered intravenously has not been determined. Presently, in the United States, either 10 ml of a 5% solution or 5 ml of a 10% solution are commonly administered to adults without reference to their height, weight or blood pressure. Since a more voluminous solution requires a longer injection time than a concentrated solution, one might expect the more concentrated solution to arrive at the fundus as a more discrete bolus, thereby defining the end point of arm-retina circulation time and possibly enhancing the resolution of microangiopathic areas within the retina. To determine if a more concentrated solution of fluorescein would be more desirable for diagnostic purposes than the currently available preparations, a controlled, prospective, double blind study is currently underway at our institution comparing 10% fluorescein solution (Alcon Fluorescite® 10%) and 25% fluorescein solution (Alcon Fluorescein Injection 25% [AL01088]).

Preliminary studies comparing the side effects of 10% and 25% have failed to demonstrate any significant difference in the incidence of adverse reactions to the fluorescein solutions.

The patients included in today's report include five normal volunteers and twenty patients referred to Georgetown University Medical Center for diagnostic fluorescein angiography. The final series will consist of 60 patients. The subject's height, weight, pre-injection and post-injection blood pressures as well as any signs or symptoms of adverse, including delayed, reactions were recorded on standard forms. Each participant received at random either a 5.0 ml injection of 10% fluorescein or a 2.0 ml injection of the 25% fluorescein solution. A photographic record was made using the TOPCON TRC-F3 High Speed Retinal Camera with Spectrocin #4 excitation filter and Spectro #5 barrier filter. The injection was administered through an antecubital vein by a Dyonics 2020 fully automatic injector usually at a pressure of 50 pounds per square inch, and without any additional saline flush. Precise time and duration (0.3-0.5 sec.) of injection and all subsequent photographs were recorded simultaneously on a Sanborn 7700 automatic recorder. Initially, a rapid sequence was employed at 3 fps. But, in order to be able to study also later events such as duration of bolus

100

and capillary filling, the frequency was soon decreased to 1 fps. The subjects returned for repeat injection with the second concentration of fluorescein solution five to ten days later. Informed consent was obtained from all participants in the study. Following development of the film, the unlabeled angiograms were studied to determine arm-choroid circulation time, arm-retina circulation time, bolus time (beginning decrease of fluorescence in a retinal artery minus arm-retinal circulation time), and beginning of maximal perifoveal capillary fluorescence. The angiograms were compared subjectively for overall quality of resolution and focus and rated as excellent, average, adequate (for diagnosis) or poor. The observers were unaware of the concentration of dye used in each angiogram. The mean circulation times for each of the above parameters were determined and compared using the 'Paired T-Test' and regression coefficients were computed to establish whether a relationship existed between arm-retina circulation time and the subject's height, weight, height and weight, systolic blood pressure, diastolic blood pressure, pulse pressure or mean blood pressure.

RESULTS

Adverse reactions

There were no serious complications incurred by any participants in this study. Table II lists the minor complications following each injection of fluorescein.

Table II. Adverse reactions following fluorescein injections (25 patients)

	10% solution No. of Patients	25% solution No. of patients
Nausea	2	4
Nausea and vomiting	1	1
Light headedness	1	0

Arm-choroid circulation time

The arm-choroid circulation time ranged between 4.7 sec. and 16.1 sec. with a mean time of 11.3 ± 2.9 seconds for the 10% solution. For the 25% solution, it ranged between 8.2 sec. and 17.0 sec. with a mean arm-choroidal circulation time of 11.6 ± 2.3 seconds. The arm-choroidal circulation times for the two concentrations were compared by the 'paired T-Test' and at the 0.05 significance level, there was no significant difference in the arm-choroidal circulation times with either solution.

Arm-retina circulation time

The range of the arm-retina circulation time was between 8.2 seconds and 20.0 seconds for the 10% solution. The mean arm-retinal circulation times were 12.0 ± 2.8 sec. and 11.8 ± 2.3 sec., respectively. There was no significant difference between these two values.

Bolus time

The bolus time was defined as the difference between the arm-retina circulation time and the time at which the peak fluorescence within the same artery first could be observed to diminish. The true end of the bolus could not be observed satisfactorily on any of the angiograms because of dilution. Of 24 cases in which the bolus could be determined, the range for 10% solution was 4.0 sec. to 14.6 sec. and for 25% solution, 5.0 sec. and 18.5 sec. The mean values were 8.42 ± 3.02 sec. and 9.18 ± 3.67 sec., respectively. By application of the 'paired T-Test', there was no significant difference between these two values.

Perifoveal capillary filling

An estimate was made of the frame in each angiogram in which the perifoveal capillaries could first be seen in their maximal fluorescence. Of the 20 cases in which these vessels could be studied, the range for 10% and 25% solutions was 12.4-30.0 sec. and 15.3-27.7 seconds, respectively. The mean perifoveal capillaries time for these arteries was 21.7 ± 5.7 seconds and 20.1 ± 6.8 sec., respectively. This difference was barely significant at the 0.05 levels.

Regressions of arm-retinal circulation time compared with height, weight, height and weight, blood pressure

Table III shows some of the single and multiple regressions performed comparing arm-retinal circulation time with height, weight, both height and weight, systolic blood pressure, diastolic blood pressure, mean blood pressure and pulse pressure. There was no linear correlation between arm-retinal circulation time and blood pressure. While there seems to exist a general tendency for arm-retina circulation time to increase with increasing weight and height (Figures 1 and 2), the sample size is still too small to draw any definite conclusion.

Table III. Correlation factors of arm-retina circulation times with regressions against height, weight, blood pressure

Arm-Retina Circulation Time	10%	25%
vs. Height	$r = 0.509$	0.308
vs. Weight	0.407	0.368
vs. Height and Weight	0.539	0.395
vs. Systolic Blood Pressure	-0.40	0.249
vs. Diastolic Blood Pressure	0.024	0.412
vs. Pulse Pressure	-0.081	-0.038
vs. Mean Blood Pressure	-0.026	-0.340

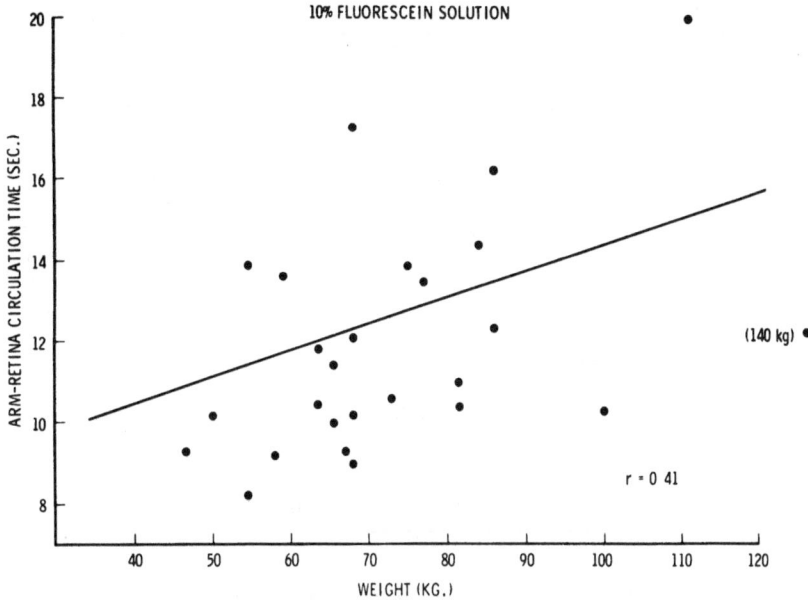

Fig. 1. Arm-to-retina circulation times against weights of patients after injection of 5 ml of 10% fluorescein solution. The correlation is relatively weak.

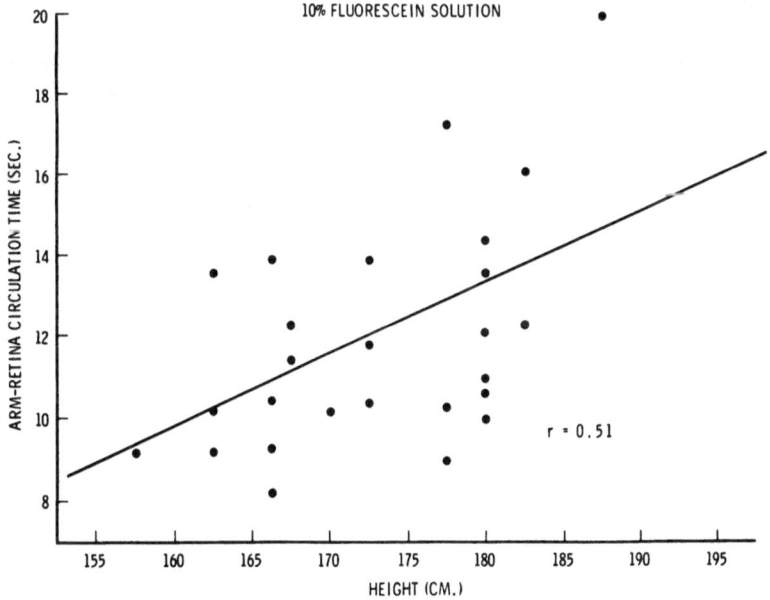

Fig. 2. Arm-to-retina circulation times against body heights of same patients as in Fig. 1 after 10% fluorescein. The correlation is slightly better.

Table IV. Resolution and focus ratings

| | 10% | | 25% | |
	Resolution	Focus	Resolution	Focus
Excellent	9	9	13	13
Average	8	11	6	9
Adequate	5	4	5	2
Poor	3	1	1	1

Table V. Overall quality of 10% solution compared to 25% solution

	Resolution	Focus
10% > 25%	4	3
10% = 25%	12	12
25% > 10%	9	10

Overall quality of resolution and focus

To determine if either solution seemed to give superior photographic results, a qualitative estimate was made of each fluorescein angiogram with special emphasis on the perifoveal capillaries. Each angiogram was rated excellent, average, adequate or poor, and was compared to the other solution. (Tables IV and V).

From this small sample, it would seem that the resolution and overall quality depend on the focus rather than the fluorescein concentration. Figures 3a and b through 8a and b represent a few examples in point.

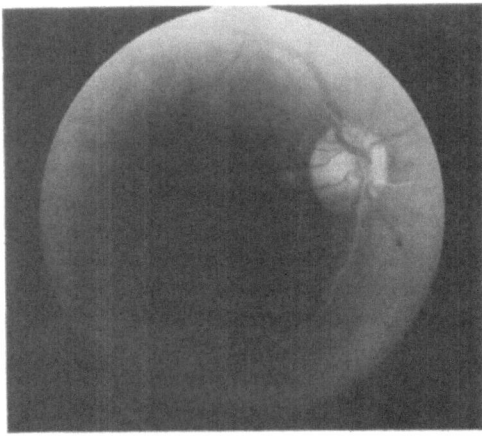

Fig. 3a.   Control, age 25 yrs; 9.05 seconds after 5 ml of 10% fluorescein.

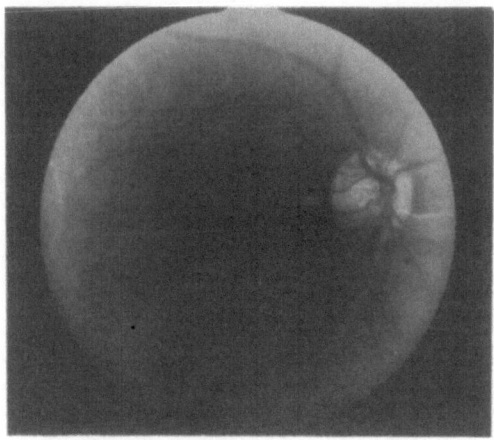

Fig. 3b. Same eye one week later; 9.65 seconds after 2 ml of 25% fluorescein. Minimally better resolution of prelaminar capillaries.

DISCUSSION

Although blood pressure level differences between patients, including hypertensives, did not show any correlation with the arm-to-retina times, this should not be taken to imply that especially a precipitous drop in blood pressure in a given individual would not influence his usual arm-to-retina appearance time. Quite to the contrary, as has been stressed by others in the past, such an occurrence will lead to a profound delay in arm-to-retina circulation time, as illustrated in Figures 9a and b.

Another experience gained in the ongoing study is that at least with the Topcon TRC F-3 one cannot at all rely on the exposed timer on the film. Without the multi-channel Sanborn recording of the entire procedure or some other absolutely reliable time control, any time-dependent investigation is doomed to doubts and disappointment. Discrepancies between the presumable film time and the Sanborn recording were frequently of such magnitude that it was finally decided to exclude all angiograms from the series without complete Sanborn recordings of both injections and photographic sequences. Although the standard deviations with cineangiography become markedly smaller, it is feasible to use the clinical set-up for simple but informative quantitative studies such as this.

Our preliminary findings suggest no significant difference in the arm-retina circulation time with either solution. In addition, the bolus time appears the same for both concentrations. The statistically slightly significant difference in perifoveal filling times may not be corroborated when our study is completed. It seems that there is a certain relationship of arm-retina circulation time to the combination of height and weight with its corollary implications for the evaluation of carotid occlusive diseases. It does appear reasonable to exclude blood pressure as a factor in arm-retinal circulation time so long as it is stable during the procedure.

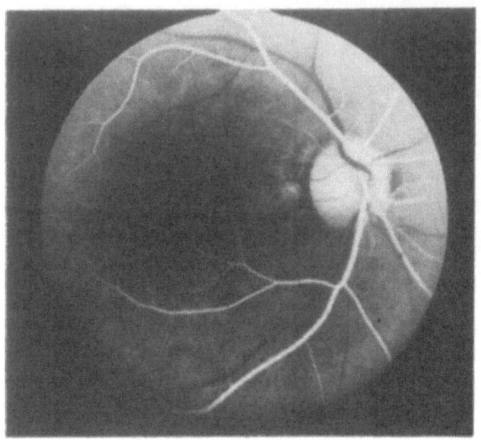

Fig. 4a.   Same run; 10.9 seconds after 10% fluorescein.

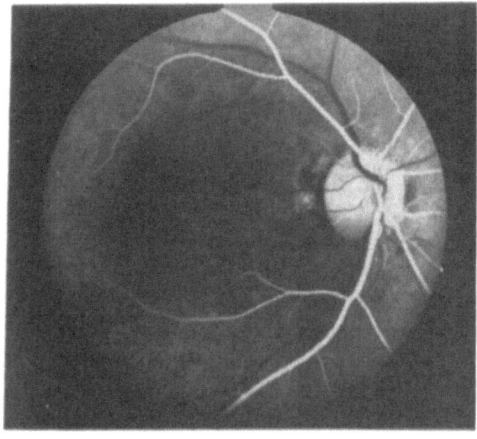

Fig. 4b.   Continued from 3b; 11.1 seconds after 25% fluorescein.

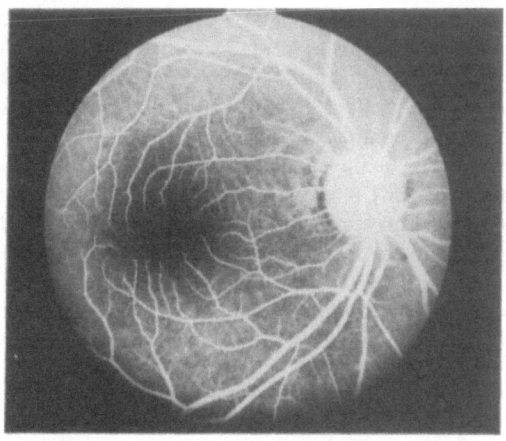

Fig. 5a.   Same run; perifoveal capillaries 15.2 seconds after 10% solution.

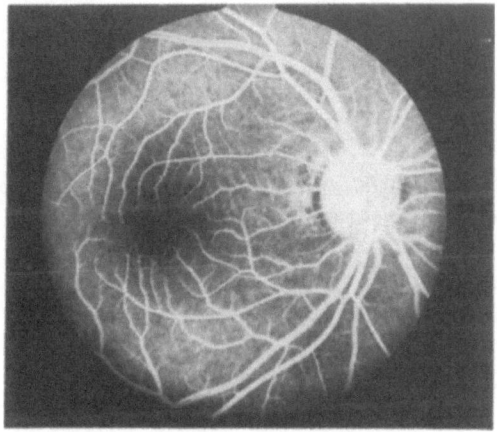

Fig. 5b.   Perifoveal capillaries 15.5 seconds after 25% solution with almost identical resolution as in Fig. 5a.

The occasional impression that the 25% solution seems to give an improved overall quality of resolution remains to be confirmed. Subjective impressions may lead to erroneous conclusions. The improved resolution seen with 25% fluorescein may reflect nothing more than a chance occurrence of sharper focus by the photographer.

The present study is being carried out with readily available clinical angiography equipment. But it must be pointed out that the much greater detail, better reproducibility and outstanding time control of fluorescein cineangiography continue to make it the method of choice whenever available for quantitative studies of this nature. Demonstration of a few examples of compromised blood flow in incomplete central retinal vein thrombo-

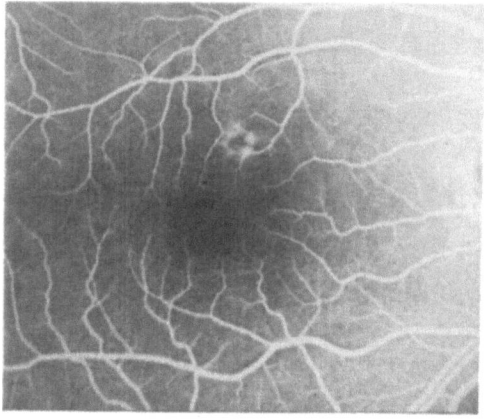

Fig. 6a. Localized pigment epithelial lesion in 63 year old Negro, 15.0 seconds after injection of 2.0 ml of 25% fluorescein.

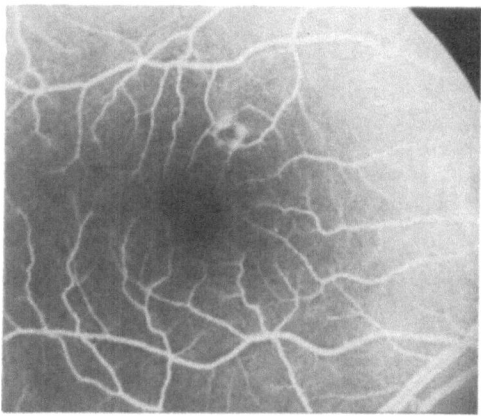

Fig. 6b. Same eye two weeks later, 15.3 seconds after injection of 5.0 ml of 10% fluorescein solution.

108

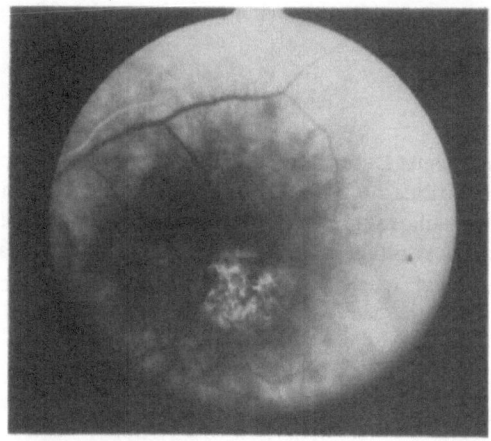

Fig. 7a. Stargardt's disease in 47 year old Caucasian 10.3 seconds after injection of 5.0 ml of 10% fluorescein.

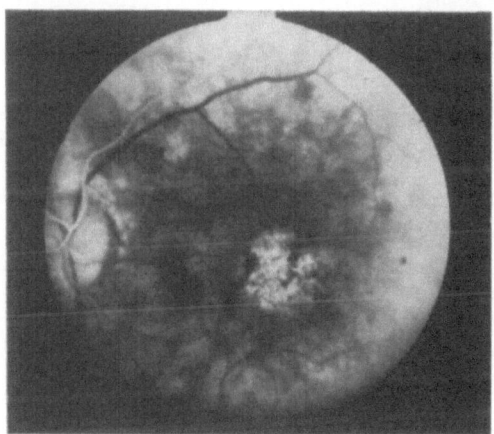

Fig. 7b. Same eye one week later, 11.0 seconds after 2.0 ml of 25% fluorescein injection.

ses and other circulatory problems by cine technique with 20 fps. concludes this discussion.

SUMMARY

Various quantitative aspects of fluorescein angiography are presented in which fluorescein solutions of 10% and 25% are administered intravenously and compared for arm-choroid circulation time, arm-retina circulation time, bolus time and perifoveal filling in 25 patients. The arm-to-retina circulation time is probably related to patient's height, less to his weight and not normally to his blood pressure. Comparison of the quality of fluorescein

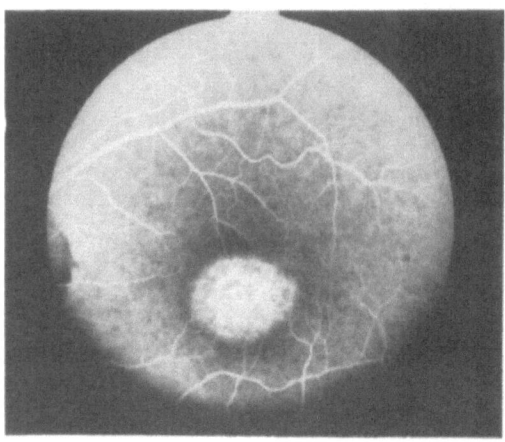

Fig. 8a.   Same run as in Fig. 7a; 17.8 seconds after 10% fluorescein.

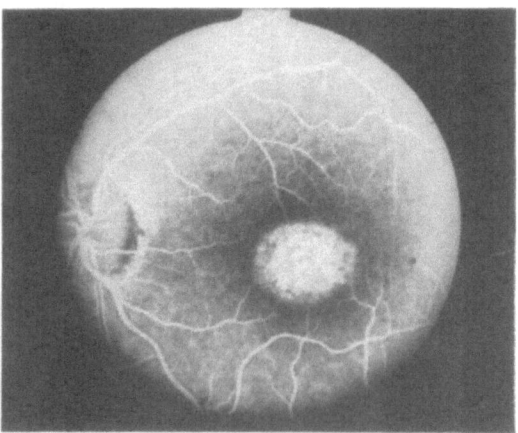

Fig. 8b.   Same run as in Fig. 7b; 16.9 seconds after 25% fluorescein.

110

angiograms obtained with each concentration is carried out, but no preliminary conclusions can be drawn regarding whether either solution gives superior results. Details of the completed study will be reported elsewhere in the near future, including statistical data on inter-observer variability.

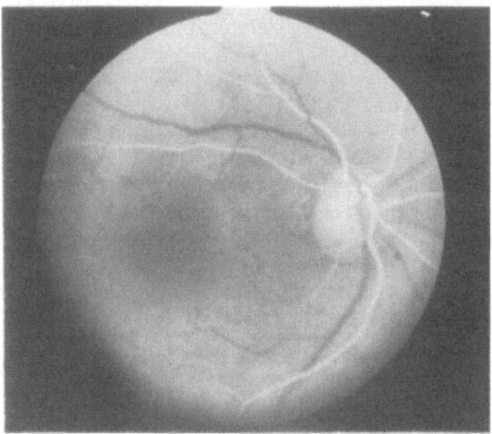

Fig. 9a. 48 year old Negro, normal control. Early arterial phase 15.2 seconds after very painful injection of 2.0 ml of 25% fluorescein. This individual's arm-to-retina circulation time was known from previous cineangiography studies to average about 10 seconds. His pre-injection blood pressure was 125/75 mm Hg. Immediately after the procedure, it had dropped to 104/56 mm Hg, explaining the delay in d; e appearance.

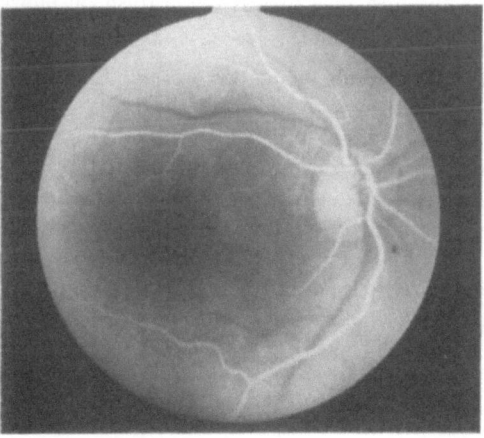

Fig. 9b. Same volunteer 2 weeks later showing comparable arterial phase already 10.25 seconds after injection of 5.0 ml of 10% fluorescein. Blood pressure before and after procedure stable with 130/65 mm Hg. This time, no unusual pain or profuse perspiration connected with the injection.

REFERENCES

DOLLERY, C.T. Dynamic aspects of the retinal microcirculation. *Arch. Ophthal.* 79: *536-539* (1968).

EVANS, P.Y. & WRUCK, J. Macular circulation times. *Exc. Med. Internat. Congress Series* No. 222: *891-897* (1970).

EVANS, P.Y. SANTORO, J., YOUNG, C., LIMAYE, S.R., KOT, P. & WRUCK, J. Arteriolar flow studies by retinal cineangiography. Fluorescein Angiography, pp. *27-31.* Tokyo, Igaku Shoin Ltd. (1974).

FLOCKS, M., MILLER, J. CHAO, P. Retinal circulation time with aid of fundus cinephotography. *Am. J. Ophthal.* 48: *3-6* (1959).

HICKAM, J.B., FRAYSER, R. & ROSS, J.C. A study of retinal venous blood oxygen saturation in human subjects by photographic means. *Circulation* 27: *375* (1963).

HICKAM, J.B. & FRAYSER, R. A photographic method for measuring the mean retinal circulation time using fluorescein. *Invest. Ophthal.* 4: *876* (1965).

OBERHOFF, P., EVANS, P.Y. & DELANEY, J.F. Cinematographic documentation of retinal circulation times. *Arch. Ophthal.* 74: *77-80* (1965).

SHIMIZU, K., YOKOCHI, K. & OKANO, T. Fluorescein angiography of the choroid. *Jap. J. Ophthalmol.* 18: *97-108* (1974).

Authors' address:
Georgetown University
3800 Reservoir Road N.W.
WASHINGTON D.C. 20007
USA

DISCUSSION

Dr Laux: I would like to ask Dr Evans: you compared the influence of different dye concentrations on picture quality and circulation times and I think you followed the injection by a saline flush. I just wonder if you have any information on the influence of this saline flush on image quality and circulation times?

Dr Evans: The study and results which we presented today did intentionally *not* include saline flush; we did look at the results quantitatively and qualitatively before and did not find any definite difference between the two techniques except for the duration of the bolus. This was shorter, and its head and tail better defined, with a small 5 to 7 ml saline flush following the automatic fluorescein injection, but otherwise the data with or without saline flush were very much the same. In order to make the results more applicable to the generally used routine, the protocol did therefore not include the saline flush (which we continue to use for all our cineangiography studies).

ARTERIOVENOUS MEAN CIRCULATION TIME IN THE HUMAN RETINA

C.E. RIVA, W.P. ROBERTS, J.W. MCMEEL & I. BEN-SIRA

(Boston, Massachusetts, USA)

Determination of retinal blood flow is fundamental to the understanding of pathophysiological processes in the fundus. Until now, blood flow in segments of the human retina has been estimated by the photographic fluorescein dilution technique (BULPITT & DOLLERY, 1971), which is slow and cumbersome. A new instrument, a two-point fluorophotometer (RIVA & BEN-SIRA, 1975), allows on-line recording of dilution curves from an artery and a vein of the retina. This makes it possible, for the first time, to use this technique as a routine clinical procedure.

RELATION BETWEEN FLUORESCENCE INTENSITY AND FLUORESCEIN CONCENTRATION

The output of the instrument is a curve (Fig. 1) representing the time course of fluorescence intensity $I(t)$. In this normal subject injected with only 20 mg of dye, $I(t)$ appears quasi-simultaneously in the artery and the vein, reaches a maximum, decreases, and then rises again slightly, due to recirculation. To determine the arteriovenous Mean Circulation Time (MCT) one needs the time course of the dye concentration, $\bar{c}(t)$. Obviously, $\bar{c}$ cannot be measured. One can use $I(t)$ instead, if $I(t) = a \, \bar{c}(t)$, where a = constant, over the entire course of the curves, as others have assumed (BULPITT & DOLLERY, 1971; KQHNER, 1974). However, a varies in time because of the combined effect of two factors: the optical absorption by blood of the excitation and fluorescent light, and the non-uniform, time-varying spatial distribution of the dye within the vessel cross section (HICKAM & FRAYSER, 1966). As a result, $I(t)$ is only a distorted representation of $\bar{c}(t)$. We have evaluated this distortion using the following assumptions: the vessels are round; the light is transmitted through blood according to Beer's law; the flow of the dye in an artery is laminar with parabolic velocity profile; and the streamline flow of the dye in a vein is such that the stream occupies a thin band across the vessel with the dye uniformly distributed within the full depth of this band. The calculations show that the distortion is negligible for the arterial curve and practically independent of the size of the vessel, the hematocrit, and the configuration of the aperture collecting the fluorescence. For a venous curve the shape of the aperture does make a difference, but this distortion can be minimized by using a round aperture slightly larger than the vein.

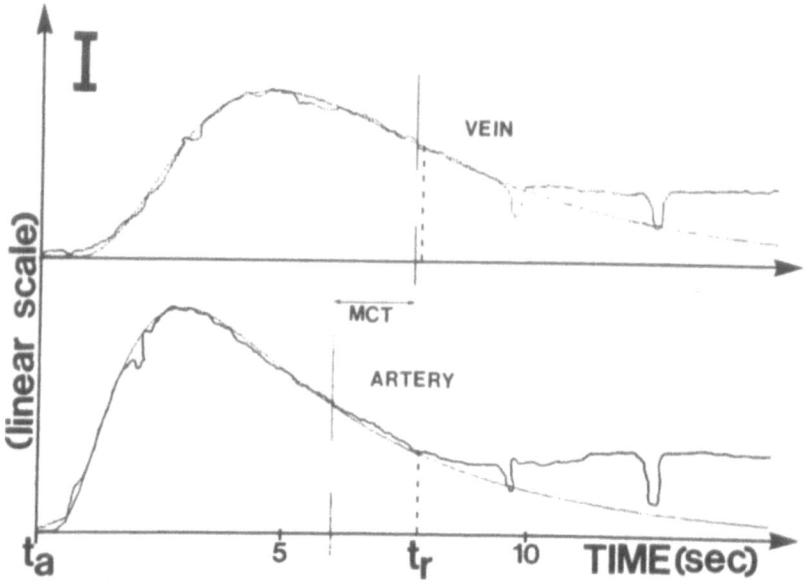

Fig. 1. Arterial and venous fluorescence intensity curves, I(t), from the superior temporal segment of a normal subject. t_a = first appearance of the dye, t_r = first appearance of the recirculation. The smooth curves are a log-normal fit of the recorded curves. MCT = 3.2 seconds.

Correction for recirculation

Recirculation occurs generally in the late part of the downslope of an arterial dilution curve. Correction for it is done by extrapolation, assuming that the downslope decays exponentially. Previous authors (HICKAM & FRAYSER, 1966; BULPITT & DOLLERY, 1971; KOHNER, 1974) have applied this method to the venous curve also, indicating incorrectly that recirculation in a large vein is also a late event. However, recirculation in a large vein begins, in fact, at practically the same time as in an artery, because the first appearance of the dye is quasi-simultaneous with that in the artery. We found that, in general, recirculation in a vein is so early that the extrapolation method of correction becomes very inaccurate. Therefore, it is more accurate, in this case, to use the method of STOW & HETZEL (1954) and fit the whole curve up to the recirculation with a log-normal distribution function. This method makes use also of the ascending portion of the curve and simplifies the calculations of MCT. Log-normal fits of the recorded arterial and venous curves are shown in Fig. 1 as an example.

Using our instrument and the log-normal fitting procedure, we have determined the MCT in 24 normal subjects (35 eyes), age 22 to 49 and in 20 diabetic patients (23 eyes), age 19 to 63, with no or mild retinopathy as defined by KOHNER (1974). Figure 2 is a histogram of the results. The MCT in most of the subjects is an average of two or more consecutive measurements.

114

ACKNOWLEDGEMENTS

This work was supported by Public Health Service grants EY-00227 and 1-ROI-EY-01242-01 from the National Eye Institute, National Institutes of Health and by Research to Prevent Blindness, Inc. — William Friedkin Award.
We thank Drs. G.T. Feke and F.C. Delori for helpful discussions. Ms.

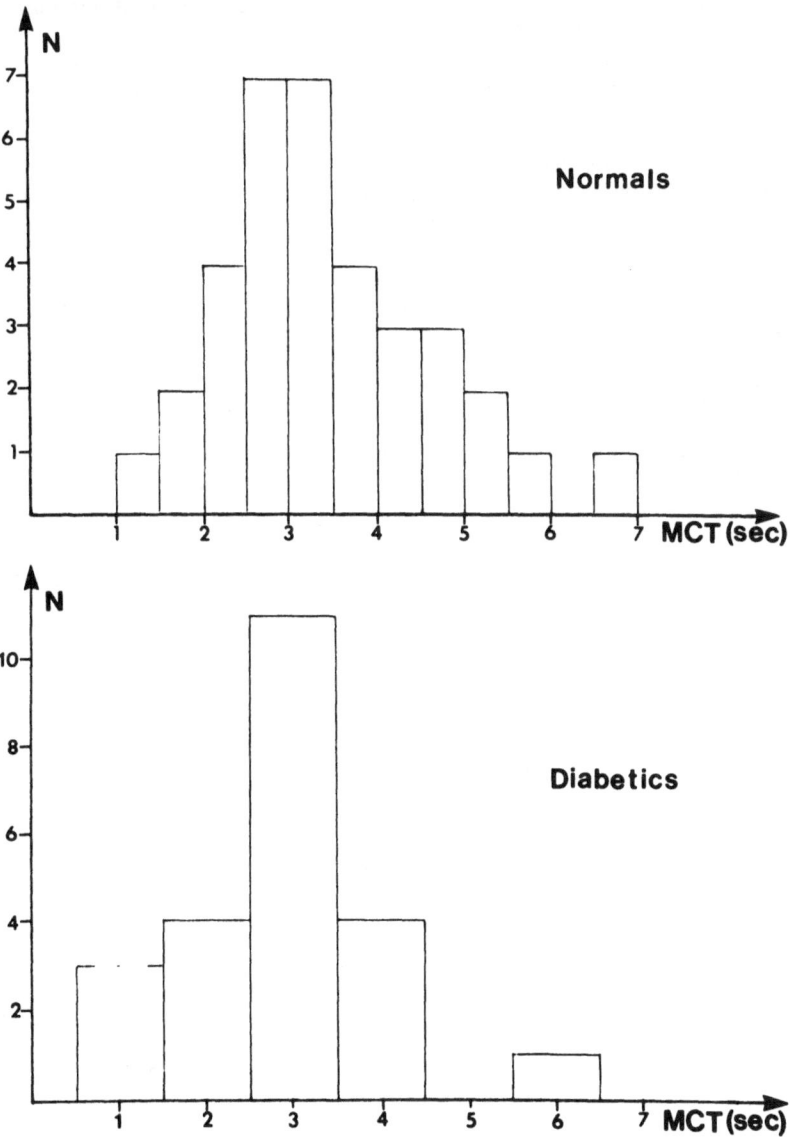

Fig. 2. Histogram of the MCT's obtained from the temporal segment in 24 normal subjects and 20 diabetics.

M.D. Gonzalez assisted in analysis of the data. Ms. S.F. Blackwell provided editorial assistance.

REFERENCES

BULPITT, C.J. & DOLLERY, C.T. Estimation of retinal blood flow by measurement of the mean circulation time. *Cardiovasc. Res.* 5: *406-412* (1971).

HICKAM, J.B. & FRAYSER, R. Studies of the retinal circulation in man: observation on vessel diameter, arteriovenous oxygen difference, and mean circulation time. *Circulation* 33: *302-316* (1966).

KOHNER, E. Retinal blood flow in diabetes mellitus. In: Diabetic Retinopathy. Lynn, J.R., Snyder, W.B. & Voiser, A. (eds.). New York, Grune and Stratton. p. *71* (1974).

RIVA, C.E. & BEN-SIRA, I. Two-point fluorophotometer for the human ocular fundus. *Appl. Optics* 14: *2691-2693* (1975).

STOW, R.W. & HETZEL, P.S. An empirical formula for indicator-dilution curves as obtained in human beings. *J. Appl. Physiol.* 7: *161-167* (1954).

Author's address:
Eye Research Institute of Retina Foundation
20 Staniford Street
Boston, Mass. 02114, USA

Reprint requests to
Editorial Sevices Unit
Eye Research Institute of Retina Foundation
20 Staniford Street
Boston, Mass. 02114, USA

THE COMPUTERIZED ELABORATION OF FLUOROANGIOGRAPHIC DATA ON RETINAL VASCULARIZATION

R. BRANCATO, L. DEL CARO, G. RAVALICO & G. SICURANZA

(Trieste, Italy)

The visualization of the vessels of the ocular fundus by fluorescein enabled us to study the vascularization of the retina and of the optic disc in their smallest details.

On one hand, fluorescein angioscopy and cine and T.V. shootings enable us to investigate ocular haemodynamics, on the other hand fluorescein angiography, with its serial photography, shows us the vascular pattern at rather close-spaced intervals. Considering the resolution of the film we employed, the latter method permits a more accurate study of the finer details.

The criteria of evaluation of each element of the retinogram depend on two basic graphic characteristics: the border and the level of grey peculiar to the structure under investigation. The comparison of the same detail in subsequent frames usually depends on subjective factors which, after all, go back to the two above-mentioned ones — that is, border and level of grey.

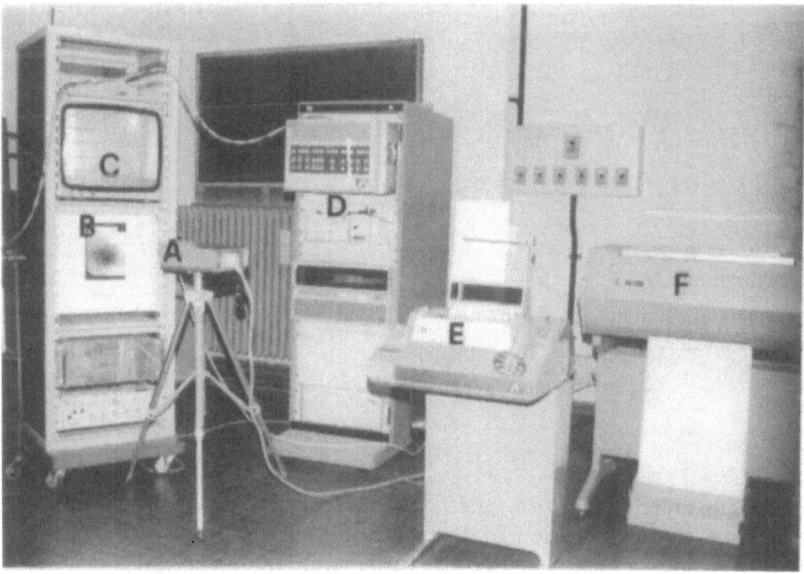

Fig. 1. Equipment for electronic elaboration of fluoroangiographic data: A. camera; B. diaphanoscope; C. monitor; D. computer; E. console teletype; F. printer.

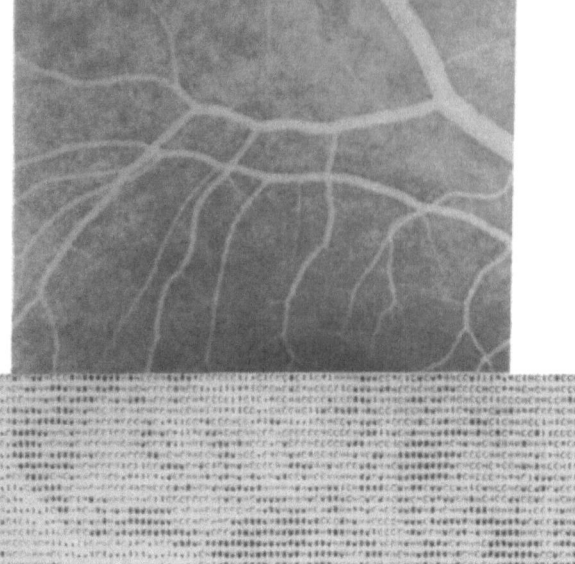

Fig. 2. Printer-computerized representation of a detail of the retinal vascularization in a normal subject.

Focusing, reflections, film grain, are all elements which play a determining role in the precision of the evaluation. Therefore, we thought it useful to employ a computer in order to elaborate fluoroangiographic data, thus receiving them free of the collateral disturbance elements which may be considered as 'noise'.

118

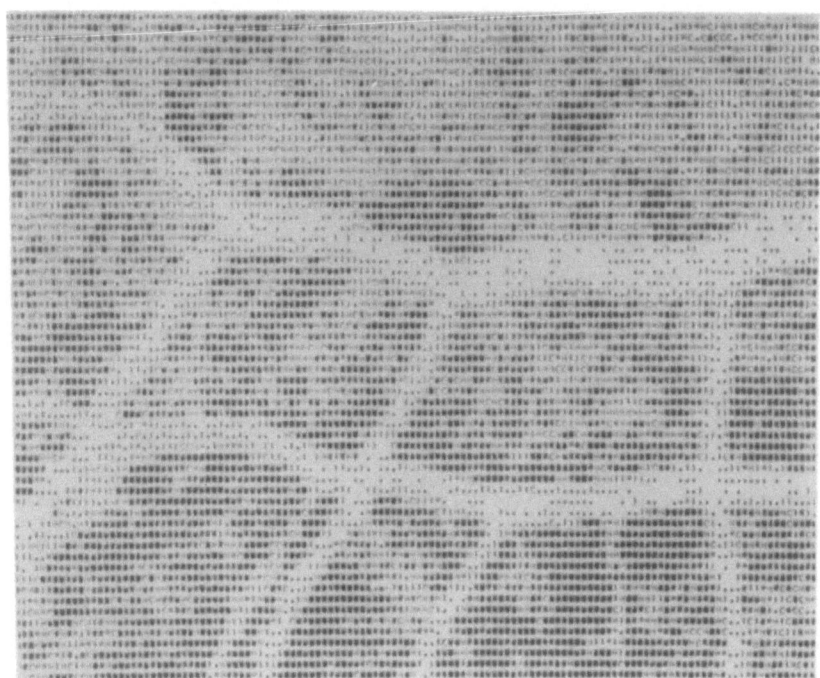

Fig. 3. The same detail of Fig. 2 elaborated by equalization.

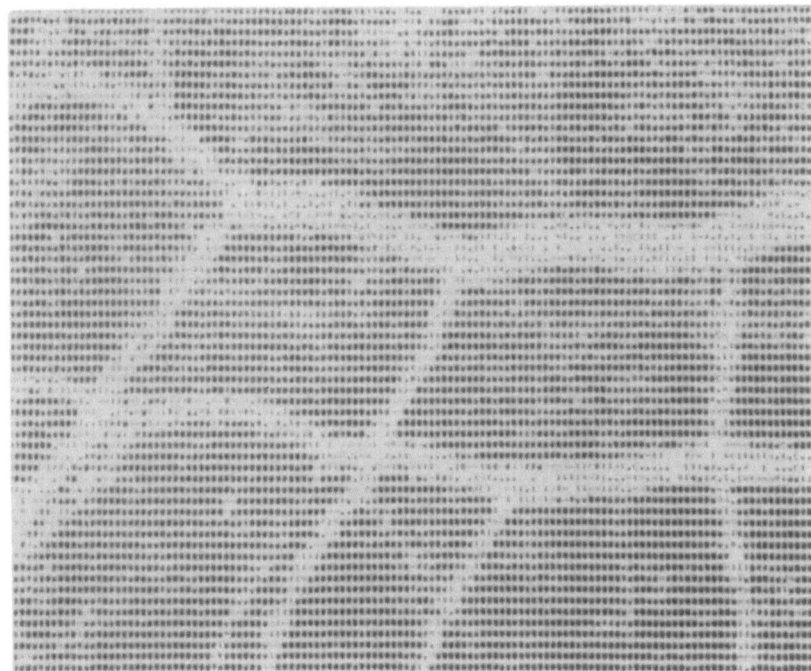

Fig. 4. The same detail of Fig. 2 elaborated by expansion of 0.6 level.

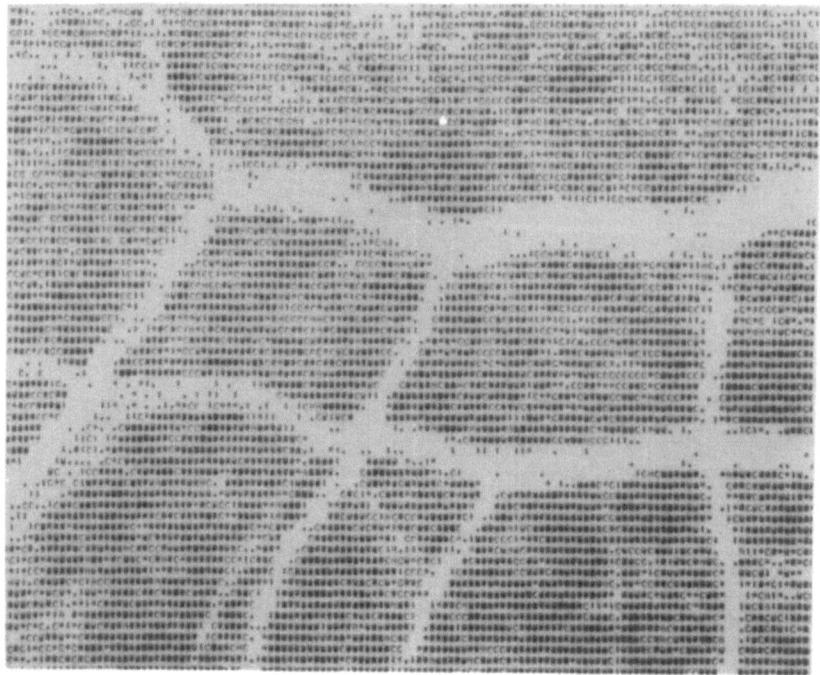

Fig. 5. The same detail of Fig. 2 elaborated by compression of blacks.

TECHNIQUE

The great versatility of the elaboration systems makes it possible to obtain a definition and a stress on some details that would otherwise get mixed up or lost. For the elaboration of data we used a Philips LDH 150/08 T.V. camera with a Schneider-Kreuznach Xenon 1:0.95/25 lens, which takes a fluoro-angiographic image. This is printed on photomechanic paper and illuminated by diaphanoscopy. The T.V. signal is sampled on 625 rows at 600 points per row, giving a total of 375,000 points. The data regarding the different levels of grey in the image are introduced in the computer (HP 2100 A) and entered in a magnetic record. Each level of grey is quantified with values between 0 and 255. As the minicomputer we employed has a limited memory (32K of 16 bits), it is only possible to elaborate an area of the image made up of 256 per 256 points maximum. The computer is supplied with the co-ordinates of the zone (window) by the console teletype (Fig. 1).

The data relevant to the levels of grey of that area are then read on the magnetic record and elaborated according to a method which makes use of the fast Fourier transform. The user sets the required types of elaboration always by console teletype, modifying as needed the representation of the various levels of grey. After elaboration, the new data are re-entered in the record. The data relevant to the chosen film trap can be sent to a printer, which records the image on normal paper, representing the various levels of

120

grey by overprints of the required characters; they can also be transmitted to a display directly connected with the computer.

With this technique we could measure the caliber of retinal vessels with absolute precision (Fig. 2).

Of all the possible elaborations of the fluoroangiographic image, we are going to show some examples of equalization, of expansion and of compression. Equalization aims at the representation of each level of grey by a constant number of points (Fig. 3).

By expansion, we choose a certain level of grey and stress its details, expanding its representation and saturating its extreme levels (Fig. 4).

By compression, which may be done towards any of the levels of grey, we carry out the operation opposite to expansion, and tend to bring to the chosen level most of the points of the nearest levels (Fig. 5).

This seems to be the best method for the evaluation of vessel caliber in subsequent examinations, and possibly after drug-induced modifications of the caliber itself.

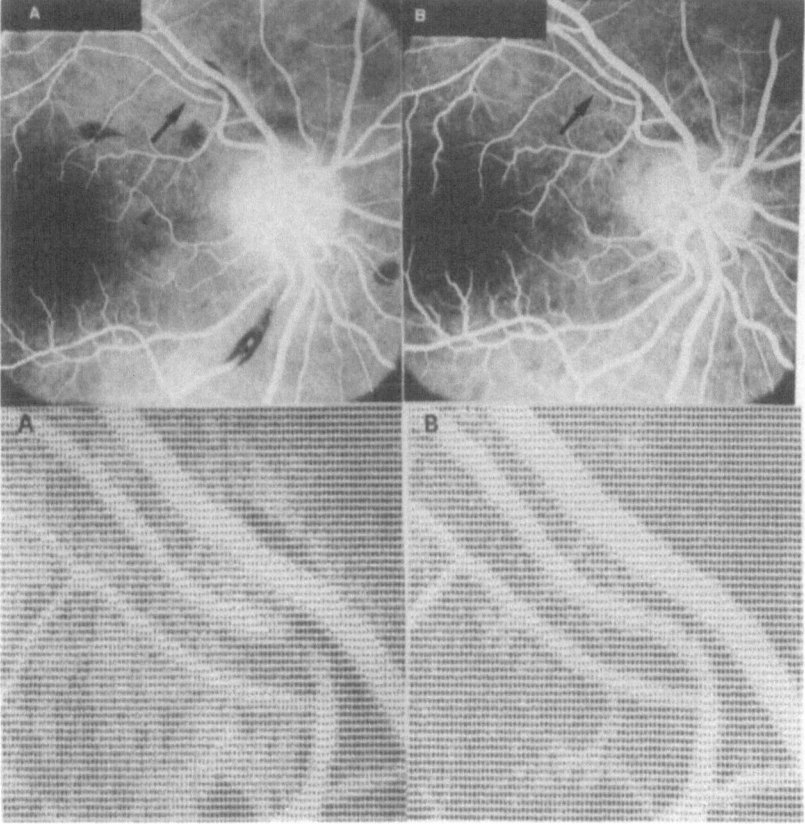

Fig. 6. Fluoroangiographic appearance and computerization of a detail in a subject with accelerated hypertension and end-stage kidney, before and after 4 months' treatment with dialysis.

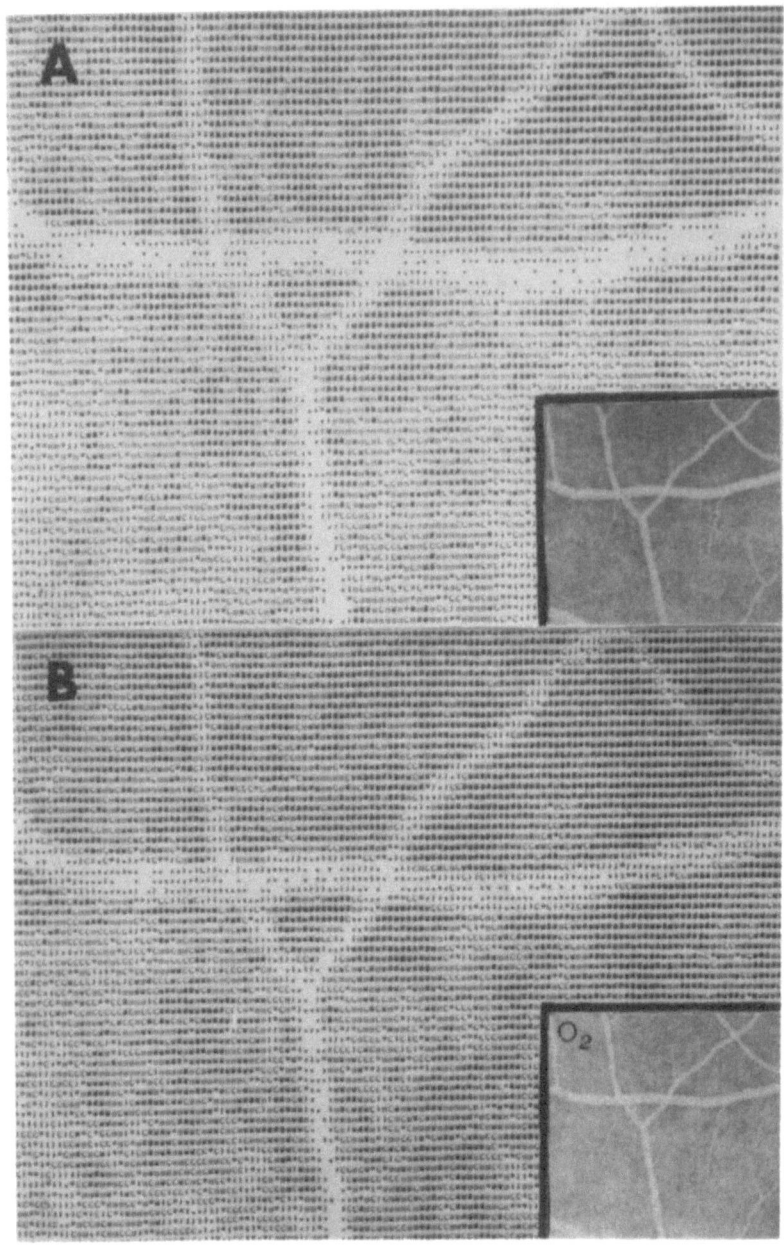

Fig. 7. A: Elaborated fluoroangiographic detail in a normal subject.
B: The same detail after inhalation of oxygen for 30 minutes.

To eliminate all possible evaluation errors related to vessel caliber changes between systolic and diastolic phase, we connected the retinograph to an electrocardiograph recording the ECG of the patient under examination. The QRS complex formed the signal which released each frame, so that each shooting was taken always in the same circulatory phase.

The two fluorescein angiographies were taken on the same film, to avoid possible errors due to the development technique.

In Fig. 6 two subsequent fluorescein angiograms of a subject with accelerated hypertension and end-stage kidney can be seen. The control was taken after 4 months' dialysis; the changes in vase-caliber can be evidenced in the computerized graphic representation.

Fig. 7A represents a detail of the vascularization during the venous phase in a computerized fluorescein angiography. Fig. 7B represents the same detail after inhalation of 60% oxygen for 30 minutes. The computerized representation of the fluoroangiographic image permits a quantitative evaluation of the oxygen-induced narrowing of retinal vessels.

To conclude, the computerized elaboration of fluoroangiographic data permits:

1. A numerically exact representation of the retinal vascular structures examined, so that they may be compared in subsequent periods.

2. An elaboration of the image by programmes which stress or suppress the various levels of grey, according to the representation needed.

REFERENCES

BRANCATO, R., D'AMORE, A., DEL CARO, L., RAVALICO, G. & SICURANZA, G. An attempt towards a new technique for the computer analysis of fluorescein angiography. *Bull. Hellen. Ophth. Society* (Suppl) 45: *529-535* (1975).

HALE, J.A.G. & SARAGA, P. Digital image processing. *Optoelectronics* 6: *333-348* (1974).

LATO, K., MATSUI, M. & MATSUMOTO, K. Fluorescein angiographic studies on retinal vascular changes in Systematic Hypertension. Photography in Ophthalmology. Int. Symp. Fluorescein Angiography. Miami, Fla. 1970. *Mod. Probl. Ophthal.* 9: *83-89* (1971).

Authors' addresses:
R. Brancato & G. Ravalico
Clinica Oculistica dell' Università
Ospedale Maggiore
34129 Trieste
Italy

L. Del Caro & G. Sicuranza
Istituto di Elettronica ed
Elettrotecnica dell'Università
34129 Trieste
Italy

TELEVISION PHOTOMETRIC TECHNIQUE FOR RECORDING FLUORESCEIN DILUTION CURVES (DROMOFLUOROGRAMS)

S. FONDA, B. BAGOLINI & M. PEDUZZI

(Modena, Italy)

INTRODUCTION

Measurements on blood flow of retinal vessels may have important clinical significance. Accurate measurements have been performed in animals (e.g. FRIEDMAN et al., 1964; ALM & BILL, 1973) with techniques usually not applicable to man.

Fluoroangiography has given impetus to the study of retinal blood flow, and photographic or photoelectric methods have been variously applied in the examination of different aspects of retinal circulation. The clinical application of both photographic and cinematographic methods presents problems dealing mainly with the maximum sampling frequency and illuminating power (HICKAM & FRAYSER, 1965, 1966; HILL, 1968; BULPITT & DOLLERY, 1971; EVANS et al., 1973; WESSING, 1974; HILL et al., 1974).

In the case of photoelectric methods on the other hand, we need to perform numerous fluorescein injections in order to record dilution curves in various vessels and to obtain information on blood flow (TROKEL, 1964; NIESEL & GASSMAN, 1972; BEN-SIRA & RIVA, 1973; NIESEL, 1974), and this is a serious limitation of the technique. We have therefore attempted to combine certain advantages of the two techniques by using a television tape-recording of the fundus sequences in much the same way as was done by L'Esperance and coworkers (L'ESPERANCE et al., 1974) but with different aims and techniques. Thus, photometric measurements of fluorescent vessels can be performed directly on a television screen and fluorescein dilution curves recorded for all chosen retinal vessels or areas by simply replaying the tape-recording.

Further advantages of the television technique are that it requires 40 to 60% less illuminating power than is necessary in cinematography and affords higher frame rates (50 Hz or 60 Hz).

The time variations of dye concentration in a vessel are normally represented and defined as dilution curves. However, the variations of fluorescein concentration in the blood are different from those one finds for a dye dilution in stagnant fluids, for they are facilitated by the blood flow, which is in a sense an 'active' phenomenon. Moreover, the fluorescein dilution curves are not fully representative of the flow of all blood components but principally of plasma. So, we should like to call the fluorescein dilution curves 'dromofluorograms' (DFG).

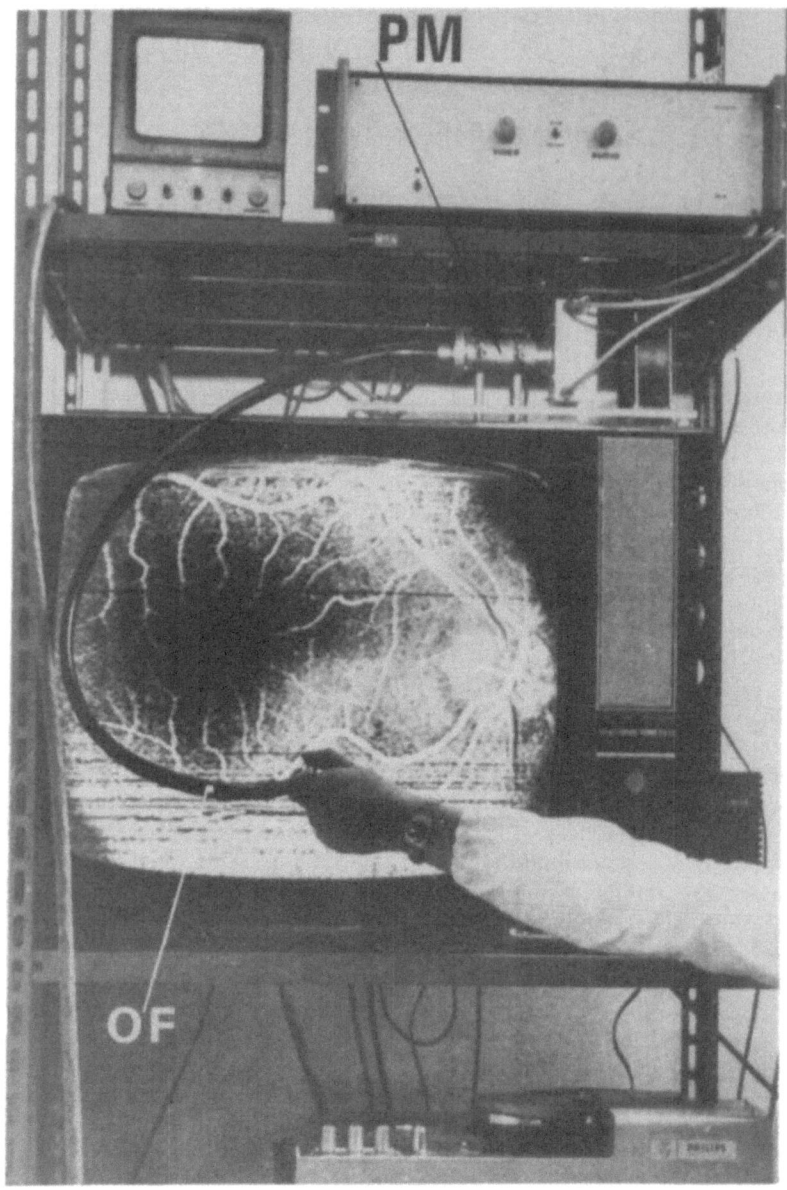

Fig. 1. Representation of the system used for recording DFG's. The photomultiplier (PM) receives the light from the fluorescent vessel through an optical fibre (OF) handled by operator.

126

MATERIALS AND METHODS

In order to obtain satisfactory television fluoroangiography recordings, we used a Zeiss Fundus camera modified according to Wessing (WESSING, 1974; BARBARO et al., 1974). We used two television cameras at the same time: one to record the fundus images (Philips LDH 0151/00; control unit LDH 0160/02, equipped with high-sensitivity plumbicon tube), the other to record time from a digital timer. The output of the cameras (after mixing) is connected to a video-tape recorder (Philips EL 3402). During first playback of the television recording the precise point at which the photometric measurement will be taken is chosen; during second playback its luminance is transmitted to a photomultiplier PM (XP 1117, Philips) by means of an optical fibre (Fig. 1). The diameter of the optical fibre was 10 mm and could be decreased by a diaphragm. The vessel diameters on the video screen were never larger than 10 mm.

The output of the PM is a compound signal. It contains a 50 Hz component, the amplitude of which is modulated by a signal at much lower frequency. The 50 Hz component comes from the frame rate of the television system and the low-frequency signal is linearly related to the fluorescein dilution curve. It is possible to filter out the high frequency component and have at the output only the biological signal related to the dilution curve; a low-pass filter with cut-off characteristics of 40 Db/dec ranging from 0.5 to 0.8 Hz gives a good recording of the dye dilution curves. The filtered signal is amplified × 2 and recorded on a strip-chart recorder. The video luminance never reached saturation during experiments and was linearly related to fluorescein concentrations.

Dye injection time was about 1.5 sec. During the recording of the television fluoroangiography two impulses were recorded in the audio channel of the video tape recorder, one at the beginning of injection, and one at the end. During playback they were picked up from the loudspeaker output and superimposed over the photometric signal. They provided a good reference signal for the start and duration of injections. The injections were always performed by hand by the same trained person who recorded the reference signals with a microphone.

In order to obtain premilinary results regarding the sensitivity of this technique we examined some normal subjects of different ages and two patients affected by hypertensive retinopathy and diabetic retinopathy. Normal subjects were divided into three groups: the first consisted of two subjects aged 20 years, the second of six subjects aged 30 to 40 years and the third of two subjects aged 65 years. The patient affected by hypertensive retinopathy was a 45 year-old man with blood pressure of 230/150; the patient affected by diabetic retinopathy was a 46 year-old woman with initial neovascularization in the papillary area and blood pressure of 150/90.

By means of an averager (Ortec 4620-4621-4623) we calculated the arterial and venous dromofluorograms for every group of normal subjects, the actuating signal (trigger) for the averager being given the moment the curve rose above zero.

In this way we obtained three couples of mean normal dromofluorograms for the three age groups in question.

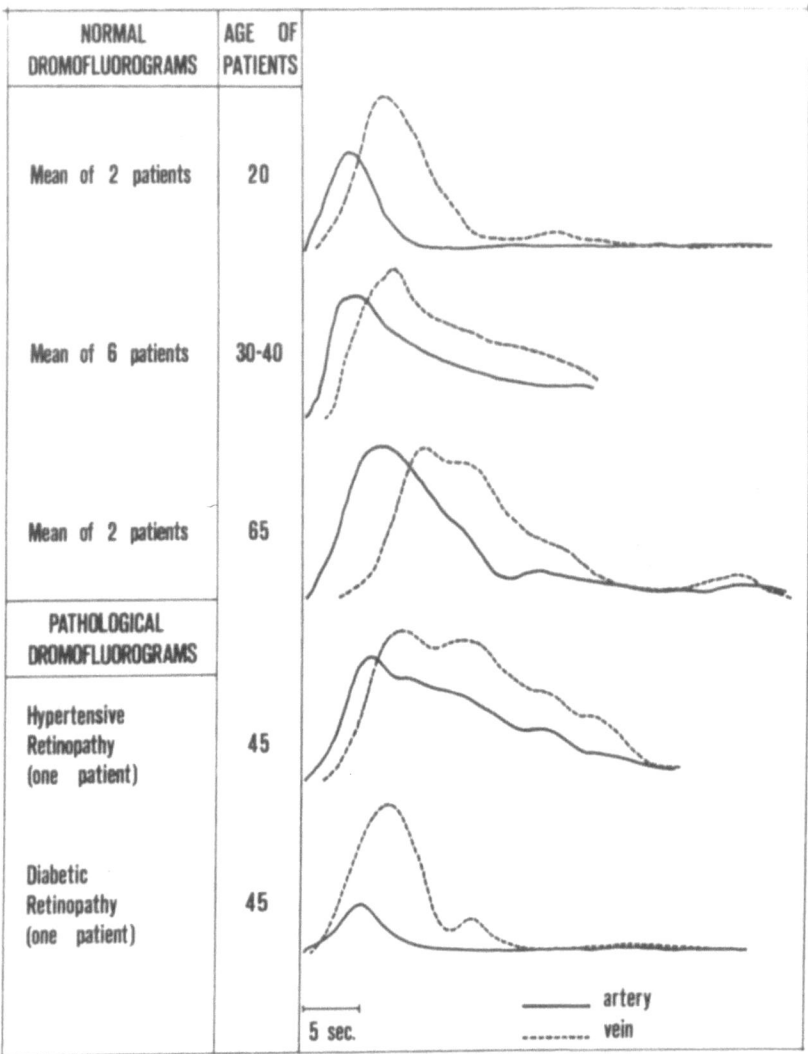

NORMAL DROMOFLUOROGRAMS	AGE OF PATIENTS
Mean of 2 patients	20
Mean of 6 patients	30-40
Mean of 2 patients	65
PATHOLOGICAL DROMOFLUOROGRAMS	
Hypertensive Retinopathy (one patient)	45
Diabetic Retinopathy (one patient)	45

5 sec.   ———— artery   ·········· vein

Fig. 2. Mean normal and pathological DFG's. Normal DFG's have been obtained by averaging single curves, the number of which is indicated on the left. Only in the first couple of DFG's (top of the Figure) recirculation can be clearly seen. The wavelets present in the other curves are artifacts due to movements of the eye and blinking.

All the DFG's were plotted in such a way that all arterial initial times were vertically aligned, and all the venous DFG's had the same amplitude. Consequently, all couples of DFG's are comparable because in every normal or pathological case the arterial and venous records were performed in the same experimental conditions. Figure 2 shows that the arterial DFG varies in amplitude from the venous DFG.

Following the scheme of Fig. 3, we measured certain parameters from the curves for every single subject. The definition of the parameters is as follows:

1. t_i — being the initial time taken for the curve to rise 0.5 mm above the base line*;

2. t_m — being the time taken for the dromofluorogram to reach maximum level;

3. T_i — being the time interval between the arterial initial time (t_{ia}) and the corresponding venous initial time (t_{iv}) expressed at $T_i = t_{iv} - t_{ia}$;

4. T_m — being the time interval between the maximum amplitude of the arterial and corresponding venous curves, t_{ma} and t_{mv}, respectively, expressed as $T_m = t_{mv} - t_{ma}$;

5. t_r — being the rising time, or the time necessary for the curve to rise from 10% to 90% of its maximum value.

These are not the only parameters one can consider; we propose in a future paper to calculate velocity, mean transit time, flow and volume according to the Steward-Hamilton method (ZIERLER, 1962). The mean values and the standard deviations of the normal parameters have been plotted vs. age (Fig. 4); for comparison, values of pathological parameters have also been plotted in the same form.

RESULTS AND DISCUSSION

The aim of the present work was to arrive at a working knowledge of the waveform variations of DFG's at different ages. We also tested the sensitivity of this technique in the detection of variations of some parameters of retinal blood circulation in markedly pathological cases.

The waveform variations of DFG's in all the subjects tested reveal two significant features (Fig. 2):

1. Only in the third group (65 years) of normal subjects is the arterial DFG amplitude slightly larger than the venous DFG; in all other cases (mean normal and pathological) the reverse is true.

2. The decaying time is considerably longer in hypertensive retinopathy if compared with all other cases examined.

The behaviour of T_i, T_m, t_{ra}, and t_{rv} in the different age groups (20, 30-40, 65 years) is represented in Fig. 4.

In normal subjects each parameter increases the older the subject is. This probably indicates (a) a tendency for the vessels to decrease in patency, and/or (b) diminished blood flow. Extremely large standard deviations can be observed for T_m, t_{ra}, t_{rv} in the second and third groups (30-40 and 65 years) of normal subjects. This could depend on different factors:

1. technical artifacts, due for example to ocular movements or blinking;

2. the relatively small number of examined subjects;

3. experimental error, calculated to be ± 0.30 sec. for T_i, ± 0.38 sec. for T_m, ± 0.15 sec. for t_{ra} and ± 0.30 sec. for t_{rv} (FONDA & BAGOLINI, 1976).

On the other hand, large standard deviations in elderly people are to be

---

* This point is arbitrary; it was chosen so that the curve could be measured with sufficient accuracy.

129

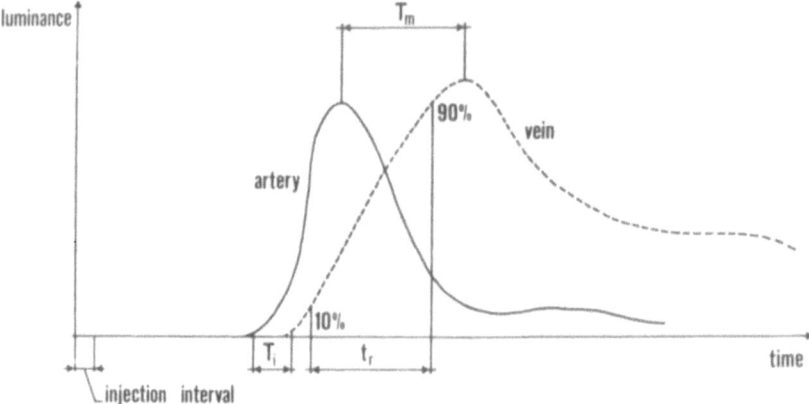

Fig. 3. Scheme defining the measured time parameters of .the arterial and venous DFG's.

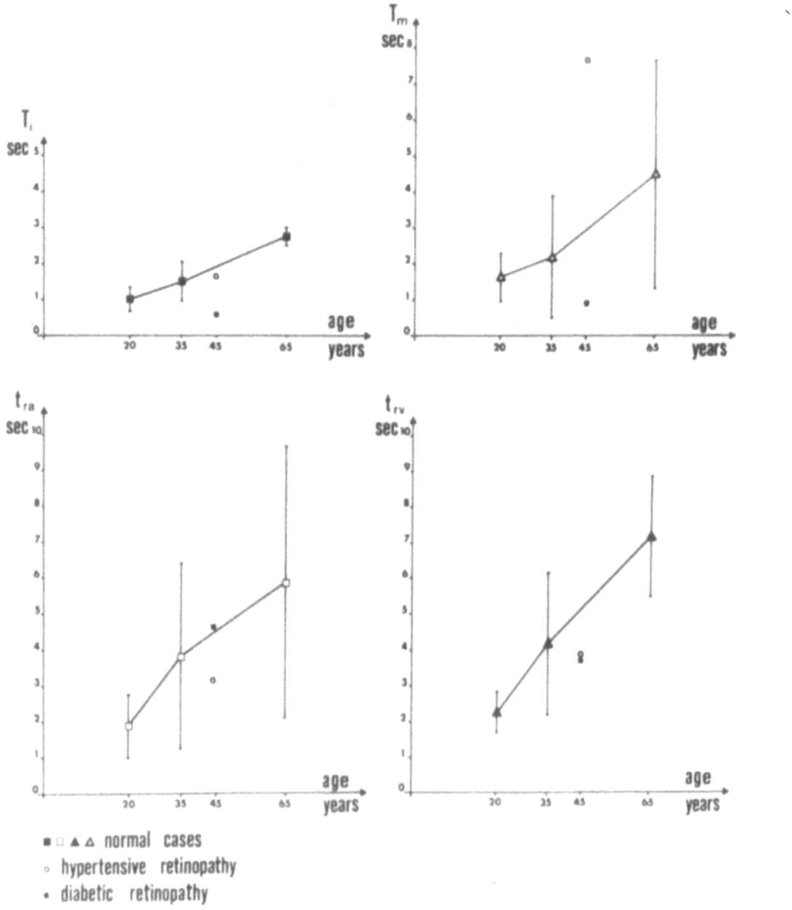

■ □ ▲ △ normal cases
○ hypertensive retinopathy
• diabetic retinopathy

Fig. 4. Plots of the measured time parameters vs. age.

130

expected in view of the many factors normally affecting blood circulation in senility.

The extremes of the standard-deviation intervals also increase with age, with the exception of the lower extreme of the S.D. interval in the second group (30-40 years) in the plot of T_m, which is lower than the corresponding one for the first group (20 years). This would appear to confirm the validity of the results.

In pathological cases, further observations can be made.

In hypertensive retinopathy, the most significant features are the very large value of T_m, and the approximately normal value of T_i; t_{ra} and t_{rv} are both less than normal but are probably within the standard deviation interval.

In diabetic retinopathy, T_i and T_m are much shorter than the corresponding normal mean values, and this, in our opinion, may indicate arteriovenous shunts; t_{ra} is nearly the same as normal, while t_{rv} is slightly less than normal, probably without exceeding standard variability. In the case of diabetic retinopathy, this technique and its results could be compared and combined with the vitreous fluorophotometry technique of Cunha-Vaz and others (CUNHA-VAZ et al., 1975).

A proper interpretation of the various physiological parameters of the DFG is necessary if we are to establish a good criterion of comparison between normal and pathological cases. From the technical point of view we have one reservation to make: during recording many wavelets are often superimposed on the DFG; they are caused by ocular movements and blinking which are in turn due to the strong light that we must still use in the excitation of fluorescein. The best way to eliminate this cause of error in recording is to use a more sensitive camera tube.

We also think that the technique must be tested over a wide cross-section of clinical cases in order to enable the true significance of the parameters to be definitively assessed.

REFERENCES

ALM, A. & BILL, A. Ocular and optic nerve blood flow at normal and increased intraocular pressures in monkeys (*Macaca irus*): A study with radioactively labelled microspheres including flow determinations in brain and some other tissues. *Exp. Eye Res.* 15: *15-29* (1973).

BARBARO V., FONDA, S., NERONI, M. & NOVATI, M. Fluoroangiografia televisiva. Tecnica e possibilità. *Atti Soc. Oftalm. Lombarda* 29: *199-205* (1974).

BEN-SIRA, I. & RIVA, C.E. Fluorophotometric recording of fluorescein dilution curves in human retinal vessels. *Invest. Ophthalmol.* 12: *310-312* (1973).

BULPITT, C.J. & DOLLERY, C.T. Estimation of retinal blood flow by measurement of the mean circulation time. *Cardiovascular Res.* 5: *406-412* (1971).

CUNHA-VAZ J., FARIA DE ABREU, J.R., CAMPOS, A.J. & FIGO, G.M. Early breakdown of the blood-retinal barrier in diabetes. *Brit. J. Ophthal.* 59: *649-656* (1975).

EVANS, P.Y., SHIMIZU, K., LIMAYE, S., DEGLIN, E. & WRUCK, J. Fluorescein cineangiography of the optic nerve head. *Trans. Am. Acad. Ophthalmol. Otolaryng.* 77. *260-273* (1973).

FONDA, S. & BAGOLINI, B. Data to be published.

FRIEDMAN, E., KOPALD, H.H. & SMITH, T.R. Retinal and choroidal blood flow determined with Krypton-85 in anesthetized animals. *Invest. Ophthalmol.* 3: *539* (1964).

HICKAM, J.B. & FRAYSER, R. A photographic method for measuring the mean retinal circulation time using fluorescein. *Invest. Ophthalmol.* 4: *876-884* (1965).

HICKAM, J.B. & FRAYSER, R. Studies of the retinal circulation in man; observation on vessel diameter, arteriovenous oxygen difference, and mean circulation time. *Circulation* 33: *302-316* (1966).

HILL, D.W. The W. Mackenzie Centenary Symposium on 'The ocular circulation in health and disease' Glasgow, 1968, J. Stanley Cant, London 1969, Henry Kimpton, p. *53*.

HILL, D.W., GRIFFITHS, J.D. & YOUNG, S. Retinal blood flow measured by fluorescein angiography. *Trans. Ophthalmol. Soc. U.K.*: *325-332* (1973).

L'ESPERANCE, F.A. JR., JAMES, W.A., MC GUFFIN, R.P. & FLEISCHMAN, J.A. The evaluation of pathological retinal hemodynamics. *Trans. Amer. Acad. Ophth. and Otolaryng.* 78: *126-147* (1974).

NIESEL, P. Probleme der Durchblutungsmessungen am Auge. *Adv. Ophthalmol.* 29: *131-140* (1974) Karger Basel.

NIESEL, P. & GASSMANN, H.B. Direkte Fluorometrische Untersuchung am Augenhintergrund. *Ophthalmologica* 165: *297-302* (1972).

TROKEL, S. Photometric study of ocular blood flow in man. *Arch. Ophthalmol.* 71: *528-530* (1964).

WESSING, A. Filmaufnahmen vom Augenhintergrund und Fluorescenzangiographie. I. Historische Übersicht. *Albrecht V. Graefes Arch. Klin. Exp. Ophthal.* 192: *227-233* (1974).

WESSING, A. II. Eigenes Gerät und Lichtenergetische Untersuchungen. Same volume pp. *235-245*.

ZIERLER, K.L. Circulation times and the theory of indicator dilution method for determining blood flow and volume. In: Handbook of Physiology, American Physiological Society. Washington D.C. 1962, sect. 2 Vol. I: Circulation, p. *585*.

Authors' address:
Clinica Oculistica
Università di Modena
Via E. del Pozzo 71
41100 Modena
Italy

DISCUSSION

Dr Riva: In relation to the last paper: We have to be very careful to take the right parameters when we want to conclude about flow or mean circulation times. The only parameter which can be used to measure flow is the mean circulation time, because the time between the artery and the vein is very much dependent on the sensitivity of your system. The fact that you found that with age the time increases is for the following reason: with age less intensity reaches the fundus because of the scattering of the blue light at the lens so that you have in fact less blue light at the fundus. This decreases the sensitivity of your system and as the sensitivity of first appearance decreases the time increases. At least in our case, using a much more sensitive method we never found that this time increases with age. But I would like to say that many mistakes have already been made by using the first appearance time to conclude on flow. This first appearance time or any time which is not the mean circulation time or mean transit time can, in my opinion, lead to wrong conclusions.

Dr Fonda: No conclusions have been reached on blood flow. We only wanted to present preliminary results about the technique. Secondly, the sensitivity of the method depends on the sensitivity of the plumbicon tube of the TV camera. You could note that the venous dromofluorograms had all the same amplitude and the amplitudes of the dromofluorograms could be varied with the variation of the luminance of the videoscreen. So the photomuliplier saw different luminances from the videoscreen, from case to case, in such a way that D.F.G.'s could be comparable.

Dr Henkind: We seem to have two separate papers not dealing with the question. I would like to ask a question, however. I think it would be difficult to state on the basis of just one exam of the diabetic, but I would like to ask Dr. Peduzzi, on the basis of your single examination, you seemed to have concluded that it is the AV shunting in the diabetic retina that is responsible for this alteration.

Were you able to actually see AV shunting in the fundus and how can you be sure that it is the AV shunting that is altering your parameters?

Dr Peduzzi: I agree with Dr Henkind that we cannot make any statement on the basis of a single observation. Therefore, what we say about the effect of AV shunting in the diabetic retina must not be assumed as a statement, but as a pure hypothesis proposed in order to suggest a proper interpretation of the dromofluorogram in this case.

Dr Henkind: I personally tend to doubt it. Are their any other questions, Dr Kohner?

Dr Kohner: It seems that from what Dr Riva and Dr Peduzzi said that the method we used in London some time ago is really not all that good or not all that valid. I do not want to defend our method. The only reason we did it that way was that we did not have anything better and we wish that Dr Riva comes and works with us and develops easier methods for us. But what I would like to ask: even if we had mean transit times by whatever method we obtained it, it really gives an estimated value of blood flow and when we have much more accurate methods of measuring this and Dr Riva has laser-doppler measurements, can we really get useful information from this type of study?

Dr Henkind: For those in the audience, the question that Dr Kohner asked is: even if we refine our methods do they mean anything?

Dr Riva: Are you questioning the usefulness of the dye dilution curve technique?

Dr Kohner: The only thing is that they estimate flow, they never give accurate flow volumes.

Dr Riva: This is true, what we want to measure, in fact, is flow rather than transit time or circulation time. I cannot see how we can arrive at absolute measurements of flow with this method.

We cannot estimate the volume. But first I want to say that your method is not at all imperfect, but I think it is cumbersome. It takes a long time to do the picture and we would like to do someting faster. This method is also useful for other purposes. I have shown not only results in diabetics but there are a lot of measurements which can be done for example on occlusions. We have measured quite a number of patients with venous occlusion, arterial occlusion. If you want to follow the effect of treatment in these patients I think it is a valuable method.

THE PATHO-PHYSIOLOGY OF RETINAL
VEIN OCCLUSION

EVA M. KOHNER

(London, England)

In a short communication it is clearly not possible to deal with all aspects of the patho-physiology of vein occlusion. The aim of this paper therefore is to indicate the early changes which follow occlusion, and to show that these changes are due solely to the obstruction of outflow.

Central and branch vein occlusion are considered together, since they have similar features. The differences are due to the difference in the site of the outflow obstruction, and therefore of the area involved.

Outflow obstruction has two immediate effects:
1. Rise in intravascular pressure and
2. Stagnation of blood flow.

All clinical features are the result of these simultaneously occurring changes.

1. RISE IN INTRAVASCULAR PRESSURE

The rise in intravascular pressure is immediate. The vessels most vulnerable to the pressure rise are the terminal venules, since their wall structure is similar to that of capillaries, but they have a larger diameter. As the wall tension necessary to balance a given transmural pressure is related directly to its radius ($T = P_{TM} \times R$), they will have a tension two or three times as great as that found in the capillaries. Large vessels with their muscular and fibrous wall are more capable or resisting pressure. However they too will be affected in more severe outflow obstruction.

Increased intravascular pressure has four effects:
a. Vascular dilatation
b. Oedema and haemorrhages
c. Endothelial cell damage
d. Opening up of collaterals.

a. *Dilatation and increased tortuosity* of the larger veins is seen in the early stages after occlusion. Capillary dilatation is also well demonstrated on fluorescein angiograms.

b. *Increased intravascular pressure* rapidly exceeds the osmotic pressure of plasma proteins. Fluid is then forced out of the vessels and *oedema* results. Haemorrhage probably indicates that the endothelial cell lining has been interrupted, but we were unable to demonstrate this in the early stages following occlusion.

Fluorescein angiograms demonstrate the leakage; most marked in the terminal venules as would be expected.

c. *Endothelial cell damage* is caused by increased intravascular pressure only if this is extreme or accompanied by ischaemia. The early changes are functional ones. Leakage of fluorescein is seen within minutes of vein occlusion. In the most severe cases of outflow obstruction all vessels from capillaries to veins are affected, though arterial leakage is never observed in the early stages of vein occlusion.

Electron microscopy demonstrates the leakage of peroxidase from capillaries which have apparently intact endothelial cells. Thus again functional damage is indicated. Three to seven days after occlusion widespread damage to endothelial cells is seen, but this is usually associated with 'stagnation'. The changes are progressive.

d. *Opening up of collaterals* at the edge of the area supplied by the obstructed vein is immediate. As Archer observed (ARCHER et al. 1976) these are capillary collaterals and over the first 72 hours they remain of capillary size. Capillary collaterals form as a result of the intravascular pressure differential between the area drained by the occluded vein compared with adjacent normal area.

In experimental animals fully developed collaterals are seen after about 3 weeks. At this time collaterals are effective in restoring the total blood flow. In human retinal branch vein occlusion collaterals are only rarely effective in restoring normal circulation. In central retinal vein occlusion cilio-retinal 'by-pass channels' can restore normal appearance and function. Since the resistance in vessels is dependent on the inverse of the fourth power of the radius (Poiseuille's law) many collaterals will have to form with a total crossectional area well above that of the vein occluded to restore flow, unless a really large one, as seen occasionally in cilio-retinal bypass channels.

2. STAGNATION OF BLOOD FLOW

Stagnation of blood flow is the result of outflow obstruction. If obstruction was complete the pressure in the vein would rise rapidly to arterial level and flow would cease. This is not usally the case in vein occlusion. Delayed and reduced perfusion of the affected area is immediate (KOHNER et al., 1970, ARCHER et al., 1976). Recent work by ROSEN (ROSEN et al., 1976) using radioactive microspheres in monkeys indicates that during the first hours of occlusion the flow in the affected segments is less than 25% of that seen in the same segment of the control eye. This gradually returns to normal in 3 weeks. In humans there is some indication that flow is progressively reduced in those patients with central retinal vein occlusion whose outflow obstruction increased (i.e. they deteriorate).

Stagnation of flow is clinically demonstrated by dark blood in the veins, which may become almost blue. Fluorescein angiogram demonstrates the granular flow and clumping of cells.

Stagnation is important for two reasons:

a. it causes ischaemia and
b. results in occlusion of small vessels.

a. *Ischaemia*

Increased flow and intravascular pressure alone cause endothelial cell proliferation as seen in collateral channels, but added ischaemia will result in severe endothelial cell damage which is often irreversible. The endothelial damage produced takes 1-3 days to develop. After 5 weeks many capillaries disappear altogether.

b. *Thrombosis*

Occlusion of capillaries was not seen in the experimental animals in the acute stages. After 3-7 days, however, many small vessels were seen to be filled with red blood cells and disintergrating platelets. If large areas of such capillaries formed — these were usually associated with large haemorrhages.

Stagnation and resulting capillary non-perfusing depends clearly on the completeness of outflow obstruction. It appears from recent work (RING et al., 1976) that increased viscosity may also play an important role, since patients with predominant capillary occlusion were found to have a higher blood viscosity than those who had predominant dilatation of capillaries, or only small areas of non-perfusion.

Capillary non-perfusion is of importance because in over 60% of cases it leads to new vessel formation or thrombotic glaucoma.

ACKNOWLEDGEMENTS

This work was supported by the Wellcome Trust and the M.R.C. My co-workers were Drs. Hamilton, Hockley, Rosen and Bird. I am grateful for their help.

REFERENCES

ARCHER, D.B., ERNEST, J.T. & MAGUIRE, C.F.J. In: Vision and Circulation. ed. J.S. Cant. p. *229*. H. Kimpton (1976).
KOHNER, E.M., DOLLERY, C.T., SHAKIB, M., HENKIND, P., PATERSON, J.W., DE OLIVEIRA, L.N.F. & BULPITT, C.J. *Amer. J. Ophthal.* 69: *778* (1970).
RING, C.P., PEARSON, T.C., SANDERS, M.D. & WETHERLY-MEIN, G. (in press).
ROSEN, D., MARSHALL, J., KOHNER, E.M. & HAMILTON, A.M. (in preparation).

Author's address:
Hammersmith Hospital & Institute of Ophthalmology
Du Cane Road   Judd Street
London W12 OWS   London W.C.1
England   England

DISCUSSION

Dr Archer: Perhaps I could start the discussion by asking Dr Kohner about these newly formed intra-retinal vessels. Do you really think that these vessels are true neovascularisation, that is, vessels that leak fluorescein, have poor tight junctions, and expand irregularly.

Dr Kohner: I think that they are newly formed vessels because they are in areas where for weeks we have nothing, no capillary perfusion, and then we get perfusion eventually. John Marshall, who did electron microscopy of these vessels found three types of capillaries: One type is what I showed, when there is a complete replacement of the capillary by glial elements and these are obviously closed capillaries. Then a second group of capillaries, where you could see macrophages within the basement membrane tube and we assumed that in these vessels there was a revascularization of a pre-existing basement membrane tube. There was a third type of capillaries which for all intents and purposes look like normal capillaries in an area where there were no capillaries before or, indeed, sometimes where you would not expect capillaries, like around arteries, and we assumed that these are proper, newformed capillaries but I do not know why they do not leak.

Dr Archer: Have you found that any of these newly formed capillaries extend beyond the internal limiting membrane in the experimental animal?

Dr Kohner: No, we have not.

NATURAL COURSE AND CLASSIFICATION OF PATIENTS WITH BRANCH RETINAL VEIN OBSTRUCTION

D.B. ARCHER

(Belfast, N. Ireland)

One hundred and sixty patients with branch retinal vein obstruction were investigated to determine the response of the retinal microvasculature to an acute segmental interruption in outflow. Patients who demonstrated no other significant fundus disease were followed for periods of one to five years following the acute vein obstruction. The rearrangement and reorganisation of the retinal capillary network in the territory of the obstructed vein were documented by ophthalmoscopy, fundus biomicroscopy, and fluorescein angiography. In selected cases suction cup ophthalmodynamometry in conjunction with fluorescein angiography was used to estimate the level of intraocular pressure at which the various arteries and arterioles to the obstructed area filled.

The patients were classified into four broad groups according to the efficiency of the arterial perfusion, competence of the retinal microvasculature in the territory of the obstructed vein and severity of retinal ischaemia.

GROUP I – NORMAL RETINAL PERFUSION AND MICROVASCULAR COMPETENCE

Sixteen patients in Group I were characterised by almost complete recovery. Arterial perfusion to the affected sector was judged to be normal, and the corresponding retinal microvasculature noted to be well perfused and competent on angiography. Residual minor alterations in capillary structure and architecture persisted for many years, however. These included dilated and deformed capillaries, well compensated collaterals, and microaneurysms. Many of these well compensated occlusions affected small order veins and were extra-foveal in distribution. In such cases the area of obstructed microvasculature was small in relation to its circumference where effective collaterals could develop and maintain good perfusion and normal circulation times. Major vein obstructions falling within this group were either incomplete or had well developed bypass systems at or near the site of obstruction. There was no significant decompensation of the retinal microvasculature on follow-up, although a gradual remodelling of the affected capillary bed occurred. Alterations in capillary calibre, variations in the number and size of microaneurysms and staining of some defective endothelial cells on angiography were typical findings. Visual acuities were nor-

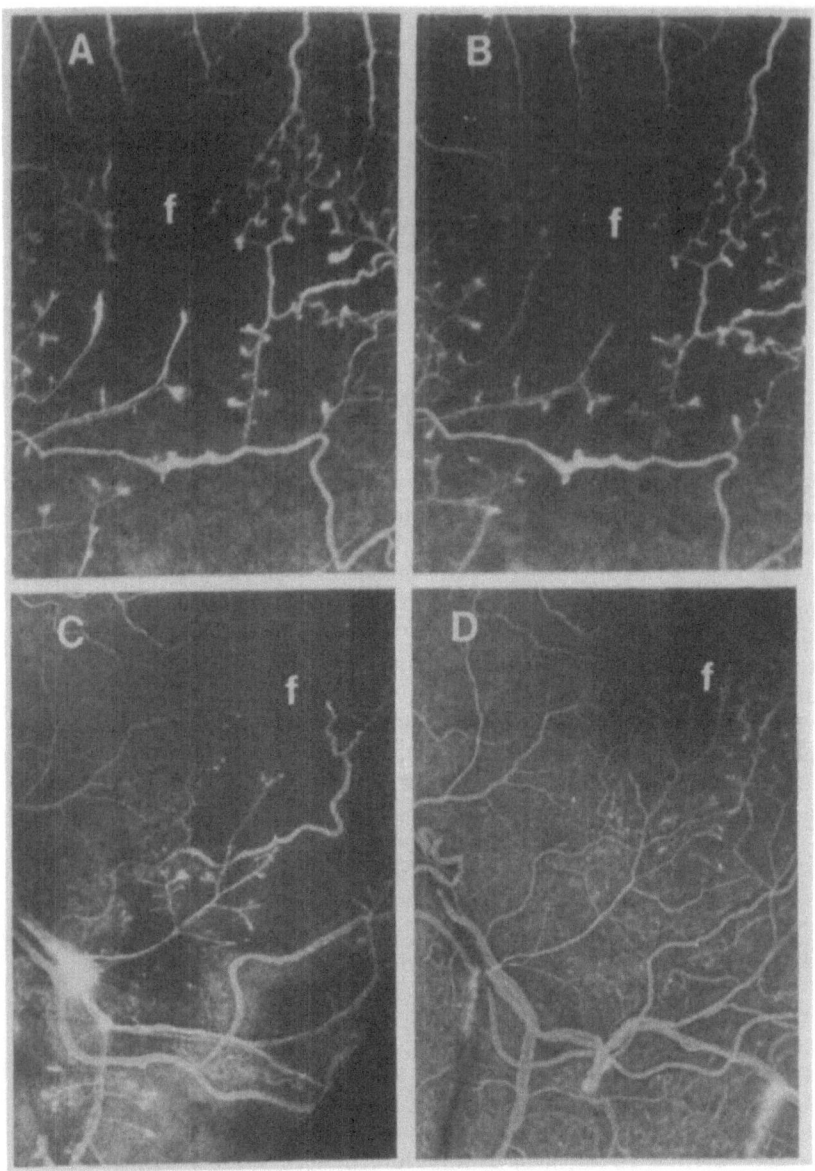

Fig. I A and B. Macular circulation of patient with left infero-temporal branch vein obstruction. New intraretinal vessels are present adjacent to the fovea (F), and show alterations over a one year period (B).

Fig. I C and D. Macular circulation of patient with left infero-temporal branch retinal vein obstruction. Extensive new intraretinal channels have formed over a one year period adjacent to the fovea (F).

mal or near normal (Table I) and visual fields were either full or demonstrated only small paracentral relative scotomata.

GROUP II – NORMAL RETINAL PERFUSION WITH SOME DEGREE OF MICROVASCULAR INCOMPETENCE

Thirty-five patients in this group demonstrated integrity of arterial flow to the obstructed area of retina and a well perfused capillary network. The affected capillaries nevertheless remained irregularly dilated, demonstrated microaneurysms and were incompetent to fluorescein. Alterations within the affected microvasculature usually stabilised within the first six months following obstruction by which time numerous well developed collaterals had formed.

The area of vascular imcompetence as estimated by fluorescein angiography was either focal or corresponded to the entire distribution of the obstructed vein. Generally there was little alteration in the microvascular pattern over the years, although collaterals decreased in size and capillary dilatation became less obvious. Visual functions accurately reflected integrity of the immediate parafoveal capillaries. Eighteen patients in whom the incompetent capillaries were extrafoveal had visual acuities of 6/9 or better. Seventeen patients with foveal involvement had acuities ranging between 6/12 and 6/60, depending on the extent of the oedema or the presence of microcystoid degenerative changes. Extensive foveal oedema generally indicated that most of the parafoveal vasculature had been implicated from the outset and that the visual prognosis was poor.

Visual fields demonstrated reduced sensitivity in the area characterised by dilated capillaries and fluid accumulation. The most pronounced field defect corresponded to the centre of the obstructed venous field where stasis was most marked. Absence of arcuate field defects suggested that no substantial infarction of the nerve fibre layer had occurred.

GROUP III – IMPAIRED ARTERIAL PERFUSION, CAPILLARY INCOMPETENCE AND NON-PERFUSION

Group III included patients in whom the arterial perfusion was impaired, and the retinal microvasculature incompletely perfused and incompetent. As the natural course of the disease was determined by the degree of retinal ischaemia, the patients were divided into two sub groups which reflected the area of capillary non-perfusion.

Subgroup A – Focal capillary closure

Twenty-nine patients were characterised by small areas of capillary closure within the territory of the obstructed vein. The zones of capillary non-perfusion varied from $\frac{1}{2}$ to 3 disc diameters in size and were bordered by irregular and dilated capillaries studded with multiple microaneurysms and incompetent to dye during angiography. Sequential angiograms taken over several years demonstrated that affected capillary beds remained dilated and that non-perfused retina altered little in area or character apart from the

Branch Retinal Vein Obstruction – Recovery of Visual Acuity*

		Patient No.	Visual Acuity							
			6/6	6/9	6/12	6/18	6/24	6/36	6/60	6/60
Group I		16	16	-	-	-	-	-	-	-
Group II		35	13	5	2	6	-	3	1	5
Group III	A	29	3	3	5	5	2	3	5	3
	B	63	18	13	6	13	1	2	7	3
Group IV		17	1	3	1	-	4	1	2	5

*Minimum Follow Up Period 1 Year Post Obstruction

disappearance of an occasional capillary radical and alterations in the number of microaneurysms. It was unusual for the area of capillary incompetence to extend beyond its original limits. There was only minimal evidence of intraretinal revascularisation of ischaemic retina and no case demonstrated pre-retinal or papillary neovascularisation.

Visual acuity depended on whether the macular capillary bed was part of the drainage bed or collateral system of the obstructed vein, and whether the parafoveal capillaries formed part of the ischaemic zone (Table I). Six patients with foveal involvement developed intraretinal oedema, lipid deposits and cystoid degenerative changes. Visual fields demonstrated scotomata that closely matched the area of non-perfused retina. Small arcuate scotomas in some instances indicated infarction of nerve fibre bundles.

Subgroup B — Widespread capillary closure

Sixty-three patients had extensive areas (greater than 4 disc diameters) of capillary non-perfusion in the distribution of the obstructed vein, often amounting to a sector of retina. The arteries subserving the affected quadrants were attenuated and filled at lower levels of intraocular pressure than their counterparts in neighbouring unobstructed areas of the retina. The affected microvasculature demonstrated extensive structural abnormalities and incompetence to dye during angiography. On follow-up a gradual refashioning and reorganisation of the microvasculature occurred in those areas adjacent to the non-perfused retina. Some capillaries, venules and arterioles developed outgrowths which extended into the ischaemic retina and in some instances forged new links with adjacent capillary beds. These new channels were intraretinal, narrow, straight, and frequently formed loops and secondary bifurcations (Fig. 1). The terminal dilated portions of these new capillaries were characteristically hyperfluorescent on angiography, probably reflecting both circulatory stasis and staining of immature endothelial cells at their advancing edge.

Pre-retinal neovascularisation occurred in the neighbourhood of major retinal veins and their tributaries and was charateristically located near the watershed zone between perfused and non-perfused retina. Surface neovascularisation appeared to develop from retinal veins, venules and newly formed intraretinal channels, which were usually situated in the neighbourhood of a major retinal vein or venule. New vessels initially grew along the surface of the retina, but eventually extended towards the vitreous cavity following detachment of the vitreous. It was unusual to observe retinal neovascularisation at less than one year following the acute obstruction, although such foci were observed as early as four months post obstruction. The development of fresh areas of neovascularisation occurred over the years, often accompanied by further closure of retinal capillary beds. In this subgroup fifty patients developed surface neovascularisation, and 24 patients developed papillary neovascularisation. Characteristically, the papillary fronds grew towards the ischaemic area of retina. Thirty-eight patients with neovascularisation had vitreous haemorrhages, three of which permanently obstructed vision. Other complications included macular oedema, microcystoid degenerative changes, premacular fibrosis and macular pigmen-

143

tation. Retinal holes occasionally occurred in ischaemic retina, often close to a nidus of neovascularisation, and in two instances led to retinal detachments. Visual acuity was closely related to the integrity of the parafoveal vasculature (Table I). Thirty-one patients with at least partially intact parafoveal capillaries had visual acuities of 6/12 or better despite widespread ischaemia. There were well defined visual field defects in this group of patients. The ischaemic zones produced large absolute scotomata usually with an arcuate character or component often amounting to a sector or a quadrant of the retina.

GROUP IV – SEVERE RETINAL ISCHAEMIA

Group IV encompassed seventeen patients with gross arterial insufficiency, widespread retinal ischaemia and neovascularisation. The basic pathology appeared to be arterial stasis and secondary vein thrombosis. The sites of venous obstruction did not necessarily occur at arteriovenous junctions and venous collaterals were often not a feature. Widespread areas of capillary non-perfusion were present and pre-retinal neovascularisation was uniform.

Papillary neovascularisation occurred in all but one case. Visual acuity was usually poor due to macular oedema, ischaemia, or persistence of vitreous haemorrhage. Four patients, however, with intact foveal microvasculature retained central visual functions of 6/9 or better (Table I). Field defects similar to those noted in Group IIIB were present.

Author's address:
Royal Victoria Hospital
Department of Ophthalmology
Grosvenor Road
Belfast BT12 6BA
Northern Ireland

COTTON-WOOL SPOTS IN RETINAL VEIN THROMBOSIS

K. ASAYAYAMA, M. UYAMA, S. UENO, A. NEGI & M. INOUE

(Kyoto, Japan)

Retinal vein occlusion exhibits various ophthalmoloscopic appearances. In some cases, retinal hemorrhages are manifest, in others, cotton-wool spots are dominant and retinal hemorrhages are rarely seen. The significance of the occurrence of these cotton-wool sponts in retinal vein thrombosis is discussed. Data in our study covers patients who were seen in our clinic during the last 5 years and were followed up for at least 6 months.

Each patient was examined by binocular indirect ophthalmoscopy, colour photography and fluorescein angiography, and the corrected visual acuity was assessed. They were treated medically with anticoagulants and cortico steroids. Photocoagulation was employed as required.

Patients were divided into three groups according to the ophthalmoscopic findings.

Group I: Predominant cotton-wool spots in the infarcted area with minor retinal hemorrhage.

Group II: Retinal hemorrhage with several cotton-wool spots.

Group III: Retinal hemorrhage with no cotton-wool spots.

The clinical results were analysed with reference to the three groups.

RESULTS

Forty-nine patients were divided into three groups (Table 1). The average age of the patients at the first visit was 59.5 years. There were no significant differences between the groups in sex incidence, affected eye or site of obstruction.

Table I. General information

Group	I	II	III
No. of patients	♂ 4 ⎱ 9 ♀ 5 ⎰	♂ 10 ⎱ 21 ♀ 11 ⎰	♂ 6 ⎱ 19 ♀ 13 ⎰
mean age	49	54	49
site of obstruction			
branch vein	7 (78%)	13 (62%)	12 (63%)
central vein	2 (22%)	8 (38%)	7 (37%)

The time required for complete absorption of the retinal hemorrhages was 41, 31 and 45 weeks respectively (Table II); however, there was no

145

Table II. Clinical course

Groups	I	II	III
Absorption of retinal hemorrhage (weeks)	41w	31w	45w
Disappearance of macular edema (weeks)	16w	28w	45w

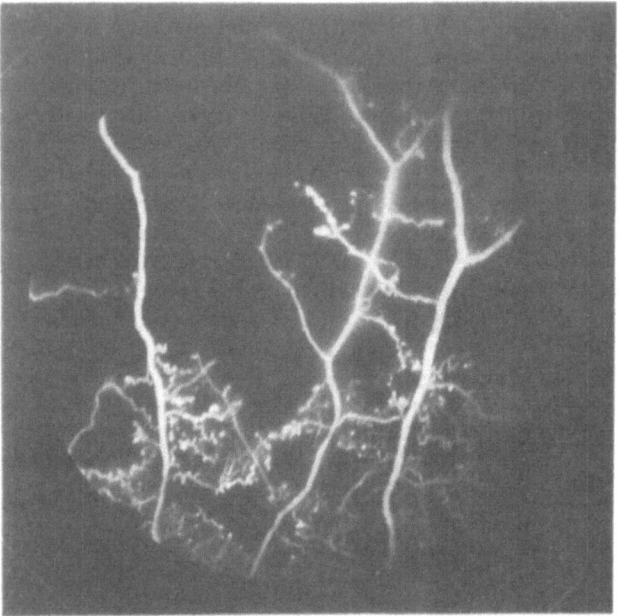

Fig. 1. Angiogram of a man aged 37. Capillary closure is revealed.

statistically significant difference between the groups. The time required for complete absorption of macular edema is shown in Table II; these differences were statistically significant. Edema of the macular area was absorbed faster in patients with cotton-wool spots, especially in those in whom cotton-wool spots were predominant, and prognosis for central visual acuity was better in the first group than in the others.

In many patients with cotton-wool spots, fluorescein angiography revealed a widespread closure of the capillary bed in the occluded area.

Case 1

The patient is a man aged 37 (Fig. 1). This is a case of occlusion of upper temporal branch vein. Cotton-wool spots were seen among the massive retinal hemorrhages on the first visit. Fluorescein angiography revealed wide spread capillary closure within the occluded area shown by dark patches in

146

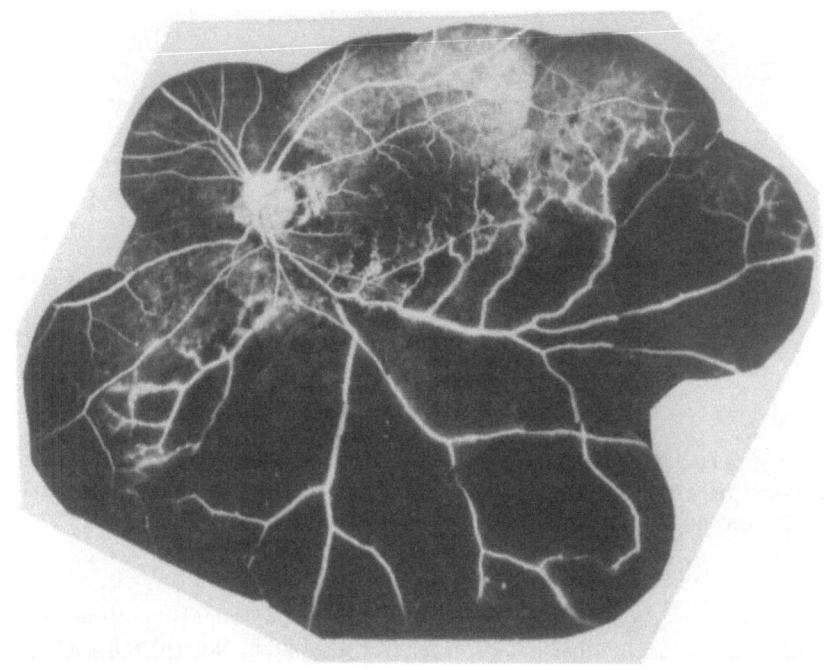

Fig. 2. Angiogram of a woman aged 44. Capillary closure area has spread to more than one quadrant. Widespread capillary closure is revealed.

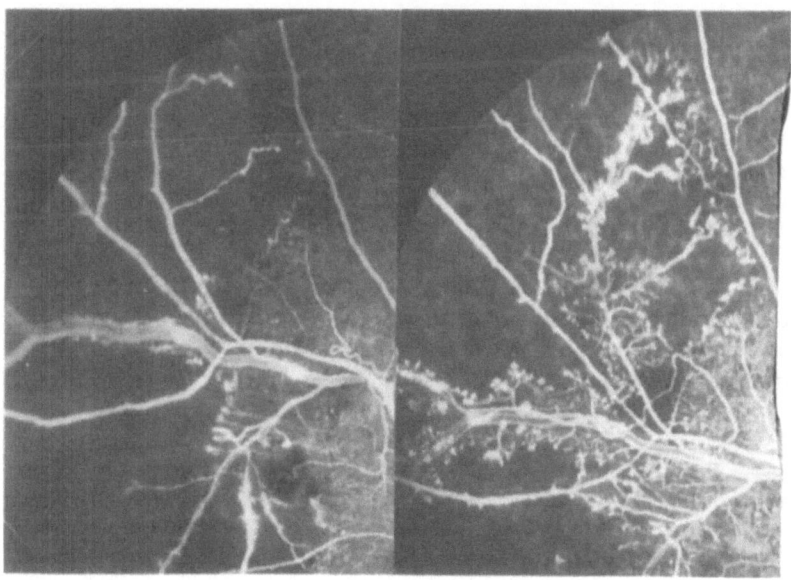

Fig. 3. Angiogram of a woman aged 37. Frame to the right was taken 3 months after that to the left. Neovascularization has developed in the areas of capillary closure.

147

Table III. Occurrence of neovascularization

Groups	I	II	III
Occurrence	78%	50%	42%

Table IV. Occurrence of capillary closure in fluorescein angiography

Groups	I	II	III
Occurrence	88%	70%	10%

the figure (Fig. 1). Six months later, vitreous hemorrhage due to neovascularization occurred, and photocoagulation was perfomred. His final visual acuity was 20/20.

Case 2

This patient is a woman aged 44. This is a case of predominant cotton-wool spots with minor retinal hemorrhage. Her angiogram showed remarkably widespread capillary closure (Fig. 2). Massive retinal hemorrhage from neovascularization in the area of capillary closure occurred 8 months later, treated by photocoagulation.

Case 3

This is a case of predominant cotton-wool spots found in a woman aged 37 (Fig. 3). The angiogram showed widespread capillary closure with neovascularization in the dark areas.

The occurrence of widespread capillary closure was found in 88% and 77% of group I and II patients respectively; however, the rate was only 10% in group III (Table III). The difference was significant.

With regard to retinal neovascularization, the frequency of occurrence is shown in Table IV. The rate was statistically higher in patients with cotton-wool spots.

Vitreous hemorrhage from these newly formed vessels was often encountered during the long course of the disease. Six intravitreal hemorrhages occurred in this study. Five were in patients with cotton-wool spots and one was in a patient without cotton-wool spots.

DISCUSSION

In this study of retinal vein occlusion, it became evident that the occurrence of the widespread capillary closure in the angiograms was higher in patients with cotton-wool spots, than without. Development of non-perfused capillary bed may be due to the following factors:
1. Low arterial blood pressure due to arterial insufficiency.
2. Blood stream stasis due to venous occlusion.

148

3. Increase of tissue pressure as a result of retinal edema. HAYREH (1965, 1971) and others stressed that arterial insufficiency was an important cause of retinal vein occlusion. In the present study, however, capillary closure was seen less frequently in cases with predominant retinal hemorrhages and no cotton-wool spots. This may be attributed to the fact that arterial insufficiency was not severe and only hemorrhagic infarction occurred.

ASHTON (1963) reported that the cause of the cotton-wool spots was a focal ischemia due to arterial insufficiency, so arterial insufficiency is more severe in patients with cotton-wool spots and the tendency is high in cases of capillary closure.

When cotton-wool spots are encountered in clinical retinal vein occlusion, the possibility of arterial insufficiency should be investigated.

SUMMARY

The significance of cotton-wool spots in retinal vein occlusion was discussed. Data for 49 patients were reviewed.

In most cases with cotton-wool spots, widespread capillary closure was seen in the occluded area on fluorescein angiography; however, in cases with no cotton-wool spots, such findings were rarely seen.

The presence of cotton-wool spots was associated with neovascularization leading to vitreous hemorrhage.

It was concluded that retinal vein occlusion with severe arterial insufficiency presents with cotton-wool spots on ophthalmoscopy.

REFERENCES

ASHTON, N. & HARRY, J. The pathology of cotton-wool spots and cytoid bodies in hypertensive retinopathy and other diseases. *Trans. Ophthalmol. Soc. U.K.* 83: *91-114* (1963).

ERNEST, J.T. & NEWELL, F.W. Classification of branch retinal vein obstruction. *Trans. Am. Acad. Ophthalmol. & Otol.* 78: *148-165* (1974).

FUJINO, T. et al. Experimental central branch vein occlusion. *Tr. Am. Ophthal. Soc.* 66: *318-406* (1968).

GASS, J.D.M. A fluorescein angiographic study of macular dysfunction secondary to retinal vascular disease: Retinal vein obstruction. *Arch. Ophthal.* 80: *550-568* (1968).

HAYREH, S.S. Occlusion of the central retinal vessels. *Brit. J. Ophthalmol.* 49: *626-645* (1965).

HAYREH, S.S. Pathogenesis of occlusion of the central retinal vessels. *Am. J. Ophthalmol.* 72: *998-1011* (1971).

HILL, D.W. & GRIFFITH, J.D. The prognosis in retinal vein thrombosis. *Trans. Ophthalmol. Soc. U.K.* 90: *309-322* (1970).

KOHNER, E.M. et al. Experimental retinal branch vein occlusion. *Am. J. Ophthalmol.* 69: *778-* (1970).

PATON, A., RUBINSTEIN, K. & SMITH, V.H. Arterial insufficiency in retinal vein occlusion. *Trans. Ophthalmol. Soc. U.K.* 84: *559-586* (1964).

Authors' address:
Department of Ophthalmology
Faculty of Medicine
Kyoto University
Kyoto, Japan

PROGNOSTIC SIGNIFICANCE OF FLUORESCEIN ANGIOGRAPHY IN CENTRAL RETINAL VEIN OCCLUSION

L. LAATIKAINEN & E.M. KOHNER

(Helsinki, Finland/London, England)

In order to study the prognostic value of fluorescein angiographic findings in central retinal vein occlusion (CRVO), 75 patients with a recent CRVO were followed up regularly for at least one year after their first symptoms.

Sixty of the 75 cases had their initial examination during the first month, 37 of them during the first week, and 15 cases during the second and third months after the onset of symptoms. After the initial presentation most patients were re-examined at 3, 6 and 12 months. In addition to clinical examination, colour photographs and fluorescein angiography were done during each visit whenever possible.

On the basis of the predominant feature in the initial fluorescein picture the eyes were separated into two groups: (1) those with capillary dilatation and abnormal permeability of blood vessels, and (2) those with retinal capillary closure.

Fifty of the 75 cases belonged to the first group. The final outcome in these eyes is presented in Table 1.

On fluorescein angiogram the abnormal permeability response is easy to demonstrate and to localise. It was found that prognosis was better when leakage was restricted to veins and terminal venules than if capillaries were affected as well. Some capillary leakage in the macula in the acute stage was, however, seen in 5 of the 28 eyes which eventually showed complete or partial resolution. In most cases, leakage from the perifoveal capillaries resulted in chronic cystoid macular oedema (maculopathy).

Table I. The final condition in eyes with capillary dilatation and abnormal permeability response (initial study)

Final condition	No. of eyes
Full resolution (VA 6/9 or better)	16
Partial resolution (VA 6/12 – 6/18)	12
Maculopathy (VA 6/24 or worse)	18
Thrombotic glaucoma	2
Retinitis proliferans	1
Preretinal fibrosis	1
Total	50

Table II. The final condition in eyes with predominant capillary closure (initial study)

Final condition	No. of eyes with capillary closure	
	Moderate	Severe
Full or partial resolution (VA 6/18 or better)	–	–
Maculopathy (VA 6/24 or worse)	6	–
Thrombotic glaucoma	3	8
Retinitis proliferans	1	5
Preretinal fibrosis	–	2
Total	10	15

Perifoveal capillary leakage is often related to a broken perifoveal capillary arcade, although 11 of the 24 eyes which developed chronic macular oedema had an apparently intact arcade.

Results of this study show that a broken perifoveal capillary arcade impaired the visual prognosis in CRVO. Only one of the 13 eyes with a broken arcade and capillary leakage recovered good vision, whereas the others developed maculopathy. These results are similar to those demonstrated for retinal branch vein occlusion by CLEMETT and co-workers (1973).

Some earlier fluorescein angiographic studies have revealed a considerable lengthening of the retinal circulation time in many cases of CRVO (HILL, 1968; VON SALIS, 1968). In the present work the prognostic significance of this finding was estimated by comparing the initial macular transit time to the final condition of the eye. The macular transit time was counted from the first dye appearance in the retinal arteries to its reappearance in the macular venules. At the initial examination the macular transit time was found to be within normal limits in almost two-thirds of the eyes with an abnormal permeability response, and there was no significant difference between the eyes developing maculopathy and those resolving.

Three of the 50 eyes with an initially good capillary perfusion developed extensive capillary closure during the first 3 months after the occlusion with a final result of thrombotic glaucoma in 2 cases and retinitis proliferans in 1 case. At the initial examination these eyes did not differ from the others with an abnormal permeability response.

Twentyfive of the 75 eyes had moderate or extensive capillary closure at the initial examination. Table 2 represents the final condition in these eyes.

All eyes with an extensive capillary nonperfusion became blind (final VA 6/60 or worse). In addition to capillary closure most smaller venules and arterioles were also obliterated in these retinae and the remaining vessels – at first the veins, but later the arteries as well – leaked fluorescein. Retinal circulation was very slow in all cases. In most eyes capillary closure was already obvious on the initial angiogram although retinal oedema and haemorrhages sometimes made the interpretation difficult. In fluorescein pictures no differentiating features could be found between the eyes developing the different complications of thrombotic glaucoma, retinitis proliferans or preretinal fibrosis.

This study showed that in 73 out of 75 eyes (98%) the final visual outcome could be accurately predicted on the basis of the 3 months examination, while the correct prognosis could be given in only 38 of 60 eyes (63%) during the first month after the onset of symptoms.

According to these results fluorescein angiography undeniably gives more information about the prognosis of CRVO than can be obtained from the ophthalmoscopic picture alone, and by differentiating cases with various types of retinal response it gives better guidelines for planning the possible therapy in an individual eye.

ACKNOWLEDGMENTS

This work was supported by the Wellcome Trust and by the Francis and Renee Hock Foundation.

REFERENCES

CLEMETT, R.S., KOHNER, E.M. & HAMILTON, A.M. The visual prognosis in retinal branch vein occlusion. *Trans. ophthal. Soc. U.K.* 93: *523-535* (1973).

HILL, D.W. Fluorescein studies in retinal vascular occlusion. *Brit. J. Ophthal.* 52: *1-12* (1968).

VON SALIS, R. Fluoreszenzretinographie. Bestimmung der Arm-Retina-Zeit bei Normalen, bei Zentralvenenthrombosen und Periphlebitiden. *Schweiz. med. Wschr.* 98: *41-46* (1968).

Authors' addresses:
Lohenpyrstö 2C
00650 Helsinki 65
Finland

Hammersmith Hospital
Du Cane Road
London W12 OHS, England

DISCUSSION

Dr Hayreh: The last two papers were of great interest to me and I think that they are very instructive from a prognostic point of view. I have been investigating patients with central retinal vein occlusion. I divide the cases into two categories (this division is extremely important): In the first group, on fluorescein angiography, there is no capillary closure; while in the second group, there is capillary closure in the retinal vascular bed. These are two different entities and unless we divide these cases into the two distinct categories, their prognosis, therapy, and the incidence of thrombotic glaucoma in them get confused. This is the reason why we find different figures are given by different authors of complications and of the response to various treatment in central retinal vein occlusion.

I have called the first category as venous stasis retinopathy, i.e., when there is no capillary closure. These patients may have fairly good vision or may present with a marked fall of central visual acuity; they do not have extensive retinal hemorrhages and have almost normal visual fields — with Goldmann perimetry quite often we can record the fields with 1/2 — associated often with a relative central scotoma.

On the other hand, the second category is that with hemorrhagic retinopathy, i.e., with capillary closure; in them the visual acuity is very poor, usually counts finger or even much worse than that; there are extensive hemorrhages and a lot of cotton-wool spots and a typical picture of ischemic retina. In the second group, the outcome is extremely poor, with capillary closure, neovascularization, vitreous hemorrhages, retinitis proliferans, thrombotic glaucoma and loss of the eye.

It is a progressive disease. In contrast to that the venous stasis retinopathy is almost always a benign, self-limiting condition, its main complication is macular edema and that is what brings the patient to an ophthalmologist. The macular edema mostly results in a cystoid macular degeneration, with the loss of central vision. In hemorrhagic retinopathy, the incidence of thrombotic glaucoma is very high; whereas in venous stasis retinopathy it is practically none — at least I have not seen it so far. I was surprised to find that in Dr Laatikainen's series two of the patients with venous stasis retinopathy had developed glaucoma but I think these are the two who either initially were misdiagnosed or they progressed on to the second group. In my series, in about 5-6% so far my initial impression was that they had venous stasis retinopathy but later, on the basis of fluorescein angiography, I had to transfer them to the other group and I felt either the thrombotic occlusion of the central retinal vein had progressed all the way forward into the optic disc to produce hemorrhagic retinopathy or my initial diagnosis was incorrect. Prognosis and the response to treatment is decided by the amount of ischemia, and the amount of capillary closure. That is why unless we divide our cases into the two groups we are not going to get a clear picture of this disease; from that point of view, I thought the paper by Drs Laatikainen and Kohner was excellent, and it stressed exactly what one should look for and divide these cases into the two groups before really proceeding any further.

Dr Kohner: The two patients who developed thrombotic glaucoma later, are patients in whom the clinical picture changed. This is the whole point we are making: that on the initial examination if the patient presents within the first months we can give prognosis to those who had predominant non-perfusion, but in those who had good capillary perfusion, things may change in the next 6 weeks. But after three months we were able to give prognosis for vision in about 98% of our patients. Now whether these patients with initially good perfusion who later deteriorate, develop a second episode of outflow obstruction we do not know, but they certainly deteriorate and even retrospectively we could not have diagnosed them differently at the first visit.

TRAITEMENT DES OCCLUSIONS VEINEUSES RETINIENNES

GABRIEL COSCAS

(Créteil, France)

OCCLUSIONS DE LA VEINE CENTRALE DE LA RETINE

1. *Les anti-coagulants* associés ou non aux anti-inflammatoires, n'ont pas fait la preuve de leur efficacité, ni pour obtenir la régression des symptômes, ni pour empêcher le passage d'un stade initial à un stade majeur de l'obstruction.

Dans notre étude, l'évolution est restée imprèvisible, soir vers la régression, soit vers l'aggravation progressive et ce traitement semble jouer un rôle non significatif statistiquement sur l'occlusion elle même. Par contre, nous avons retrouvé un rôle de prévention du glaucome néovasculaire: sur 37 cas d'occlusions de la veine centrale de la rétine avec un recul de 1 à 5 ans, nous avons observé seulement deux cas de glaucome néovasculaire, donc un pourcentage de 5,5%, nettement plus bas que toutes les statistiques d'évolution spontanée.

2. *Les fibrinolytiques* (et surtout l'Urokinase) malgré de grands espoirs, n'ont pas fait la preuve d'une efficacité plus grande.

Certes, on a observé quelques cas heureux qui ouvrent des perspectives encourageantes. Il faut noter cependant:

— leur efficacité retardée sur les angiographies pendant quelques jours malgré l'amélioration franche de l'acuité (persistance des signes angiographiques après Urokinase, malgré une récupération importante subjective et objective de l'acuité visuelle).

— le retard du remplissage veineux persiste souvent après normalisation de l'acuité et de l'angiographie.

L'hypothèse retenue dans l'utilisation des fibrinolytiques (toujours associés d'ailleurs aux anti-coagulants), est de permettre de passer une phase critique et de faciliter ainsi, la recanalisation ou la constitution d'une circulation de suppléance satisfaisante.

Notre étude randomisée n'est cependant pas encore significative car le nombre de patients est trop petit (37) pour pouvoir tenir compte des différents facteurs en jeu: le terrain, l'age, la cause de l'occlusion et surtout, le siège et l'étendue de l'obstruction par rapport à la lame criblée, ainsi que la possibilité anatomique de développement d'anastomoses optico-ciliaires. Au stade actuel de notre étude, les meilleurs résultats sont observés chez les sujets jeunes et chez ceux qui avaient encore une bonne acuité visuelle initiale.

3. *La photocoagulation* ne paraît avoir, dans les occlusions du tronc de la veine centrale de la rétine, que des indications limitées.

Son utilisation repose, comme chez le diabétique, sur des applications à type de photocoagulation pan-rétinienne (P.P.R.) qui ont pour but, de diminuer l'oedème rétinien et d'éviter la constitution de proliférations vasculaires pré-rétiniennes et pré-papillaires avec leur risque d'hémorragie dans le vitré.

Les résultats que nous avons observés sont satisfaisants: régression de l'oedème dans tout le champ rétinien périphérique, normalisation du calibre veineux et disparition des néo-vaisseaux pré-rétiniens.

Toutefois, le problème de la dégénérescence maculaire ne semble pas actuellement résolu d'une manière satisfaisante par cette technique de traitement: nous n'avons jamais obtenu de modification d'un oedème maculaire cystoïde déjà installé.

Le rôle préventif du glaucome néo-vasculaire par la photocoagulation panrétinienne, vu la relative rareté de cette complication est difficile à apprécier actuellement. Toutefois, l'angiographie systématique de l'iris semble indiquer la possibilité de dépister précocément l'évolution vers ce glaucome néo-vasculaire; une photocoagulation précoce pourrait alors avoir un effet favorable.

La photocoagulation conserve donc des indications limitées dans les occlusions de la veine centrale de la rétine puisqu'elle apporte seulement une amélioration fonctionnelle, surtout dans le champ visuel périphérique.

LES OCCLUSIONS DE BRANCHE VEINEUSE RETINIENNE

Nous avons eu la possibilité d'étudier et de suivre 76 cas d'occlusions de branches veineuses rétiniennes avec un recul de 1 à 5 ans. Dans le déclenchement de ces occlusions, deux facteurs dominent tous les autres:
— la sévérité de l'atteinte artérielle générale et de l'hypertension artérielle;
— la sévérité des lésions au niveau du croisement artério-veineux rétinien.
1. *Les traitements médicaux.* Sur le plan thérapeutique, les fibrinolytiques n'ont que peu d'indications et dans nos essais (12 cas) nous avons constaté qu'il existe toujours un retrécissement vrai de la colonne sanguine qui persiste après la perfusion d'Urokinase et ceci même dans les formes régressives.

Les anti-coagulants et anti-agrégants ont été essayés pour tester leur efficacité dans la lutte contre le passage de l'occlusion incomplète à l'obstruction majeure. Cependant, dans ces cas les progrès sont lents et très peu quantifiables: dans notre série de 76 patients, un tiers a reçu des anti-coagulants et anti-agrégants isolément; les pourcentages d'amélioration, d'aggravation et de stabilisation y sont égaux et identiques au groupe témoin (aussi bien pour l'acuité visuelle que sur les angiographies).
2. *Les indications de la photocoagulation* se déterminent par rapport aux deux facteurs essentiels du pronostic:
— le siège de l'obstruction par rapport au drainage maculaire,
— et dans l'évolution ultérieure, le développement des néo-vaisseaux,

2.1 Le siège de la lésion:

L'évolution spontanée a mis en évidence d'une manière absolue la différence de pronostic visuel selon qu'il y ait ou non atteinte des veinules de drainage

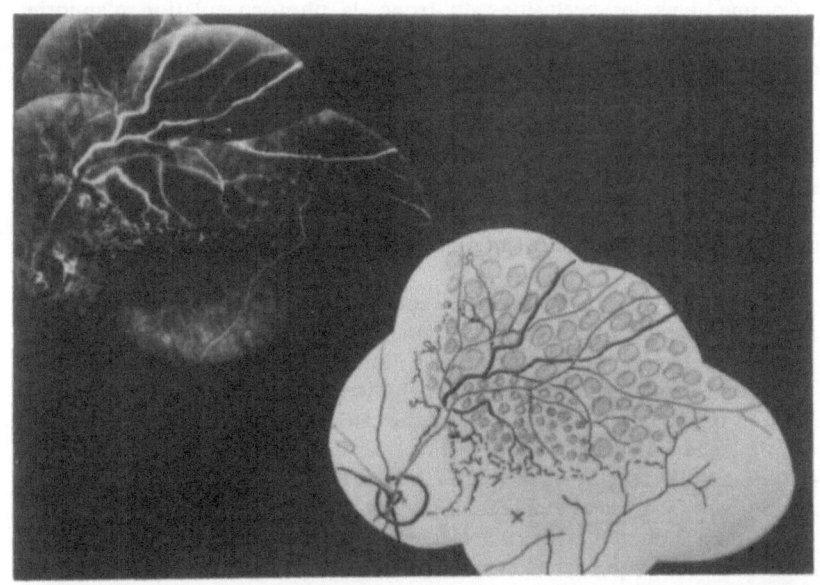

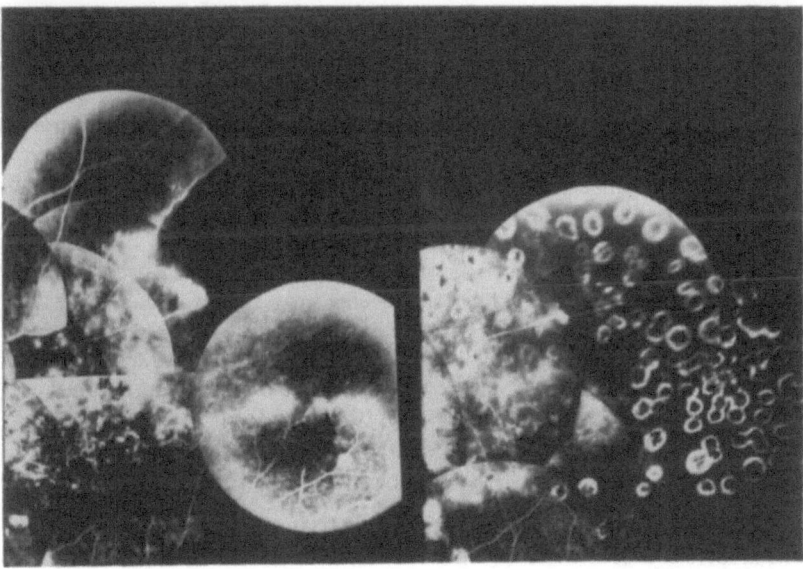

de la région maculaire, quel que soit le site exact de l'obstruction: la disposition anatomique est évidemment pré-existante et ne peut être modifiée par aucune thérapeutique.

Le pronostic visuel reste bon, dans l'evolution spontanée, toutes les fois que le réseau capillaire périvoféolaire est respecté, sauf dans les cas d'aggravation secondaire du degré d'obstruction avec extension des lésions vers la fovéola.

Comme dans les occlusions du tronc, la photocoagulation n'apporte guère de progrès dans la dégénérescence cystoïde du tissu rétinien secondaire à un oedème trainant.

Toutefois, à un stade précoce, elle peut être utile: il est devenu indispensable d'opposer les lésions avec *exclusion spontanée* du lit capillaire rétinien, sans oedéme et les formes comportant une *dilatation majeure* des capillaires avec diffusions, oedème et baisse rapide de l'acuité:
— la photocoagulation devrait détruire tous les capillaires pathologiques qui laissent diffuser le colorant — jusqu'à l'arcade anastomotique si nécessaire.
— La photocoagulation doit détruire tout le secteur exclu car hypoxique et ischémique, depuis le site de l'occlusion jusqu'à la périphérie, à la manière d'une photocoagulation pan-rétinienne, limitée au secteur malade (Fig. 1).
— Elle doit cependant respecter la circulation de suppléance qui entoure ce secteur et qui va se modifier et se simplifier au cours de l'évolution.
— Enfin, elle ne sera pas trop précoce, car elle est dangereuse et souvent douloureuse. Il est nécessaire d'attendre les 8 à 12 semaines utiles à la résorption des hémorragies et à l'établissement des suppléances.

En tenant compte de tous ces éléments, dans notre série, la dégradation visuelle a été identique dans les cas traités ou non traités.

2.2 Le développement des néo-vaisseaux:

L'étude angiographique de l'évolution spontanée tardive montre, dans un certain nombre de cas, l'apparition de néo-vaisseaux et de formations télangiectasiques ₁plus ou moins volumineuses et qui font courir un grand risque d'hémorragies récidivantes dans le vitré.

Elles laissent diffuser très abondamment la fluorescéine même s'il est assez fréquent qu'elles soient perfusées assez lentement par le colorant.

En voici quelques exemples (Fig. 2).

La photocoagulation sectorielle, associant les applications pan-rétiniennes sur tout un secteur et les applications locales sur les néo-vaisseaux et les télangiectasies, est indispensable dans ces cas: elle diminue de manière considérable le risque d'hémorragies récidivantes du vitré et améliore ainsi nettement le pronostic éloigné des occlusions de branches veineuses rétiniennes (2/10 cas d'hémorragies dans le lot traité contre 6/10 dans le lot témoin avec recul de 1 à 4 ans).

CONCLUSION

La photocoagulation des occlusions veineuses trouve ses indications majeures dans la lutte contre le développement des néo-vaisseaux — non pas tant dans les occlusions du tronc et le glaucome néo-vasculaire, que pour les séquelles néo-vasculaires tardives des occlusions de branches veineuses avec risque hémorragique. Les autres traitements médicaux n'ont pas fait la preuve de leur efficacité.

Adresse de l'auteur:
Service d'Ophtalmologie de Créteil
Université de Paris-Val de Marne
40 Avenue de Verdun
94010 Créteil, France

MACULOPATHY AND VISUAL PROGNOSIS
IN RETINAL VEIN OCCLUSION

J.A. OOSTERHUIS, S.C. SEDNEY & H.S. WIJNANDS

(Leyden, The Netherlands)

Slowing down of the bloodstream in retinal vein occlusion leads to ischaemia of the retinal tissue, ischaemia causes retinal oedema which in turn causes a decrease of visual acuity.

Occlusion of small branches of the retinal vein causes only a slight oedema of part of the macula, which is consistent with maintaining a fair or even good visual acuity. Occlusion of large branch veins causes a more marked macular oedema, spreading over most or all of the macular area; visual acuity is diminished and may even be poor. In occlusion of the central retinal vein a very intense macular oedema is always present all over the macular area and visual acuity is always poor, less than 0.1. Thus, there is a close correlation between intensity of the macular oedema and the loss of central vision. Therefore, restoration of visual acuity after regression of the macular oedema is good when secondary macular lesions have not developed, whereas the prognosis of visual acuity is moderate to poor when macular oedema has led to secondary macular lesions such as cystoid macular oedema, pigmentepithelial dystrophy, macular fibrosis and circinate exudates. This is clear from our results, summarized in Table I and Table II.

It appears that the first sign of degeneration, being a cystoid macular oedema, is not as harmless in retinal vein occlusion as it is for instance in the Irvine-Gass syndrome. After regression of the macular oedema following

Table I

Cystoid macular oedema and pigment-epithelial dystrophy
before and after photocoagulation in branch vein occlusion

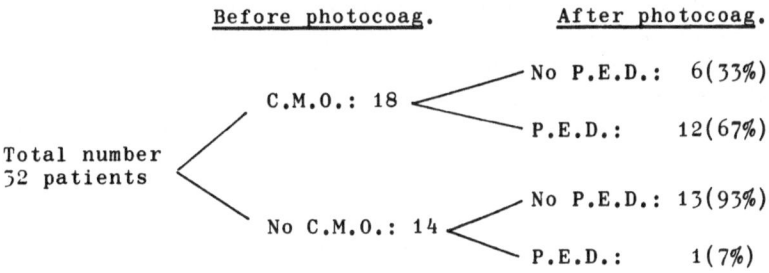

(C.M.O.: cyst.mac.oedema;   P.E.D.: pigment-epith.dystrophy)

Table II

Number of patients	Macular condition		Average VA	
	Before treatment	End follow-up	Before treatm.	End follow-up
13	Macular oedema	No mac.oedema	0.18	0.71
6	Cyst.mac.oedema	No mac.oedema	0.24	0.47
12	Cyst.mac.oedema	Pigm.epith.dystr.	0.16	0.34
31				

In 1 patient the cystoid structure persisted.

photocoagulation treatment pigment-epithelial dystrophy developed in 12 (67%) out of 18 patients with cystoid macular oedema, but in only 1 (7%) out of 14 patients with macular oedema without a cystoid structure (Table I). The relation between macular degeneration and final visual outcome is shown in Table II. In 13 patients with macular oedema only, which cleared without damage to the macular area, the average visual acuity improved from 0.18 prior to photocoagulation to 0.71 at the end of the control period. In 6 patients who showed cystoid macular oedema, which cleared without ophthalmoscopically visible signs of macular damage, the visual acuity improved from 0.24 to 0.47. In the 12 patients in whom the cystoid macular oedema eventually induced the development of pigment-epithelial dystrophy the average visual acuity rose from 0.16 to only 0.34. From these results we may conclude that it is of utmost importance for the visual prognosis that macular oedema regresses before a cystoid structure in the macular area has developed, which may easily lead to a pigmentary degeneration in the macular area.

There is a distinct time-intensity relationship, as shown in Fig. 1. All 13 patients with central retinal vein occlusion showed an extremely intensive macular oedema and already a distinct cystoid macular structure at the first examination; all patients developed pigmentepithelial dystrophy later on, in part of them associated with a fibrotic macular scar. On the other hand, a slight oedema may exist for many months or even longer without inducing signs of secondary degenerations; after collateral circulation has developed and macular oedema has regressed macular function may be restored spontaneously and photocoagulation is not indicated in these cases. Therefore, criteria for photocoagulation should depend on:
1. intensity of the macular oedema as indicated by the decrease of visual acuity;
2. duration of the macular oedema which is related to the intensity of the macular oedema, as has been shown in Fig. 1;
3. presence of signs of secondary degeneration, cystoid macular oedema being the first to appear; the easiest and most reliable method of assessing the presence of cystoid macular oedema is with the aid of the slitlamp and fundus contactlens.

The favourable results of photocoagulation treatment are shown in Table III (SEDNEY, 1976). The difference between 84.4% improvement in the 32 photocoagulation-treated eyes and the 26% and 52% improvement in the anticoagulant-treated and non-treated patients, respectively, is statistically significant. As decrease of visual acuity is related to the development of macular oedema and as photocoagulation generally rapidly leads to a regression of macular oedema, the favourable results of photocoagulation are to be attributed to the favourable effect on the macular area, as in these patients macular oedema regressed before it had induced the development of secondary macular degeneration.

Thus, we should closely follow the condition of the macular area so as, on the one hand, not to let the favourable period for performing photocoa-

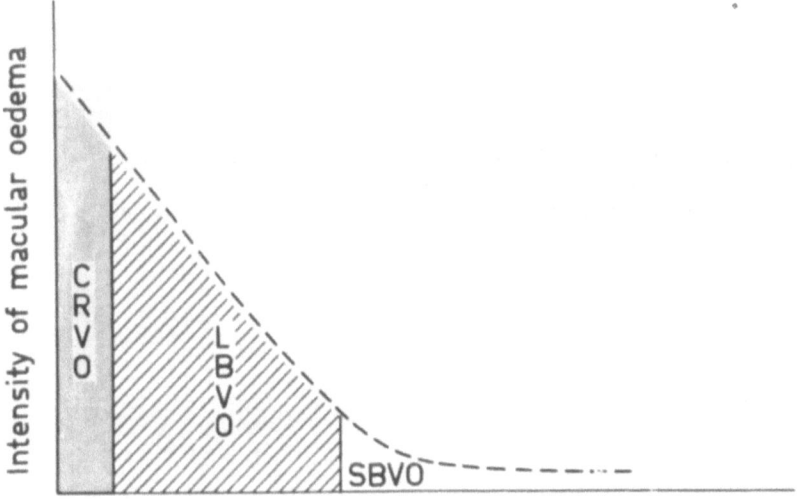

Duration of oedema

– – – – – Development of cystoid macular oedema

Fig. 1. CRVO = central retinal vein occlusion; LBVO = large branch vein occlusion; SBVO = small branch vein occlusion.

Table III

Comparison of results in three groups of patients with branch vein occlusion

	Number of eyes	Improved	Unchanged	Deteriorated
Without treatment	25	13(52%)	8(32%)	4(16%)
Anticoagulant treatm.	19	5(26%)	7(37%)	7(37%)
Photocoag. treatment	32	27(84.4%)	4(12.5%)	1(3.1%)

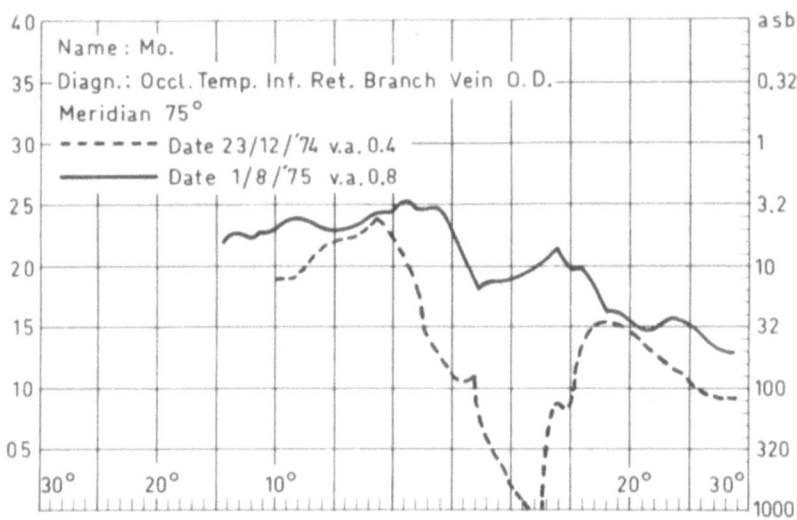

Fig. 2. Static perimetry curves in a patient with retinal branch vein occlusion.
- - - - - : at the first examination
———— : 7 months later after spontaneous almost complete regression of the fundus lesions

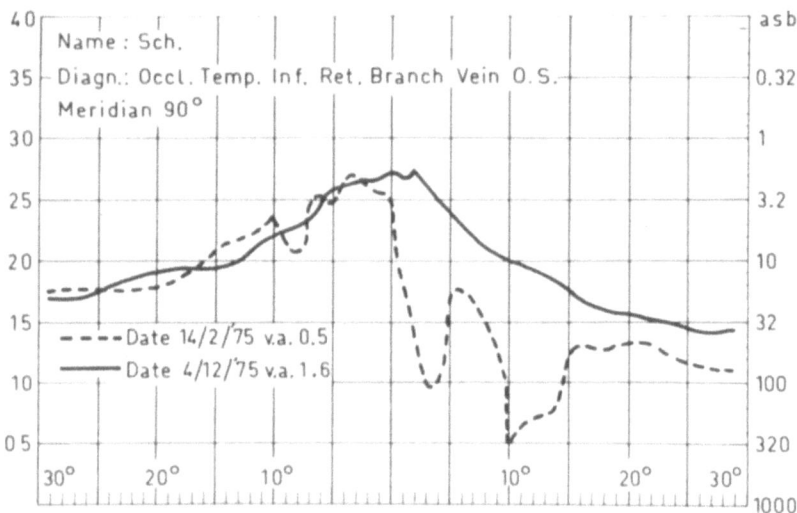

Fig. 3. Static perimetry curves in a patient with retinal branch vein occlusion.
- - - - - : at the first examination
———— : 9 months later after spontaneous almost complete regression of the lesions

gulation pass and, on the other hand, not to perform photocoagulation unnecessarily.

Apart from the visual acuity being indicative of the condition of the posterior pole, quantitative perimetry by means of the Tübinger perimeter gives an exact registration of the loss of light sensitivity of the whole macular area. Figs. 2 and 3 show the curves of quantitative perimetry in 2 patients. In view of the gradual improvement of macular function, for which the quantitative perimetry was a better parameter than the visual acuity and the macular oedema on the fluorogram, no photocoagulation was performed.

Finally, there is a relation between macular oedema and capillary non-perfusion, as both are related to ischaemia. However, areas of non-perfusion in the macular region may be associated with a fair visual acuity, two examples being given in Fig. 4 and 5 with visual acuity of 0.8 and 0.6, respectively. As both fluorograms show, macular oedema is absent. There-

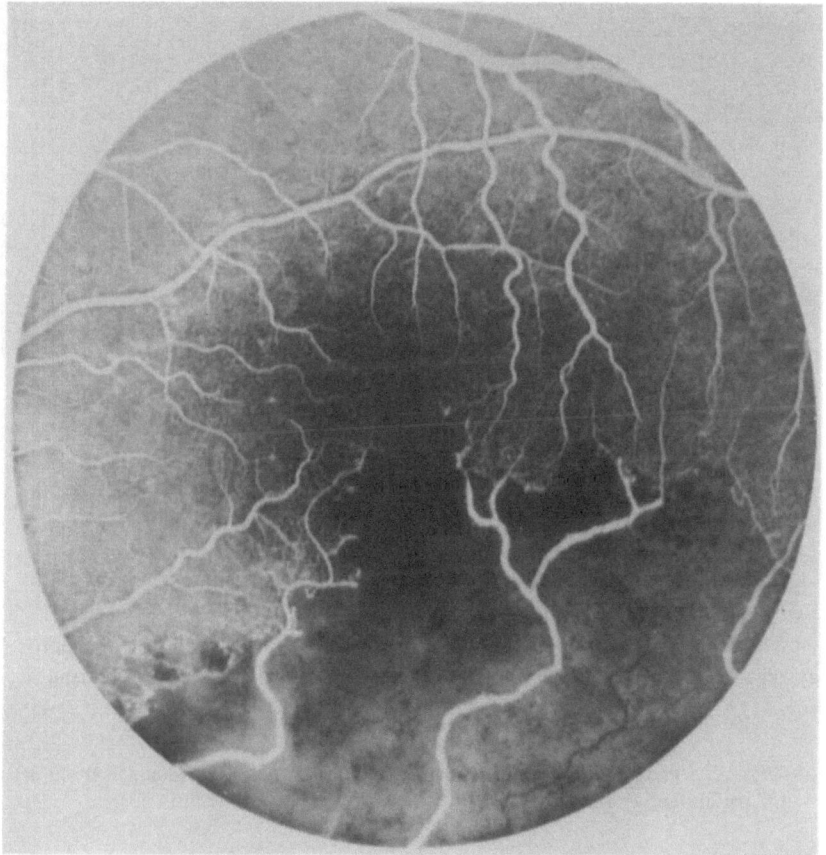

Fig. 4. Retinal branch vein occlusion with considerable arteriolar occlusive component. Large areas of non-perfusion are anoxic, as macular oedema is absent visual acuity is still 0.6.

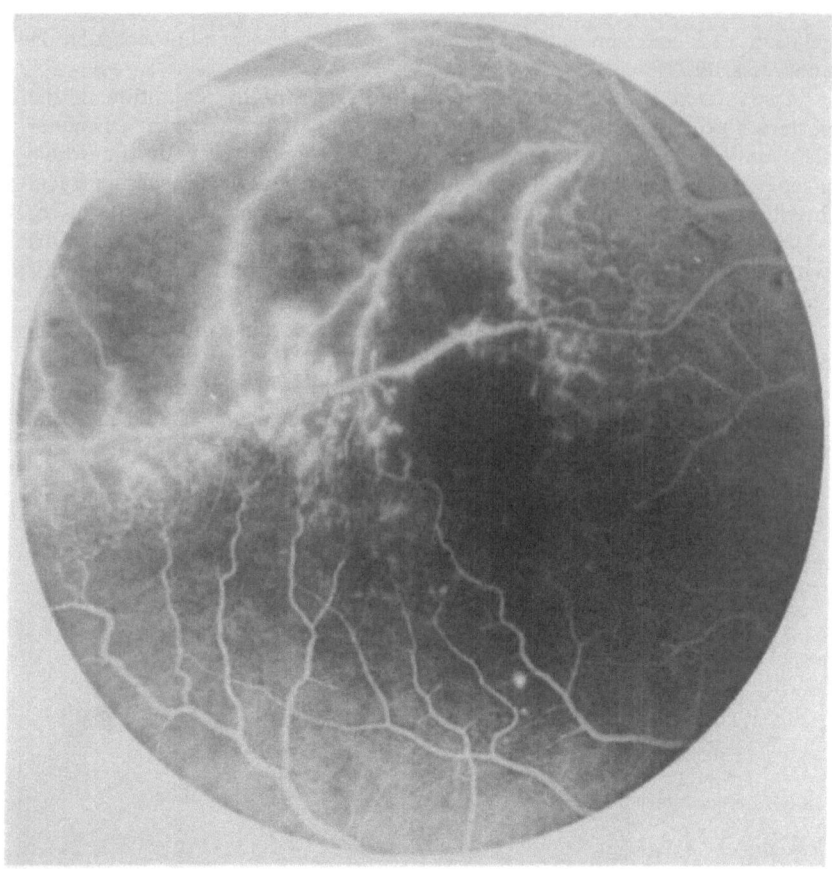

Fig. 5. Retinal branch vein occlusion. As the areas of non-perfusion are anoxic, they do not induce macular oedema and thus visual acuity is still 0.8.

fore, loss of vision is more related to macular oedema and the ensuing secondary degenerations than to capillary non-perfusion in the macular area, as in this region the metabolism of the retina is mainly served by the choroidal circulation and not by the retinal circulation, which in this area has only one layer of capillaries.

Thus, we may conclude that macular oedema is the all important factor as regards visual prognosis and indication for photocoagulation treatment.

REFERENCE

SEDNEY, S.C. Photocoagulation in retinal vein occlusion. Thesis, Leiden. Dr. W. Junk B.V. Publishers, The Hague (1976).

Authors' adress:
Oogheelkundige Kliniek
Academisch Ziekenhuis
Leyden, The Netherlands

A COMPARATIVE STUDY OF TREATED AND NON–TREATED CASES OF CENTRAL RETINAL VEIN OCCLUSION

GEORGE THEODOSSIADIS

(Athens, Greece)

Light coagulation has hitherto been used for the treatment of central retinal vein occlusion (ZWENG et al. 1974, WETZIG & THATCHER 1974, THEO-DOSSIADIS et al. 1974), although the etiology and natural course of the disease remain unknown. In order to investigate the efficacy of light coagulation in central retinal vein occlusion, two groups of patients were used. The first group of 25 eyes was subjected to light coagulation with xenon arc (Zeiss/Oberkochen) and argon laser (Optics Technology), while the 18 eyes of the second group served as controls. This latter group consisted mainly of patients who had refused the proposed treatment and had therefore been treated with anticoagulants (CLEMENTS et al. 1968, DUFF et al. 1951). The follow-up of our cases varied from one to six years. At the first examination all patients a) were 52-75 years of age, b) presented the hemorrhagic retinopathy type with venous distension, hemorrhages distributed throughout the area of affected venous drainage and swelling of the optic disc, c) had visual acuity at the first examination varying between light perception and 20/400, d) had delayed fluorescein appearance in the main retinal vessels (16″ and more), and e) showed oedema of the macula or/and hemorrhage. The onset had occurred 6-70 days before. Diabetics and patients with chronic simple glaucoma in the affected eye were excluded. Most of the patients of both groups had hypertension and their retinal arteries showed alterations. During the first and the follow-up examinations all patients were subjected to routine check-up, which included the taking of color photographs, fluorescein angiography, ERG and, wherever possible, examination of the visual field and color perception. The follow-up consisted of monthly examinations for half a year after the onset and subsequently every three months until the 18th month. Some of the patients were followed up beyond the 18th month, once a year.

LIGHT COAGULATION TECHNIQUE

This involved three sessions. During the first session light coagulation was applied along the upper and lower temporal vein and their branches. The other two sessions followed in fortnightly intervals and covered the remaining retinal veins.

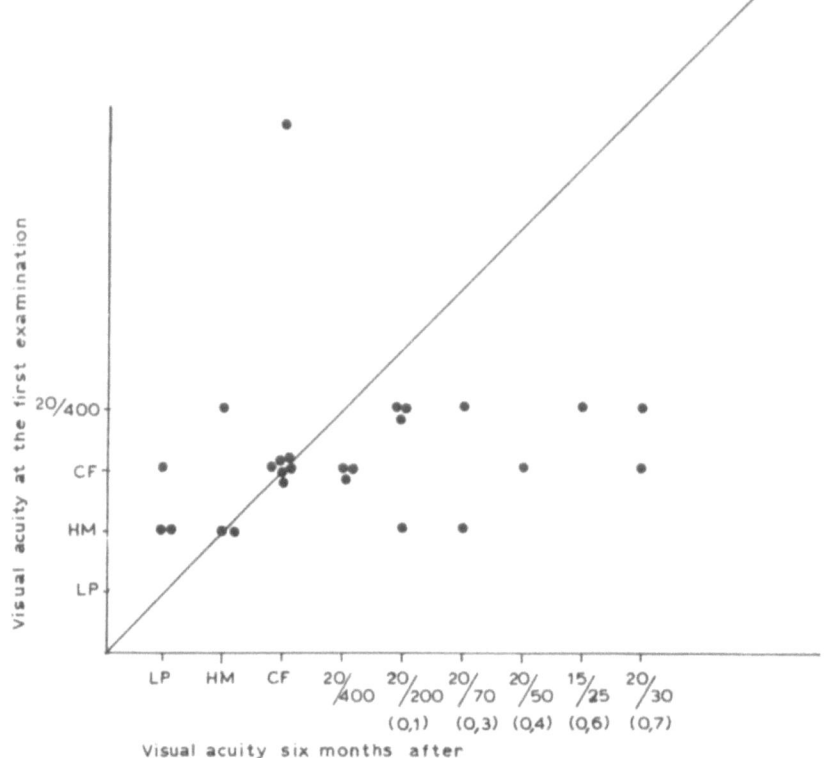

Fig. 1. Group with light-coagulation (Argon Laser or Xenon Arc)

RESULTS

I) Visual acuity

Visual acuity acquired after 6 months following treatment in the light-coagulated group and after 12 months in the control group is set forth in Figs 1 and 2. From these it will be seen that a) in the light-coagulated group visual acuity improved in 14 out of 25 patients, deteriorated in 5 and remained unchanged in 6, and that b) in the control-group, out of 18 patients 4 showed improvement, 9 deterioration and 5 no change in visual acuity.

II) Condition of retinal vessels, especially of the veins

a) *Light-coagulated group* (3 months to 1 year after): 23 out of the 25 patients showed a notable lessening of vein calibre and vein engorgement with a consequent diminution of the retinal oedema and of hemorrhages, especially at the posterior pole of the eye fundus. New vascular formation at the optic head nerve or in the macular area was observed in 4 out of the 25 patients.

166

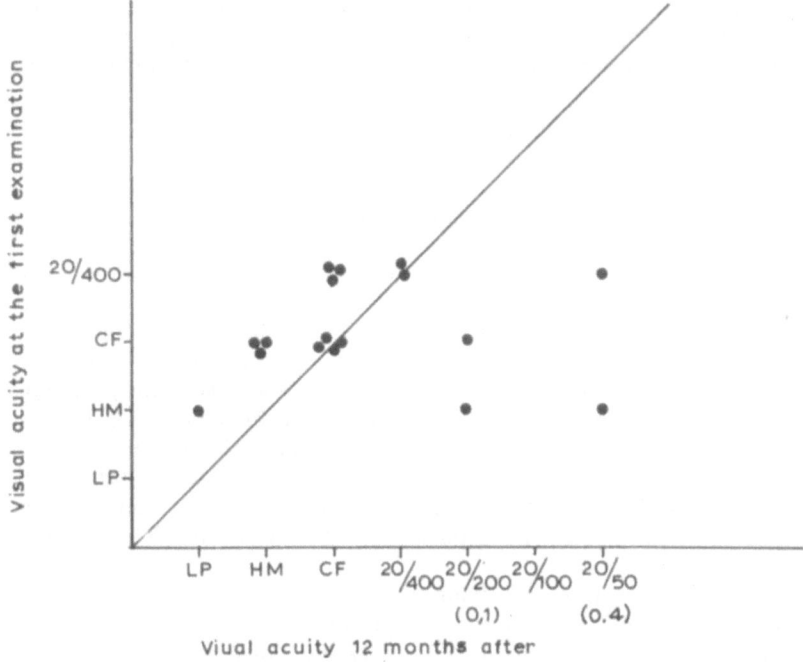

Fig.2. Control group

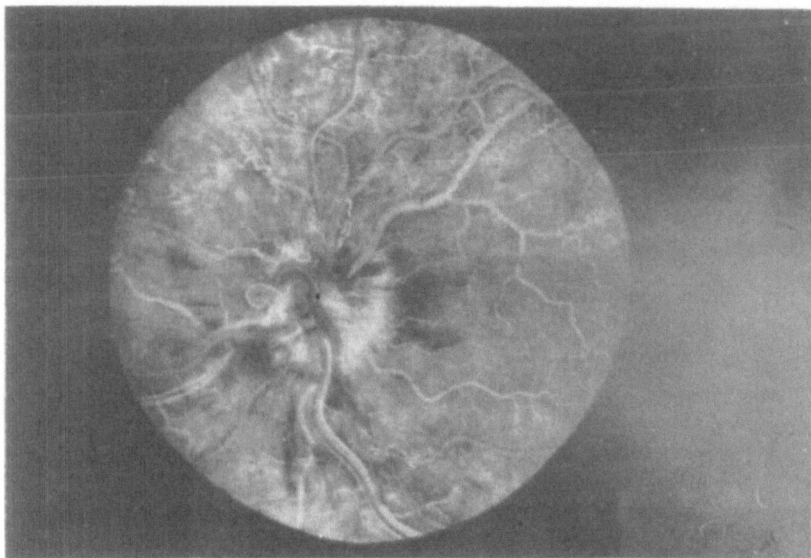

Fig. 3. Control-group patient, 1 year after: Poor fluorescein circulation, neovascularisation and sinuous course of the veins.

167

b) After three months the *control patients* did not show any change in the clinical picture of the fundus. After one year their picture varied, presenting mainly: vascular obstructions of varying degree, poor fluorescein circulation (HILL & GRIFFITHS 1970), sheathing of the veins, neovascularisation, decrease of the vein calibre but continuing sinuous course of the veins (Fig. 3) (OOSTERHUIS 1968).

III) Time of fluorescein appearance

a) *Light-coagulated group* (3 months to 1 year after): In this group the time of dye appearance in the vessels of the optic head nerve showed a marked improvement in 22 out of the 25 cases, compared to conditions before light coagulation. Besides in most cases a restoration of retinal circulation was noted, which coexisted, however, with a leakage at the posterior pole. In some cases there was a delay of fluorescein circulation. The fluorescein picture remained virtually the same after the lapse of one year.

22 out of the 25 patients presented one year after light coagulation varying degrees of degenerative changes in the macula, such as alterations of pigment epithelium, pigment deposits, macroaneurism formation, slight oedema (Fig. 4).

b) *Control group*: Wherever fluorescein angiography was feasible, the results after 3 moths to 1 year varied. Stagnant circulation continued, while new vascular formations with a leakage of dye were observed. In some cases retinal blood circulation was restored, even where the function of the eye was lost (Fig. 5).

IV) Occurrence of hemorrhagic glaucoma

a) *Light coagulated group*: None of the patients of this group showed hemorrhagic glaucoma during the entire follow-up period.

b) *Control group*: 3 out of the 18 patients suffered hemorrhagic glaucoma 57-110 days after the onset of the disease.

Secondary criteria such as color perception and ERG (1 year after): The 100 hue test for color perception revealed in the patients of both groups having a visual acuity of 20/400 or more mainly yellow defects and a displacement towards red. The extent of the color vision defect was related to the decline of visual acuity. The ERG-curve during the onset was linear, whereas after 6 months and beyond, the curve reappeared in the patients of both groups with visual acuity of 20/400 and more, but was lower than normal.

DISCUSSION

Improved visual acuity was established in a comparatively greater number of patients treated with light coagulation, although this improvement was statistically not significant. Wherever an amelioration of visual acuity was achieved, this became manifest after the third session, the best results being observed about 6-8 months after light coagulation. In the control group,

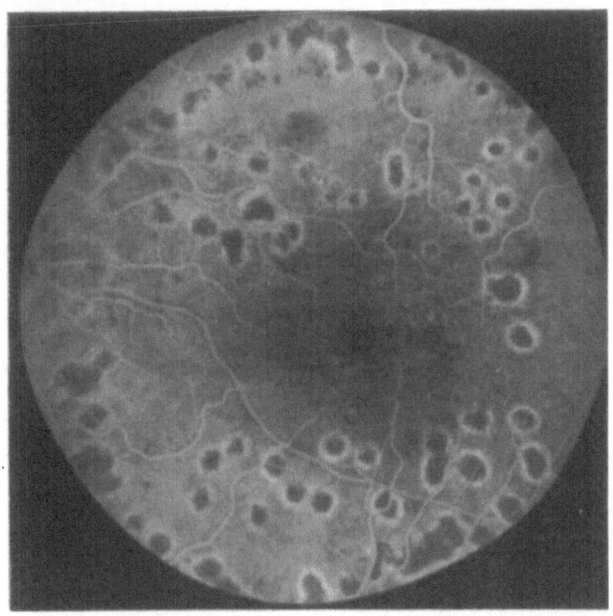

Fig. 4. Patient of light-coagulated group, 6 months after: Alterations of pigment epithelium, microaneurism and slight macular oedema.

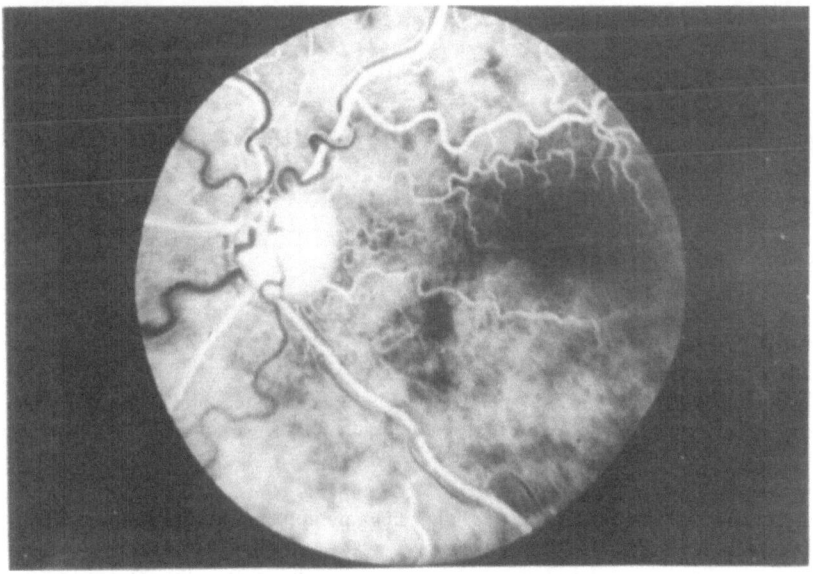

Fig. 5. Control-group patient, 1 year after: Retinal blood circulation restored, but atrophy of the optic nerve head is evident. There is no light perception.

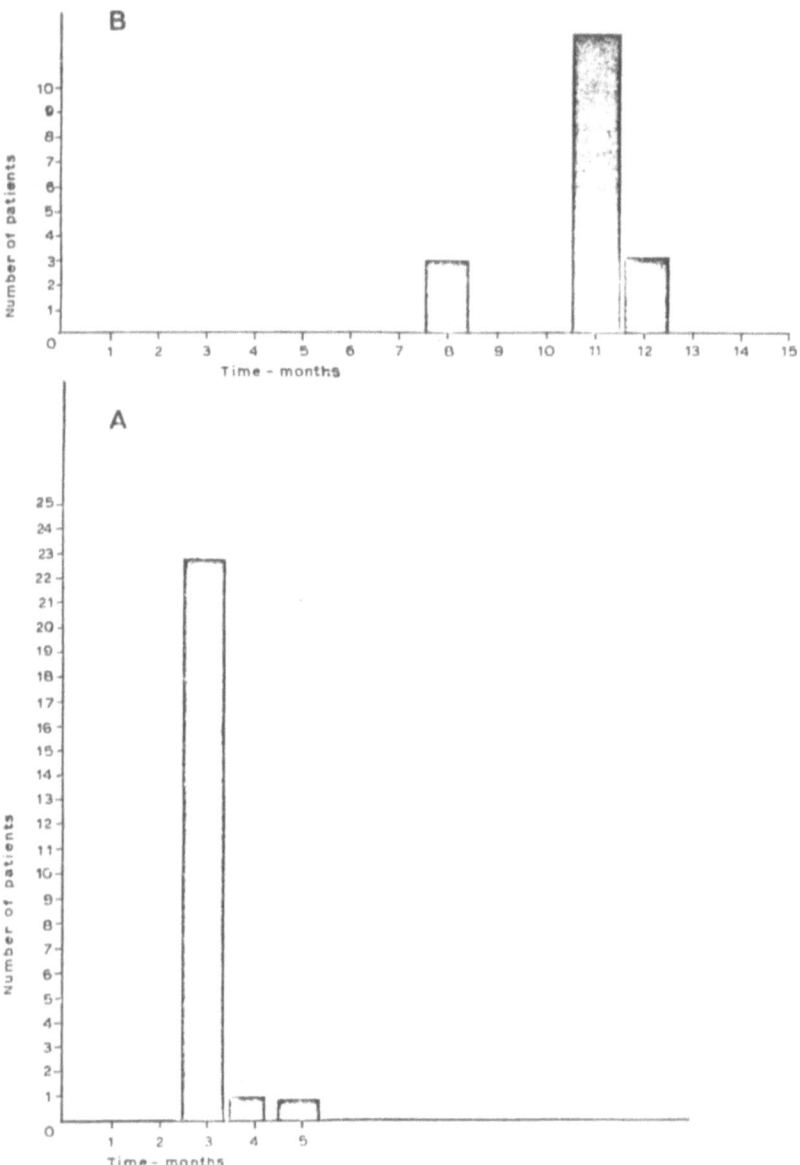

Fig. 6. Lessening or absorption of the retinal oedema (diminution of vein calibre and vein engorgement). A. With Argon Laser light-coagulation. B. Without light-coagulation.

wherever an improvement ensued, this became apparent approximately one year after the onset.

In the light coagulated group the visual acuity eventually attained was dependent on: 1) The time lapse between onset and treatment, the best results being achieved upon relatively early treatment, 2) The presence of

170

extensive hemorrhage or blood clots in the macular area at the time of treatment, and 3) The presence of cystoid degeneration in the macular area at the time of treatment. In instances 2) and 3) visual acuity did not improve.

In the treated group there was a pronounced regression of the retinal oedema, especially at the posterior pole, about 3 months after light coagulation. This was accompanied by a decongestion of the retinal blood circulation, i.e. a diminution of the calibre of the retinal vein and a lessening of its engorgement. On the other hand, where decongestion was obtained in the control group patients, this became apparent after 8 months and later. Fig. 6 demonstrates graphically that treatment shortened the duration of retinal oedema, while lessening the engorgement of the retinal veins and their calibre in a statistically significant proportion ($p > 00.1$).

Quite generally the application of light coagulation did not prevent the occurrence of alterations of the macula, which were noted in 22 of the 25 patients. These alterations varied as to their gravity and became more marked with fluorescein angiography. It would appear that light coagulation prevents the occurrence of hemorrhagic glaucoma in cases of central retinal vein occlusion, since this complication was not encountered in any of the light-coagulated patients. This circumstance might be attributed to the fact that the destruction of hypoxic areas of the retina by means of light coagulation eliminates hypoxic factors which would otherwise stimulate new vascular formation (ZWENG, WISE, ASHTON).

Late complications occurred in both groups. In the light coagulation group 4 out of 25 patients showed macular oedema after 2, resp. 3 years and neovascularisation, which were managed with further light coagulation. Among those control group patients who did not develop hemorrhagic glaucoma, 3 out of the 14 patients suffered a hemorrhage of the vitreous or the retina due to neovascularisation. Paleness of the optic nerve head was observed in some cases of both groups.

CONCLUSION

Visual acuity

In the light coagulation group an improvement of visual acuity was noted in a greater number of cases, although this improvement was statistically not significant.

Vascular condition

After light coagulation there was a pronounced recession of retinal oedema accompanied by a lessening of the calibre of the retinal vein and of the engorgement. In the control group patients these results occurred in fewer cases and relatively much later.

Macula

Light coagulation did not prevent various degrees of degenerative macular changes in the majority of cases.

No case of this was recorded in the light coagulation group. On the contrary, there were 3 cases of hemorrhagic glaucoma among the 18 patients of the control group.

REFERENCES

ASHTON, N. Neovascularisation in ocular disease. *Trans. Ophthal. Soc. U.K.* 81: *145-161* (1962).

CLEMENTS, D.B. et al. Retinal vein occlusion. A comparative study of factors affecting the prognosis, including a therapeutic trial of Atromid S in this condition. *Brit. J. Ophthal.* 52: *111-116* (1968).

DUFF, I.F. et al. Anticoagulant therapy in occlusive vascular disease of the retina. *Arch. Ophthal.* 46: *601-617* (1951).

HILL, D.W. & GRIFFITHS, J.D. The prognosis of retinal vein thrombosis. *Trans. Ophthal. Soc. U.K.* 90: *309-322* (1970).

MICHAELSON, I.C. Retinal circulation in man and animals (Thomas, Springfield, 1954).

OOSTERHUIS, J.A. Fluorescein fundus photography in retinal vein occlusion. In: Henkes, Perspectives in Ophthalmology. (Excerpta Medica, Amsterdam, 1968).

THEODOSSIADIS, G. et al. Behandlungsergebnisse der Lichtkoagulation bei Ast-und Zentralvenenverschluss. *Klin. Mbl. Augenheilk.* 164: *713-721* (1974).

WETZIG, P.C. & THATCHER, D.B. The treatment of acute and chronic central venous occlusion b; light coagulation. In: Limitations and Prospects for Retinal Surgery. *Mod. Probl. Ophthal.* 12: *247-253* (Karger, Basle, 1974).

ZWENG, H.Ch. et al. Argon laser photocoagulation in the treatment of retinal vein occlusin. In: Limitations and Prospects for Retinal Surgery. *Mod. Probl. Ophthal.* 12: *261-270* (Karger, Basle, 1974).

Author's address:
54 Omirou Street
Athens 135r-
Greece

SURGERY FOR VASCULAR OBSTRUCTIONS
OF THE RETINA (POSADA'S TECHNIQUE)

C.F. BARSANTE, H. ROCHA & P. GALVAO

(Belo Horizonte, Brazil)

A.F. ASPECTS

The aim of the technique presented by VASCO POSADA at the Chilean Congress of Ophthalmology in 1968 was to promote revascularization in cases of vascular obstruction in the posterior segment of the eye. Therefore, the posterior scleral ring and canal, probably the site of possible obstruction of the vascular trunk, is incised.

In 1969, one of us performed Posada's technique in a case of posttraumatic arterial obstruction and followed the recanalisation with fluorescein angiography. The marked revascularisation 24 hours after surgery justified the use of this technique for other cases of vascular obstructions, arterial as well as venous. We have treated 35 cases.

The technical details, our results and comments on the operation will be presented at the fifth European Congress of Ophthalmology (Hamburg).

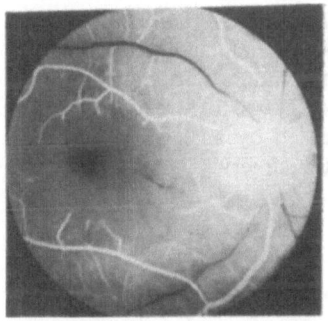
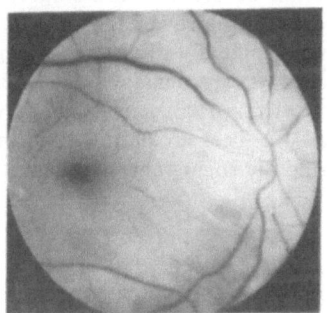
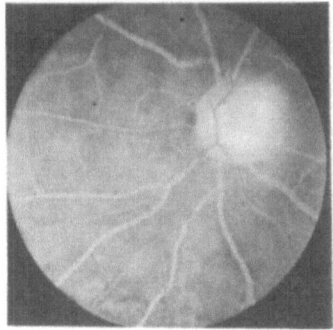

Fig. 1. Occlusion of the central retinal artery.
A. REC system.
B. Arterial phase.
C. Venous granulous stream.

Our purpose here is to discuss the fluoroangiographic aspects before and after the operation.

In cases of prethrombosis of the central retinal vein, with reasonable good visual acuity, the circulation is more rapidly normalized after surgery. The veins become significantly narrower, the retinal edema and the hemorrhages are more rapidly reabsorped and the circulation through the veins becomes easier. It is interesting to note that reabsorption of hemorrhages takes longer than reabsorption of retinal edema.

Patients with a recent complete obstruction of the central retinal vein or with a prethrombosis evoluating to thrombosis, recuperate more rapidly after surgery than patients with an older thrombosis, which is quite logical.

In case of obstruction of the central retinal artery, we can better visualize the radiated epipapillar capillaries (REC-Shimizu), because the peripapillary system (RPC) is also occluded (Fig. 1). The retinal edema is extensive, mainly in the posterior pole (cherry-red spot) (Fig. 2). 24 hours after surgery the edema is reduced and the arterial circulation is perfectly seen. The venous circulation normalises. A macular branch of the inferior temporal artery remains spastic for some days. A few months later an optic atrophy is noticed.

In central retinal vein obstruction, control fluoroangiographies 24 to 48 hours after surgery demonstrate clearly an increase in rate of flow in the vein. The diameter of the veins quickly diminishes in many cases; the papilledema progressively lessens as well as the retinal edema and the hemorrhages.

As an example we documented a case (Fig. 3). It gives evidence of the venous obstruction before Posada's surgery was performed. 48 hours after surgery, the veins are narrower (Fig. 3 C). 30 days later the hemorrhages and edema have completely disappeared (Fig. 4). The radiated peripapillary capillary network is very marked and presents shunts and obstructions (Fig. 5, arrows). The visual acuity which was 20/400 before operations, improved to 20/40. The circulation time increased by an average of 8 to 10 see, comparing the angiograms before and after surgery.

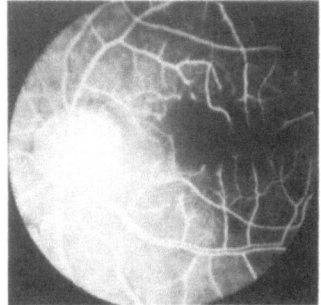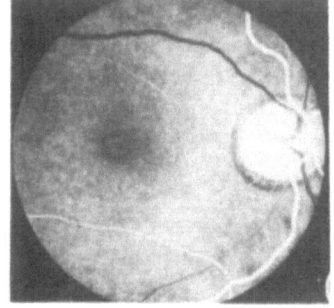

Fig. 2. A. Same case 48 hs after the surgery, with arterial branch spasm.
B. Optic atrophy and macular degeneration 3 months after the surgery.

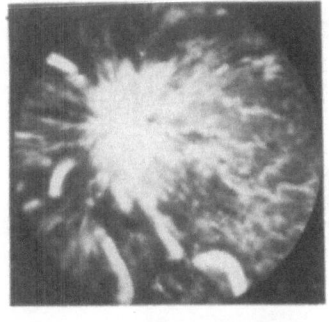
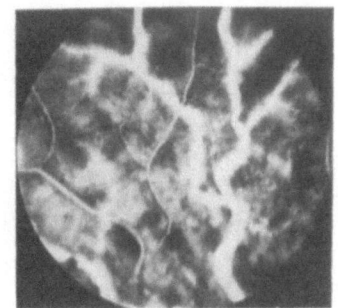

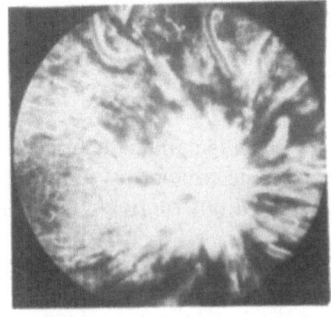

Fig. 3. Occlusion of the central retinal vein.
A. and B. Before the surgery.
C. 48 hs after the operation.

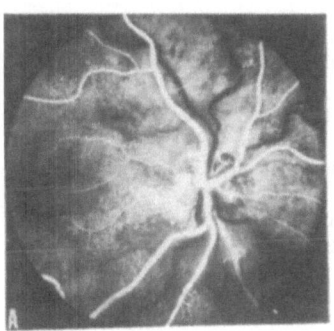
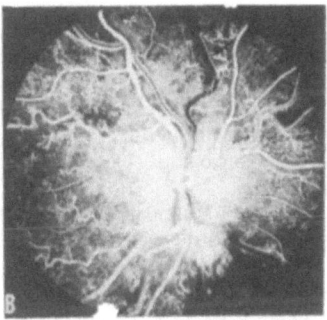

Fig. 4. A. and B. Same case after 3 months.

Recently we have been operating on patients with diabetic retinopathy, with marked venous congestion and pronounced edema. All five cases treated with this technique showed an unquestionable improvement. This allowed xenon arc or argon laser coagulation in the following days. The follow-up is still too short but the first results look very promising.

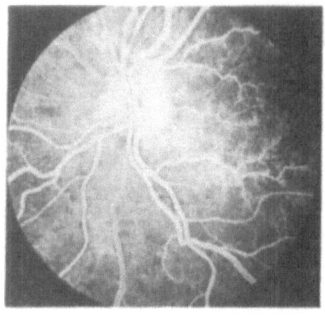 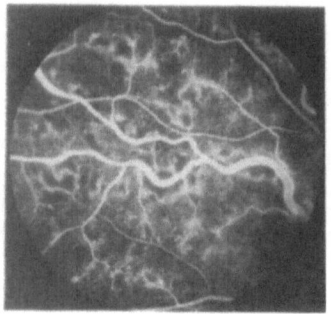

Fig. 5.   A. and B.   Same case after 6 months.

CONCLUSION

Fluoroangiographies of patients operated on by Posada's technique demonstrate in most cases and unequivocal improvement of the circulatory status 24 to 48 hours after surgery. This is primarily so in recent obstructions.

REFERENCES

BARSANTE, C., SOARES, E.F. & GALVAO, P.G. Obstrução da rêde capilar pré-vascular comprovada pela angiografia fluoresceínica em casos de trombose da veia central da retina. XVII Congresso Brasileiro de Oftalmologia I (abstract): *283* (1973).

GASS, J.D. M-A fluorescein angiographic study of macular dysfunction' secondary to retinal vascular disease. II. Retinal vein obstruction. *Arch. Ophthal.* 80: *550-568*ᐧ (1968).

ROCHA, H., GALVÃO, P., SOARES, E. & SOARES, E. Avanços Cirúrgicos em Oftalmologia. Livro Jubilar do Prof. Hilton Rocha – Pongetti (Rio) (1971).

SHIMIZU, K. Microangiografia Fluoresceínica del Fondo Ocular, JIMS' (Barcelona) (1975).

VASCO POSADA, J. Revascularizacion del Segmento Anterior e Posterior del Ojo. XXI Concilium Ophthal (México) 11: *1561-1569* (1970).

Authors' address:
Department of Ophthalmology
Medical School
Federal University of Minas Gerais
Belo Horizonte
Brazil

ANATOMICAL CORRELATION OF THE NORMAL
FLUOROANGIOGRAPHY OF THE FUNDUS

M. SPITZNAS

(Essen, Germany)

Before going into the discussion of the anatomical basis of typical fluorescein angiographic findings, some basic remarks have to be made. Tissues are
composed of cells and intercellular spaces. Passive movement of substances
across tissues is termed diffusion. Where diffusion is blocked, we talk about
a diffusion barrier. The structures allowing diffusion are called 'leaky' and
the ones impeding diffusion are termed 'tight'. Normally, cells are tight,
thus representing an obstacle to perfusion. An exception are the leaky pores
of fenestrated capillaries which are covered by portions of the cell membrane, while the cytoplasm is missing. The intercellular spaces are normally
leaky, i.e. they are open to diffusion. An exception are regions, where the
outer leaflets of neighbouring cells fuse, thus obstructing the intercellular
spaces. These tight structures are called 'zonulae occludentes'. The behaviour of fluorescein in the ocular tissues is determined by these simple laws
of diffusion and all fluorescein angiographic findings can be explained as an
interaction between diffusion and healthy or diseased anatomical structures.
In the following, I will therefore try to correlate angiographic facts to the
underlying morphology. Because of the shortage of space the illustrations of
the original presentation are not reproduced.

Fact no. 1:   Retinal vessels are tight to fluorescein

Explanation

The lumen of the vessels is entirely encompassed by the bodies and the
cytoplasmic prolongations of endothelial cells. Where two endothelial cells
meet, the intercellular space is occluded by zonulae occludentes.

Exception

Conditions which are accompanied by a transient or permanent disruption
of endothelial zonulae occludentes or by a loss of endothelial cells. This is
the case in inflammations or other disorders such as diabetic retinopathy,
Coats' disease, Eales' disease and/or neovascularization.

Fact no. 2: Choroidal vessels are leaky to fluorescein

Therefore the choroid stains diffusely during angiography.

177

Explanation

The lumen is encompassed by endothelial cells and their prolongations. Where two endothelial cells meet, the intercellular space is occluded by zonulae occludentes. However, the thin prolongations of the endothelial cells carry numerous pores, which allow the passage of some fluorescein.

Exception

Inflammations, which lead to a transient disruption of the zonulae occludentes, thus causing a focal increase of leakiness.

Fact no. 3: In spite of the leakiness of the choroidal capillaries choroidal fluorescence is barely seen

Explanation

Visualization of choroidal fluorescence is blocked by the melanin granules in the overlying retinal pigment epithelium.

Exception

Conditions with loss or lateral displacement of melanin. An example for a loss of pigment are the pigmentary defects of maculopathy or larger, so-called 'punched out', lesions with almost total loss of pigment. An example for the lateral displacement of pigment are Drusen of Bruch's membrane. They have a fenestration effect which allows better visualization of choroidal fluorescence.

Fact no.4: Bruch's membrane is leaky to fluorescein

Explanation

Bruch's membrane is a loose structure without cells and junctions. Only in perpendicular light microscopic sections Bruch's membrane appears as a solid structure. Electron microscopic pictures and flat sections reveal that it is in fact a loose meshwork. Therefore, breaks in Bruch's membrans, as they occure in angioid streaks, do not primarily increase the diffusion of fluorescein from the choroid toward the retina. However, they have a fenestration effect so that the choroidal fluorescence is seen better.

Fact no. 5: The pigment epithelium is tight to fluorescein

Explanation

The apical portions of the intercellular spaces are closed by zonulae occludentes. This is nicely demonstrated by perfusion studies with electron dense tracers such as peroxidase. Material entering the intercellular space from the choroid is stopped at the basal end of the zonulae occludentes, and

178

material approaching the intercellular space from the retinal side is stopped at the apical end of the zonulae occludentes so that the postzonular intercellular space remains free.

Exception

Disruption of one or more zonulae occludentes, as seen in central serous retinopathy. Through these disruptions fluorescein can now diffuse under the sensory retina, were it stains the subretinal accumulation of exudate present in such cases.

Fact no. 6: The margin of chorioretinal scars is leaky to fluorescein, while the center is tight

Explanation

In the chorioretinal scar, the retinal pigment epithelium is replaced by scar tissue which lacks zonulae occludentes. In the center of the scar, the choroidal capillaries are closed or missing. Therefore, there is no perfusion with and thus no leakage of fluorescein. At the margins, however, the choroidal capillaries are open. Here, fluorescein penetrates the capillary pores described above and diffuses freely through the intercellular spaces of the scar tissue toward the surface of the retina.

Fact no. 7: The sensory retina is leaky to fluorescein

Any dye leaving diseased retinal blood vessels spreads within the retina.

Explanation

The intercellular spaces of the sensory retina are not occluded by zonulae occludentes. This again can be shown microscopically by the diffusion of tracer material which has been injected into the vitreous cavity. After a few seconds all the intercellular spaces of the sensory retina are filled with electron dense tracer material.

Fact no. 8: Fluorescein does not usually form bullous accumulations under the retinal pigment epithelium

Explanation

The numerous basal infoldings of the retinal pigment epithelium are firmly bound to one another and to Bruch's membrane by so-called hemidesmosomes, which serve as attachment devices.

Exception

Pigment epithelial detachment. Here the close relationship between the pigment epithelium and Bruch's membrane shows a focal interruption,

179

resulting in an elevation of the pigment epithelium and an accumulation of dye under the pigment epithelium. This accumulation of dye is visible through the uninterrupted retinal pigment epithelium, indicating that the pigment has been displaced or lost.

When the retinal pigment epithelium cannot withstand the pressure from behind and ruptures, a picture identical to central serous retinopathy with a circumscribed leakage point is superimposed over the pigment epithelial detachment.

Fact no. 9: A number of disorders, namely presumed histoplasmosis, exudative senile maculopathy and Fuch's spot in high myopia are characterized by an accumulation of vessels under the sensory retina. These vessels leak fluorescein

Explanation

Such accumulations of vessels consist of displaced choroidal capillaries, which do not only retain the distribution pattern typical for the choriocapillaries. They also retain the choroidal capillary pores which leak fluorescein.

In conclusion, I hope that this short synopsis of the anatomical basis of some typical findings will help toward better understanding and safer interpretation of fluorescein angiography.

Author's address:
Universitàts-Augenklink
Hufelandstrasse 55
4300 Essen
B.R.D.

THE DEVELOPMENT OF THE CHOROIDAL VASCULAR SYSTEM

K. HEIMANN

(Cologne, Germany)

In the early years of this century VERSARI laid the foundations of research into the development of choroidal vascular system; he prepared the choroidal vessels by injecting Prussian blue. Other authors have since contributed to this field, notably FUCHS, DEDEKIND, SEEFELDER, BARBER and MANN. In current handbooks the chapters dealing with the development of the eye in man usually describe the development of choroidal vascular system as occurring in three phases during the first four months of gestation, corresponding to the three distinct layers of vessels in the adult choroid.

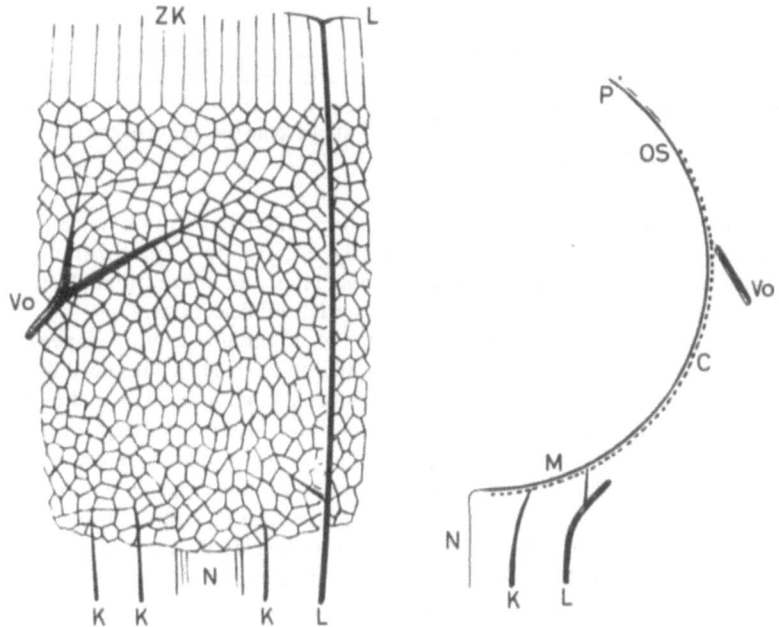

Fig. 1. Choroidal vasculature at the end of the 2nd month. K = Short posterior ciliary arteries; L = long posterior ciliary arteries; N = optic nerve; VO = vortex vein; Zk = level of what will become the ciliary body; M = region that will become the macular zone; C = choriocapillaris; OS = region that will become the region of the ora; P = pigment epithelium. (HEIMANN, 1972, 1974).

181

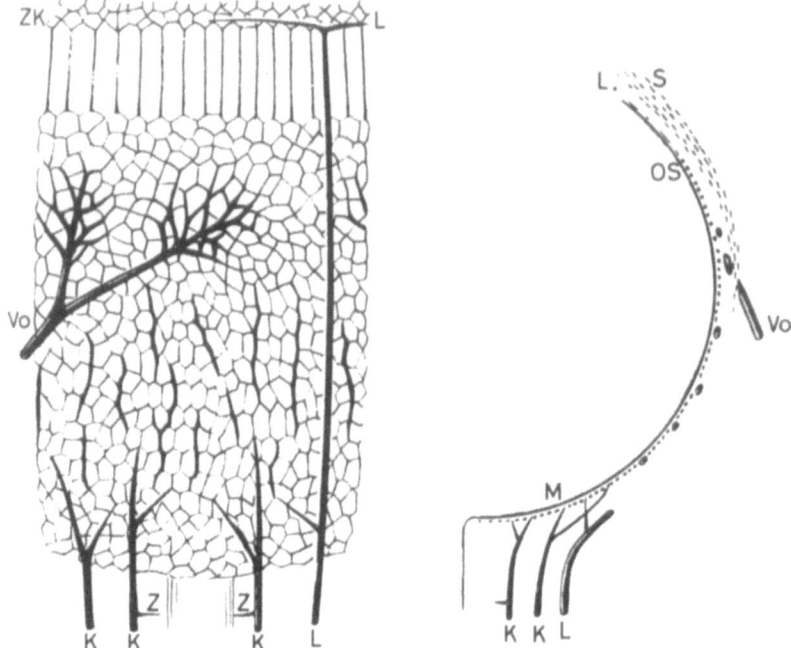

Fig. 2. Choroidal vasculature at the end of the 3rd month. K = Short posterior ciliary arteries; L = long posterior ciliary arteries; Z = initial stage of the formation of the circle of Haller-Zinn; Vo = vortex vein; Zk = level of the ciliary body" M = region that will become the macular zone; OS = region that will become the region of the ora; S = sclera. (HEIMANN, 1972, 1974).

We have studied the development of choroidal vasculature covering an age span from the end of the second month of gestation to parturition by means of injection of Indian ink and neoprene latex and conventional histology preparing sagittal but also flat and tangential serial sections.

Towards the end of the second month (Fig. 1) there is only one layer of vessels in the region of what will eventually be the choroid: a dense capillary meshwork, the primitive choriocapillaris. Several small arterial branches of the inner ophthalmic artery and the two long posterior ciliary arteries descend directly and perpendicularly into the posterior region of the capillary meshwork. At least some of these minute arterial twigs later develop into short posterior ciliary arteries. The primitive choriocapillaris is drained via larger venous vessels which arise near the middle of the globe and enter the infra- and supra-orbital venous plexuses. Arteries are of a narrow, veins of a wider calibre, the veins are separated from the surrounding mesoderm by one endothelial layer only.

In the course of the 3rd month the vessels of the choriocapillaris are more sharply defined and the endothelial nuclei become grouped towards the peripheral side of the vessels. During this time the sclera is formed, starting in the anterior part of the periocular mesoderm. Injections of Indian ink showed that at the end of the 3rd month the choroidal vasculature has

182

reached the following stage (Fig. 2): Six to eight trunks of the posterior ciliary arteries approach the sclera from behind in a region surrounding the optic nerve head; they penetrate the sclera and divide immediately afterwards. About three short posterior ciliary arteries run parallel to the optic nerve. These supply the peripapillary zone of the choroid and begin to form a ring in the sclera round the optic nerve as an early stage in formation of the circle of Haller-Zinn. One short arterial trunk supplies the region which later becomes the submacular zone of the choroid. The branches of the remaining trunks of the posterior ciliary arteries do not reach beyond the posterior third of the globe and enter the primitive choriocapillaris directly.

We can substantiate VERSARI's observation that the two long posterior ciliary arteries too, send some isolated branches towards the posterior part of the choriocapillaris. We could not observe these twigs in later stages, but ERNEST localized also in choroids of adults recurrent branches of the temporal long posterior ciliary arteries which supply the submacular zone. The long ciliary arteries fork out in the distal third, their terminal branches forming a circle above the region that will become the ciliary body.

The system of vortex veins has reached the following stage: in the anterior part of the choroid some of the widest capillaries merge to form fascicles running in an anterior-posterior direction. The fascicular vessels themselves merge to form a vortex vein which then perforates the sclera.

The primitive choriocapillaris shows a slightly different pattern in different segments of the globe. In the posterior segments the meshes are square, whereas those in the middle segments are rhombic. Between the larger venous trunks they form a polygonal pattern; further away from the region of the venous vessels the capillaries run parallel in a meridional direction and finally break up into an irregular network in the region where the ciliary body will form. Those capillaries which run meridionally through the choriocapillaris are then shifted outwards the meshwork of the choriocapillaris closing again underneath them. From this stage on a definitive choriocapillaris is being established (Fig. 3).

This change proceeds gradually from the posterior regions of the choroid towards the anterior parts, so that the definitive choriocapillaris does not reach its final position at the ora until the last months of gestation. The vessels which are excluded from the choriocapillaris are venous and join with the system of vortex veins formed earlier but which up to this stage had only connected with the anterior part of the choriocapillaris. Between the veins there are branches of the short posterior ciliary arteries that reach up to the level of the equator.

This process, i.e. the formation of what will be Haller's layer of large vessels, occurs mainly during the fourth month, although it is initiated during the third month, and there are veins and arteries simultaneously right from the beginning.

Towards the end of the 4th month the anterior ciliary arteries have also formed and take part in forming the major arterial circle of the iris, together with branches of the long posterior ciliary arteries. It is mainly during the 5th month that the layer of small and medium vessels forms between the layer of large vessels and the definitive choriocapillaris in all parts of which now exhibit a uniformly polygonal pattern. With the increase in size of the

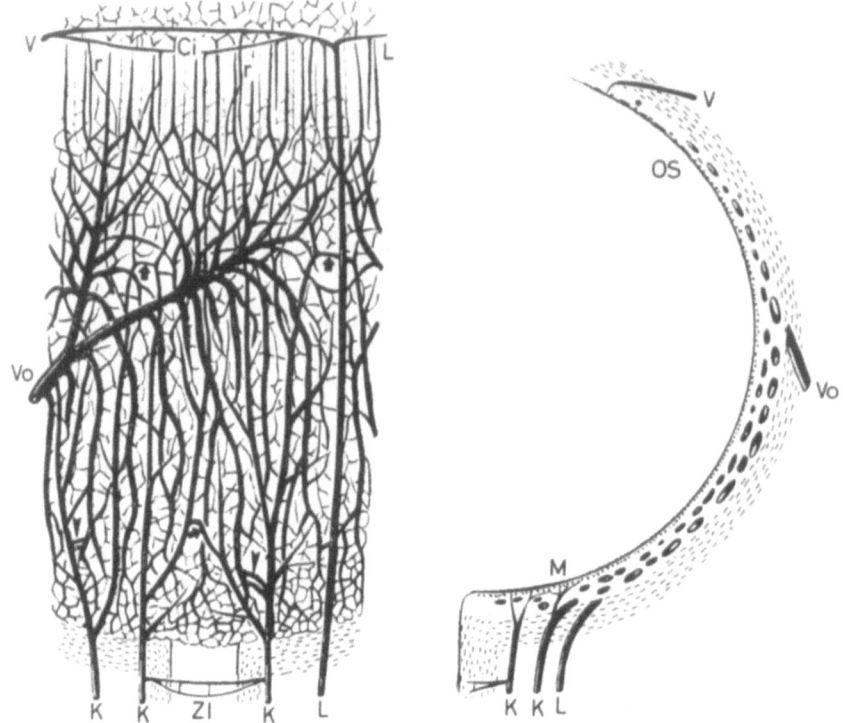

Fig. 3. Choroidal vasculature at the end of the 4th month. K = Short posterior ciliary arteries; L = long posterior ciliary arteries; ZI = formation of the circle of Haller-Zinn; Vo = vortex vein; V = anterior ciliary artery; Ci = beginning of the formation of the major arterial circle of the iris; M = region that will be the macular zone; OS = region that will be the region of the ora; H = Haller's layer. (HEIMANN, 1972, 1974).

globe and the choroid there is a corresponding increase in the number and length of the connections between the larger vessels and the choriocapillaris. There are thus a considerable number of typically arched venules arising from the choriocapillaris, running under the large vessels and finally entering a vein. These connections will eventually form Sattler's layer which also contains both veins and arteries from the beginning. Towards the end of the 5th month all three vascular layers of the choroid have formed and are evident in the posterior half of the choroid, anteriorly there are only two layers of vessels between the equator and the ciliary body. The remaining four months show increasing density and differentiation of the vascular system, which permits us to make some interesting observations on the anatomy:

Neoprene casts give us valuable information on the stage of development of the choroidal vasculature reached in the sixth month (Fig. 4).

There is a dense network of vessels in three layers from the optic nerve-head to the equator. Some branches of the short posterior ciliary arteries reach up to the region of the ora. Behind the equator the vessels gradually merge into two layers, only this cast did not demonstrate the system of vortex veins. A retrograde filling of the vortex veins in the 9th month demonstrated the formation of the ampullae, but we did not find the 'bulbiculi' that KISS & ORBAN described.

In all regions of the fetal choroid there are numerous interarterial anastomoses between branches of the short posterior ciliary arteries in both parts of the vascular layer. In the peripheral choroid the short posterior ciliary arteries that advance from the posterior region form arcade-like anastomoses, from which more small vessels branch out perpendicularly towards the periphery. There are fewer of these interarterial anastomoses in mature fetuses, and some can be demonstrated even in neoprene casts of young adults. Their number decreases with advancing age. Presumably in the fetal period and the early childhood there is not such a strong functional segmental distribution in the choroid as in the adults, where choroidal arteries behave as endarteries as we know by fluoresceinangiography. The formation of recurrent arterial branches arising from the major arterial circle of the iris and supplying the anterior part of the choroid can be observed from the 6th to 9th months. There are considerable differences between casts as to the clarity of definition of these recurrent arterial branches but we have not

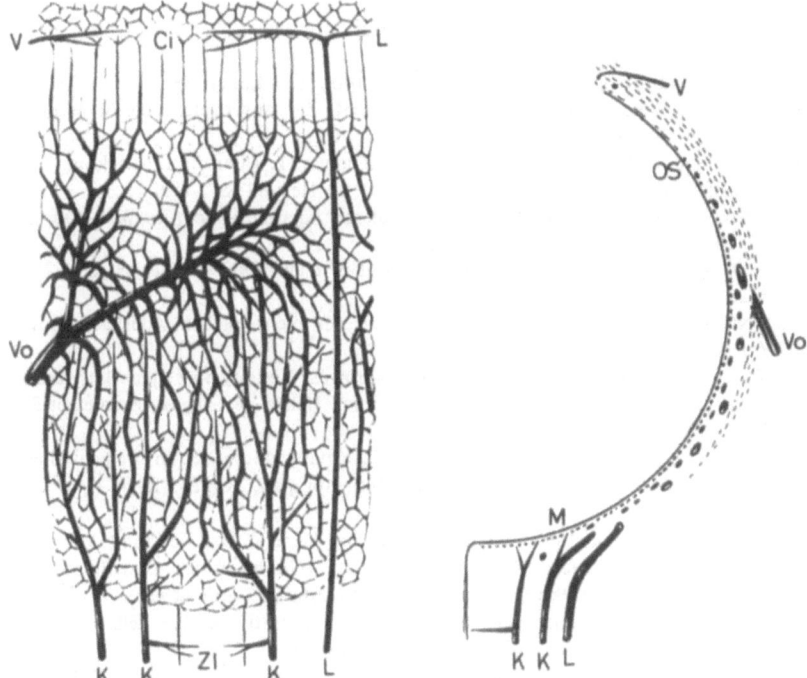

Fig. 4. Choroidal vasculature in the middle of the 6th month. K = Short posterior ciliary arteries; L = long posterior ciliary arteries; ZI = circle of Haller-Zinn; Vo = vortex vein; V = anterior ciliary artery; Ci = major arterial circle of the iris; R = recurrent branches; M = region that will be the macular zone; OS = ora serrata; (   ) = inter-arterial anastomosees; H = Haller's layer; S = Sattler's layer. (HEIMANN, 1972, 1974).

185

been able to find any case of direct end-to-end anastomosis between a recurrent arterial branch and a short posterior ciliary artery in fetal choroids as in the adult. The circle of Haller-Zinn has completely anastomosed in the 6th month.

Up to now the study of the submacular choroidal vascular pattern is of a special interest. If in fetuses of the last trimenon those vessels that run over the posterior pole are dissected, you can see that the submacular zone is supplied through small arterial branches, having in most cases one to three trunks which branch out in star-shaped tufts and thus differ from other choroidal arteries, which divide dichotomously in anterior direction. One is led to believe that in such a region there must exist haemodynamic conditions different from those in the remaining part of the choroid. The characteristic run of these vessels may be observed when the choroid and the short posterior ciliary arteries are photographed from the side. The macular choroidal artery is practically covered by a tent formed by the other ciliary arteries.

In recent studies by means of neoprene injection and staining the choroidal vessels after Krey's method we also found this special course of the submacular arteries in adults' eyes.

REFERENCES

BARBER, N. Embryology of the human eye. Kimpton, London (1955).
DEDEKIND, F. Beitrage zur Entwicklungsgeschichte der Augengefäße des Menschen. *Anat. Hefte* 38: *1* (1909).
FUCHS, H. Entwicklungsgeschichte des Wirbeltierauges. 1. Über die Entwicklung der Augengefäße des Kaninchens. *Anat. Hefte* XXVIII, Heft 84: S. *1* (1905).
HEIMANN, K. Zur Gefäßentwicklung der macularen Aderhautzone. *Klin. Mbl. Augenheilk.* 157: *636-642* (1970).
HEIMANN, K. The development of the choroid in man. *Ophthal. Res.* 3: *257-273* (1972).
HEIMANN, K. Untersuchungen zur Entwicklung der menschlichen Aderhaut. *Adv. Ophthal.* 28: *30-47* (1974).
KISS, F. & T. ORBAN. A szem elülsó felének keringési Viszonyai az újabb kutatások alapján. (Zirkulationsverhältnisse in der vorderen Hälfte des Auges). Szemészet 3: (1951).
KREY, H. Die selektive Anfärbung der Chorioidalgefäße durch den histochemischen Nachweis der alkalischen Phosphatase am Flächenpräparat. *Graefes Arch. Ophthal.* 192: *65-72* (1974).
MANN, J. The development of the human eye. British Medical Ass., London (1964).
SEEFELDER, R. In: Schieck & Bruckner, Kurzes Handbuch der Opthalmologie, vol. 1: Anatomie. Entwicklung, Mißbildungen, Vererbung. Berlin (1930).
VERSARI, R. Alla conoscenza della morfogenesi degli strati vascolari della coroide. Ric. Lab. Anat. umana norm. R. Univ. Roma 8 (1901).
WEITER, J.J. & J.T. ERNEST. Anatomy of the choroidal vasculature. *Am. J. Ophthal.* 78: *583-590* (1974).

Author's address:
Universitäts-Augenklinik
Joseph-Stelzmannstrasse 9
5 Köln 41
B.R.D.

FLUORESCEIN ANGIOGRAPHY AND
ANGIOARCHITECTURE OF THE CHOROID

KOICHI SHIMIZU & KAZUYOSHI UJIIE

(Maebashi, Japan)

The term fluorescein angiography has frequently been used as synonymous to fluorescein angiography of the retina. Angiography of the choroid has been difficult because of the dense three-dimensional distribution of choroidal vessels, absence of barrier in the choroidal vessel wall which allows rapid diffusion of fluorescein throughout the extravascular space of the choroid, and the filter effect of the pigment epithelium which interferes with the direct observation of choroidal fluorescence. After a rather early phase on, the fluorescence from the dye in the choriocapillaris effectively mask the underlying choroidal vessels.

When working with retinal fluorescein angiography, one can study the order of dye filling or hemodynamic aspects of retinal circulation as well as actual perfusion defects in pathological conditions. Considerable confusion has resulted from the lack of sharp discrimination between these two concepts in the interpretation of choroidal fluorescence. Choroidal filling 'delay' induced by artificial ocular hypertension was frequently and erroneously interpreted as choroidal filling 'defect'.

A more detailed fluorescein angiographic study of the choroid has become possible through two approaches. One is the study of eyes with defective retinal pigment epithelium and/or the choriocapillaris as in the case of retinitis pigmentosa or choroidal sclerosis. We can see the distribution and hemodynamics of the larger choroidal vessels. The other approach is the use of rapid sequence angiographic technique which allows the evaluation of choroidal circulation before dye entered the retinal vessels.

Typical dye-filling pattern and arrangement of choroidal vessels are seen in a case of choroideremia (Fig. 1 & 2). Dye initially appears in choroidal arteries emerging just temporal to the fovea. One of these arteries seems to be the long posterior ciliary artery. Arteries irrigating the upper and lower choroidal sectors then fill by the dye. These choroidal arteries bifurcate forming an acute angle as they run toward the periphery. Rarely do they cross one another so that they appear to be end arteries similar to the retinal arteries.

The macular vessels show a peculiar pattern. Firstly, dye inflow into the macular choroid takes place later than the extramacular choroidal area. Secondly, they form a bush-like arrangement in sharp contrast to the curvilinear pattern of the extramacular choroidal vessels. Thirdly, the papillomacular choroidal area appears to be far less vascularized than other chor-

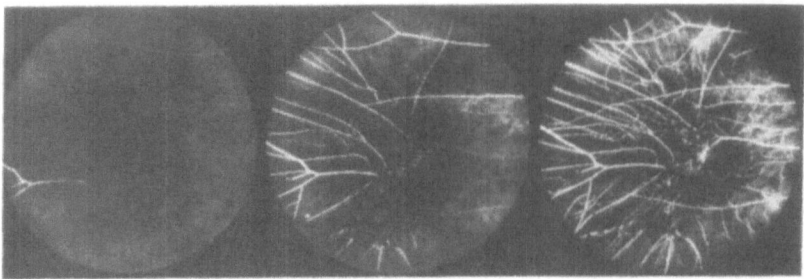

Fig. 1. Order of dye filling in the choroid in a case with choroideremia (left: 13″, middle: 15″, right: 17″). Dye initially appears in choroidal arteries temporal to the fovea (left). Arteries running toward the upper and lower periphery then fill by the dye (middle). Vessels in the submacular choroid show bush-like structure (right).

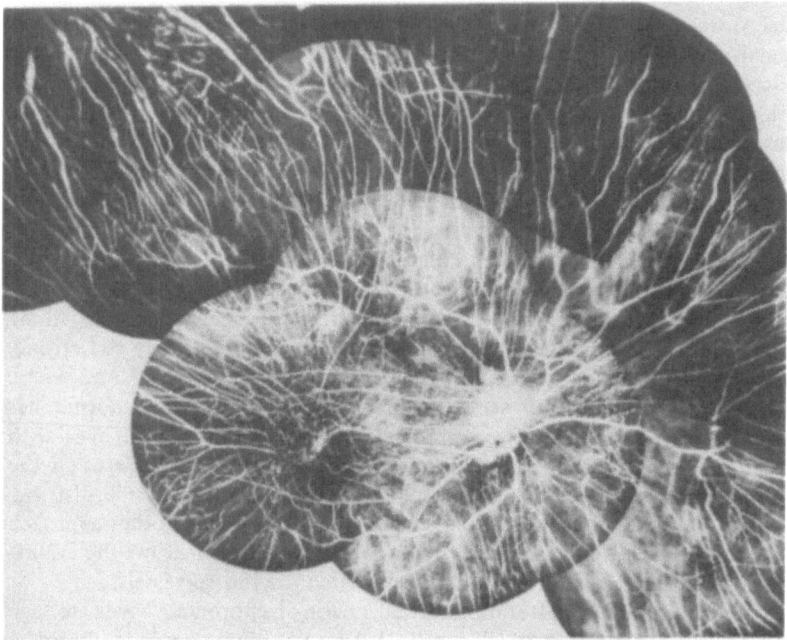

Fig. 2. Composite angiogram of the same case as in Fig. 1. The choroidal arteries run in curvilinear pattern and bifurcate at acute angles, excepting what appears to be the long posterior ciliary artery. The choroidal arteries seem to emerge at the edge of an oval area surrounding the macula and the disc.

oidal areas. These features were also regularly observed in a number of eyes with advanced retinitis pigmentosa.

We shall now discuss the typical angiographic pattern of the choroid in normal eyes when studied with the following standard technique. Five ml of 10% fluorescein was injected rapidly and and in less than one second. Sequence angiography at the rate of 3 frames per second was started 6 seconds after the start of injection. This technique facilitated a proper documentation of choroidal fluorescence during the earliest angiographic phases. We obtained following values for arm-to-choroid and arm-to-retina circulation times in normal subjects (SHIMIZU et al., 1974).

In our series of 124 normal subjects, the onset of choroidal fluorescence was usually earlier and not later than the dye inflow into the central retinal artery at the optic nervehead except one single instance. The arm-to-choroid circulation time (ACCT) averaged 8.0 ± 1.0 seconds. The arm-to-retina circulation time (ARCT) averaged 8.8 ± 1.0 seconds. The difference between ACCT and ARCT averaged 0.8 ± 0.4 seconds. For the estimation of ARCT, the first 'trickle' of dye was disregarded and we waited till the appearance of the actual head of dye bolus in the central retinal artery.

The pure 'choroidal phase' was thus of a relatively long duration persisting for two to three consecutive frames and allowed us a good insight into the vessel pattern and hemodynamics of the choroid. Typically, the course of larger vessels in the outer choroidal layer became visible in the earliest angiograms. This tasselated pattern was soon replaced by coarsely

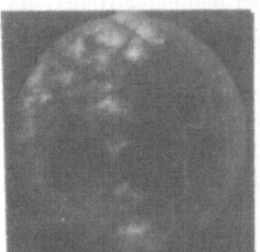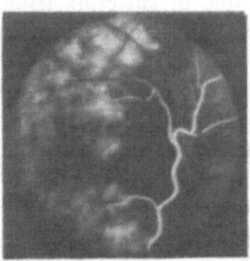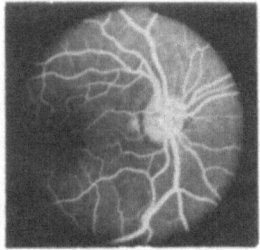

Fig. 3. Sequence angiogram of a normal eye (left: 9.6″, middle: 10.3″, right: 31.3″). The temporal hemisphere is the first to fill by the dye, followed by dye filling in the choroidal hemisphere nasal to the disc. Uniform choroidal fluorescence results after maximum dye filling is reached (right).

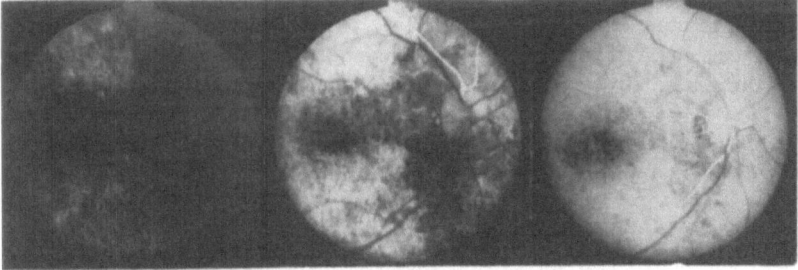

Fig. 4. Sequence angiogram of an eye with advanced retinitis pigmentosa (left: 8.5″, middle: 10.3″, right: 13.1″). Larger choroidal arteries in the temporal hemisphere are initially angiographed (left). Seconds later (middle), more uniform choroidal fluorescence appears due probably to choriocapillaris dye filling. Uniform choroidal fluorescence results in spite of the initial sector-shaped dye filling pattern (right).

189

granulated fluorescent patches apparently representing dye inflow into the choriocapillaris. These patches of choroidal fluorescence were various in size and shape. They had well-defined borders and were sharply demarcated from neighboring still non-fluorescent areas.

This irregular choroidal fluorescence in the early angiograms was a regular phenomenon. While we got the impression that it occurred in an exaggerated way in eyes with supposed delay in choroidal circulation, e.g. ocular hypertension, some forms of choroiditis and papilledema, its presence could be recorded as a rule in normal eyes whenever suitable fluorescein angiographic technique was employed.

The longitudinal choroidal zone just temporal to the disc was one of the chief areas that showed delayed dye inflow (Fig. 3, 4). This initial nonperfusion occasionally involved the optic disc sector adjacent to the choroidal zone (Fig. 5). This phenomenon was explained by the fact that both the involved choroidal and disc sectors are irrigated by arterial branches of the same choroidal arterial trunk (Fig. 6). We could record the presence of such a cilio-papillar artery connecting the peripapillar choroidal artery and the prelaminar capillaries of the disc in 46 eyes (SODENO, 1974). While these eyes were either myopic or suffering from peripapillar atrophy, its frequency led us to suppose that this was probably a regular feature in normal eyes.

The initial irregular choroidal fluorescence, even if impressive it may be, turned into uniform fluorescence at the maximum choroidal filling phase a few seconds later. This fact strongly indicated that the initial irregular choroidal fluorescence merely reflected a difference in the topological order of arterial inflow in various choroidal areas and not the actual presence of non-perfusion or diminished circulation of the involved area. The sharply demarcated border of the fluorescent patches in the early-phase angiogram suggested that the choroidal arterial supply was sectorial in nature and that each functional unit of the choriocapillaris possessed a rather well-defined borderline.

In order to correlate the above fluorescein angiographic facts with morphology, we conducted a series of animal studies by means of plastic cast of choroidal vessels in monkeys (*Macaca irus*). We opened the neck of the anesthetized animal and perfused the carotids with plasma-substitute solution which contains 6% hydroxyethyl starch and electrolytes to match the human plasma. After circulating blood was sufficiency washed out, glutaraldehyde was added to the perfusing fluid. Thereafter, liquid plastic monomer (Mercox) was injected into the carotids. This plastic material polymerized in about 10 minutes without appreciable change in volume. Thereafter, the eyeball was removed together with the orbital content and was dissolved by immersing in 20% potassium hydroxide solution for a few days. The corrosion-resistant vessel cast was washed, desired portion was dissected and dried. The plastic cast was coated with gold particles by ion spattering and was examined by scanning electron microscope.

By means of this plastic cast technique, we could observe the choroidal vessels in minute detail and in stereoscopic view. The choroidal specimen could be studied either from behind (scleral view) or from the front (retinal view).

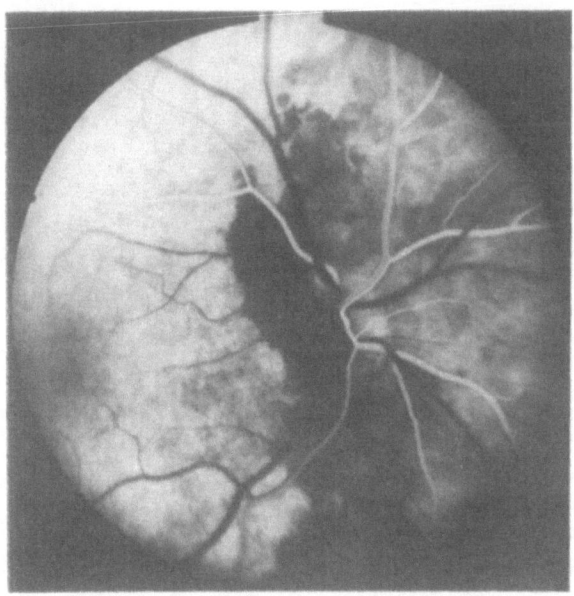

Fig. 5. Sector-shaped choroidal filling delay in a normal eye (10.6"). The longitudinal non-fluorescent zone is demarcated by sharp irregular borderline from the surrounding dye-filled area. The temporal disc sector also shows absent dye filling. A uniform due filling of the choroid and the disc occurs 3 seconds later.

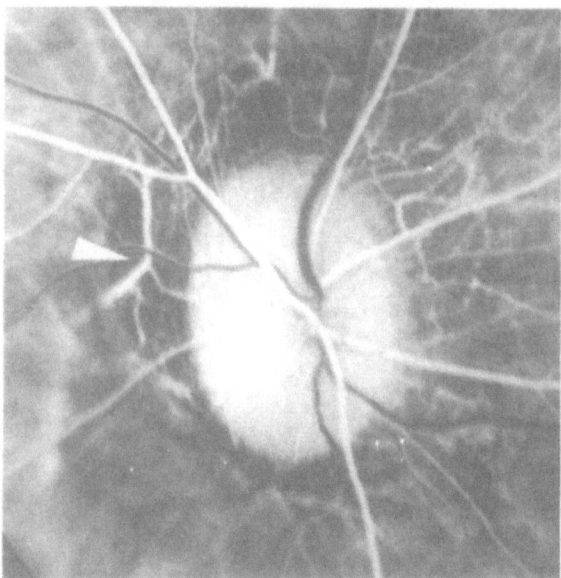

Fig. 6. Fluorescein angiogram showing the presence of a feeder vessel to the prelaminar capillaries of the disc. This 'cilio-papillar artery' originates from a choroidal artery which extends ot the upper and the lower peripapillary choroid. The delayed dye filling in Fig. 5 is explained by assuming the presence of such an artery.

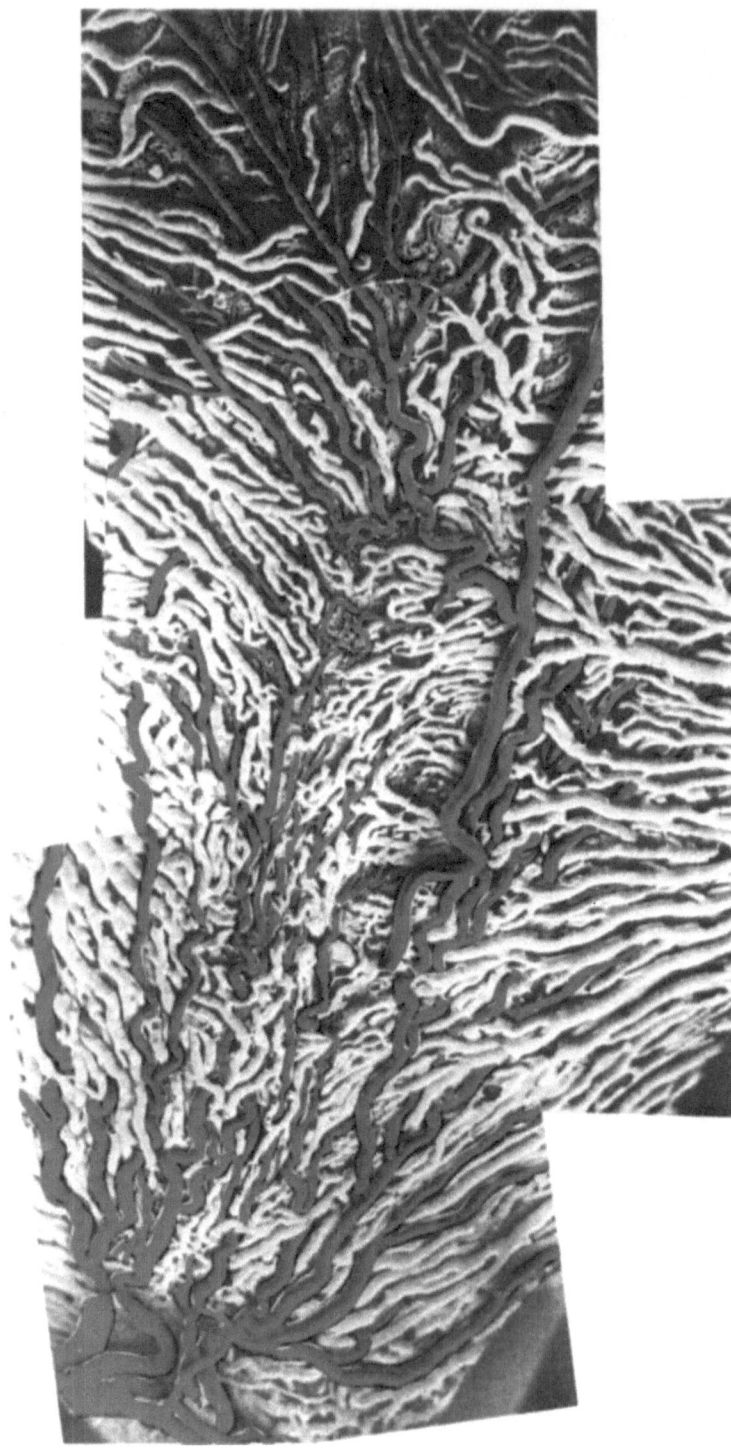

Fig. 7. Composite plastic cast of the monkey choroid as seen from behind. A group of short posterior ciliary arteries enter the choroid near the site of entrance of the optic disc (upper left). The proximal portion of the long posterior ciliary artery was broken. It gives a massive branch to irrigate the choroidal sector temporal to the macula. The macular choroid has a plural arterial supply coming from the nasal and temporal directions. The SPCA's are initially located in the outer choroidal layer and gradually shift to the inner choroidal layer.

A composite microphotograph of the posterior choroid is shown in Fig. 7. A group of short posterior ciliary arteries (SPCA's) are seen as they enter the choroid by piercing the sclera temporal to the optic nerve. The macula is located approximately in the center of the composite angiogram. This finding reminds us of the fact that the choroid is a very richly vascularized tissue. It would almost appear as if the choroid consisted solely of vessels.

We painted the choroidal artery in red in order to differentiate the arteries from veins in Figure 7. The identification of arteries could be done with relative ease by adopting the following rules. For one, major arterial trunks could be traced downstream starting from the site of entrance of SPCA's. Further, arteries were characterized by the presence of constriction at the site of bifurcation if the form of annuli. Also, the choroidal arteries were distributed in a fan-shaped pattern radiaging from around the optic disc. They reduced their caliber as they ran toward the periphery. In contrast to this rule, the veins increased their caliber as they approached the vortex veins. They showed greater variability in caliber and lacked annuli-like constrictions at the site of merging of vessels.

The site of entrance of long posterior ciliary artery (LPCA) is seen lower to the macula in Fig. 7. Its proximal portion is broken probably because the missing portion was located intrasclerally for a considerable length before entering the choroid. The LPCA gives off a big branch which actively participates in the arterial irrigation of a large, fan-shaped choroidal sector temporal to the macula.

The branches of the SPCA's are initially located in the outer choroidal layer and posterior to the choroidal veins. After they coursed a certain distance, approximately the length between the disc and the macula, they gradually move to the inner choroidal layer and therefore anterior to the veins.

The pattern of distribution of choroidal arteries, as they appear on the plastic cast, is generally segmental. The choroidal arteries appear to be end arteries on macroscopic view. Because of the active participation of LPCA in the local choroidal circulation, the upper and lower choroidal hemispheres seem to form functionally separate units.

A unique exception to the end-arterial nature of choroidal vasculature is observed in the macular choroid (Fig. 7). This particular area is supplied by arteries coming from the nasal side and also by recurrent branches originating from the lower temporal LPCA and the upper temporal SPCA. The macular choroid thus seems to be plurally supplied by a number of arterial branches that happen to be in the paramacular area.

There are also numerous arterio-arterial anastomoses and probable arterio-venous communications in the macular choroid (Fig. 7). The venous drainage from the macula is directed into both upper and lower directions. The two-directional venous drainage is secured by well-built veno-venous anastomosis. This feature well contrasts with the temporal peripheral choroid, where the venous drainage is conducted strictly in one direction, namely either toward the upper- or lower-temporal vortex vein. The LPCA in the temporal meridian serves as watershed zone for the venous drainage in the temporal periphery.

Another cast model of the choroid together with the anterior portion of the optic nerve is shown in Fig. 8. The central retinal artery and vein are shown in the center of the cut surface of the optic nerve. The optic nerve itself appears to be highly vascularized. Medium-sized arteries, most of which are branches of the SPCA's, run posteriorly and parallel to the axis of the optic nerve. The intrascleral portion of the SPCA's are tortuous and constricted.

The macular choroid and the choriocapillaris of the eye shown in Fig. 8 is presented in magnified view as Fig. 9. The terminal arterioles enter the choriocapillaris at a right angle. They show a marked constriction just where they join the latter. The number of feeder arterioles are overwhelmingly greater than that of veins. It is apparent that numerous feeder arterioles are responsible for a given small area of the choriocapillaris in the macular choroid.

That the feeder arterioles seem to be much more numerous than venules in the posterior choroid is illustrated in Fig. 10. A big knotty collector vein is seen rising perpendicularly from the choriocapillaris. The blood in the choriocapillaris is first collected into three venules which immediately join to enter the venous trunk. The feeder artery, on the other hand, enter the choriocapillaris via narrower but longer arterioles which run, for a short distance, parallel to and in apposition to the choriocapillaris. A focal constriction is present where the terminal arterioles join the choriocapillaris.

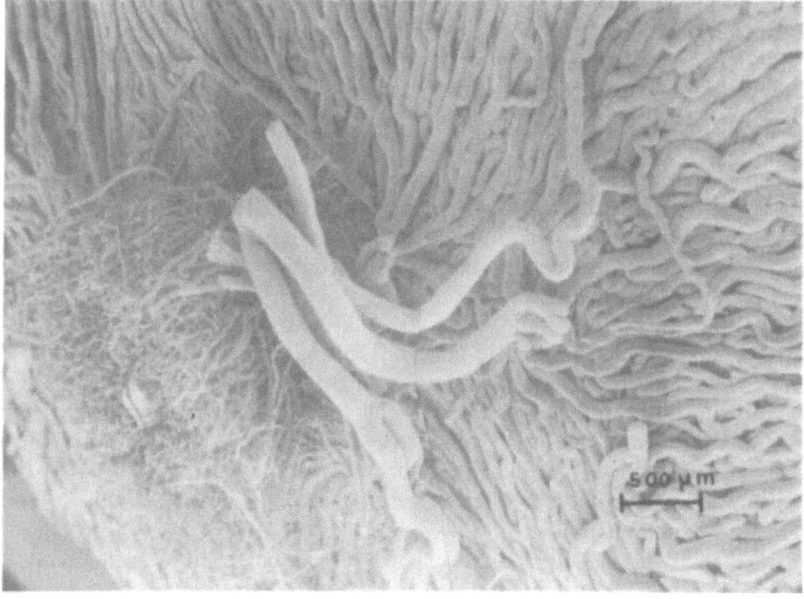

Fig. 8. Plastic cast of the anterior portion of the optic nerve and the peripapillary choroid (scleral view). The optic nerve is richly vascularized by network of capillaries. The central retinal artery and vein are seen in the center of the cut surface of the optic nerve. Numerous arterioles run posteriorly surrounding the optic nerve. The SPCA's enter the choroid temporal to and near the optic nerve.

194

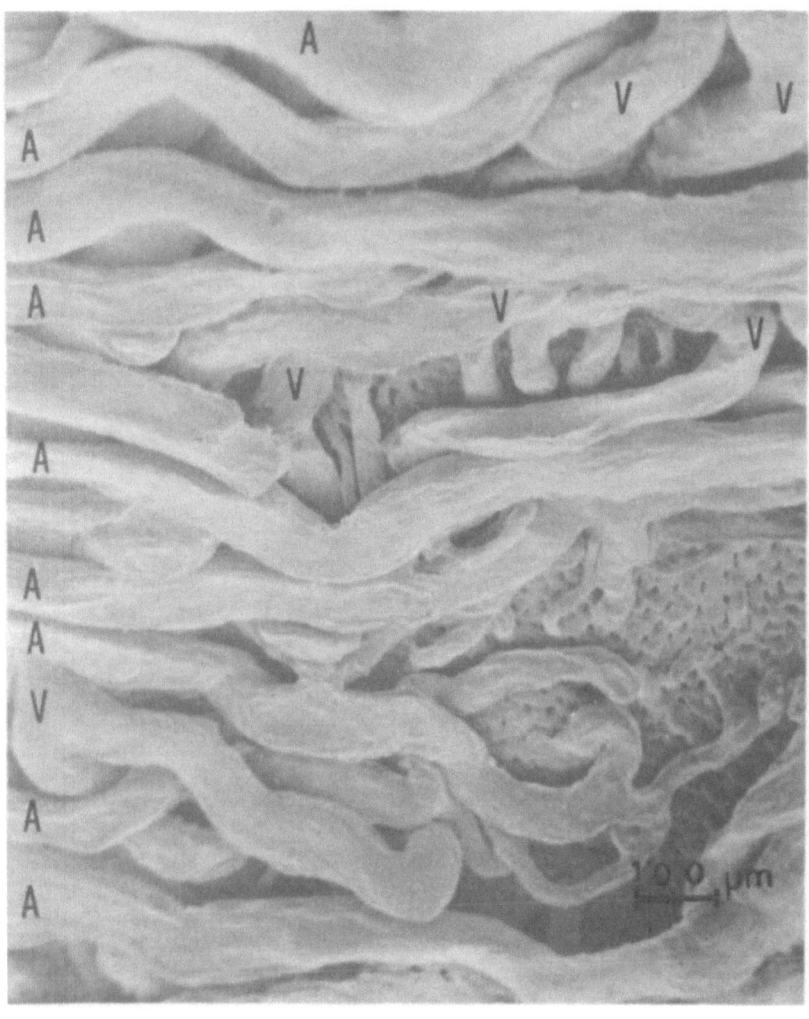

Fig. 9. The macular choroid in the same eye as Fig. 8. Arteries are much more numerous than veins. They either make a sharp right-angle bending or give arteriolar branches
to feed the choriocapillaris. There is a radical shift in caliber between the parent artery
and the feeder arteriole. A focal constriction is present where the arterioles join the
choriocapillaris.

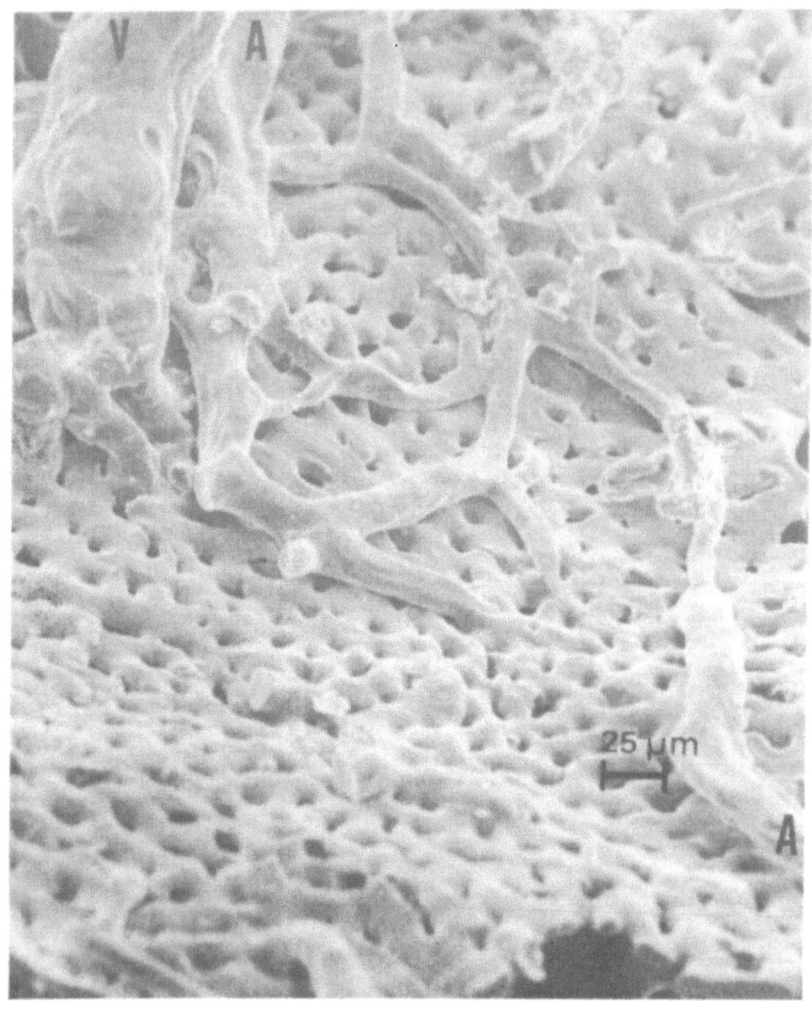

Fig. 10. Paramacular choroid showing feeder arterioles, veins and the choriocapillaris (scleral view). There are abundant interarterial intercommunications. Terminal arterioles show a constriction as they join the choriocapillaris.

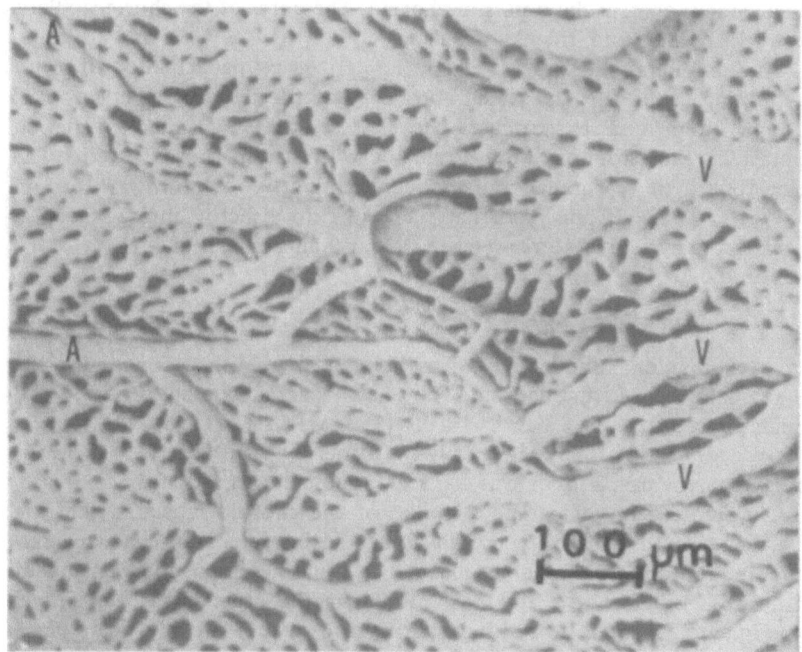

Fig. 11. Peripheral choroid (scleral view). The arteries and veins run close to and in apposition to the choriocapillaris. They are less cylindrical. An interarterial anastomosis is seen in the center. The transition from artery to choriocapillaris to vein is less clear-cut than in the macular choroid. The choriocapillaris shows coarser and more irregular network.

There are numerous interarterial anstomotic communications. Such an interarterial anastomosis has been a frequent feature in other specimens. It seems that the terminal choroidal artery is not strictly end-arterial in nature but that a group of terminal arteriolar branches contribute to the irrigation of the choriocapillaris unit.

The peripheral choroid shows an essentially different pattern of angioarchitecture besides the fact that the choroid is thinner and is less densely populated with vessels. The choroidal arteries run close to and parallel to the choriocapillaris (Fig. 11). The terminal arteries are fewer in number so that a single feeder artery irrigates a larger choriocapillaris area than in the posterior choroid. Also, multiple arterial supply to a given small choriocapillaris area is almost an exception. The transition from terminal arteriole into choriocapillaris is much subtler. The arterioles are less cylindrical and are flattened in shape.

The veins in the peripheral choroid show features similar to the arteries (Fig. 11). They are flattened and the transition from choriocapillaris to vein is very subtle. The choroidal veins lie almost in the same level as the choriocapillaris. Because of this feature, the choroidal arteries are generally located outer to the veins in the peripheral choroid. The choriocapillaris itself is also

197

much coarser than in the posterior choroid. The pores of the choriocapillaris network are large and irregular in shape.

The peripheral choroid was also characterized by participation of recurrent branches of the LPCA and probably of the anterior ciliary arterial system. Interarterial anastomoses became less and less frequent, while, on contast, rich anastomoses were formed between parent choroidal veins. The veins took a more parallel course directed either up- or downward to join the vortex veins. It appeared that there was no effective interconnection between the upper and lower veins in the far temporal meridian.

DISCUSSION

An overwhelming number of works have been published concerning the angioarchitecture of the choroid. They have been adequately reviewed and summarized by KOLMER & LAUBER (1936), ROHEN (1964), AMALRIC (1969, 1971) and HEIMANN (1974). Works by ASHTON (1952, 1953) using neoprene cast also serve as classical monuments in this area.

Our fluorescein angiographic studies of the choroid indicated that the SPCA's seem to enter the choroid along the border of an oval area surrounding the optic disc and the macula. Our findings are in good agreement with those by ASHTON and AMALRIC. On the other hand, our animal experiments using plastic cast have clearly shown that the SPCA's do penetrate the sclera in the vicinity of the entrance of optic nerve. We can explain the apparent discrepancy between the anatomical and clinical findings by assuming the following model.

The SPCA's are initially located in the outermost choroidal layer and outer to the choroidal veins after entering the choroid. After they coursed a certain distance, they gradually move to the inner choroidal layer and therefore anterior to the veins. Thus, the majority of the SPCA's are not visible on fluorescein angiograms in the papillomacular region because they lie behind a dense layer of choroidal veins that mask the arteries. That the SPCA's seem to enter the choroid along an oval around the disc and the macula is just an apparent phenomenon and has to be interpreted upon the above anatomical basis.

The presence of a 'macular artery' has been a disputed topic. Our plastic cast studies have demonstrated that the macular choroid is not irrigated by a single artery but by a number of arteries that happen to be near by. In one of our specimens (Fig. 7), even the LPCA participated in the arterial supply to the macula via recurrent branches. This plural arterial supply seems to be unique to the macular choroid and forms a sharp contrast to the end-arterial nature of the extramacular choroidal vasculature.

The macular choroid was also characterized by the richness and the perpendicular course of feeding arterioles to the choriocapillaris. There were also numerous interarterial communications. Their shape and their impressive frequency seemed to indicate that they play an important role in the hemodynamics of the choroid and that they were probably functioning in balancing the blood pressure at the arteriolar level. They would also contribute to the maintenance of adequate perfusion of the choriocapillaris by providing a plural and alternate route of arterial blood supply. The almost regular presence of interarterial anastomoses would necessitate the view that the end-arterial nature of the choroid holds only in regard to the interconnected arterioles as a group and not the individual terminal arterioles.

The unique exception of the macular choroid from end-arterial nature finds its counterpart in the nature of venous drainage. The macular blood can be drained in either, upper or lower, direction thanks to the presence of veno-venous anastomosis.

It is already known that the transition from choroidal artery to arteriole and then to choriocapillaris does not take place in a continuous and subtle way but in abrupt stages. Our findings are in accord with the accepted view.

The posterior choroid consists of big arteries which occupy the outermost layer, arterioles which are located in the middle layer and which are directed perpendicular to the place of the choriocapillaris, and the choriocapillaris proper. There is a radical shift in the caliber and the direction at each of the three stages. A sharp constriction was universally present as the arterioles entered the choriocapillaris. A similar constriction was almost regularly found at the site of bifurcation of big choroidal arteries. We still do not know the significance and the anatomical basis for these constrictions. It might appear that these constrictions are mere artefacts during the process of plastic casting and that the site of constrictions indicate where the vessels withstood the pressure of perfusion fluid. While admitting that this is a possible explanation, we feel that the constrictions actually do exist. A similar constriction has also been observed as a regular feature in plastic casts and on fluorescein angiograms of the retina.

Our plastic cast studies of the choroidal vessels are thus in good agreement with what has been found by means of fluorescein angiography in human eye. Our method using the new plastic material has the advantage that the choroidal vessels can be examined in both retinal and scleral view. A detailed and three-dimensional study is possible with the use of scanning electron microscopy. The chief value of our present observations seems to lie in corroborating what has been stated by earlier workers through more concrete and irrefutable evidences.

REFERENCES

AMALRIC P. & BONNIN, P. L'angiographie fluorescéinique. *Bull. Soc. d'Opthalm. France.* Rapport Annual: *177-186,* 200-207 (1969).

AMALRIC, P. Circulation choroïdienne. C.R. Symp. int. angiographie fluorescéinique, Albi, 1969, pp. *193-203.* Karger, Basel (1971).

ASHTON, N. Observations on the choroidal circulation. *Brit. J. Ophthal.* 36: *465-481* (1952).

ASHTON, N. Central areolar choroidal sclerosis. A histo-phathological study. *Brit. J. Ophthal.* 37: *140-147* (1953).

HEIMANN, K. Untersuchungen zur Entwicklung der menschlichen Aderhaut. *Adv. Ophthal.* 28: *30-77* (1974).

KOLMER, W. & LAUBER, H. Handbuch der mikroskopischen Anatomie des Menschen. Vol. 3, Pt. 2. Auge, pp. *93-105.* Julius Springer, Berlin (1936).

ROHEN, J.W. Handbuch der mikroskopischen Anatomie des Menschen. Vol. 3, Pt. 4. Das Auge und seine Hilfsorgane, pp. *177-185.* Springer, Berlin (1964).

SHIMIZU, K., YOKOCHI, K. & OKANO, T. Fluorescein angiography of the choroid. *Jap. J. Ophthalm.* 18: *97-108* (1974).

SODENO, Y. Cilioretinal artery and the microcirculation of the optic disc. *Acta Soc. Ophthalm. Jap.* 78: *561-575* (1974).

Authors' address:
Department of Ophthalmology
Gunma University
School of Medicine
3-39-15 Showamachi
Maebashi 371
Japan

DISCUSSION

Dr Bonnet: Est-ce que M. Shimizu pourrait me dire par quel moyen il parvient à différentier les artères des veines sur ses moulages en plastique?

Dr Shimizu: There are several features with which we can tell if a given vessel is an artery or a vein. In the composite angiogram you can trace the entrance of the short ciliary artery near the optic disc. If you trace it further to the periphery you can tell exactly which vessels are arteries. This is one point. You can also do it the other way round. You start from the periphery and there you have the ampulla of the vortex vein and you can trace the veins towards the center. After you have done a certain number of such exercises you get to know if it is a vein or an artery just by looking at a small portion of the vessel in question. A choroidal artery regularly shows a sphincter-like constriction at the site of bifurcation, although I am not quite sure if it is a real finding or an artefact. A similar constriction has been also found where the artery joins the choriocapillaris. Another criterion: an artery becomes narrower and narrower as it approaches the periphery, while the vein merges and increases in caliber as it nears the peripheral choroid.

PHYSIOLOGICAL ANATOMY OF THE
CHOROIDAL VASCULATURE

SOHAN SINGH HAYREH, M.D., Ph.D., F.R.C.S.

(Iowa City, USA)

The Choroidal Vasculature has been extensively studied in the past by post-mortem injection techniques (ASHTON, 1952; RUSKELL, 1961; RING & FUJINO, 1967; VILSTRUP, 1952; WYBAR, 1954a, b). However, fluorescein angiographic studies in the living eye have revealed that the post-mortem studies did not give us correct information about the physiological anatomy of this vascular bed. Fluorescein angiography can truthfully be said to have made the major contribution so far in the study of the choroidal circulation in health and disease.

I studied the physiological anatomy of the choroidal vasculature by fluorescein fundus angiography experimentally (in rhesus monkeys) and clinically (in the human). The findings are described in detail elsewhere (HAYREH, 1969, 1970, 1973, 1974a-d, 1975; HAYREH & BAINES, 1972a, b, 1973) and are briefly summarized here.

ARTERIAL SUPPLY OF THE CHOROID

Posterior ciliary arteries (PCAs) and their subdivisions

There is a good deal of confusion about their nomenclature and number. The various posterior ciliary arteries can be divided into the following categories:

a. Main posterior ciliary arteries

In man 2 (in 48%) or 3 (in 39%) posterior ciliary arteries arise from the ophthalmic artery (HAYREH, 1962). The artery which goes to the nasal choroid is called the Medial Posterior Ciliary Artery (MPCA) while the one to the temporal choroid is the Lateral Posterior Ciliary Artery (LCPA). Sometimes there may be a Superior Posterior Ciliary Artery.

b. Short posterior ciliary arteries (SPCAs)

These are the various subdivisions of the main posterior ciliary arteries seen outside the eyeball, and may be 10-20 in number.

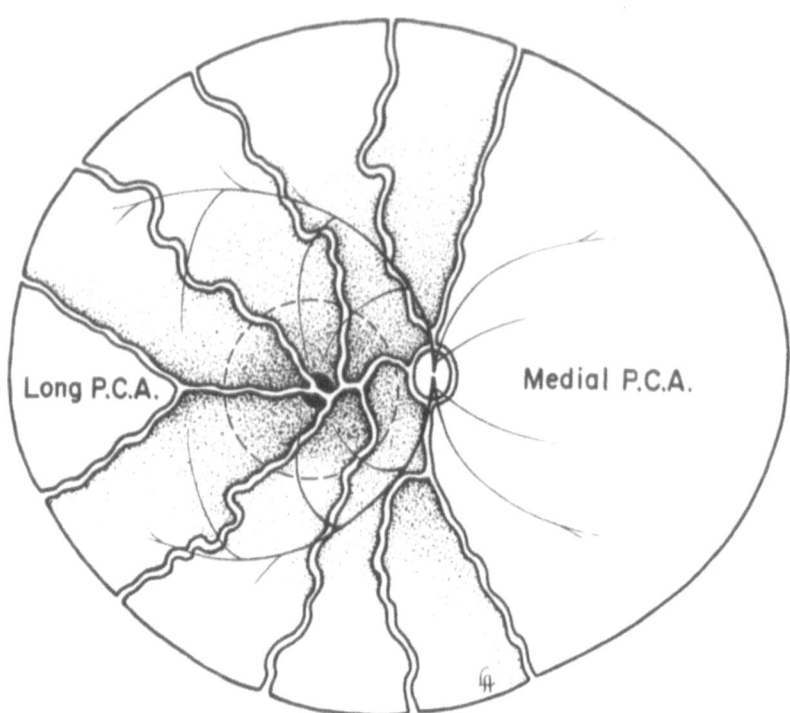

Fig. 1. Diagrammatic representation of distribution by various temporal SPCAs and their watershed zones in posterior part of fundus. Dotted circle in region of distribution of temporal SPCAs represents macular region. Areas of supply by medial PCA and temporal long PCA are also shown.

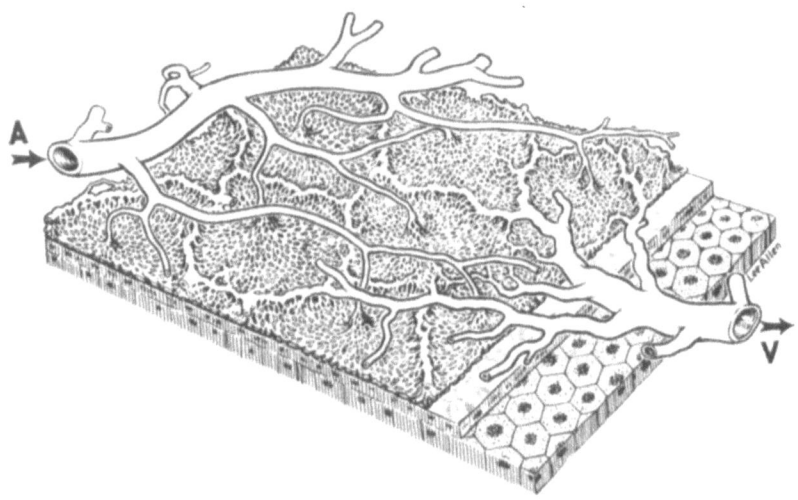

Fig. 2. Three-dimensional schematic representation of choriocapillaris flow pattern. A choroidal arteriole; V choroidal vein.

202

c. Long posterior ciliary arteries

These are usually two-one on the medial and the other on the lateral side. Each long posterior ciliary artery is one of the multiple branches of the main posterior ciliary artery.

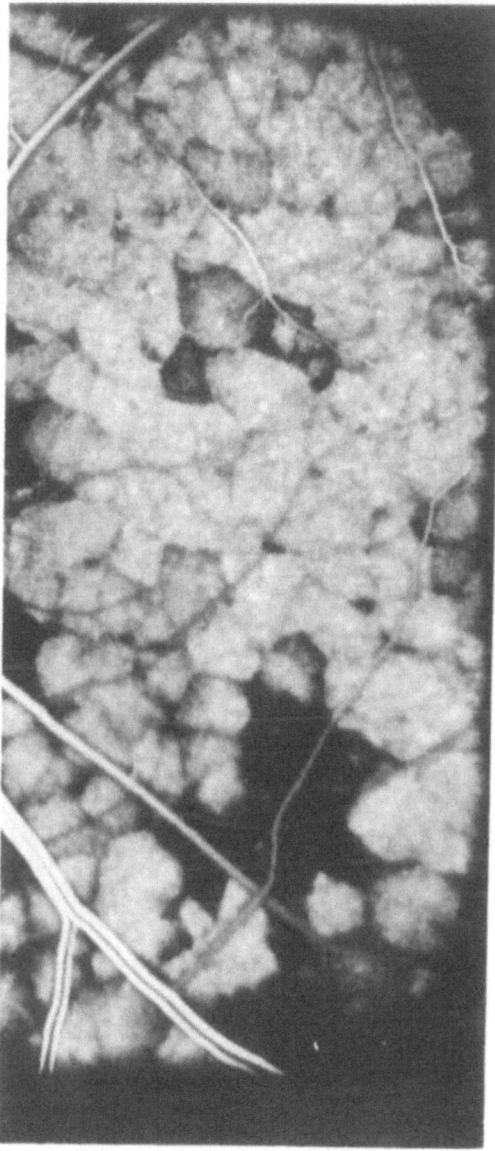

Fig. 3. Choriocapillaris pattern in fluorescein fundus angiogram of monkey eye, showing various units of choriocapillaris mosaic (each unit supplied by terminal choroidal arteriole): note presence of some empty units among normally filled units.

The Medial Posterior Ciliary Artery and Lateral Posterior Ciliary Artery usually supply the nasal and temporal halves of the choroid respectively, with the boundary between them generally passing through the optic disc (Fig. 1). The Short Posterior Ciliary Arteries supply segments of the choroid extending radially from the posterior pole to the periphery; each segment varies greatly in size, shape and location and has irregular borders (Fig. 1). Smaller subdivisions of the Short Posterior Ciliary Arteries supply still smaller segments of irregular shape and size. Ultimately each terminal choroidal arteriole supplies a small segment of choriocapillaris (Fig. 2, 3). There is a marked spatial variation in the filling of the various choroidal segments so that on fluorescein angiography well-defined geographical filling defects are commonly seen in the normal choroid in both man and monkey (Fig. 3).

The temporal long posterior ciliary artery invariably supplies a sector of the choroid, extending radially and temporally, starting almost immediately from the point where the artery joins the choroid temporal to the macular region (HAYREH, 1974d) (Fig. 1).

Choriocapillaris

Fluorescein angiographic studies have shown that each terminal choroidal arteriole supplies an independent segment of the choriocapillaris, with the

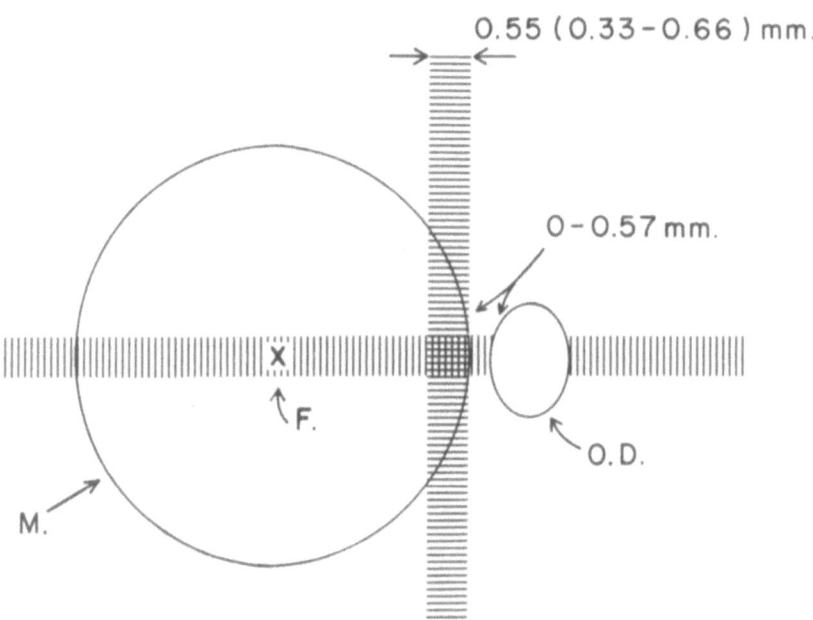

Fig. 4. Diagrammatic representation of watershed zones of vortex veins. F and X fovea; M macular region; OD optic disc.

arteriole joining the segment at about its center; the draining venules lie around the periphery of this segment (HAYREH, 1974b((Fig. 2). This supports observations by other authors on the vascular pattern in the choriocapillaris (DOLLERY et al., 1968; TORCZYNSKI & TSO, 1976; WEITER & ERNEST, 1974) but contradicts those of KREY (1975). Each segment is a functionally independent unit, usually of polygonal shape with no anastomoses with the adjacent segments *in vivo* (Fig. 3). The various segments are arranged like a mosaic.

VENOUS DRAINAGE OF THE UVEAL VASCULATURE

My *in vivo* studies revealed (HAYREH & BAINES, 1973) that each vortex vein has a well-defined functional segmental distribution extending throughout the entire antero-posterior length of the uveal tract, involving the veins in the corresponding segment of the iris, ciliary processes and the choroid. There is poor communication between the adjacent venous segments. The watershed zones between the various vortex veins therefore extend anteroposteriorly through the entire length of the uveal tract – a horizontal watershed between the upper and lower vortex veins passes through the optic disc and macular region, while a vertical watershed between the temporal and nasal vortex veins passes in between the optic disc and macular region (Fig. 4).

Choroidal anastomoses

My *in vivo* studies revealed that choroidal arteries do not anastomose at any level with any neighbouring artery, and are functional end-arteries (HAYREH, 1969, 1970, 1975; HAYREH & BAINES, 1972a). Thus the main posterior ciliary arteries and their various subdivisions right down to the terminal choroidal arterioles and the choriocapillaris have a segmental distribution. The border between any two neighbouring vessels, from the main posterior ciliary arteries right down to the terminal choroidal arterioles, forms a watershed zone. The watershed zone between the main posterior ciliary arteries usually passes through the optic disc. In man, the watershed zone between the Medial Posterior Ciliary Artery and Lateral Posterior Ciliary Artery usually lies between the optic disc and the macular region (Fig. 5) and this has been reported by other authors as well (YOKOCHI et al., 1973). The watershed zones between the various temporal short Posterior Ciliary Arteries and also those of the temporal long posterior ciliary artery are shown schematically in Fig. 1.

This finding of a segmental distribution by the posterior ciliary arteries and their subdivisions seems to conflict with the experience of that clinical or experimental occlusion of these arteries may produce only small patchy choroidal infarcts or even none at all (HAYREH, 1973, 1975; HAYREH & BAINES, 1972b). The subject is discussed elsewhere (HAYREH, 1975). Briefly, this is because the segment of the choroid supplied by an artery does not correspond exactly with the segment drained by a big choroidal vein; there is always a certain amount of overlap between the adjacent

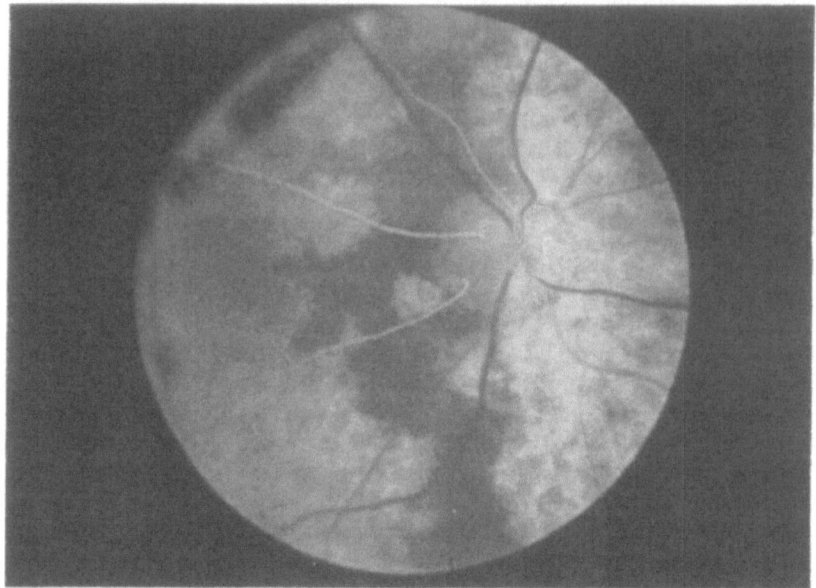

Fig. 5. Fluorescein fundus angiogram of right eye of 66-year-old man with old central retinal artery occlusion but patent cilio-retinal arteries. Note filling of choroid on temporal and nasal sides with watershed zone between them still not filled. Small isolated island of choriocapillaris is filling inferotemporal to optic disc. There are two cilio-retinal arteries on temporal side.

arterial segments via the veins. Thus there is a certain amount of reflux of blood into the choriocapillaris of the occluded segment from veins draining occluded as well as unoccluded segments of the choroid (Fig. 6). Most probably this reflux of blood from a big vein into the occluded segment is due to the pumping action produced by ocular pulsation. Moreover, the venous blood in the normal choroid has a very high concentration of oxygen, so that even a slow trickle of venous blood in the occluded zone is enough to supply the required amount of oxygen. Experimental choroidal infarcts were seen in only those areas which did not have any such reflux of blood for a considerable length of time.

Submacular choroid

My *in vivo* studies in monkeys (HAYREH, 1974c) revealed that the submacular choroid had no special artery; this confirms previous observations by various authors (RING & FUJINO, 1967; WYBAR, 1954a) but is contrary to some claims about having seen such an artery (WEITER & ERNEST, 1974). This part of the choroid seems to be supplied by small recurrent branches arising from the various temporal Short Posterior Ciliary Arteries soon after their joining the choroid. While the Short Posterior Ciliary Arteries run radially towards the periphery from the macular region, the macular branches most probably run towards the center of the macular region. Each Short Posterior Ciliary Artery supplies a segment of the sub-macular choroid (Fig. 1). My studies also showed that the macular region is the meeting point not only of many watershed zones of the various Short Posterior Ciliary Arteries (Fig., 1), but also of all the watershed zones of the vortex veins (HAYREH, 1974c).

It is well known that an area where watershed zones meet is highly vulnerable to ischemic disorders in any generalized chronic ischemic disorder. In view of this, it is postulated that senile macular degeneration, and allied macular disorders are most probably due to this unusual pattern of the sub-macular choroid, compared with the rest of the choroid. The subject is discussed in detail elsewhere (HAYREH, 1975).

Peripheral part of the choroid

Watershed zones between the Short Posterior Ciliary Arteries and the Anterior Ciliary Arteries are located in this region. This may be responsible for pigmentary and other degenerations seen in old persons in this part of the fundus.

The normal filling pattern of the choroidal vascular bed on fluorescein angiography

Choroidal filling usually starts before the dye fills the retinal arterioles on the optic disc (the time interval being up to 2 seconds in normal healthy

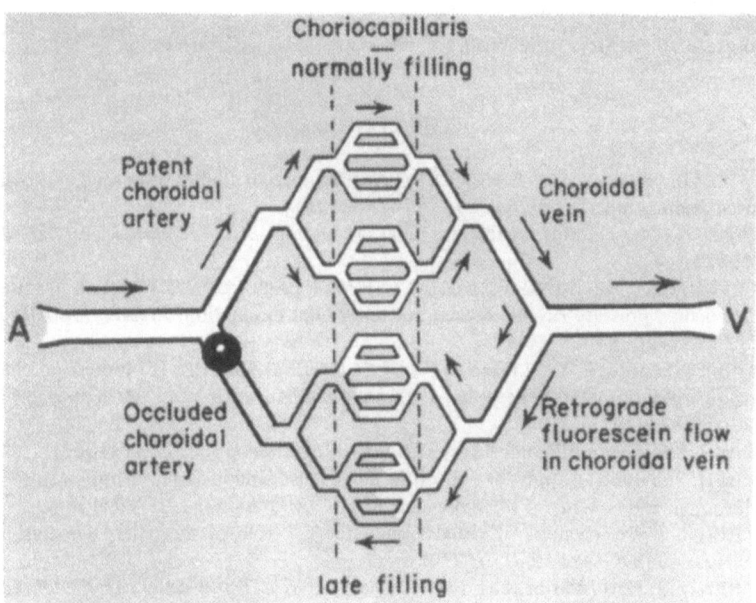

Fig. 6. Diagrammatic representation of mechanism of retrograde filling of choroid in area of an occluded short PCA.

persons – 0-1.5 sec. (EVANS et al., 1973), 0.8 ± 0.4 sec. (SHIMIZU et al., 1974)). However, the retinal and choroidal circulations may some time start to fill simultaneously, or even occasionally the retinal before the choroidal in normal eyes. The early filling of the choroid occurs because its blood flow is faster than that in the retina, since the wide-lumen choriocapillaris offer much less resistance to blood flow than the retinal capillaries. The normal choroidal vascular bed always shows irregular, well-defined, geographical filling defects, varying in size and shape, in the choriocapillaris; they are commonly seen in the peripapillary choroid but may occur anywhere. These physiological spatial filling defects almost always last only a few seconds (1-2 sec. (OOSTERHUIS & BOEN-TAN, 1971), 2 sec. (HYVARINEN et al., 1969), 2.8 (1.8-3.9 sec. – giant-sized filled within 1.8-2.5 sec.) sec. (EVANS et al., 1973), up to the early retinal arteriovenous phase (ARCHER et al., 1970)) and only very rarely persist after the major retinal veins start to fill with fluorescein, i.e., the beginning of the retinal arterio-venous phase (HAYREH, 1974a). This fact is extremely important in distinguishing physiological spatial defects from pathological defects; the latter are seen when the perfusion pressure in the choroidal vascular bed falls as in glaucoma, low-tension glaucoma and allied disorders. The concept presented by EVANS et al. (1973) and SHIMIZU et al. (1974) that *all* choroidal filling defects on angiography are a physiological phenomena is not only wrong but also highly misleading. Localized pathological filling defects or circulatory delays in the choroid are distinct and important entities, not to be confused with morphologically identical physiological defects.

ACKNOWLEDGEMENTS

I am grateful to Mrs. Julie Wolf for her secretarial assistance.

REFERENCES

ARCHER, D., KRILL, A.E. & NEWELL, F.W. Fluorescein studies of normal choroidal circulation. *Amer. J. Ophthal.* 69: *543-554* (1970).

ASHTON, N. Observations on the choroidal circulation. *Brit. J. Ophthal.* 36: *465-481* (1952).

DOLLERY, C.T., HENKIND, P., KOHNER, E.M. & PATERSON, J.W. Effect of raised intraocular pressure on the retinal and choroidal circulation. *Invest. Ophthal.* 7: *191-198* (1968).

EVANS, P., SHIMIZU, K., LIMAYE, S., DEGLIN, E. & WRUCK, J. Fluorescein cineangiography of the optic nerve head. *Trans. Amer. Acad. Ophthal. & Otolaryng.* 77: OP *260-273* (1973).

HAYREH, S.S. The ophthalmic artery. III. *Brit. J. Ophthal.* 46: *212-247* (1962).

HAYREH, S.S. Blood supply of the optic nerve head and its role in optic atrophy, glaucoma, and oedema of the optic disc. *Brit. J. Ophthal.* 53: *721-748* (1969).

HAYREH, S.S. Pathogenesis of visual field defects – role of the ciliary circulation. *Brit. J. Ophthal.* 54: *289-311* (1970).

HAYREH, S.S. Occlusion of the posterior ciliary arteries. *Trans. Amer. Acad. Ophthal. & Otolaryng.* 77: OP *300-309* (1973).

HAYREH, S.S. Recent advances in fluorescein fundus angiography. *Brit. J. Ophthal.* 58: *391-412* (1974a).

HAYREH, S.S. The Choriocapillaris. *Albrecht v. Graefes Arch. Ophthal.* 192: *165-179* (1974b).

HAYREH, S.S. Submacular choroidal vascular pattern. *Albrecht v. Graefes Arch. Ophthal.* 192: *181-196* (1974c).

HAYREH, S.S. The long posterior ciliary arteries. *Albrecht v. Graefes Arch. Ophthal.* 192: *197-213* (1974d).

HAYREH, S.S. Segmental nature of the choroidal vasculature. *Brit. J. Ophthal.* 59: *631-648* (1975).

HAYREH, S.S. & BAINES, J.A.B. Occlusion of the posterior ciliary artery. I. Effect on choroidal circulation. *Brit. J. Ophthal.* 56: *719-735* (1972a).

HAYREH, S.S. & BAINES, J.A.B. Occlusion of the posterior artery. II. Chorio-retinal lesions. *Brit. J. Ophthal.* 56: *736-753* (1972b).

HAYREH, S.S. & BAINES, J.A.B. Occlusion of the vortex veins. An experimental study. *Brit. J. Ophthal.* 57: *217-238* (1973).

HYVARINEN, L. MAUMENEE, A.E., GEORGE, T. & WEINSTEIN, G. Fluorescein angiography of choriocapillaris. *Amer. J. Ophthal.* 67: *653-666* (1969).

KREY, H.F. Segmental vascular patterns of the choriocapillaris. *Amer. J. Ophthal.* 80: *198-202* (1975).

OOSTERHUIS, J.A. & BOEN-TAN, T. N. Choroidal fluorescence in the normal human eye. *Ophthalmologica* 162: *246-260* (1971).

RUSKELL, G.L. Choroidal vascularization in the rabbit. *Amer. J. Ophthal.* 52: *807-815* (1961).

RING, H.G. & FUJINO, T. Observations on the anatomy and pathology of the choroidal vasculature. *Arch. Ophthal.* (Chicago) 78: *431-444* (1967).

SHIMIZU, J., YOKOCHI, K. & OKANO, T. Fluorescein angiography of the choroid. *Jap. J. Ophthal.* 18: *97-108* (1974).

TORCZYNSKI, E. & TSO, M.O. The architecture of the choriocapillaris at the posterior pole. *J. Ophthal.* 81: *428-440* (1976).

VILSTRUP, G. Studies on the choroid circulation. Edit. Ejnar Munksgaard, Copenhagen (1952).

WEITER, J.J. & ERNEST, J.T. Anatomy of the choroidal vasculature. *Amer. J. Ophthal.* 78: *583-590* (1974).

WYBAR, K.C. A study of the choroidal circulation of the eye in man. *J. Anat.* (London) 88: *94-98* (1954a).

WYBAR, K.C. Vascular anatomy of the choroid in relation to selective localization of ocular disease. *Brit. J. Ophthal.* 38: *513-527* (1954b).

YOKOCHI, K., MARUYAMA, H. & SODENO, Y. Microcirculation of the disc and peripapillary choroid. *Acta Soc. Ophthal. Jap.* 77 (10): *1534-1542* (1973).

Author's address:
Department of Ophthalmology
University of Iowa Hospitals & Clinics
Iowa City, Iowa 52242
USA

CHOROIDAL ARTERIAL OCCLUSIVE DISORDERS

SOHAN SINGH HAYREH M.D., Ph.D., F.R.C.S.

(Iowa City, USA)

Having previously given the background information on the physiological anatomy of the choroidal vasculature (HAYREH, 1976), I would like very briefly to discuss the various lesions seen in choroidal arterial occlusive disorders. These I have discussed in detail elsewhere (HAYREH, 1974a, b, 1975a, b; HAYREH & BAINES, 1972a, b). The choroid supplies the overlying pigment epithelium and the outer retina, which comprises the layer of rods and cones, the outer nuclear and plexiform layers, and the whole thickness of the foveal retina. In eyes with a cilioretinal artery, a variable area of the inner retina is also supplied. Although the peripapillary choroid also takes part in the blood supply of the anterior part of the optic nerve, I do not propose to discuss nerve lesions here, as I have dealt with them at length elsewhere (HAYREH, 1975b).

Choroidal arterial occlusive lesions can conveniently be divided into two categories:

I Lesions due to occlusion of the posterior ciliary arteries or their subdivisions.

II. Lesions due to localized occlusion of choriocapillaris units.

I. LESIONS DUE TO OCCLUSION OF THE POSTERIOR CILIARY ARTERIES OR THEIR SUBDIVISIONS

Experimental occlusion of the posterior ciliary arteries in rhesus monkeys (HAYREH & BAINES, 1972a) produced patchy fundus lesions situated posterior to the equator and in the region of supply by the occluded artery, i.e., in the temporal part in lateral posterior ciliary artery occlusion, in the nasal part in medial posterior ciliary artery occlusion, and in both temporal and nasal parts in occlusion of all the posterior ciliary arteries (Fig. 1). The lesions were of all shapes and sizes, usually triangular, wedge-shaped, geographical or sectoral, and varying from tiny spots corresponding to an individual choriocapillaris segment to large ones involving a considerable area (Fig. 2, 3); the intervening fundus appeared normal. Lateral posterior ciliary artery occlusion produced more extensive lesions than medial posterior ciliary artery occlusion. The color of the lesions depended upon their stage of evolution — fresh patches seen within 24 hours after the occlusion were well-defined and homogeneously white in color (Fig. 1a, 2, 3), due to infarc-

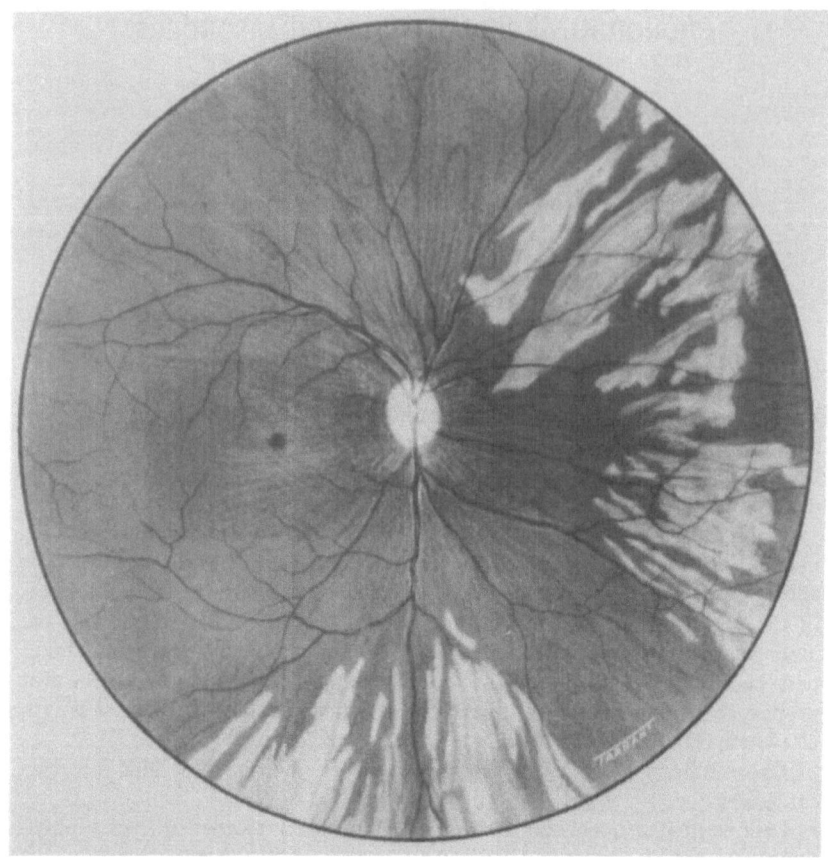

Fig. 1. Fundus appearances in rhesus monkey after experimental occlusion of all posterior ciliary arteries.
a. After 4 days.

tion of the pigment epithelium and outer retinal layers (Fig. 4); after 2-3 weeks they assumed a granular, greyish, depigmented appearance, with areas of hyperpigmentation around them (Fig. 1b). Occasionally no depigmented patches were visible, and the fundus showed areas of hyperpigmentation only. In Fig. 3 the narrow strips of normal-looking fundus between the white lesions were mostly overlying large choroidal veins; this would indicate that diffusion of oxygen through the thin-walled choroidal veins is enough to prevent ischemic damage to the overlying tissue. The fluorescein angiographic pattern of the choroidal lesions depends upon the age of the lesion. In fresh white lesions no background choroidal fluorescence was usually seen during the transit of the dye, but during the late phase the necrotic tissue stained with fluorescein (Fig. 5a). In old lesions there was mottled hyperfluorescence with hypofluorescent spots corresponding to the pigmented areas during the transit of the dye, with no late staining (Fig. 5b). ANDERSON & DAVIS (1974) confirmed these experimental observations. BUETTNER et al. (1973), by similar studies, found pigment epithelial changes as early as one hour after posterior ciliary artery occlusion and, in 24 hours, necrosis of the pigment epithelium and photoreceptor cells.

Clinically, similar wedge-shaped chorioretinal degenerative patches, with the apex of the wedge towards the posterior pole and the base towards the periphery of the fundus (Fig. 6), have been described in a large number of conditions. The earliest description seems to be that of HEPBURN in 1912 and 1935, who described sectoral fundus lesions in patients, starting with ill-defined areas of retinal edema, which later resolved to sectoral pigmentary changes in the pigment epithelium. AMALRIC (1971) has reported similar lesions since 1958. Their exact pathogenesis was firmly established by the experimental production of similar lesions in monkeys (ANDERSON & DAVIS, 1974; HAYREH & BAINES, 1972a). Since then many case reports have appeared in the literature describing ischemic lesions of the choroid. The various conditions in which these are seen can be classified as follows:

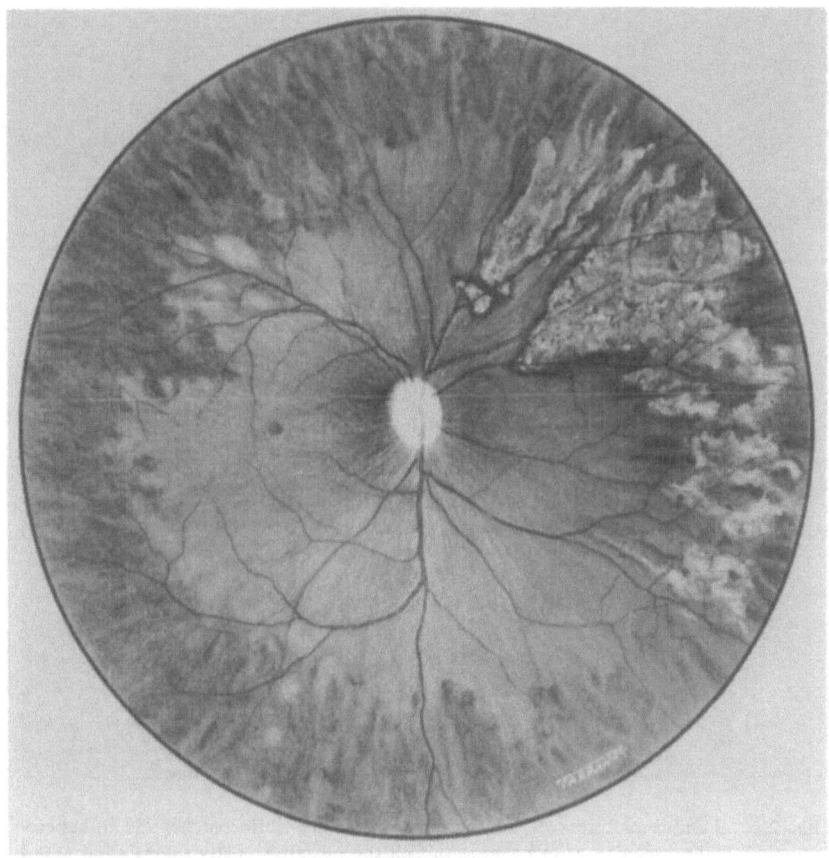

b. After 91 days.

213

a. Systemic diseases

1. Temporal arteritis (AMALRIC, 1971; FOULDS et al., 1971; HAYREH, 1975a; HAYREH & BAINES, 1972b) (Fig. 6).
2. Malignant hypertension (AMALRIC, 1971).

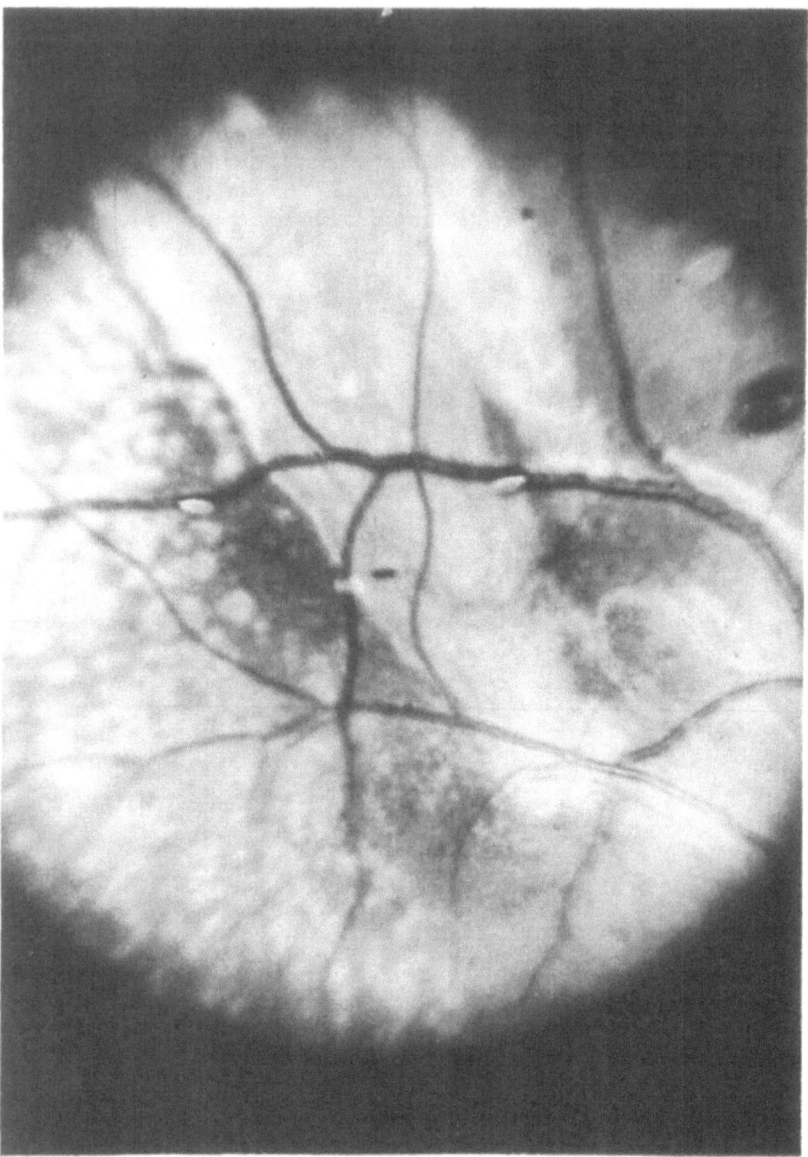

Fig. 2, 3. Fundus pictures of rhesus monkey showing white patches (2) in supero-temporal region one day after occlusion of all the posterior ciliary arteries and (3) in infero-temporal region 2 days after occlusion of the lateral posterior ciliary artery.

3. Toxemia of pregnancy (AMALRIC, 1971).
4. Chronic glomerulonephritis (AMALRIC, 1971).
5. Collagen diseases, e.g., systemic lupus erythematosus (AMALRIC, 1971), scleroderma (KLIEN, 1968), periarteritis nodosa, etc.
6. Hemorrhagic shock (AMALRIC, 1971).
7. Hematologic diseases, e.g., sickle cell disease (CONDON et al., 1973), polycythemia (AMALRIC, 1971), and cryoglobulinemia (AMALRIC, 1971).
8. Raynaud's disease (AMALRIC, 1971).

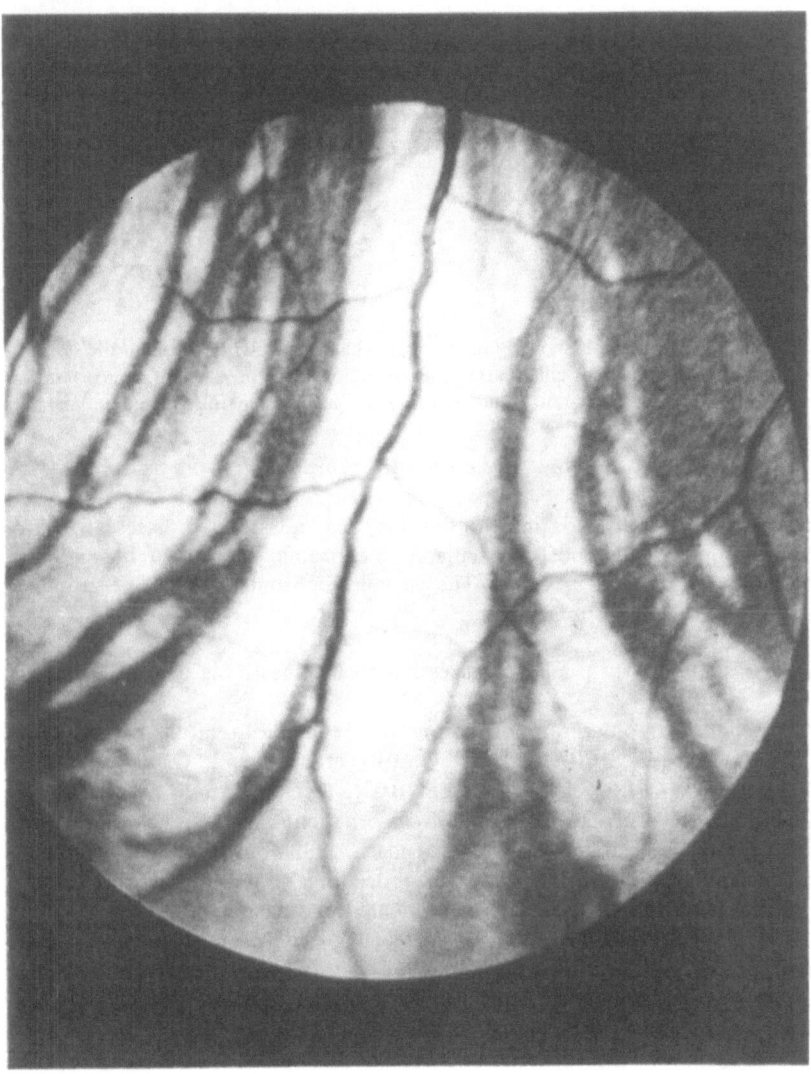

Fig. 3. For legend see Fig. 2

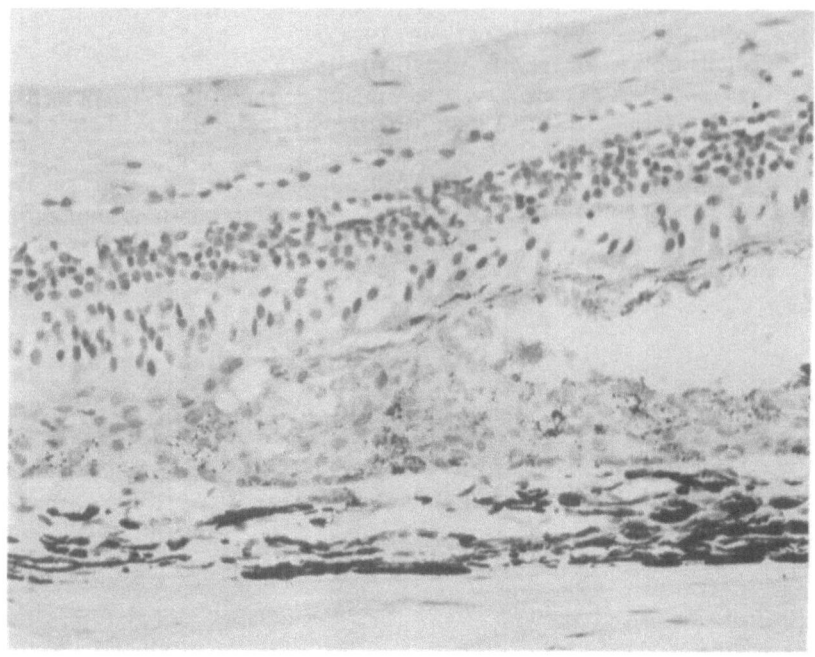

Fig. 4. Microphotograph showing microscopic changes in a white patch in the fundus, 11 days after the posterior ciliary artery occlusion. Note the presence of necrosis of the pigment epithelium, rods, cones and outer nuclear layer. Hematoxylin and eosin stain.

b. Local vascular disorders

The arterial supply to the choroid may be cut off by diseases of the carotid, ophthalmic, posterior ciliary or choroidal arteries or by embolic occlusion of the latter vessels. The various reported cases can be grouped into the following disorders:

1. Ocular compression during anesthesia

A large number of case reports are available in the literature (AMALRIC, 1971; CARR & SIEGEL, 1973; GAVIO et al., 1962; GILLAN, 1953; GIVNER & JAFFE, 1950; HOLLENHORST et al., 1954; JAMPOL et al., 1975a; SLOCUM et al., 1948) in which a patient had his eye compressed during anesthesia, either by the face mask or by the head rest (as in the sitting position used in neurosurgical procedures); in some cases this situation was made worse by associated systemic hypotension.

Since in almost all cases there is associated central retinal artery occlusion as well, the retinal changes masked the underlying lesion, misleading earlier authors into considering that the visual loss and fundus lesions were due to occlusion of the central retinal artery, although the associated chorioretinal pigmentary degeneration could not be explained on the basis of the central retinal artery occlusion alone. Some of these cases were even in-

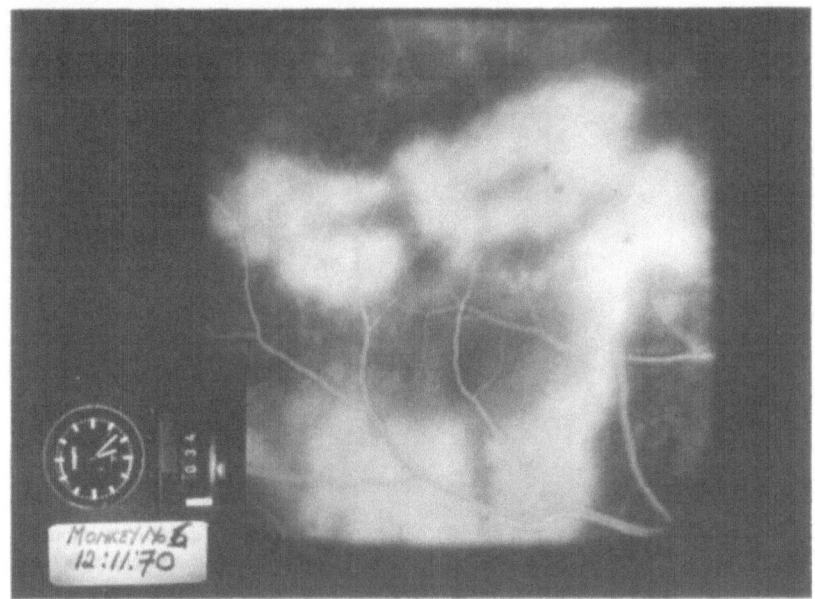

Fig. 5. Fluorescein angiograms of a rhesus monkey fundus in the macular region and the area temporal to it after lateral posterior ciliary artery occlusion.

a. 2 days after the occlusion showing late fluorescence of the white patches.

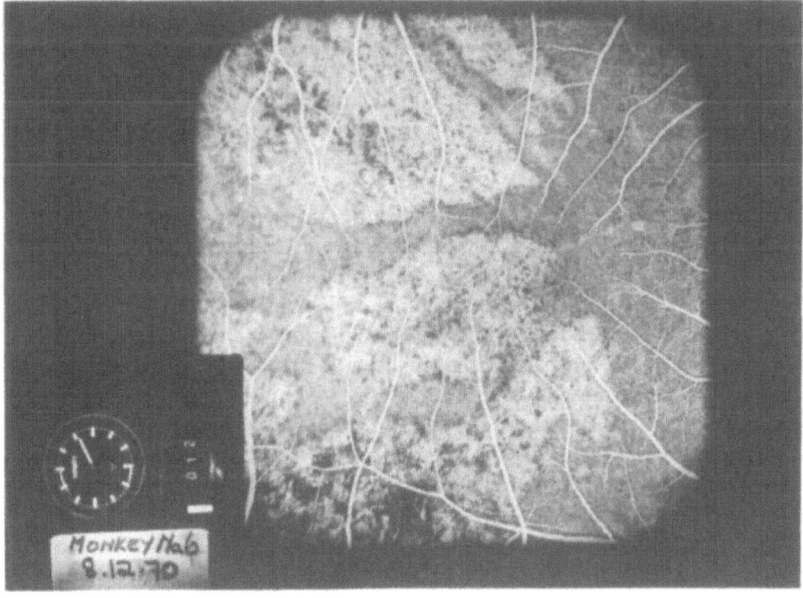

b. Same after 26 days after the occlusion, showing unmasking of the choroidal fluorescence.

217

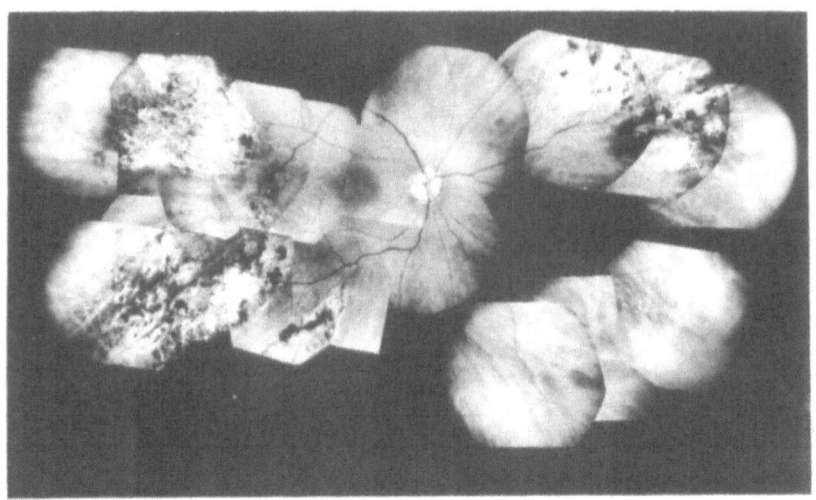

Fig. 6. Chorioretinal lesions in a 68-year old man with temporal arteritis 12 months after the onset. The patient had no perception of light because of anterior ischemic optic neuropathy in both eyes, and had bilateral extensive chorioretinal lesions.

cluded in the category of retinitis pigmentosa (CARR & SIEGEL, 1973) because of the close ophthalmoscopic resemblance between the two.

2. Carotid artery disease

Atheromatous lesion, stenosis, or occlusion of the carotid arteries (AMAL-RIC, 1971) or their involvement by phycomycosis (BULLOCK et al., 1974) have been reported to cause choroidal ischemic lesions.

3. Photocoagulation

In the treatment of various types of retinopathy by photocoagulation the underlying choroidal arteries may be inadvertently closed. I have seen choroidal ischemic lesions produced after experimental photocoagulation of the retinal vessels in rhesus monkeys, and these lesions are usually situated in the peripheral fundus. Recently photocoagulation for proliferative sickle-cell retinopathy has been reported to be associated with acute choroidal infarcts in 17 eyes (GOLDBAUM et al., 1976); the fundus lesions were located peripheral to the photocoagulation sites. Heavy photocoagulation of the macular region, advocated by some for neovascularization in this area, could produce choroidal ischemic lesions, because all the temporal short posterior ciliary arteries initially join the choroid in that area.

4. Trauma

Traumatic lesions of the choroidal arteries or their parent trunks may produce choroidal infarction (AMALRIC, 1971).

218

5. Arteriosclerosis or atherosclerosis of the posterior
ciliary arteries or their subdivisions

In eyes of middle-aged and older patients where no obvious cause can be found for the vascular occlusion, this may be responsible for the choroidal ischemia. Presumably many segmental chorioretinal degenerative lesions of obscure etiology and some of the atypical sectoral or uniocular retinitis pigmentosas also belong to the category of choroidal arterial occlusive disorders.

Long posterior ciliary artery occlusion: Ischemic choroidal lesions in the distribution of the long posterior ciliary artery have been reported (AMALRIC, 1963; GOLDBAUM et al., 1976). They have a characteristic location in the region of supply by the artery (HAYREH, 1974b). The occurrence of anterior segment ischemia after retinal detachment surgery has been attributed in the past to interference with the long posterior ciliary arteries. My studies revealed that there is no basis for such an assumption (HAYREH, 1974b).

II. LESIONS DUE TO DISORDERS OF THE CHORIOCAPILLARIS

a. Occlusive disorders

In this group can be included lesions with well-established histopathological evidence of occlusion of the choriocapillaris, as well as those where no such proof is available as yet because of the benign nature of the lesions.

1. Small localized chorioretinal infarcts, corresponding to localized segments of choriocapillaris supplied by terminal choroidal arterioles (HAYREH, 1974a, 1975b) or vessels of similar size

These are seen in conditions associated with fibrinoid necrosis of the arterioles. This occurs in malignant hypertension (KLIEN, 1968), chronic glomerulonephritis (KLIEN, 1968), toxemia of pregnancy (GITTER et al., 1968; KLIEN, 1968), scleroderma (KLIEN, 1968), periarteritis nodosa and other collagen diseases. There is infarction of the pigment epithelium and the adjacent layers of the retina. These lesions are equivalent to the cotton-wool spots seen in the retinopathy in these diseases, the former due to occlusion of terminal choroidal arterioles and the latter to occlusion of terminal retinal arterioles. Similar chorioretinal infarcts have also been reported in Goodpasture syndrome (JAMPOL et al., 1975b). The normal pigment epithelium exercises a chorioretinal barrier which breaks down as a result of ischemic damage to the pigment epithelial cells. This seems to be responsible for the non-rhegmatogenous serous retinal detachment seen in most of the above-mentioned conditions. During the acute phase fluorescein angiography reveals a fluorescein leak from the choroid at the site of the lesion (GITTER et al., 1968); and the dye gradually accumulates in the subretinal fluid. These lesions later on resolve and leave small isolated chorioretinal degenerative lesions containing central clumps of pigment sur-

219

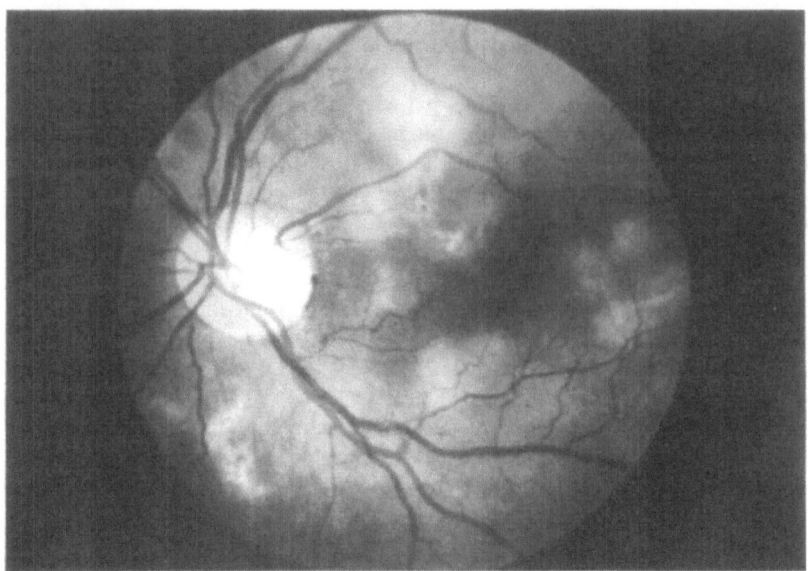

Fig. 7. In so-called 'Acute posterior multifocal placoid pigment epitheliopathy'.
a. Fundus appearances during the acute phase.

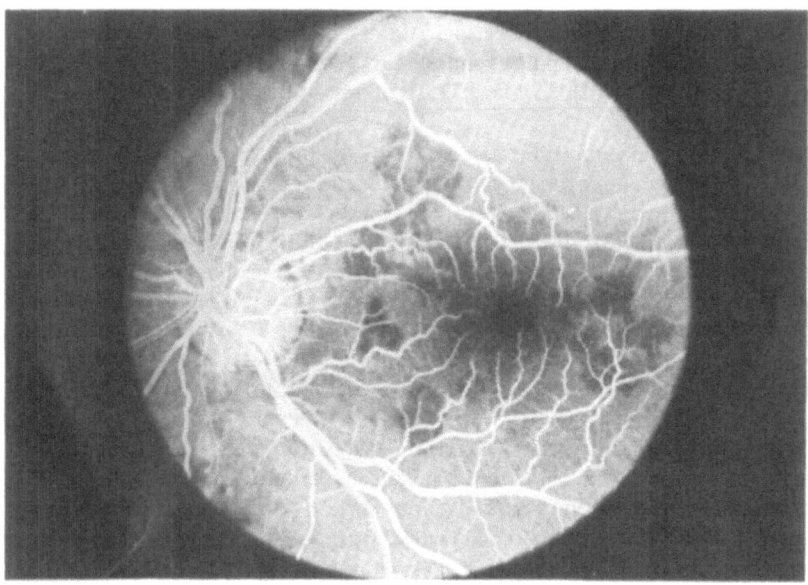

b. Fluorescein fundus angiogram during arteriovenous phase, showing localized non-filling of the choroid in the areas of the lesions.

220

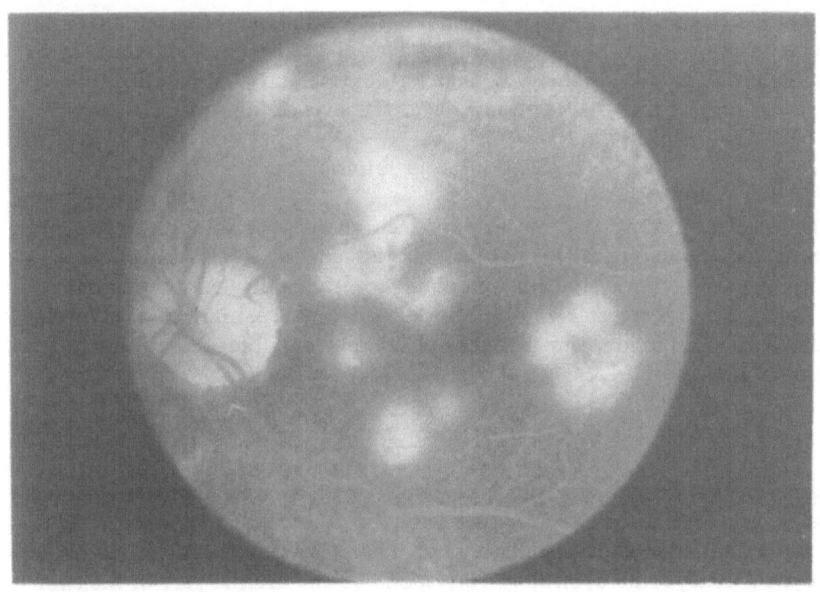

c. Fluorescein fundus angiogram during the late phase, showing fluorescein staining of the lesions (compare with Fig. 5a).

rounded by a yellowish halo (KLIEN, 1968), which have been called Elschnig's spots. Similar lesions have been produced experimentally in animals (GAY et al., 1964; GOLDOR & GAY, 1967; HENKIND, 1967).

2. So-called 'Acute posterior multifocal placoid pigment epitheliopathy' (GASS, 1968)

The ophthalmoscopic and fluorescein angiographic findings in this disease entity are highly suggestive of its being occlusive disorder of the terminal choroidal arterioles, because each focus in this disease has a close resemblance in size and shape to one or several combined units of choriocapillaris (Fig. 7). The initial whitish focus probably represents pigment epithelial infarction and the later depigmented spots indicate pigment epithelium degeneration overlying the occluded units of the choriocapillaris. However, the cause of the occlusion still remains obscure. I have recently come across several cases with markedly elevated erythrocyte sedimentation rate without any detectable systemic or ocular cause.

3. Harada's disease

During the acute phase fluorescein angiography reveals multiple fluorescent spots situated at the level of the pigment epithelium (SHIKANO & SHIMIZU, 1968) which very much correspond in size and shape to the

221

choriocapillaris units. There is associated non-rhegmatogenous serous retinal detachment due to breakdown of the barrier at the level of the pigment epithelium. Later on there is pigment epithelium degeneration. These findings suggest that the lesion may be at the level of the choriocapillaris.

4. Central serous retinopathy

The classical leaking fluorescent spot seen on fluorescein angiography and associated serous retinal detachment in this condition may be due to involvement of a choriocapillaris unit and its overlying pigment epithelium.

In 2, 3 and 4 we lack any definite histopathological information on the nature of the lesions in the choriocapillaris and the entire hypothesis remains unproven.

b. Other lesions

Some fundus lesions very much resemble choriocapillaris units in size and shape, and one is tempted to speculate that these lesions are also due to disorders of the choriocapillaris. For example, the lesions in so-called Doyne's honeycomb dystrophy correspond to the arterial part of the choriocapillaris unit (HAYREH, 1974a, 1975b) and suggest that they may be due to a disorder of the arterial segment of the choriocapillaris. In fundus flavimaculatus the shape and distribution of the 'fish tail' lesions resemble venous segments of the choriocapillaris units (HAYREH, 1974a, 1975b) and suggest that this may be a disorder of the venous part of the choriocapillaris unit. However, the inheritance pattern seen in this syndrome is hard to explain on a vascular basis.

Fluorescein fundus angiography has therefore been the chief technique responsible for giving us a great amount of new information on the physiological anatomy of the choroidal vasculature, and most of the information on the choroidal arterial occlusive disorders discussed above.

ACKNOWLEDGEMENT

I am grateful to Mrs. Julie Wolf for the secretarial help.

REFERENCES

AMALRIC, P. Le territoire chorio-retinien de l'artere ciliaire longue posterieure. Etude clinique. *Bull. Soc. d'Ophtal. Fr.* 5: *1-10* (1963).

AMALRIC, P. Acute choroidal ischaemia. *Trans. Ophthal. Soc. U.K.* 91: *305-322* (1971).

ANDERSON, D.R. & DAVIS, E.B. Retina and optic nerve after posterior ciliary artery occlusion. *Arch. Ophthal.* 92: *422-426* (1974).

BUETTNER, H., MACHEMER, R., CHARLES, S. & ANDERSON, D.R. Experimental deprivation of choroidal blood flow. *Amer. J. Ophthal.* 75: *943-952* (1973).

BULLOCK, J.D., JAMPOL, L.M. & FEZZA, A.J. Two cases of orbital phycomycosis with recovery. *Amer. J. Ophthal.* 78: *811-815* (1974).

CARR, R.E. & SIEGEL, I.M. Unilateral retinitis pigmentosa. *Arch. Ophthal.* 90: *21-26* (1973).

CONDON, P.I., SERJEANT, G.R. & IKEDA, H. Unusual chorioretinal degeneration in sickle cell disease. *Brit. J. Ophthal.* 57: *81-88* (1973).

FOULDS, W.S., LEE, W.R. & TAYLOR, W.O.G. Clinical and pathological aspects of choroidal ischaemia. *Trans. Ophthal. Soc. U.K.* 91: *323-341* (1971).

GASS, J.D.M. Acute posterior multifocal placoid pigment epitheliopathy. *Arch. Ophthal.* 80: *177-185* (1968).

GAVIO, C.A., CABANNE, G.R. & REY, H. Ceguera unilateral postanestesia general. *Arch. Oftal. B. Aires* 37: *265-267* (1962).

GAY, A.J., GOLDOR, H. & SMITH, M. Chorioretinal vascular occlusions with latex spheres. *Invest. Ophthal.* 3: *647-656* (1964).

GILLAN, J.G. Two cases of unilateral blindness following anesthesia with vascular hypotension. *Can. Med. Assoc. J.* 69: *294-296* (1953).

GITTER, K.A., HOUSER, B.P., SARIN, L.K. & JUSTICE, J. Toxemia of pregnancy. *Arch. Ophthal.* 80: *449-454* (1968).

GIVNER, I. & JAFFE, N. Occlusion of the central retinal artery following anesthesia. *Arch. Ophthal.* 43: *197-201* (1950).

GOLDBAUM, M.H., GALINOS, S.O., APPLE, D., ASDOURIAN, G.K., NAGPAL, K., JAMPOL, L., WOOLF, M.B. & BUSSE, B. Acute choroidal ischemia as a complication of photocoagulation. *Arch. Ophthal.* 94: *1025-1035* (1976).

GOLDOR, H. & GAY, A.J. Chorioretinal vascular lesions with latex microspheres (a long-term study). Part II. *Invest. Ophthal.* 6: *51-58* (1967).

HEPBURN, M.L. Inflammatory and vascular diseases of the choroid. *Trans. Ophthal. Soc. U.K.* 32: *361-386* (1912).

HEPBURN, M.L. The role played by the pigment and visual fields in the diagnosis of the fundus. *Trans. Ophthal. Soc. U.K.* 55: *434-477* (1935).

HAYREH, S.S. The choriocapillaris. *Albrecht v. Graefes Arch. Ophthal.* 192: *165-179* (1974a).

HAYREH, S.S. Long posterior ciliary arteries. *Albrecht v. Graefes Arch. Ophthal.* 192: *197-213* (1974b).

HAYREH, S.S. Anterior ischemic optic neuropathy. Springer-Verlag, New York, Heidelberg (1975a).

HAYREH, S.S. Segmental nature of the choroidal vasculature. *Brit. J. Ophthal.* 59: *631-648* (1975b).

HAYREH, S.S. Physiological anatomy of the choroidal vasculature. Proc. International fluorescein angiography symposium, *Doc. Ophthalm. Proc. Series* 10: *201-209* (1976).

HAYREH, S.S. & BAINES, J.A.B. Occlusion of the posterior ciliary artery. II. Chorioretinal lesions. *Brit. J. Ophthal.* 56: *736-753* (1972a).

HAYREH, S.S. & BAINES, J.A.B. Occlusion of the posterior ciliary artery. III. Effects on the optic nerve head. *Brit. J. Ophthal.* 56: *754-764* (1972b).

HENKIND, P. In discussion of paper by Goldor & Gay, *Invest. Ophthal.* 6: *55-58* (1967).

HOLLENHORST, R.W., SVIEN, H.J. & BENOIT, C.F. Unilateral blindness occurring during anesthesia for neuro-surgical operations. *Arch. Ophthal.* 52: *819-930* (1954).

JAMPOL, L.M., GOLDBAUM, M., ROSENBERG, M. & BAHR, R. Ischemia of ciliary arterial circulation from ocular compression. *Arch. Ophthal.* 93: *1311-1317* (1975a).

JAMPOL, L.M., LAHAV, M., ALBERT, D.M. & CRAFT, J. Ocular clinical findings and basement membrane changes in Goodpasture's syndrome. *Amer. J. Ophthal.* 79: *452-463* (1975b).

KLIEN, B.A. Ischemic infarcts of the choroid (Elschnig spots). *Amer. J. Ophthal.* 66: *1069-1074* (1968).

SHIKANO, S. & SHIMIZU, K. Atlas of fluorescence fundus angiography. pp. *125-135.* Igaku Shoin Ltd, Tokyo (1968).

SLOCUM, H.C., O'NEAL, K.C. & ALLEN, C.R. Neurovascular complications from malposition on the operating table. *Surg. Gyn. Obstet.* 86: *729-734* (1948).

Author's address:
Department of Ophthalmology
University of Iowa Hospitals & Clinics
Iowa City, Iowa 52242
USA

DISCUSSION

Dr Amalric: J'ai vu tout à l'heure des clichés de Hayreh qui m'ont un peu surpris, aussi durant la pose, j'ai demandé à ce qu'on les replace; vous allez les voir.

Dans cet exemple expérimental que nous a montré Hayreh, nous voyons sur le cliché de gauche la zone maculaire oblitérée avec une vascularisation intacte tout autour. C'est sur ce cas particulier que je voudrais demander à Mr Hayreh s'il ne pense pas que dans certains cas il puisse y avoir quelques artérioles qui correspondent à la zone maculaire centrale.

Dr Hayreh: No, I do not think so. In fact this demonstrates very well the distribution by the various segments of the short posterior ciliary arteries which are coming into this area. It also shows very well the areas of distribution by the various short posterior ciliary arteries meeting right in the fovea. Why is this filling? Well, that is because, if you remember I pointed out in my presentation the peripapillary choroid fills up from behind through its communications with the pial plexus of the optic nerve. This filling gradually extends and always fills the choroid from the macular region up to the optic disc. That is why this area is always spared. And the other fact one has to keep in mind is that here we are dealing with experimental studies in very young healthy animals, the age of which about corresponds to teenagers (about 10-12 years old) in the human. Hence they (the monkeys) have very good potentials for anastomoses, whereas in an old person of 60-70 years old we will get much more massive damage than we see in healthy animals. In addition to that, some filling also comes from the venous circulation by retrograde filling. Does this satisfy you?

Dr von Winning: I cannot readily comprehend that, following the initial infarction of the choroid and its scar formation, there is a slowly progressive course and I would ask what is the substrate of this; secondly, when there is a progressive area, if this is only inside the borders of the vascular distribution of that particular zone or if it spreads outside the original vascular zone?

Dr Hayreh: If I correctly understand, you want to know how long these lesions keep on progressing. I followed these animals mostly up to three months. There was a very mild pigmentary change. If you remember the big diagram which I showed to demonstrate the changes in the periphery of the fundus after three months, the lesion was hyperpigmented but there was no distinct chorioretinal scarring. The chorioretinal scars appear only in the area where we see infarcts to begin with. It does not get any worse than that and it also does not spread beyond the involved zone.

Dr von Winning: The progressive course is thus only for a limited period.

Dr Hayreh: Yes, only for a limited period.

Dr Heimann: Concerning the macular supply of the choroid. We injected isolated branches in different human eyebank eyes and found a segmental distribution but no watershed zone in the macular area.

Dr Gass: It seems to me that Dr Hayreh, Dr Shimizu and Dr Amalric have demonstrated quite well that there is a segmental blood supply of the choroid. I think that this is not surprising as most tissues in the body have a segmental blood supply. The important question that needs answering, and there seems to be some disagreement, is: is there a fair or good possibility for anastomotic blood flow in the choroid, and what does all this mean clinically? It seems to me that clinically we rarely see diseases, particularly in the macular region that we can attribute to choroidal arterial insufficiency. We do see diseases which reflect obstruction of the choriocapillaris. All of the anatomical evidence including that provided by Dr Hayreh shows that there is an excellent possibility for anastomosis in the choroidal circulation. Despite the fact that the choriocapillaris is arranged into little segments each supplied by a central artery and drained by peripheral venules, there would appear to be free communication across these zones. I should like to say that Dr Hayreh's argument that there is no anastomosis would be much stronger if after occluding a short ciliary artery he could show us a series of angiographic pictures made for a time greater than the arteriovenous phase. If we could see pictures for at least five to ten minutes, I believe that we would see evidence of dye spreading from the zone of perfusion into the zone of occlusion. If there is no anastomosis, why don't we see evidence of outer retinal infarction within several hours after occluding the monkey's choroidal artery? I think we have to be careful in interpreting these experimental studies where a short ciliary artery is suddenly cut and dye is immediately injected into adjacent arteries. Failure of the dye to perfuse an area during the first 30 to 60 seconds is not unequivocal evidence that there are no pathways of anastomosis between the perfused and nonperfused areas. Dr Hayreh, what do you see in those monkeys beyond 10-12 seconds following injection of the dye?

Dr Hayreh: We will have to sit up all evening if I were to give evidence for all the things Dr Gass has asked for and I do have angiograms of all these features. These eyes were not only followed for 15-20 seconds but were followed for three months and angiography was done every other day initially to follow exactly what happened and how the circulation in the occluded segments progressed. Once there is a filling defect in the choriocapillaris, it does not fill simply by extension from already filled choriocapillaris into the unfilled zone as the time passes, but the empty segments fill by a retrograde flow through the venous channels and other sources. The filling defects retain their sharp borders till late. That answers one of your questions because you wanted to know if there was any extension of filling from the filled choriocapillaris into the empty choriocapillaris.

Dr Gass: How do you explain that on the basis of your diagram? Why don't you get dye moving across, if the anatomy of the choriocapillaris is as shown in Dr Shimizu's preparation and even in your diagram?

225

Dr Hayreh: We do not know why it does not happen. We have to start with the facts which we see. The fact is that we have not seen this extension and we have not seen this in the human as well. I have no satisfactory explanation for that. I have just given you the information based on what I have seen, but I do not know the full mechanism beyond that.

Dr Gass: I think we have to accept that. I would make it much more convincing if you would include some angiograms that go up to 1 minute, 5 minutes.

Dr Hayreh: I already pointed out that if I were to cover the entire subject in detail, it would require more time than was given to me. I tried to present the maximum material in the minimum time available. What else could I do?

Dr Archer: I would agree with Dr Gass that we now have to examine more closely the pathophysiology of the retina and choroid. Dr Ernest, at the University of Chicago has utilised an oxygen micro electrode advanced into the retina to estimate choroidal blood flow. After tying off a temporal posterior ciliary artery he found there was a marked decrease in macular oxygen pressure levels although some blood flow persisted. After about 3 weeks the macular oxygen pressure levels returned to almost normal. Therefore I think function at the macula is probably not much affected due to the fairly rapid return of the macular choroidal blood supply to normal. When a temporal short posterior ciliary artery occulusion is accommpanied by ligation of a nasal vortex vein alteration in macular oxygen pressures were very much reduced therefore it would seem that blood can be shunted from one side of the choroidal venous circulation to the other.

Dr Hayreh: I would agree with that. That is what I was showing. The vortex veins act as a very important safety mechanism to prevent massive infarction of the choroid. If there was no regurgitation through the vortex veins, we would get much more extensive lesions in the choroid. And the other thing is that the macular choroid fills from the nasal side via the adjacent peripapillary choroid, the latter fills by its pial communications. The oxygen concentration is very high because only 3% of the arterial oxygen is utilised normally by the choroid and high concentration of the venous blood in the choroid is sufficient to maintain viability of the pigment epithelium and the rest of the tissue so long as some venous blood can flow into it even after 10 minutes of its entering the choroidal vascular bed.

Dr Evans: Dr Hayreh has quoted our report* of 1972 with results obtained from healthy human beings, concerning the delays in fluorescein filling of choroidal watershed zones of up to 4 seconds, as measured by cineangiography. I fail to understand why his term 'physiological filling defect' should be preferable to 'physiological filling delay'. I also cannot appreciate why a distinction of 'arterio-venous phase' (for an acceptable range of normal choroidial filling variations) as opposed to 'much later' (for true filling

---

* EVANS, SHIMIZU, et al. Fluorescein cineangiography of the optic nerve head. *Trans. Am. Acad. Ophthalm. Otolaryng.* 77: OP-260-273 (1973).

defects should be more appropiate than an accurate, simple notation of the time interval itself. The 'arterio-venous phase' refers to the retina, is vague and variable, and has no constant relation to the onset of choroidal perfusion. And 'much later' is obviously even less quantitative. Those may be semantics only. But I am particularly disturbed about Dr Hayreh's implications that we denied the existence of *any* real pathological fluorescence filling defects in the human choroid. At no time did we ever suggest that. As Dr Hayreh and we all remember, 5-6 years ago, some of the suction cup experiments resulted in claims of significance for almost any 'dark' area in the peripapillary choroid in connection with artificially increased intra-ocular pressure. It was especially against those claims that we underscored the practically universal presence of the physiological choroidal watershed areas with their delayed dye filling.

Dr Henkind: I think after discussing his findings with Dr Shimizu, and knowing Dr Hayreh's findings quite intimately, I am convinced both of them are right. The argument really should not be extrapolated to what happen in chronic pathology. What Shimizu is showing on injections of vascular pathways I think Singh Hayreh shows the same pathway involved in an acute experiment which generally has no hearing on the human situation and nobody has actually demonstrated what actually happens in the chronic situation. Where we really are lacking evidence is not on the vascular patterns anymore or the microstructure but what happens in chronic disease. Unfortunately, a paper by Dr Federman apparently was supposed to be given at this meeting. Dr Federman of Philadelphia has evidence that could be the fruit for the next ISFA meeting in 4 years. He has shown by freeze fracture techniques — and I unfortunately could not show the slides for lack of time yesterday — that the pore system in the choriocapillaris is not the same in all regions of the fundus. He is able to show that the pores differ in distribution from the macula to the equator, to the periphery. But what is even more dramatic is that the pores changes direction in various diseases, for example, over malignant melanomas the pores point towards the melanoma instead of pointing towards the retina, suggesting that the pore system itself may be a dynamic and not a constant system; one that could change depending on physiological needs. If this indeed proves to be correct then our whole emphasis on the choroid as a pretty static structure will change and I would suspect that you could explain for instance diseases like Haradas disease where you get a tremendous output of fluid not on the basis that the choroid does not normally leak but that it is leaking more because the pore system is breaking down or being altered.

ETUDE DE LA CIRCULATION CHORIO-CAPILLAIRE
DU FOND D'OEIL HUMAIN

JEAN-PIERRE AUBRY

(Albi, France)

L'étude angiographique de Fonds d'yeux normaux apporte des éléments intéressants sur la circulation choroïdienne. Nous avons voulu étudier plus spécialement deux d'entre eux, car ils nous ont paru essentiels;

En premier lieu, les clichés précoces d'angiographies de Fonds d'yeux normaux nous ont montré l'existence quasi-constante de phénomènes de retard au niveau de zones très localisées de l'épithélium pigmentaire.

Deuxièmement, l'étude de montages réalisés à partir de clichés de temps veineux nous a permis de mettre en évidence au niveau du fond d'oeil, une zone privilégiée sur le plan de la circulation choriocapillaire, et qui correspond à peu près à la partie centrale du pôle postérieur.

Sur les clichés précoces des angiographies, il existe des zones où la fluorescence de l'épithélium pigmenté est absente. Les zones restent sombres alors que le fond pigmentaire voisin s'imprègne progressivement de colorant. Leur forme et leur surface sont variables selon les sujets, mais elles ont certains caractères communs qu'il semble intéressant de dégager. Il sagit de plages à contours irréguliers, en carte de géographie, pouvant parfois prendre un aspect géométrique. Leur fréquence est maximale au niveau du pôle postérieur. Ces images sont parfaitement reproductibles d'une angiographie à une autre, et ce, quel que soit le temps qui les sépare. Elles se rencontrent surtout chez les sujets jeunes, et se localisent surtout au niveau de la région périmaculaire (La macula est difficile à explorer à cause des divers écrans pigmentaires présents à son niveau).

Nous avons fait porter notre étude sur 129 angiographies normales présentant des zones de retard circulatoires, la méthode utilisée étant de décalquer ces zones à partir des clichés angiographiques eux-mêmes.

Nous avons ainsi relevé deux grands groupes de retards, différant uniquement entre eux par leur surface.

— Les uns, petits, disposés parfois en mosaïque plus ou moins dense, gardent leurs caractères morphologiques tout au long des temps précoces; leur imprégnation uniforme et homogène par le colorant les fait disparaître prgressivement; ils se condondent alors avec les zones voisines, comblant ainsi leur retard.

— Le deuxième groupe est formé par des retards occupant une surface beaucoup plus étendue. De densité uniforme sur les premiers clichés, ils peuvent parfois se morceler en plages secondaires, identiques à celles du premier groupe. Leur vitesse d'imprégnation peut alors varier de l'une à l'autre. Mais il faut insister sur le fait que chacune de ces plages s'imprègne de façon homogène.

La rapidité de disparition de ces images est variable. Au cours de notre étude, nous avons relevé des valeurs de temps s'échelonnant entre 2 secondes et 12 secondes (différence entre le temps d'apparition de ces images et leur disparition complète). La moyenne de nos mesures se situe à 5 secondes 6/10 pour les 129 fonds d'yeux étudiés.

La répartition géographique de ces zones de retard circulatoire est résumé dans le tableau suivant:

	Parapapille	Temporal supérieur	Temporal inférieur	Périphérie et temporo-maculaire
Isolés (I)	17	143	93	29
Confluentes (II)	70	135	80	22
I + II	87	278	173	51
% isolés/confluentes	20%	51%	54%	57%
% nombre total de retards (589)	15%	47%	29%	9%

Ce tableau montre la relative rareté des retards circulatoire dans les zones parapapillaires. Il existe une plus grande fréquence de retards dans le secteur temporal supérieur, surtout par rapport aux régions temporo-maculaire et périphérique. Par contre, dans les zones équatoriales, les retards circulatoires sont très peu nombreux. Ils ont tous une surface très importante; leurs limites sont mal définies. C'est à leur niveau que les temps de disparition sont les plus longs.

Comment interpréter ces retards circulatoires?

La théorie selon laquelle ils seraient dûs à des phénomènes de non-imprégnation des capillaires rétiniens est écartée car ces images peuvent apparaître bien avant l'imprégnation du réseau circulatoire rétinien. Le rôle d'écran à la fluorescence choroïdienne joué par certaines régions de l'épithélium pigmenté semble difficile à soutenir. Nous avons d'ailleurs trouvé deux retards circulatoires au centre desquels des gros vaisseaux choroïdiens imprégnés de colorant sont parfaitement visibles grâce à un véritable 'effet fenêtre' de la couche pigmentée.

Il semble que ces retards circulatoires soient des images de groupes d'unités choriocapillaires dépendant d'une seule artériole choroïdienne. Une anomalie circulatoire durable siégeant au niveau de ce vaisseau expliqueraient ainsi le caractère parfaitement reproductible de ces images.

Alors que les retards du pôle postérieur sont toujours de faible surface et de limites marquées, ceux des zones périphériques sont toujours de larges plages, mal définies sur le plan morphologique et de disparition lente. A leur niveau la circulation choriocapillaire semble dépendre d'un nombre d'artérioles beaucoup moins important qu'au niveau des zones centrales.

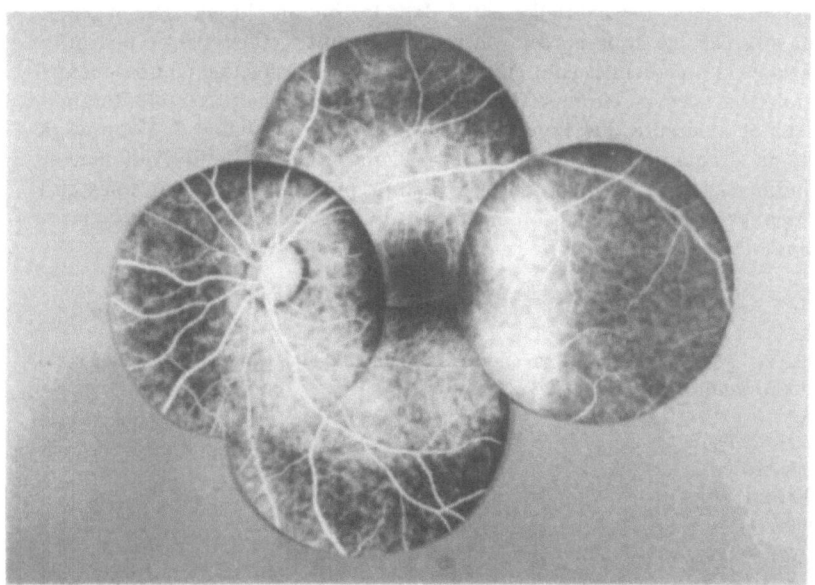

L'étude d'angiographie du pôle postérieur lors des temps veineux vient à l'appui de ces hypothèses. Sur des montages photographiques de clichés de fonds d'yeux normaux, on voit se détacher une zone hyperfluorescente, centrée sur la macula (figure I). Elle s'étend sur une surface circulaire dont le rayon dépasse la papille de I à 2 diamètres papillaires dans le champ nasal du fond d'oeil. On y trouve la quasi-totalité des retards circulatoires. C'est également à son niveau que la méthode des équidensités montre la plus grande spécificité de la circulation choroïdienne; les artérioles sont très nombreuses et chacune d'entre elles semble correspondre à une choricapillaire.

Au-delà de ce cercle, par contre, l'imprégnation pigmentaire est plus faible et les équidensités montrent un nombre limité d'artérioles choroïdiennes s'abouchant à des plages choriocapillaires étendues. Alors qu'au niveau du pôle postérieur nous rencontrons une juxtaposition d'îlots choriocapillaires dont les limites sont marquées par une progression des densités de pente forte, les études faites au niveau de la périphérie indiquent la présence de flaques choriocapillaires à limites mal définies au niveau desquelles la progression des densités prend une pente très faible. Cette différence est peut-être dûe à des communications de type anastomotique, entre des îlots choriocapillaires très peu spécialisés.

La pathologie choroïdienne semble nous donner des exemples en accord avec ces deux types circulatoires bien distincts. Citons en premier lieu l'épithéliopathie en plaques dont les lésions élémentaires couvrent très exactement la zone centrale précédemment décrite et rapellent la morphologie des îlots choriocapillaires retrouvée sur les équidensités. Par contre les zones périphériques sont le siège de lésions vasculaires beaucoup plus vastes, moins systématisées, dont le type semble être le syndrome triangulaire.

Il semble donc que la circulation choroïdienne réponde à deux systèmes différents. L'un, très spécialisé, situé dans la zone la plus centrale et répondant aux besoins de la perception visuelle la plus élaborée. A ce niveau les artérioles choroïdiennes sont en très grand nombre; chacune d'entre elles est en relation avec un nombre d'unités choriocapillaires qui semble diminuer au fur et à mesure que l'on approche la région maculaire. A l'opposé, le système circulatoire périphérique dessert une rétine à fonction uniquement campimétrique, d'où le nombre beaucoup plus faible des artérioles choroïdiennes et leur terminaison au niveau de plages choriocapillaires plus ou moins anastomotiques.

BIBLIOGRAPHIE

AUBRY, J.P. Exploration de la chorio-capillaire par le technique des équidensités. *Arch. Opht.* (Paris), 35, 3; *237-244* (1975).

Adresse de l'auteur:
26 rue Mariès
8100 Albi
France

OCCLUSION DES VEINES CHOROIDIENNES

P. AMALRIC

(Albi, France)

L'étude de la circulation du réseau veineux choroïdien ne date que de quelques années. Pendant longtemps artères et veines ont été confondues sous le nom commun de gros vaisseaux et mis à part les golfes vortiqueux, aucune étude systématique de ce réseau n'avait été entreprise. Aussi, est-on surpris lorsque l'on consulte les vieux traités de voir apparaitre des images d'atypies veineuses considérées alors comme rares. Ce réseau veineux est cependant très important puisqu'il correspond non seulement au réseau choroïdien, mais aussi aux grandes veines confluentes provenant des procès ciliaires.

Un point important dans cette étude a été réalisé le jour où l'expérimentation animale est devenue possible. Toutes les méthodes antérieures d'im-

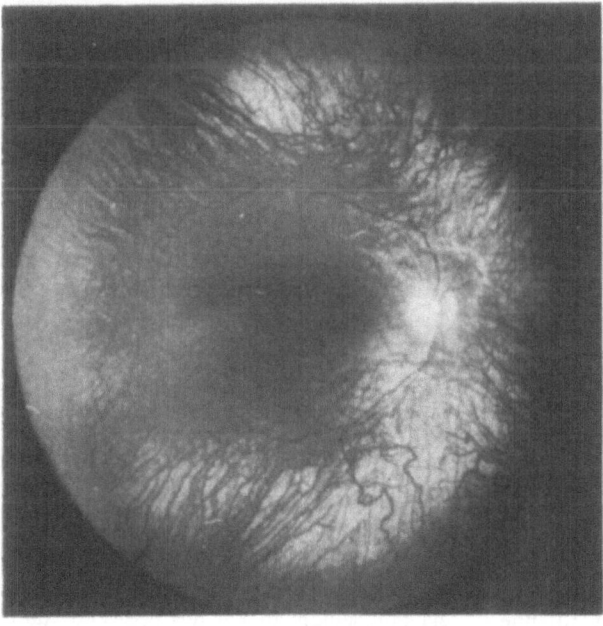

Fig. 1. Photographie grand angle du réseau vortiqueux de la région maculaire Lumière anérythre.

233

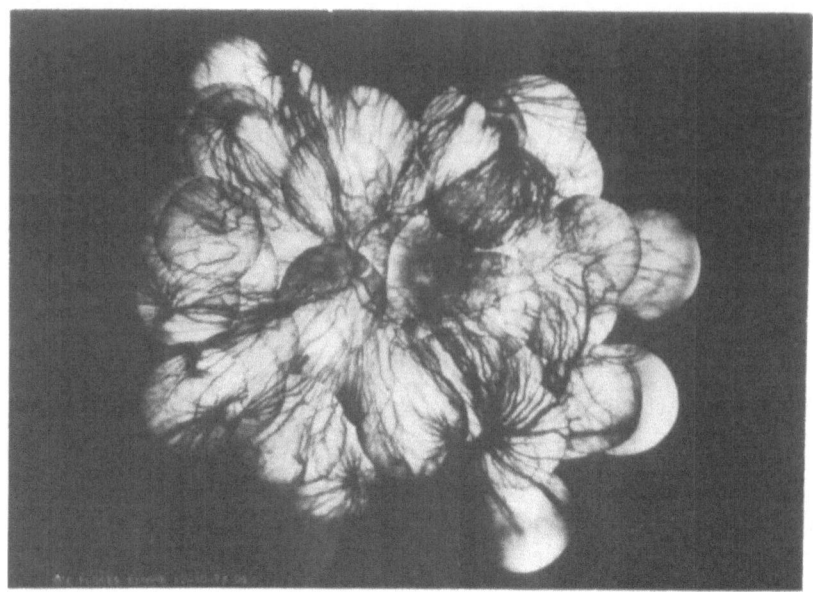

Fig. 2.   6 golfes vortiqueux chez une même malade.

prégnation au néoprène sur le cadavre, de visualisation à travers une fenêtre sclérale ou de l'étude de la circulation chez l'albinique était sur le plan morphologique acceptable, mais sur le plan dynamique elle n'apportait pas un élément d'ensemble suffisant. C'est surtout la clinique qui avec l'appui de la médecine expérimentale nous a ces derniers temps mieux fait comprendre ce problème complexe.

L'examen de la choroïde a bénéficié des améliorations de la rétinographie au cours de ces dernières années, non seulement par l'amélioration de la prise de vue avec les rétinographies grand angle (Fig. 1) qui insensiblement nous permettent d'accéder à l'extrême périphérie, mais aussi par l'adjonction de filtres nombreux. Ceux-ci suivant les cas, préciseront les grands axes et parfois les plus fins vaisseaux. Tous les filtres rouges nous paraissent les plus utiles, quoiqu'il soit difficile par eux seulement de parvenir à différencier nettement artère et veine.

L'angiographie fluorescéinique d'abord, l'angiographie à l'indocyanine ensuite, ont également leur intérêt; mais en définitive pour toute cette étude, c'est surtout la comparaison des résultats obtenus par les différentes méthodes qui nous parait le plus utile. Enfin, à l'avenir, nous croyons que la télévision apportera des éléments précieux pour étudier la dynamique circulatoire choroïdienne et cela non seulement par des prises de vue classiques transpupillaires, mais aussi par l'illumination transclérale pour l'étude de la périphérie choriorétinienne.

Les golfes vortiqueux sont les mieux connus de tout l'ensemble choroïdien. Ils le doivent à la constance relative de leur situation et à la confluence des grosses veines qui le constituent. Il faut cependant reconnaitre que les anomalies sont nombreuses et qu'en particulier il y a souvent plus de quatre sorties veineuses choroïdiennes périphériques (5, 6 et parfois 8 (Fig. 2). A l'inverse, on peut constater dans des cas qui ne sont pas rares, l'unique existence d'une seule veine pour toute l'hémichoroïde inférieure (Fig. 2). Le golfe vortiqueux siège à la partie médiane. Il réunit tout le contingent veineux inférieur du secteur temporal au secteur nasal. Ceci est important à savoir pour bien comprendre certaines complications.

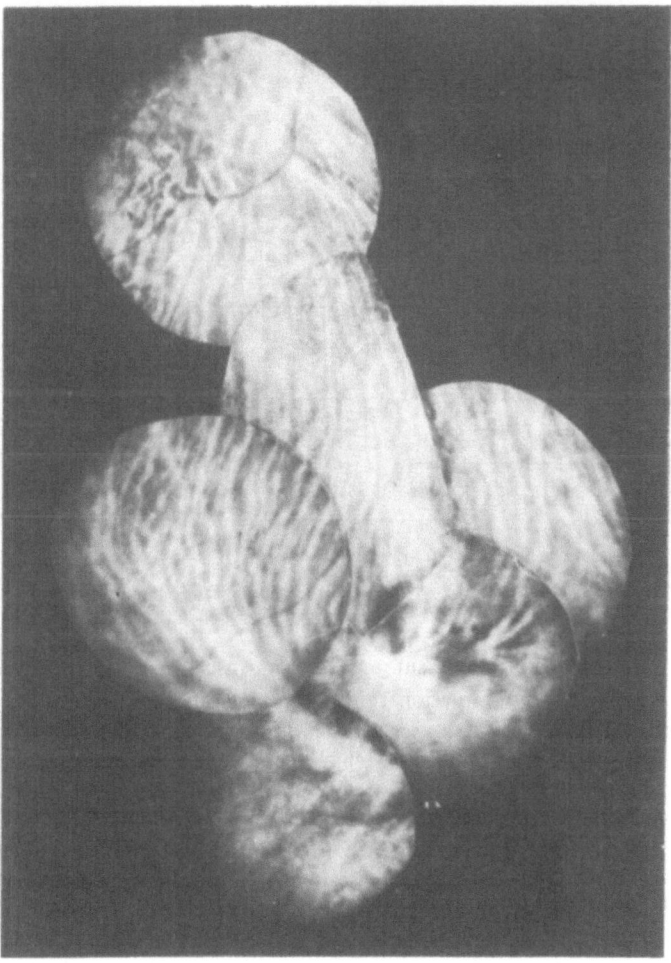

Fig. 3.   Une vortiqueuse pour toute une hémi choroïde inférieure.

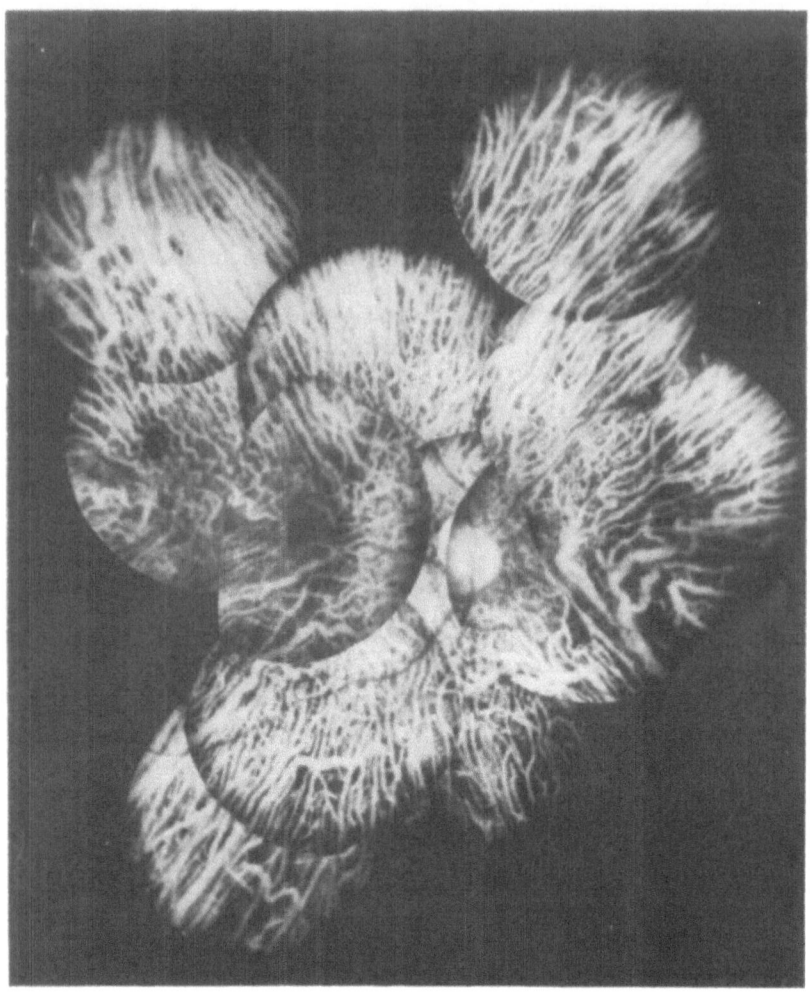

Fig. 4. Confluent vortiqueux sur le nôté nasal de la papille.

Mais ce qui n'avait pas été surement connu jusqu'à ces dernières années, c'est l'existence d'une circulation veineuse péripapillaire réalisant un axe de dérivation. Ce réseau veineux est surtout important dans le secteur nasal. Il se tient en général à distance de la papille. On peut voir en ce point une confluence veineuse (Fig. 4) servant de collecteur entre les différents réseaux vortiqueux. Cela parait logique si on pense que le coté temporal de la papille correspondant à la macula est le plus important pour l'oxygénation de celle-ci. Par voie de conséquence, la densité artérielle est plus grande en ce point, la densité veineuse étant plus importante dans le secteur nasal. Réunissant tous les réseaux veineux, on perçoit aussi de grandes voies de dérivation entre les différents systèmes vortiqueux, temporal et nasal, supérieur et inférieur. Ils siègent à distance de la papille et de la macula; leur incurvation légère ne géne en rien la rapidité du débit que leur diamètre autorise. Souvent, aussi une dérivation veineuse de gros calibre se situe entre la papille et la macula, réunissant alors le secteur temporal supérieur à la zone inférieure. Enfin, il est difficile de définir le schéma commun en raison des variations individuelles, mais nous pensons que ces quelques points que nous venons de préciser correspondent bien à l'immense majorité des cas normaux. A coté de ce schéma choroïdien régulier et harmonieux, il faut reconnaitre les extrêmes variations si nombreuses au point que l'on a pu prétendre que ces atypies vasculaires constituaient pratiquement la règle. Les faits expérimentaux (HAYREH) étaient quelque peu troublants, on pouvait se demander où se faisait la sortie veineuse lorsque les quatre vortiqueuses étaient oblitérées et que le tableau du fond d'oeil au bout de quelques semaines ne se trouvait pas modifié par une pareille occlusion. Le sang

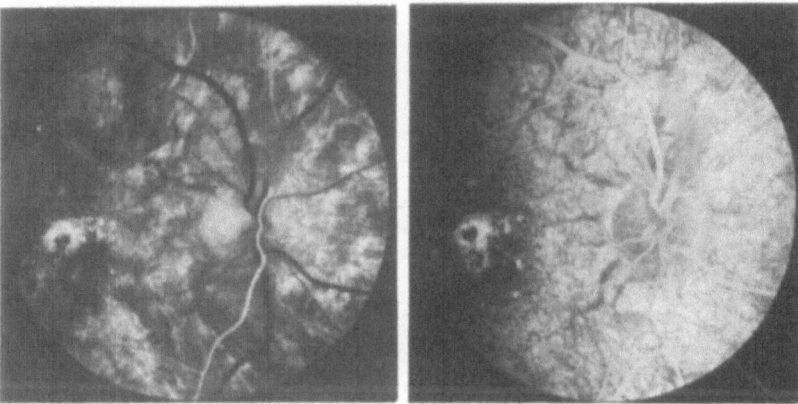

Fig. 5. Temps artériel de l'angiographie fluorescéinique.
Fig. 5bis. Temps veineux de l'angiographie fluorescéinique. Visualisation du réseau veineux choroïdien pépipapillaire.

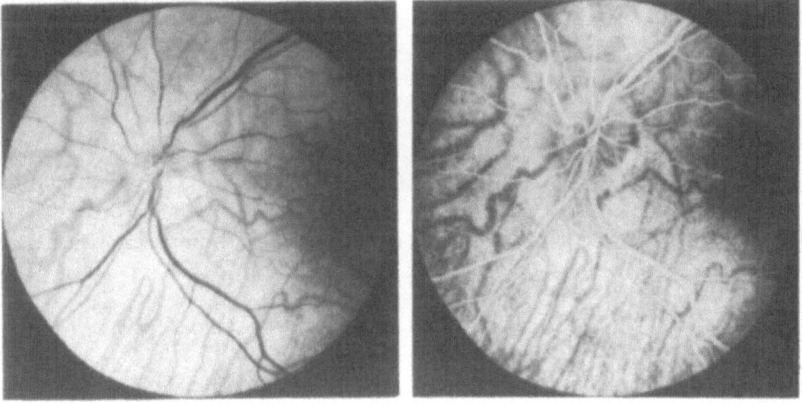

Fig. 6 + 6bis. Tronc vortiqueux sur le côté nasal de la papille.

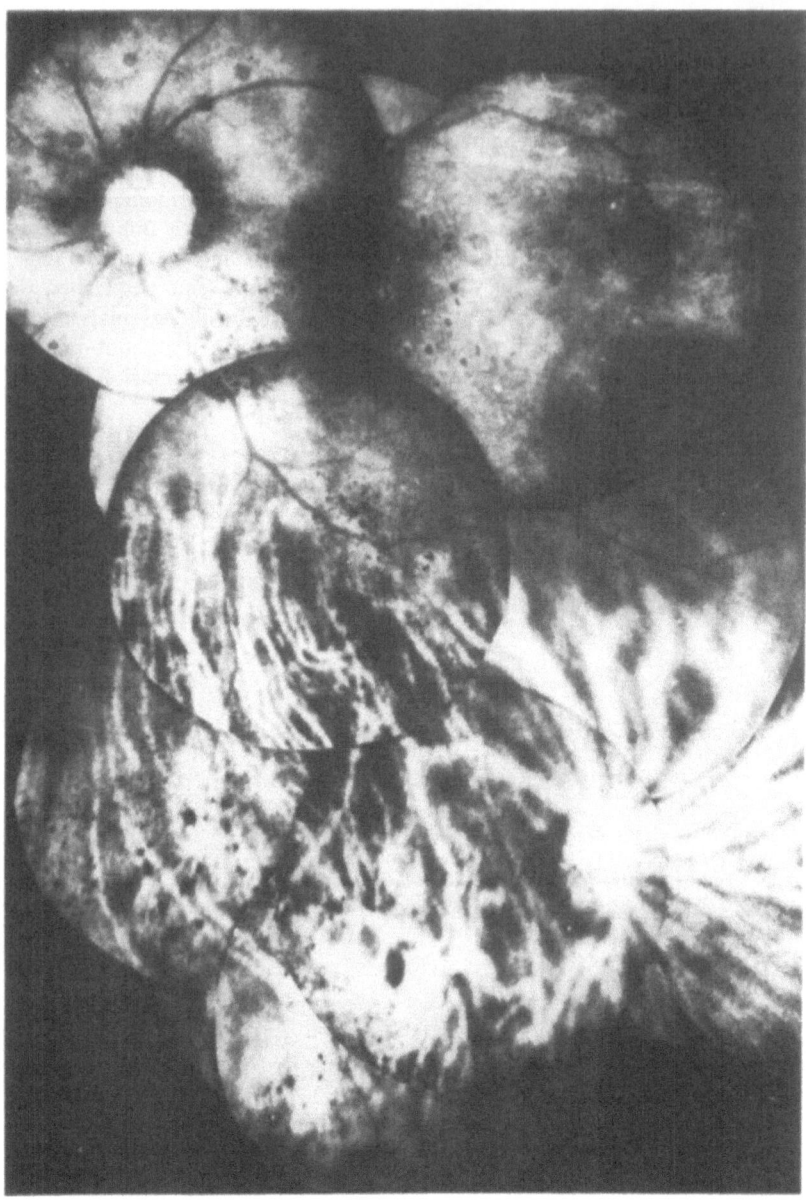

Fig. 7. Traumatisme vortiqueux avec arrêt circulatoire de plusieurs rameau veineux.

veineux à notre avis dans ce cas ne pouvait s'écouler qu'à travers le réseau veineux péripapillaire et de là par les gaines gliales regagnait les grands courants orbitaires. L'angiographie et l'infra rouge associés nous ont montré que ces sorties veineuses péripapillairs étaient extrêmement nombreuses. Il peut y avoir dans certains cas plusieurs veines formant une couronne radiaire autour de la papille et drainant une quantité importante de sang veineux (Fig. 5 et 5bis). Il peut y avoir aussi et ceci est plus fréquent, des golfes vortiqueux importants siégeant tout autour de la papille à la partie supérieure, la partie inférieure, et surtout dans le secteur nasal; quelquefois même avons nous vu un golfe vortiqueux unique intéressant le secteur nasal de la papille (Fig. 6 et 6bis).

OBLITERATIONS DES GOLFES VORTIQUEUX

La *thrombose des vortiqueuses* a été souvent évoquée à l'occasion de la chirurgie du décollement de la rétine. Elle est un facteur d'hémorragie intraoculaire parfois préoccupant, mais rarement des complications secondaires graves. Il n'est que rarement décrit de complications irréversibles.

Les *traumatismes vortiqueux* sont fréquents (Fig. 7). On voit souvent sur des rétinographies avec filtre rouge, après résorption d'une hémorragie intra-

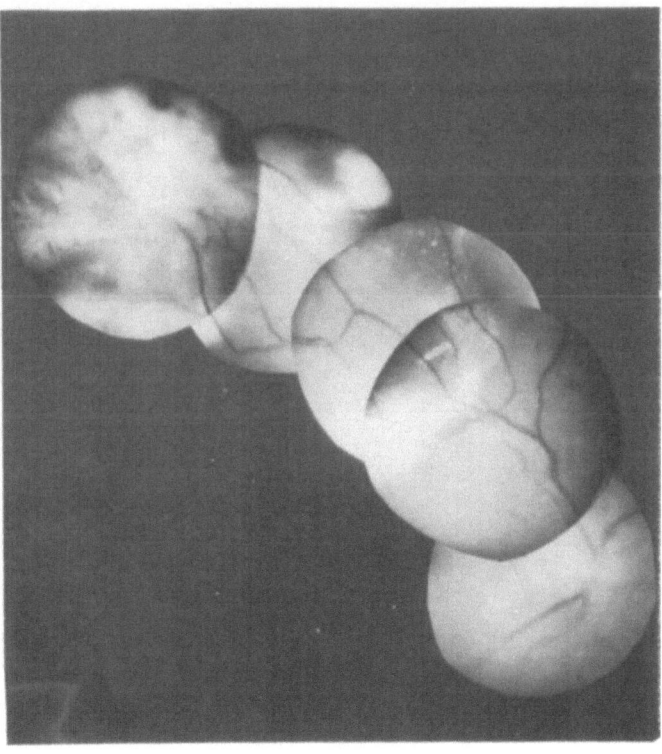

Fig. 8. Thrombose vortiqueuse.

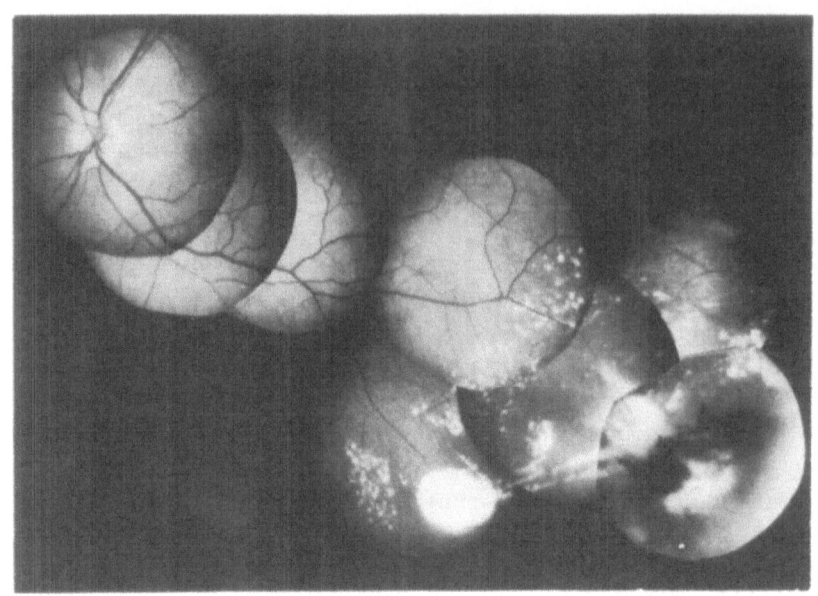

Fig. 9.   Réaction exsudative et hémorragique siégeant au niveau d'un tronc vortiqueux.

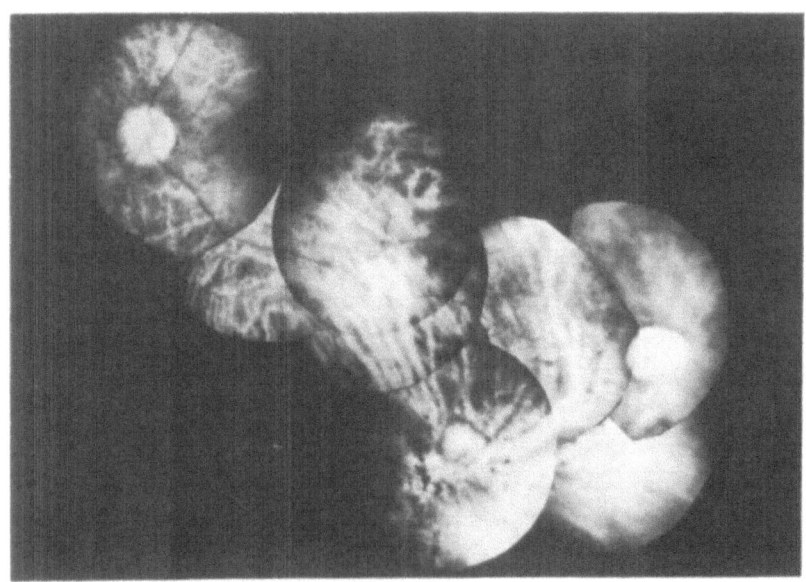

Fig. 9bis.   Reseau vortiqueux visible sur le cliché en infra rouge.

240

oculaire, des lésions veineuses importantes et des arrêts circulatoires sur plusieurs gros vaisseaux.

L'*inflammation* aiguë des troncs vortiqueux (Fig. 8) s'observe rarement. Nous en avons vu un cas chez une femme pendant un accident éclamptique. Il se traduisait par une exsudation massive de tout le fond d'oeil avec le maximum des lésions au milieu du golfe vortiqueux. L'oeil fut perdu par des lésions de fibrose choriorétinienne secondaire intense.

L'inflammation en ces points peut déterminer des réactions exsudatives qui peuvent en imposer parfois pour une néoformation. Nous en avons vu deux cas où après disparition de la réaction oedémateuse on pouvait voir sur les rétinographies en rouge que la zone pathologique se situait exactement au niveau du golfe vortiqueux (Fig. 9 et 9bis). Nous pensons que devant tout processus d'étiologie inconnue, d'allure infectieuse, vasculatoire ou

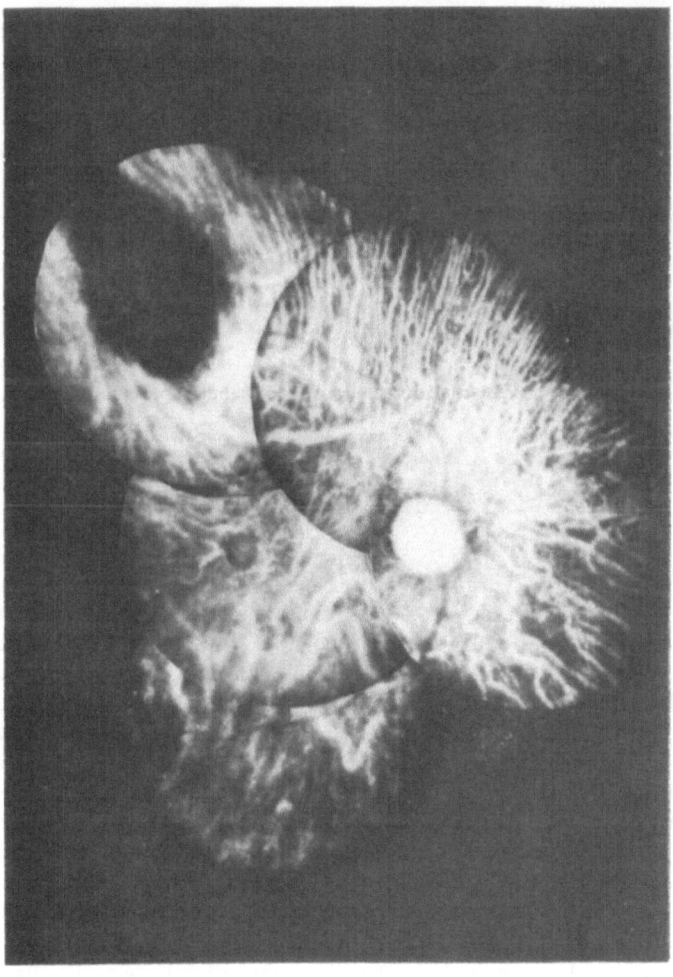

Fig. 10. Pigmentation choroïdienne centrée sur un golfe vortiqueux.

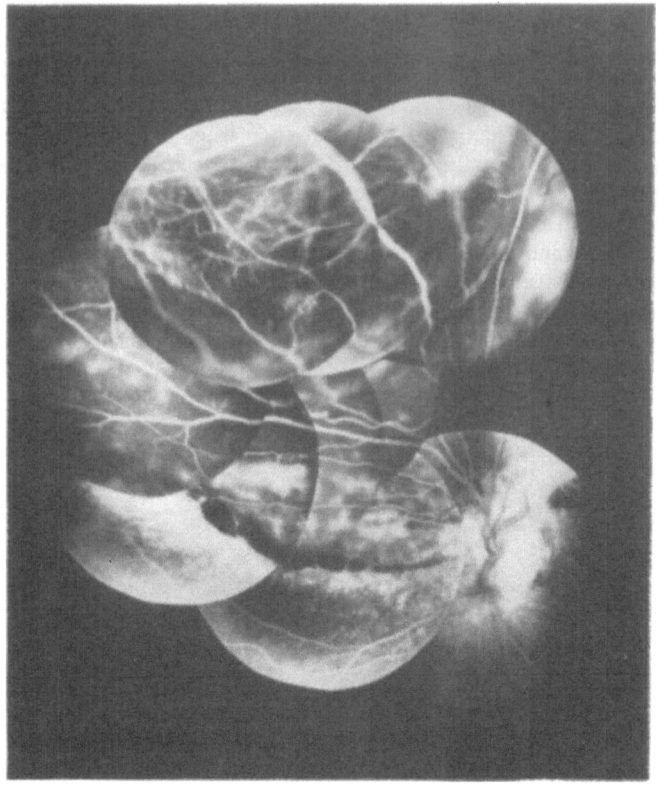

Fig. 11 et 12. Pseudo mélanome choroïdien avant et après ponction.

pseudo-tumorale, il faut toujours penser aux veines vortiqueuses et non pas seulement à une rétinite de Coats ou à une tumeur du corps ciliaire comme ce fut le cas chez les deux malades que nous vous montrons. Les larges troubles pigmentaires que la rétinographie en rouge met en évidence (Fig. 10) souvent comme des taches aboutissant aux golfes vortiqueux. Ils évoquent parfois une pseudo-tumeur que la rétinographie permettra d'éliminer. Nous avons vu un cas où le diagnostic de mélanome avait été affirmé par plusieurs et malgré que l'échographie eut révélé une réponse liquidienne pure, certains avaient proposé l'énucléation. En fait, il s'agissait d'un décollement choroïdien localisé, s'accompagnant d'une réaction inflammatoire du vitré et d'un léger tyndall de la chambre antérieure, d'un rétrécissement de l'angle et au niveau du fond d'oeil d'une vaste pseudo-tumeur noire débutant dans la région vortiqueuse nasale supérieure, mais n'allant pas jusqu'à la périphérie (Fig. 11). La ponction amena la guérison totale de ce décollement choroïdien chez un jeune (Fig. 12).

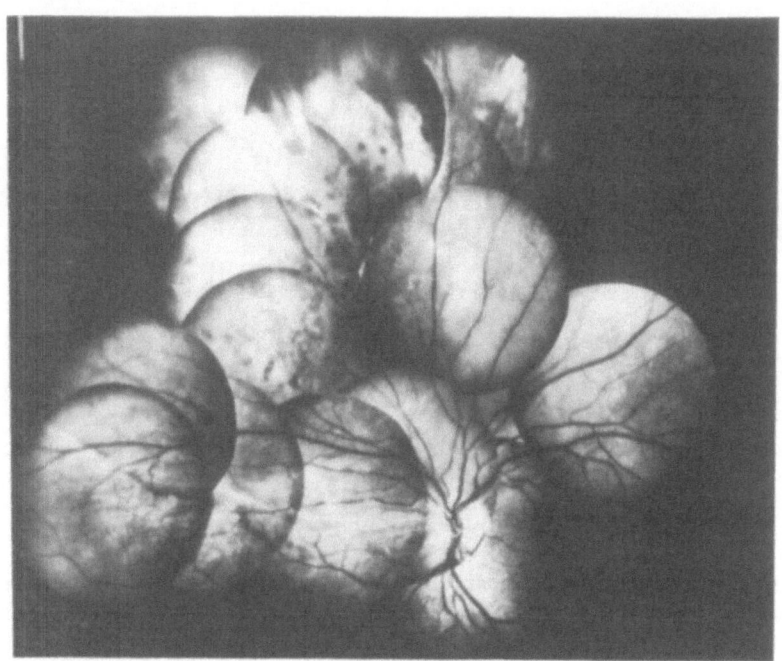

Fig. 12.

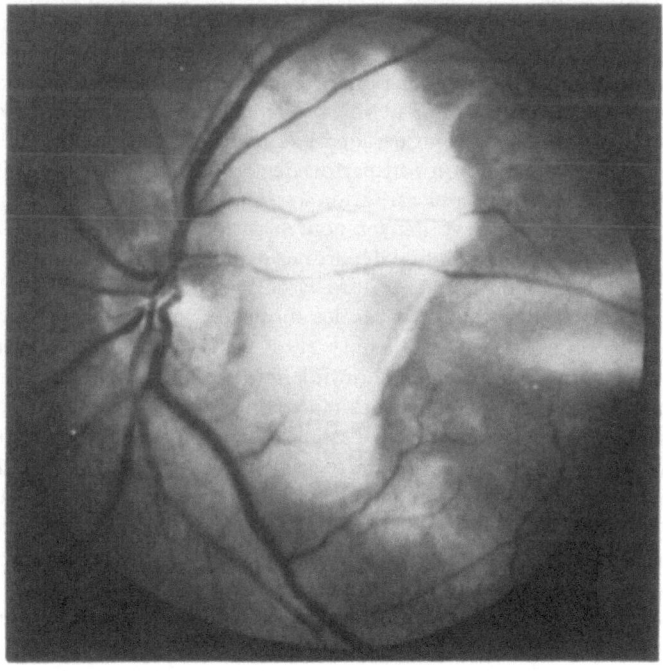

Fig. 13.   Exsudation massive péri papillaire d'origine inconnue.

243

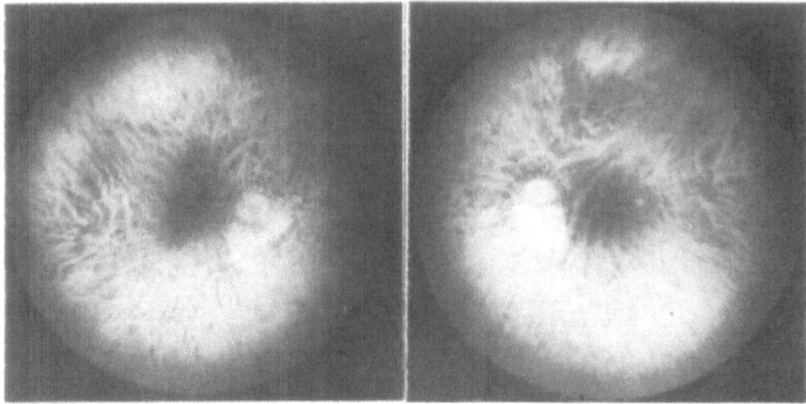

Fig. 14 et 14bis. Hémi atrophie choroïdienne bilatérale avec hémi-atrophie papillaire (Retinographie grand angle avec filtre rouge).

OCCLUSIONS VEINEUSES PERIPAPILLAIRES

Les occlusions veineuses péripapillaires sont également fréquentes. Toute la pathologie choroïdienne péripapillaire est d'ailleurs extrêmement complexe et faire la part de ce qui revient à un déficit artériel capillaire ou veineux est certainement difficile.

Cependant, les notions anatomiques que nous rappelons tout à l'heure, à savoir la corrélation étroite entre le réseau veineux choroïdien normal et la région péripapillaire, la fréquence des golfes visibles ou invisibles, la sortie veineuse du sang provenant de la région maculaire, tout cela peut dans certaines circonstances, expliquer l'importance des manifestations cliniques. Dans le domaine infectieux on peut voir survenir des exsudations massives et envahissantes prenant leur point de départ au niveau de ces plexus (Fig. 13). Dans le domaine vasculaire on voit parfois de véritables angiomatoses locali-sées bilatérales allant vers la cicatrisation après avoir semblé constituer pen-dant plusieurs mois un grave danger pour la vision de ces yeux. Certaines angiomatoses également à point de départ péripapillaire sont nettement amé-liorées par une coagulation du tissu fibro-vasculaire.

Nous voulons signaler enfin les cas des anomalies veineuses papillo-macu-laires avec modifications de la papille et dysversion de tout le système choroïdien. Ces hémiatrophies choroïdiennes sont souvent bilatérales, s'accompagnant souvent l'hémorragies maculaires des deux cotés et le point qui nous parait le plus important, c'est l'existence dans de nombreux cas d'une tache de Fuchs à la jonction entre les deux systèmes. La possibilité de réaliser dans ces cas des rétinographies grand angle pour mieux étudier l'ensemble, une étude plus précise de la dynamique circulatoire au niveau de la macula devrait (Fig. 14), dans le cadre des dystrophies de Fuchs, individu-aliser une forme à pathogénie particulière.

En résumé, après une longue période d'incertitude sur la pathologie veineuse choroïdienne, nous arrivons à mieux préciser les tableaux en nous basant non seulement sur les dispositions anatomiques de chaque système, mais aussi sur des recherches étioloques plus précises.

CLINICAL APPLICATION OF INDOCYANINE GREEN ANGIOGRAPHY

ARNALL PATZ, M.D., ROBERT W. FLOWER, MICHAEL L. KLEIN, M.D.,
DAVID H. ORTH, M.D., JAY A. FLEISCHMAN, M.D. & SCOTT MCLEOD

(Baltimore, Md, USA)

FLOWER, elsewhere in this monograph, has reviewed the fluorescence characteristics of indocyanine green (ICG) and the filter combinations and film best suited for ICG angiography. KOGURE and co-workers (1970) first studied infrared absorption angiography utilizing intra-arterial injections of ICG in monkeys. FLOWER & HOCHHEIMER (1973, 1974, 1976) further perfected ICG angiography so that intravenous injections could be utilized. This development permitted the practical clinical testing of the dye which is noted for its low incidence of side effects and toxicity. FLOWER & HOCH-HEIMER (1976) have continued their studies and made available the ICG fluorescein angiography camera for the examination of a series of patients with pigmented fundus tumors, retinal vascular and macular disorders. The present report summarizes our experience in approximately 150 consecutive patients with these conditions.

SUBRETINAL NEOVASCULARIZATION

The peak fluorescence energy of indocyanine green is in the near infrared portion of the spectrum. The better transmission qualities, through the ocular media, and through the retinal pigment epithelium, suggested as the first priority the study of subretinal (subpigment epithelial) neovascularization emanating from the choroid. ICG fluorescence passes readily through the increased pigment in the pigment epithelium in the central portion of the macula which normally blocks underlying choroidal fluorescein fluorescence. Since many subpigment epithelial new vessel membranes extend into the central portion of the macula and have the greatest impact on vision, the ability to resolve structures beneath the pigment epithelium seemed to be a logical step forward in our management of these patients. The limitations of ICG and its failure to prove clinically helpful in the diagnosis and management of subretinal new vessel membranes has been the greatest disappointment in the use of this dye in studies thus far. In only two instances in approximately 25 patients with probable subpigment epithelial neovascularization, indocyanine green permitted partial resolution of the neovascular membrane when standard fluorescein angiography did not provide resolution. Even in these two cases where a new vessel membrane was suspected on ICG dye studies, the precise borders of the neovascular membrane could not be ascertained with sufficient confidence to serve as a guide to photo-

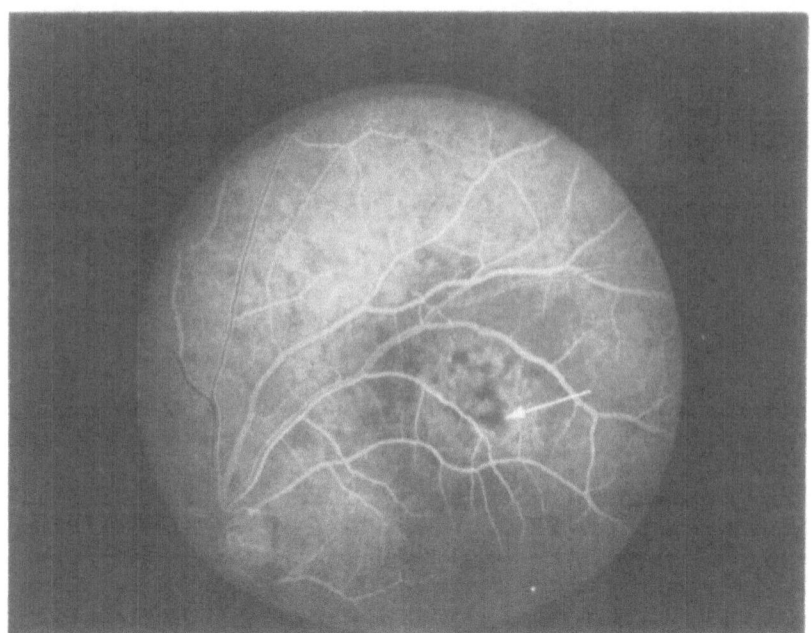

Fig. 1A. Presumed nevus of choroid showing early fluorescein transit. Note area of partially blocked fluorescence in center of lesion (arrow).

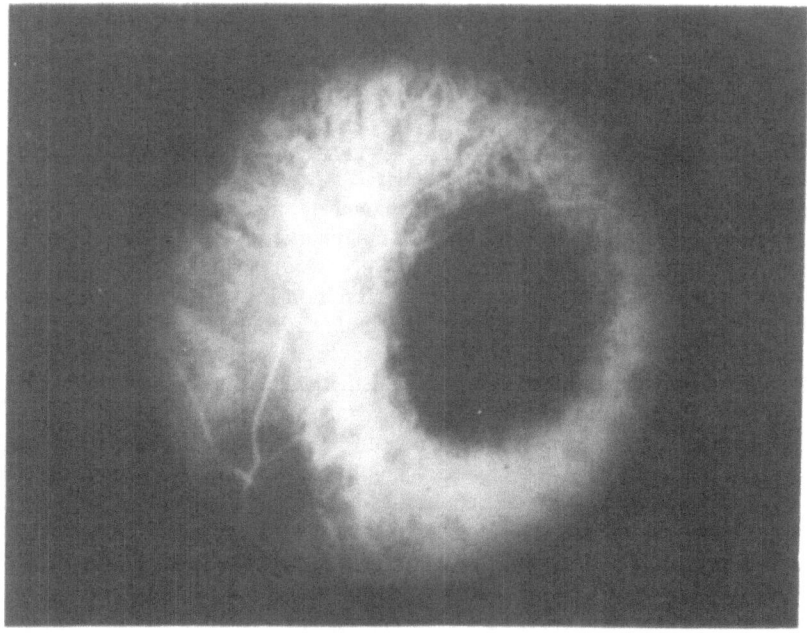

Fig. 1B. ICG fluorescent angiogram taken at the exact same time following dye injection. Note sharp delineation of pigmented tumor and resolution of choroidal vessels along border of tumor.

246

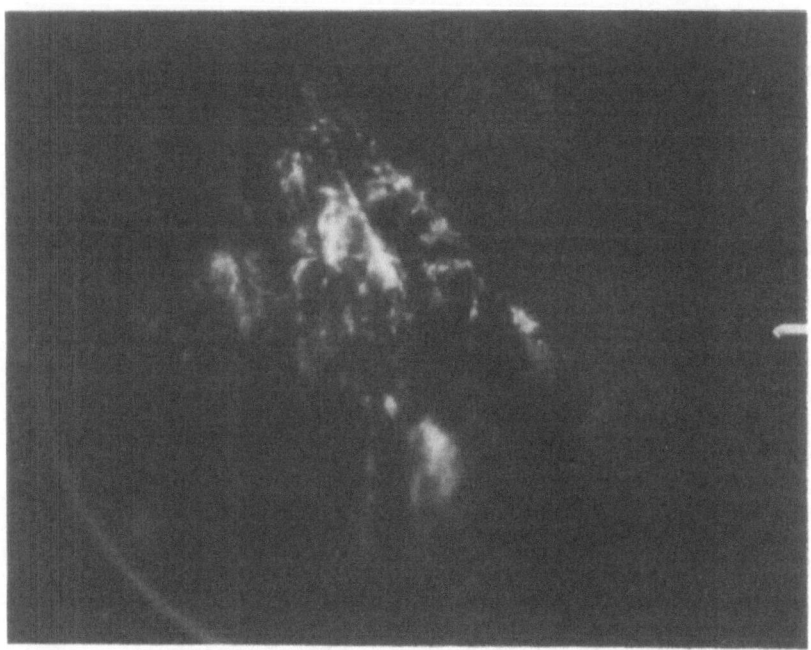

Fig. 2A. Early fluorescein angiogram of patient with mildly pigmented choroidal melanoma in the mid-periphery of the fundus.

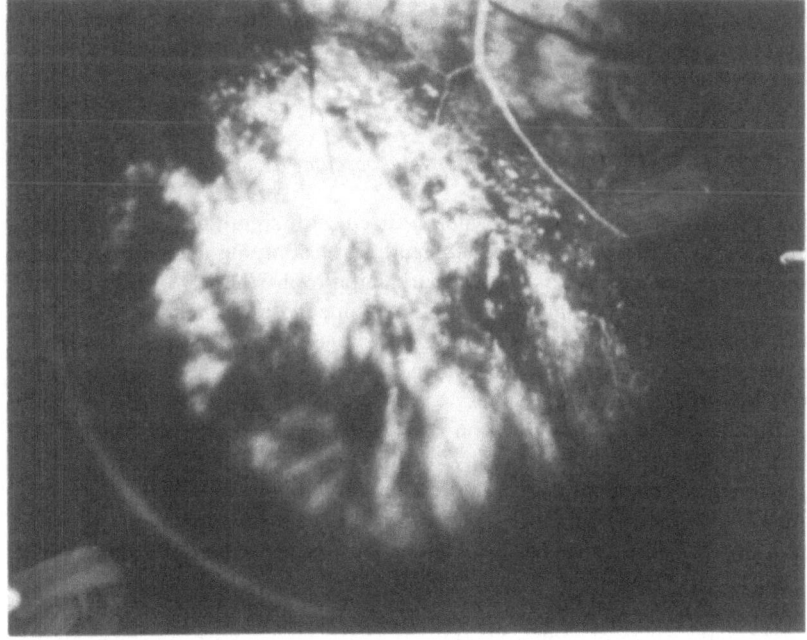

Fig. 2B. Several seconds after photograph in 2A shows diffuse leakage of fluorescein.

coagulation treatment. An example of one of these cases where the new vessel membrane could apparently be resolved by indocyanine green, but not with fluorescein, was in senile macular degeneration.

Choroidal nevi and melanomas

ICG angiography provides good resolution of the medium and larger-size choroidal vessels throughout the fundus although it does not permit resolution of finer choriocapillaris details. In the evaluation of patients with pigmented tumors to determine their growth characteristics, we have found that the ICG angiogram gives a sharp delineation of the pigmented borders of the tumor. Fig. 1A & 1B. Although we have not had sufficiently long follow-up of patients with presumed choroidal nevi vs. low-grade melanomas, a series of these patients is being followed for possible encroachment by the tumor on the adjacent choroidal vessels. Whether or not this will prove practical in the management of choroidal nevi and possible melanomas will require several years of observation of these patients.

In one lightly pigmented malignant choroidal melanoma, Figures 2A to 2D, ICG angiography permitted resolution of the larger vessels coursing through the tumor and, indeed, demonstrated for the first time in our study, staining of the vessel walls and leakage of ICG into the tumor mass. As indicated in the Introductory chapter by FLOWER, ICG does not normally leak from the choroidal vessels, including the choriocapillaris. The leakage of ICG in this patient represents a change of vascular integrity possibly related to the malignant nature of the tumor. In this patient fluorescein angiography leaked profusely from the surface of the tumor and permitted no details of the vascular pattern within the tumor, Figure 2B. In amelanotic or lightly pigmented tumors, the ability to resolve the vascular landmarks in the tumor may provide useful information to document tumor growth.

Basic studies on choroidal vascular dynamics

ICG angiography, particularly when utilized with simultaneous fluorescein angiography, provides a convenient method of studying choroidal vascular dynamics. This provides a useful experimental tool. Whether or not this will prove to have clinical application in patients with retinal and choroidal vascular diseases will require a study of a large series of patients with age-corrected normals. The method is already suitable for the experimental animal study of the two circulations.

The present clinical application of ICG angiography is quite limited. At the present time, ICG angiography technique may be considered an adjunct to standard photography and fluorescein angiography in documenting the size, and particularly the border characteristics, of pigmented ocular tumors. Also, when the tumor is not heavily pigmented, the dye permits resolution of the vascular landmarks in the tumor.

One advantage of ICG angiography over fluorescein angiography is in the patient with severe photophobia (ORTH et al. (1976). With ICG the patient perceives only a faint red light from the illumination source; therefore, there

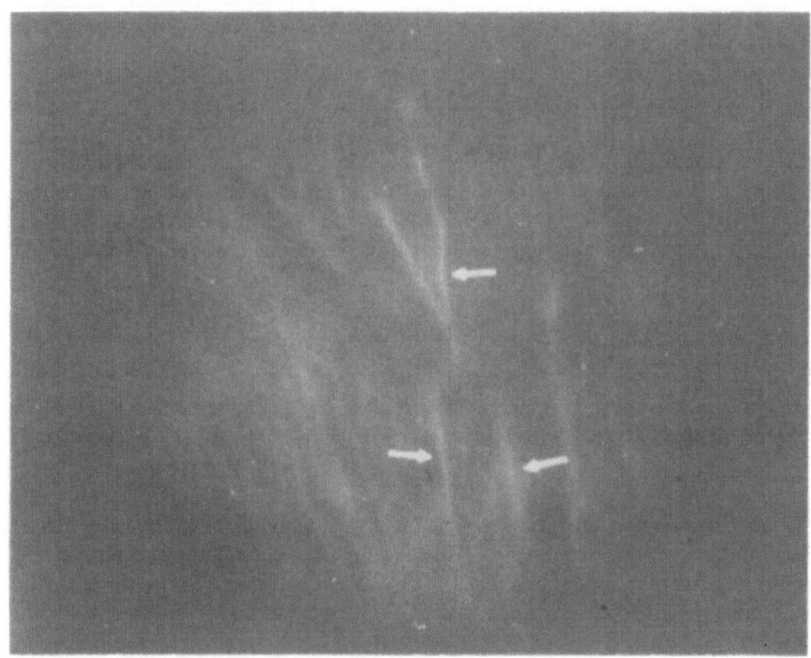

Fig. 2C. ICG photograph made at same time as fluorescein photograph in Fig. 2A. Note vessels in tumor, arrows.

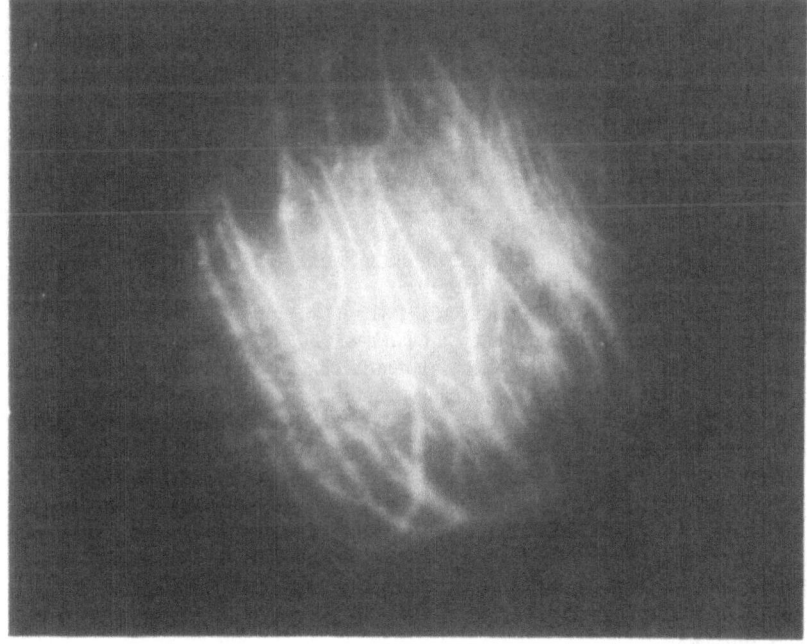

Fig. 2D. Several minutes later, further staining of vessel walls of tumor and leakage of ICG dye into the mass of tumor.

249

is no problem with patient cooperation even in the presence of severe photophobia. Furthermore, in patients with slight haze of the ocular media, ICG fluorescence passes through the hazy media better to permit resolution in some instances where fluorescein angiography is unsatisfactory. ICG, which is rapidly removed from the circulation, can be repeated within the span of a few minutes since there is no significant residual fluorescence (CHERRICK et al., 1960; WHEELER et al., 1958; KETTERER et al., 1960). In the occasional patient who has experienced adverse side effects from sodium fluorescein injections, ICG can frequently be utilized without untoward reaction. Indeed, there have been no known side effects to ICG. In our human volunteers and patients with retinal diseases, we have observed no evidence of nausea or other side effects. Two instances of mild syncope occurred from the needle injection in the arm, prior to the administration of ICG dye.

CONCLUSION

ICG angiography can*not* at the present time be recommended as a diagnostic method for routine usage. We recommend its further trial in centers having large tumor referral services — and we recommend it for the investigator studying the dynamics of the choroidal circulation.

REFERENCES

CHERRICK, G.R., STEIN, S.W., LEEVY, C.M. & DAVIDSON, C.S. Indocyanine green: observation on its physical properties, plasma decay and hepatic extraction. *Jour. Clin. Invest.* 39: *592* (1960).

FLOWER, R.W. Choroidal angiography using indocyanine green dye: a review and progress report. *Ophthal. Digest*, July (1974).

FLOWER, R.W. & HOCHHEIMER, B.F. A clinical technique and apparatus for simultaneous angiography of the separate retinal and choroidal circulations. *Invest. Ophthal.* 12: *248* (1973).

FLOWER, R.W. & HOCHHEIMER, B.F. Indocyanine green dye fluorescence and infrared absorption choroidal angiography performed simultaneously with fluorescein angiography. *Johns Hopkins Med. Journal* 138: *33* (1976).

KETTERER, S.G. WIEGNAND, B.D. & RAPAPORT, E. Hepatic uptake and biliary excretion of indocyanine green and its use in estimation of hepatic bloodflow in dogs. *Amer. Jour. Phys.* 199: *481* (1960).

KOGURE, K., DAVID, N.J., YAMANOUCH, U. et al. Infra-red absorption angiography of the fundus circulation. *Arch. Ophth.* 83: *209* (1970).

ORTH, D.H., PATZ, A. & FLOWER, R.W. Potential clinical application of indocyanine green choroidal angiography — preliminary report. *Eye, Ear, Nose & Throat Monthly*, January (1976).

WHEELER, H.O., CRANSTON, W.I. & MELTZER, I.I. Hepatic uptake and biliary excretion of indocyanine green in the dog. *Proc. Soc. Exper. Bio. & Med.* 99: *11* (1958).

Authors' address:
Wilmer Institute
Johns Hopkins Hospital
601 N. Broadway
Baltimore, Maryland 21205
USA

DISCUSSION

Dr Bonnet: Me permettrez vous à la suite de la communication du Dr. Patz de souligner l'intéret de l'angiographie au vert d'indocyanine dans le diagnostic des tumeurs de la choroide, en vous montrant quelques clichés concernant un cas d'angiome de la choroide. Il s'agit d'un homme de 40 ans qui présente cette tumeur dont le siege juxtapapillaire évoque la possibilité d'un angiome. Les clichés angiographiques sont fortement en faveur du diagnostic d'angiome de la choroide. L'angiographie au vert d'indocyanine pratiquée ici avec des films couleurs montrent une imprégnation progressive de la tumeur par le colorant, imprégnation qui augmente fortement au temps veineux où la tumeur est intensément colorée en vert. Cette imprégnation va diminuer très progressivement puisque la circulation dans ces tumeurs est très lente. Du fait d'un malentendu le médecin qui suivait ce malade a pratiqué l'énucléation avant que l'on ait donné les résultats de l'angiographie. L'examen histopathologique confirme le diagnostique d'hémangiome de la choroide. Ces données angiographiques ne doivent pas surprendre puisque le vert d'indocyanine ne diffuse pas à travers les parois vasculaires ainsi lorsque le vert d'indocyanine est visible ce ne peut être qu'à l'intérieur de cavités vasculaires. Cette tumeur est entièrement colorée puisqu'elle n'est rien d'autre qu'une juxtaposition de cavités vasculaires.

Dr Saari: I should like to contribute to the paper of Dr Patz. Indocyanin green fluorescence angiography really gives a new dimension to the evaluation of the choroid. We are very happy that it has been possible for us in the Oulu University Eye Clinic to work with Dr Flower of Johns Hopkins and Dr Hyvarinen of Helsinki in doing indocyanin fluorescence angiography. I would like to present very shortly a patient. Here we can see the right eye of a 77 year old man with central choroidal areolar sclerosis. Fluorescein angiography only shows choroidal vessels in that area were pigment epithelium has been destroyed. The indocyanin fluorescence angiogram shows the choroidal vessels through the pigment epithelium, differentiating choroidal arteries and veins as well as the superficial and deep vessels when stereo photographs are used.

WATERSHED ZONE DEGENERATION, A CLINICAL SYNDROME?

P.J.M. BOS, P.T.V.M. DE JONG & E.L. GREVE

(Amsterdam, The Netherlands)

INTRODUCTION

The purpose of this study is to interpret the clinical, angiographic and perimetric features of a group of six male patients with decrease of vision and metamorphopsia. Sometimes we found pigment mottling and oedema in the macula and around the optic disc. Angiography showed in some patients hyperfluorescent leaking spots in the macular area and in a vertical zone temporal to the optic disc. In others, only hyperfluorescence in a zone temporal to the optic disc was seen. Perimetry revealed corresponding deep scotomas.

CASE I

This healthy 41-year old man suffered from decreased vision for a few months and metamorphopsia in both eyes. Examination showed a visual acuity correctable to 6/18 in the right eye and finger counting in the left eye. In both macular regions we found pigment epithelium degeneration (P.E.D.) with oedema. The optic discs were normal. No signs of inflammation were found. In the right eye a triangular area of P.E.D. was seen in the periphery. Fluorescein angiography showed besides a normal arm-retina time, band- and sector-shaped hyperfluorescent leaking areas in a vertical plane temporal to the optic disc. In the macular region hyperfluorescent spots were seen with leakage on later pictures. There was a marked symmetry between the two eyes. Kinetic perimetry showed corresponding absolute scotomas. Clinical, biochemical and neurological examination revealed no abnormalities. The situation of both eyes took an unfavourable course, despite high doses of Prednisone. Also bilateral retinal detachment occurred, which disappeared later on.

CASE II

This 46-year old healthy man noticed decreased vision with metamorphopsia in his left eye. On examination, corrected visual acuity in the right eye was 6/6 and in the left 6/24. In the left macula there was subretinal oedema. On fluorescein angiography we found bilateral lesions in the posterior pole, almost equal to those seen in the first patient. The leakage, however, was doubtful. Perimetry showed corresponding absolute scotomas.

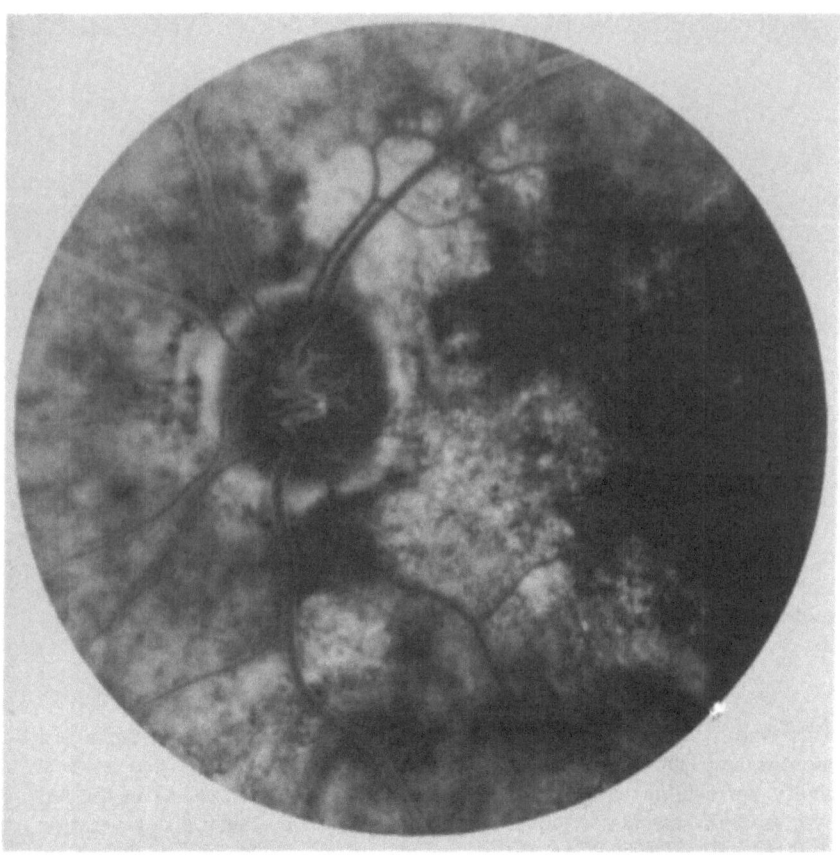

Fig. 1a. The configuration of this degenerative area is the same as that of early filling defects in normal patients.

CASE III

A 39-year old Eurasian healthy man was seen because of a central serous choroidopathy in his right eye. His corrected vision in both eyes was 6/6. In the right macula we noticed oedema; the left eye appeared normal. Fluorescein angiography revealed in both eyes large wedge-shaped areas of hyperfluorescence inferior to the optic disc with leakage and irregular patches in the macular region. Corresponding absolute scotomas were found. Up till now, the central visual function remains good.

CASE IV

This 51-year old man noticed decreased vision in his left eye. Corrected vision was 6/6 in both eyes. On the temporal side of the − normal − optic disc of the left eye pigment degeneration was noticed. Fluorescein angiography showed a prolonged arm-retina time, narrow retinal arteries and an irregularly

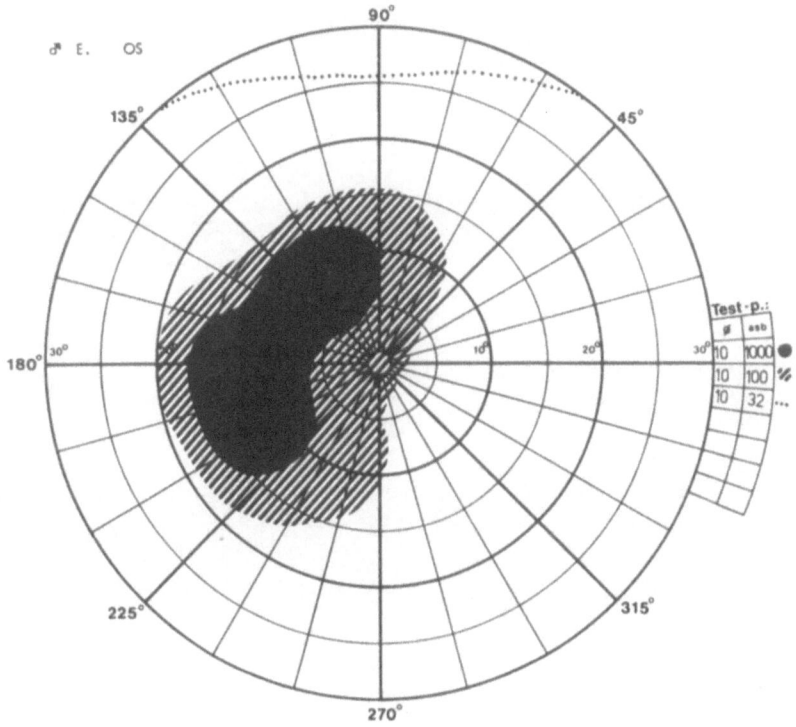

Fig. 1b.   The visual field shows a corresponding scotoma.

bordered area of P.E.D. temporal to the optic disc without leakage (see Fig. 1a). This degenerative area corresponded with an absolute scotoma (Fig. 1b).

CASE V

This 42-year old man was seen because of amaurosis fugax. He had vision 6/6 in both eyes. Around both optic discs, but mainly temporal, areas of P.E.D., suggesting clusters of Elschnig spots, were seen. Fluorescein angiography showed a prolonged arm-retina time. Ophthalmodynamography was suggestive of bilateral carotid artery stenosis.

CASE VI

This 46-year old man was referred because of decreased vision in the right eye. His history revealed a myocardial infarct in 1971. Corrected vision in the right eye was 6/12, in the left 6/6. Examination of the right eye showed P.E.D. between macula and optic disc; the left eye revealed yellow spots in the macula and so-called Siegrist streaks (1899). The affected area in the right eye was wedge-shaped without leakage on fluorescein angiography. Visual field analysis showed a relative centrocoecal scotoma.

255

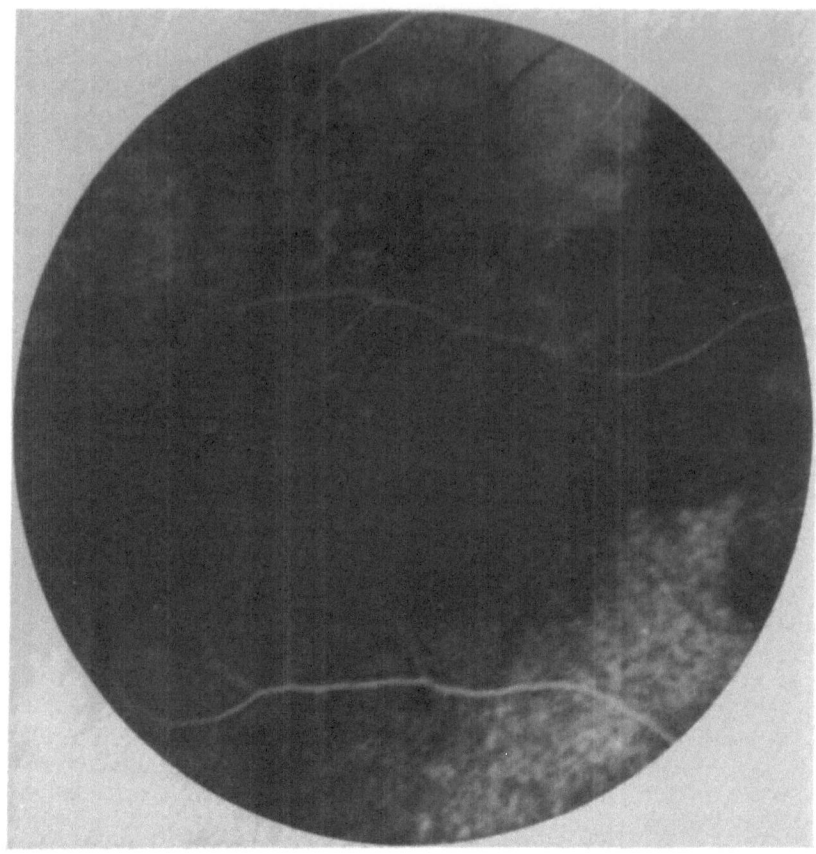

Fig. 2a. These pictures show pigment epithelium degeneration in the temporal zone of the optic disc, adjacent to a not yet filled area (watershed zone). A few seconds later this area also shows pigment epithelium degeneration (Fig. 2b).

DISCUSSION

Ophthalmoscopy suggested in cases II and III a central serous choroido-pathy as the cause for the decline of vision, but when we saw the angio-grams we were at a loss to put all signs under a single heading. Features that tally with local choroidal circulation disturbances were visible in three pa-tients: a triangular syndrome (AMALRIC, 1971, 1973; case I), Siegrist streaks (SIEGRIST, 1899; case VI) and Elschnig spots (KLIEN, 1968; case V). The myocardial infarction (case VI), bilateral carotid artery stenosis (case V) and prolonged arm-retinal time (cases IV and V) hinted at a more general vascular disorder. We were struck by the fact that the areas of P.E.D. coincided with early choroidal filling defects (see Fig. 2). Recent publica-tions on choroid circulation (HAYREH, 1972, 1975) have shown that the arterial blood supply is sectorial. The temporal part of the choroid is usually filled by the lateral posterior ciliary artery (P.C.A.), the nasal part by the

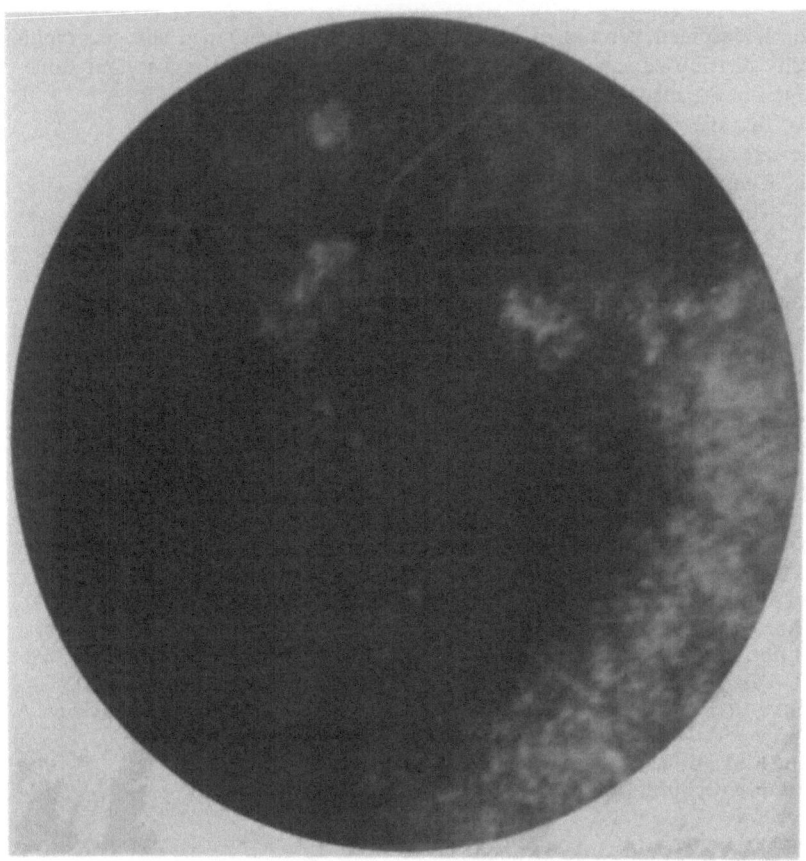

Fig. 2b.   For legend see Fig. 2a.

medial P.C.A. These two parts are separated by a so-called watershed zone (HAYREH, 1974). In man this zone is often recognizable as an early filling defect in the temporal peripapillary area (SHIMIZU, 1974). Also in the macular region these filling defects can be seen where they represent watershed zones of short P.C.A.'s.

Comparison of these data with the angiograms of our patients suggested to us the existence of a watershed zone syndrome. Also Hayreh's hypothesis that the watershed zones are the most vulnerable parts of the choroid in case of circulation disturbance, is in accordance with the general and local vascular affections in four of our patients. The visual fields point to lesions of the retinal outer layers overlying the P.E.D. areas and thus the watershed zones. On angiography the discs were normal and as we expected there were no fibre bundle defects.

SUMMARY

Six patients with pigment epithelium degeneration in the posterior pole have been discussed. The typical findings in these middle-aged men are:
1. Decrease of visual acuity and metamorphopsia.

2. Widespread patches of hyperfluorescence, wedgeshaped and geographically distributed, mainly in a vertical zone temporal to the disc, but sometimes in the macular area. A few cases show leakage.
3. In most patients the lesions are bilateral and symmetric and
4. are accompanied by large and intense scotomas.
5. They run a chronic and in one case a very unfavourable course.
6. The angiographic localization of the lesions correlates with the watershed zones.
7. Symptoms are mentioned that are suggestive for vascular disorders as a cause for this disease.

REFERENCES

AMALRIC, P. Acute choroidal ischaemia. *Trans. U.K.* 91: *305-322* (1971).

AMALRIC, P. Choroidal vessel occlusive syndromes. Clinical aspects. *Tr. Am. Acad. Ophth. & Otol.* 77: *291-299* (1973).

HAYREH, S.S. Occlusion of the posterior ciliary artery. I. Effects on choroidal circulation. *Brit. J. Ophthal.* 56: *719-735* (1972).

HAYREH, S.S. Submacular choroidal vascular pattern. *Graefes Arch. Ophthal.* 192: *181-196* (1974).

HAYREH, S.S. Segmental nature of the choroidal vasculature. *Brit. J. Ophthal.* 59: *631-648* (1975).

KLIEN, B.A. Ischemic infarcts of the choroid (Elschnig spots). *Amer. J. Ophthal.* 66: *1069-1074* (1968).

SHIMIZU, K., YOKOCHI, K. & OKANO, T. Fluorescein angiography of the choroid. *Jap. J. Ophthal.* 18: *97-108* (1974).

SIEGRIST, A. Beitrag zur Kenntniss der Arteriosclerose der Augengefässe. IX. Int. Congr. Ophthal. Utrecht, *131-139* (1899).

Authors' address:
Eye Clinic
Wilhelmina Gasthuis
University of Amsterdam
1e Helmersstraat 104
Amsterdam
The Netherlands

DISCUSSION

Dr Gass: I want to comment briefly on Dr Bos' paper. We have seen about 12 patients very similar to the one he presented, with the exception that every one of our patients had had at least in one eye a serous detachment of the retina involving the macula. And I think these cases represent a severe form of central serous retinopathy. The large areas of pigment epithelium atrophy that often have a teardrop shape may extent all the way to the periphery of the fundus and they are related to chronic, recurrent, long standing retinal detachment. Often it is outside the macular area and the patient does not know that he has it. Very often there is demonstrable leak in the upper portion of this zone. So I think it is the same disease. It is of interest that all these patients were males and middle-aged. I think these patients should be watched extremely carefully, given an Amsler grid, because these are the patients who can lose significantly pericentral as well as central vision over a period of years and should be photocoagulated if you can catch them with a detachment.

Dr Bos: We considered also the diagnosis of central serous retinopathy. However, the peripapillary degenerative areas did not present localized leaking points but did diffuse over their entire surface. These areas correspond to watershed areas. It is not proved if there is an essential difference in pathogenesis between the two diseases. Theoretically an analogous etiology (watershed zone) could be postulated for central serous retinopathy.

CONSIDERATION OF THE CILIORETINAL CIRCULATION*

J. JUSTICE, JR. & R.P. LEHMANN

(Houston, Texas, USA)

The incidence of cilioretinal arteries in 1000 consecutive patients was deter-mined by review of stereo color fundus photographs and fluorescein angio-graphs. One or more cilioretinal artery was present in 49.5 per cent of all pa-tients or in 32.1 per cent of the 2000 eyes in this series. They occurred bi-laterally in 14.6 per cent and contributed to some portion of the macular circulation in 18.7 per cent of the patients. A great deal of variability of size, number and distribution of cilioretinal vessels was observed.

Prior studies, based on direct visualization of the fundus, have noted cilio-retinal arteries in 7 per cent to 29.6 per cent of patients examined.

The careful review of stereo fundus photographs and early phase fluo-rescein angiographs aided in the observation of these vessels which, in many cases, could have gone clinically undetected. The authors contend this ac-counts for the surprisingly high incidence of cilioretinal arteries in the pre-sent series as compared with previous reports.

Authors' address:
Baylor College of Medicine
Houston, Texas
USA

* Abstract of paper presented at the Symposium

CHOROIDAL NAEVUS AND MELANOMA

J.A. OOSTERHUIS & C.H. SCHEFFER

(Leyden/Utrecht, The Netherlands)

Many papers have dealt with the characteristic features of choroidal tumours, which have been summarized by GASS (1974). Some special features will be described below.

In choroidal naevi we sometimes found that the naevus was clearly outlined by hypofluorescence in the arterial filling phase; in the choroidal filling phase, however, the visibility of the naevus diminished or even disappeared completely. In the late filling phase hypofluorescence in the area of the naevus reappeared (Figs 1a, b). This 'hide and seek' phenomenon is only observed in tumours when the choriocapillaris is free of naevus cells. The disappearance of visibility of the naevus can be explained by the fact that the naevus is shielded by the intense fluorescence of the choriocapillaris overlying the naevus.

Differentiation between naevus and melanoma in case of small pigmented tumours near the posterior pole can be extremely difficult (Table I). Generally, the melanoma is small as at an early stage it causes visual disturbance; elevation is usually slight. Subretinal exudation is not only observed in melanoma, as especially naevus with Drusen in the macular area has a tendency to develop a subretinal pooling of fluid. Therefore, also the fluorogram of both lesions can be very similar; perimetry can be of help. In case of a relative scotoma this may be caused by either naevus or melanoma; absence of a scotoma is indicative of a naevus, the presence of an absolute scotoma may be observed incidentally in a choroidal naevus but generally points to the presence of a melanoma. In these cases the most, sometimes the only, reliable test is the P32 isotope uptake test, especially when carried

Table I. Pigmented tumour posterior pole

D.D.	naevus	melanoma
Size	small	small
Elevation	slight	slight
Subretinal exudation	±	±
Fluorogram: leakage	±	±
Perimetry: scotoma	absent/ relative	relative/ absolute
P^{32} isotope uptake	−	+

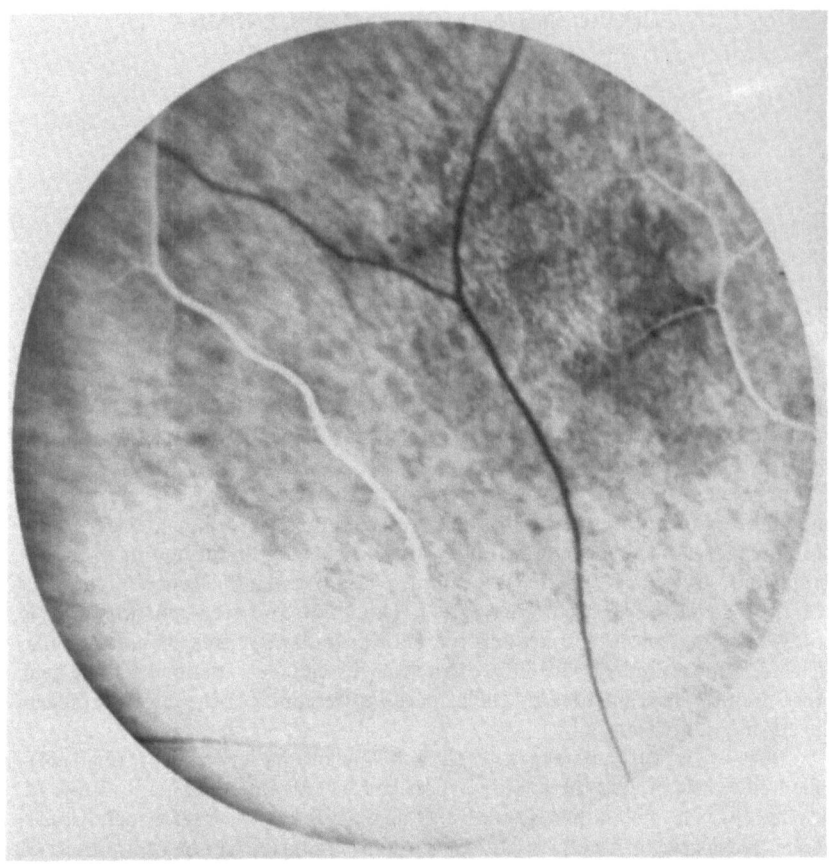

Fig. 1a. Fluorogram of a choroidal naevus in the choriocapillary filling phase. The naevus is scarcely visible as it is hidden behind the fluorescence of the overlying choriocapillaris.

out at the posterior pole by an experienced examiner.

In case the results of the various examination methods, such as ophthalmoscopy, fluorography, perimetry and isotope uptake test, are in agreement, pointing to malignancy, one should perform enucleation without delay and not wait to see whether the tumour shows signs of growing. Moreover, we found a choroidal tumour, which on the fluorogram showed a marked increase in size in the course of two years, to be a choroidal haemangioma on histologic examination. (Figs. 2a, b). Finally, MANSCHOT* demonstrated that already in very small choroidal melanomas ingrowth into the draining vessels can be observed; in these cases a waiting attitude may considerably increase the risk of metastatic disease.

We studied the frequency of characteristic features of melanoma in

* lecture before the Dutch Ophthalmological Society, March 1976.

264

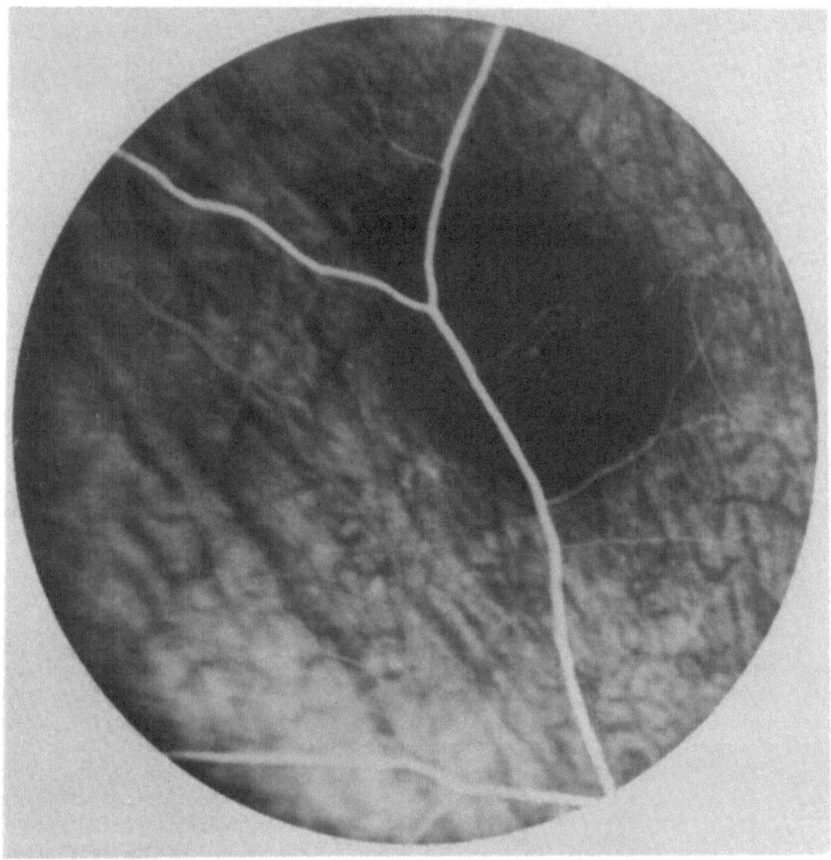

Fig. 1b. Same fundus as fig. 1a in the late venous phase shows a hypofluorescence at the site of the naevus.

117 tumours in which the diagnosis melanoma was verified on histologic examination. The results are summarized in Table II.

Hypofluorescence can be caused by hyperpigmentation of the tumour, haemorrhages at the surface of the tumour or necrosis of the tumour. Visibility of a vessel structure on the surface of the tumour was only visible in large tumours protruding through Bruch's membrane. Dilation of retinal capillaries was also mainly seen when the retina was overlying large tumours.

Table II. 117 Choroidal melanomas (histol. verified)

hypofluorescence	3 eyes (3%)
perforation Bruch's membrane	14 eyes (12%)
vessel structure	25 eyes (21%)
dilation retinal capillaries	50 eyes (43%)
fluorescent dots at the margin of the tumour	37 eyes (32%)
orange-yellow dots (lipofucine)	42 eyes (36%)

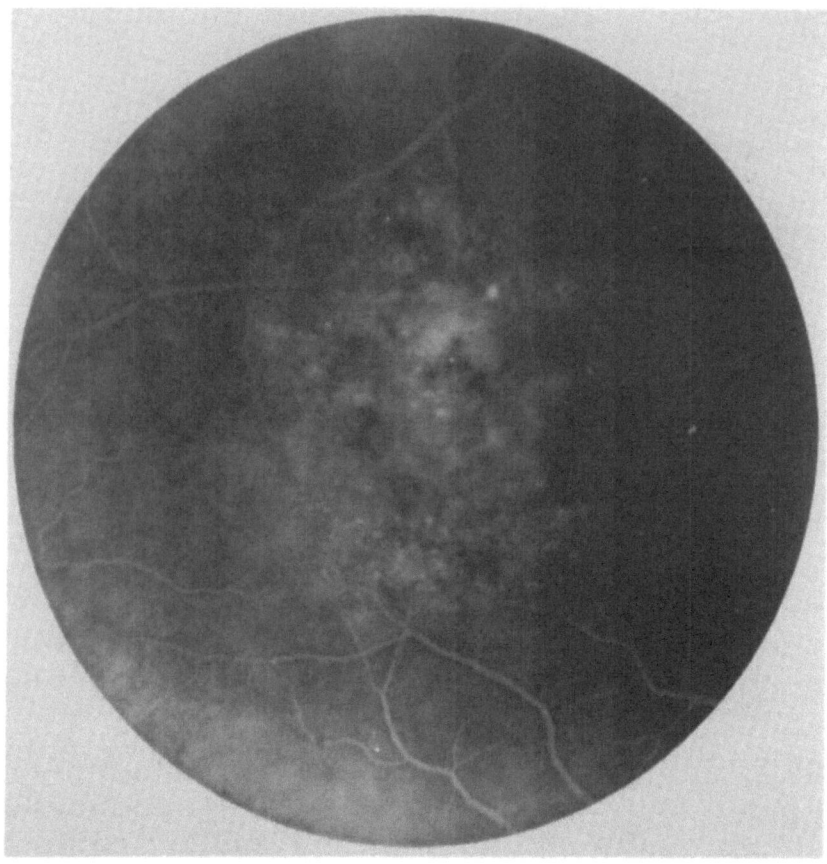

Fig. 2a. Fluorescence angiogram of a choroidal tumour presumed to be a melanoma or a haemangioma.

An interesting phenomenon was the presence of a bandshaped zone of absence of fluorescence at the periphery of choroidal melanomas. On histologic examination the choroid in these areas contained melanoma cells with intact overlying pigment epithelium.

The most surprising finding in our study was that in several eyes both on ophthalmoscopic and fluorographic study the tumour only seemed to border on the macular area but that the histologic sections revealed that the tumour had already grown behind the posterior pole. This might bear some importance with regard to the indication for photocoagulation treatment.

REFERENCE

GASS, J.D.M. Differential diagnosis of intraocular tumors. Mosby, St. Louis (1974).

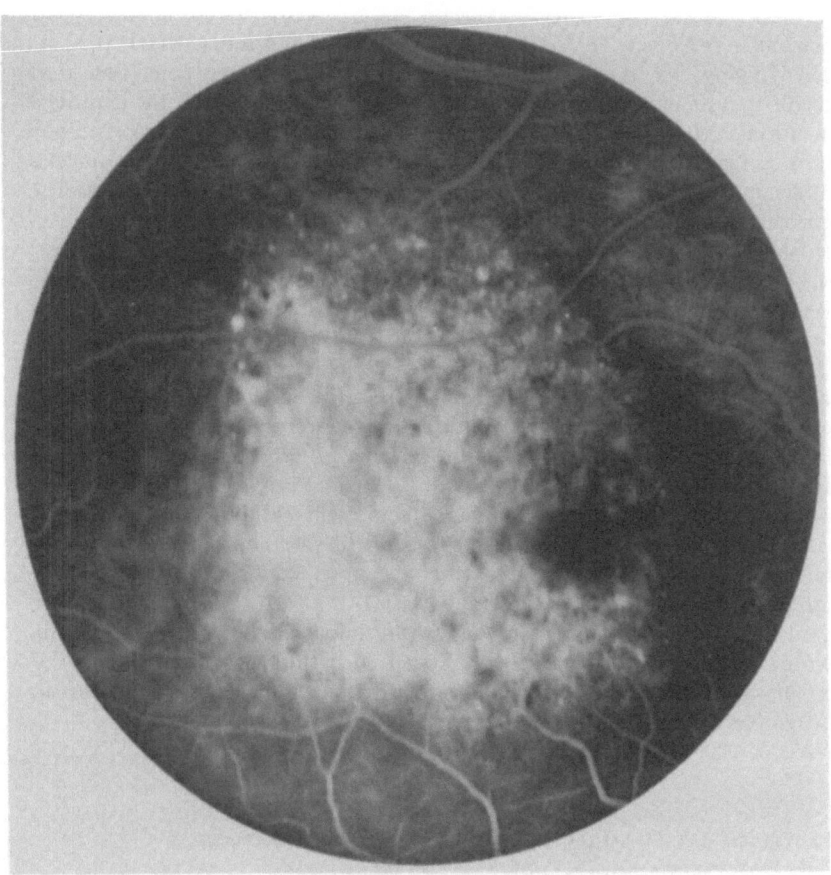

Fig. 2b. Same fundus as fig. 2a 2 years later. As the size of the tumour had increased the eye was removed but the histologic finding was a haemangioma!

Authors' addresses:
Prof. Dr. J.A. Oosterhuis
Eye Clinic
University Hospital
Leiden
The Netherlands

C.H. Scheffer, M.D
Royal Dutch Eye Clinic
Utrecht
The Netherlands

persons — 0-1.5 sec. (EVANS et al., 1973), 0.8 ± 0.4 sec. (SHIMIZU et al., 1974)). However, the retinal and choroidal circulations may some time start to fill simultaneously, or even occasionally the retinal before the choroidal in normal eyes. The early filling of the choroid occurs because its blood flow is faster than that in the retina, since the wide-lumen choriocapillaris offer much less resistance to blood flow than the retinal capillaries. The normal choroidal vascular bed always shows irregular, well-defined, geographical filling defects, varying in size and shape, in the choriocapillaris; they are commonly seen in the peripapillary choroid but may occur anywhere. These physiological spatial filling defects almost always last only a few seconds (1-2 sec. (OOSTERHUIS & BOEN-TAN, 1971), 2 sec. (HYVARINEN et al., 1969), 2.8 (1.8-3.9 sec. — giant-sized filled within 1.8-2.5 sec.) sec. (EVANS et al., 1973), up to the early retinal arteriovenous phase (ARCHER et al., 1970)) and only very rarely persist after the major retinal veins start to fill with fluorescein, i.e., the beginning of the retinal arterio-venous phase (HAYREH, 1974a). This fact is extremely important in distinguishing physiological spatial defects from pathological defects; the latter are seen when the perfusion pressure in the choroidal vascular bed falls as in glaucoma, low-tension glaucoma and allied disorders. The concept presented by EVANS et al. (1973) and SHIMIZU et al. (1974) that *all* choroidal filling defects on angiography are a physiological phenomena is not only wrong but also highly misleading. Localized pathological filling defects or circulatory delays in the choroid are distinct and important entities, not to be confused with morphologically identical physiological defects.

ACKNOWLEDGEMENTS

I am grateful to Mrs. Julie Wolf for her secretarial assistance.

REFERENCES

ARCHER, D., KRILL, A.E. & NEWELL, F.W. Fluorescein studies of normal choroidal circulation. *Amer. J. Ophthal.* 69: *543-554* (1970).

ASHTON, N. Observations on the choroidal circulation. *Brit. J. Ophthal.* 36: *465-481* (1952).

DOLLERY, C.T., HENKIND, P., KOHNER, E.M. & PATERSON, J.W. Effect of raised intraocular pressure on the retinal and choroidal circulation. *Invest. Ophthal.* 7: *191-198* (1968).

EVANS, P., SHIMIZU, K., LIMAYE, S., DEGLIN, E. & WRUCK, J. Fluorescein cine-angiography of the optic nerve head. *Trans. Amer. Acad. Ophthal. & Otolaryng.* 77: OP *260-273* (1973).

HAYREH, S.S. The ophthalmic artery. III. *Brit. J. Ophthal.* 46: *212-247* (1962).

HAYREH, S.S. Blood supply of the optic nerve head and its role in optic atrophy, glaucoma, and oedema of the optic disc. *Brit. J. Ophthal.* 53: *721-748* (1969).

HAYREH, S.S. Pathogenesis of visual field defects — role of the ciliary circulation. *Brit. J. Ophthal.* 54: *289-311* (1970).

HAYREH, S.S. Occlusion of the posterior ciliary arteries. *Trans. Amer. Acad. Ophthal. & Otolaryng.* 77: OP *300-309* (1973).

HAYREH, S.S. Recent advances in fluorescein fundus angiography. *Brit. J. Ophthal.* 58: *391-412* (1974a).

AN ANGIOGRAPHIC AND HISTOPATHOLOGIC CONFRONTATION CONCERNING THE CHORIORETINAL CHANGES IN FRONT OF A HUMAN MALIGNANT MELANOMA OF THE CHOROID (ELECTRON MICROSCOPIC STUDY)

S. LIMON & G. COSCAS

(Paris, France)

The malignant melanoma of the choroid of a fifty year old man lifting up the inferior temporal vessels is analysed by angiography. Then, after the enucleation of the eye, the light and electron microscopic study of the tumor and of the surrounding chorio-retinal region is performed.

The angiographic pictures show a double circulation with tortuous choroidal vessels within the tumor. Large deep areas of the lesion having irregular wide pools of diffusion are stained by the fluorescein. They are more or less masked by a large irregular unhomogeneous dark area. There is leakage along the inferior temporal vein which passes over the tumor. During the late stages, the fluorescein stains nearly the whole tumor and there is a persistance and an accumulation of the dye.

The light and electron microscopic study confirms the diagnosis of a malignant melanoma of the choroid which is constituted by a few fusiform cells and by numerous poorly pigmented round pseudoepithelial cells. Areas of necrosis of the tumoral tissue predominate along the chorio-retinal junction, as does also the melanin pigment which is accumulated in the macrophages. Big vessels with just a thin endothelial wall are scattered throughout the whole tumor. At the center of the lesion, the tumor ruptured the Bruch's membrane and widely invaded the retina as far as the nerve fibers layer. It is very near the inferior temporal vessels but does not surround them. The middle layers of the wall of these vessels are swollen by a slight oedema which dissociates and thickens the basement membranes, however, the endothelial cells and their junctions are normal. Many red blood cells are scattered around the vein among the nerve fibers. The visible changes in the basement membranes of the capillaries which contain many vacuoles are common in a person of this age and we cannot say that they are caused entirely by the tumor. Laterally the tumor has destroyed a part of the chorio-capillaris. Where the latter is still present, it is as dilated as the big choroidal vessels which lie in front of it. The tumor barely touches the pigmentary epithelium, but the basement membrane of the pigment epithelium is intact. There is a slight retinal detachment. At the edges of the tumoral region there is also an enormous diffuse vascular dilatation in the choroid. There are many serous detachments of the pigment epithelium basement membrane and the epithelial cells themselves. The visual retina is also detached. Just a thin layer of subretinal fluid separates the inner retinal layers from the pigment epithelium. This fluid contains some tumor cells,

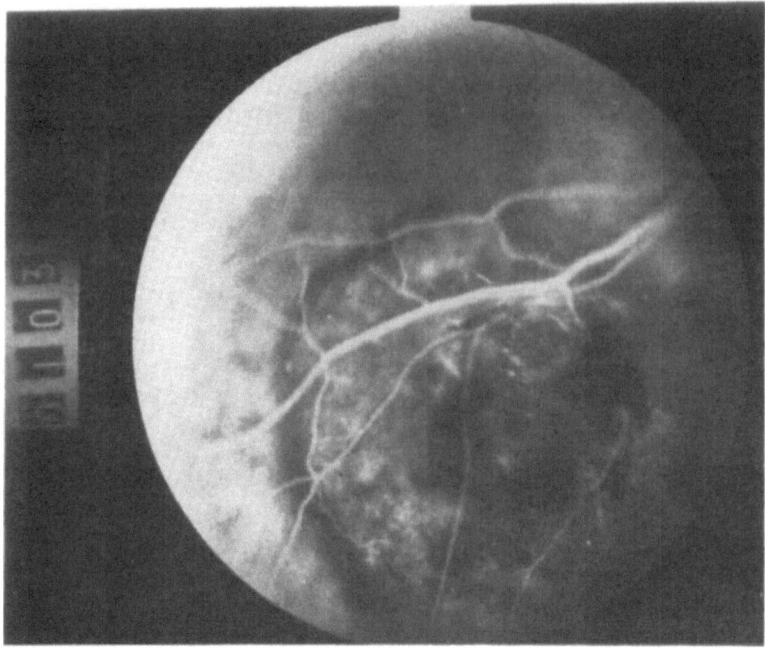

Fig. 1. Angiography of the malignant melanoma of the choroid situated under the inferior temporal vessels near the papilla. In the 103rd second.

pigmented epithelial cells and fragments of the outer segment of the photo-receptor cells. The top of their inner segment is surrounded by this fluid. The peripheral retinal detachment does not extend as far as the enormous choroidal vascular dilatation which is present far beyond the edges of the tumoral tissue.

Thus, the results of the angiographic and histological studies are typical for a malignant melanoma of the choroid, and we thought if of interest to compare them in the same case.

The double retino-choroidal vascularisation illustrates well the vascular-isation which develops inside the tumor. The precocity of the staining resulting in large fluorescent areas with blurred edges is explained by the enormous choroidal vasodilatation and the poorly pigmented tissue of the tumor. The masking process is essentially the consequence of the central haemorrhage which is evident clinically. But, in our opinion, the diffusion of the fluorescein through the wall of the inferior temporal vein seems to be more important than one would expect from the aspect of the slight changes of the different layers of this vessel. However the abundant blood extravasation confirms the increase of the vascular permeability.

On the other hand, when looking at the angiographic pictures it is more difficult to appreciate the exact role of the tumoral necrosis and of the presence and the size of the epithelial serous detachments which are them-selves hidden by the retinal detachment. Each of these processes causes the

270

image of staining with diffusion, but it is impossible to judge their effect separately.

In conclusion, it would appear to be extremely useful to perform this comparative study whenever possible, as it reveals the perfect correlation existing between the anatomical interpretation of the angiographic data and the presence of lesions as confirmed by the histological control. However, it remains difficult clinically to make a strict qualitative and quantitative analysis of several pathological processes associated in the same lesion, and which have more or less the same angiographic expression.

REFERENCES

BRIHAYE VAN GEERTRUYDEN, M. Contribution à l'étude des tumeurs mélaniques de l'uvée et de leur origine. *Docum. Ophthal.* 17: *163-166* (1963).

CALLENDER, G.R., WILDER, H.C. & ASCH, J.E. Five hundred malignant melanomas of the choroid and ciliary body followed five years and longer. *Amer. J. Ophthal.* 85: *962-965* (1942).

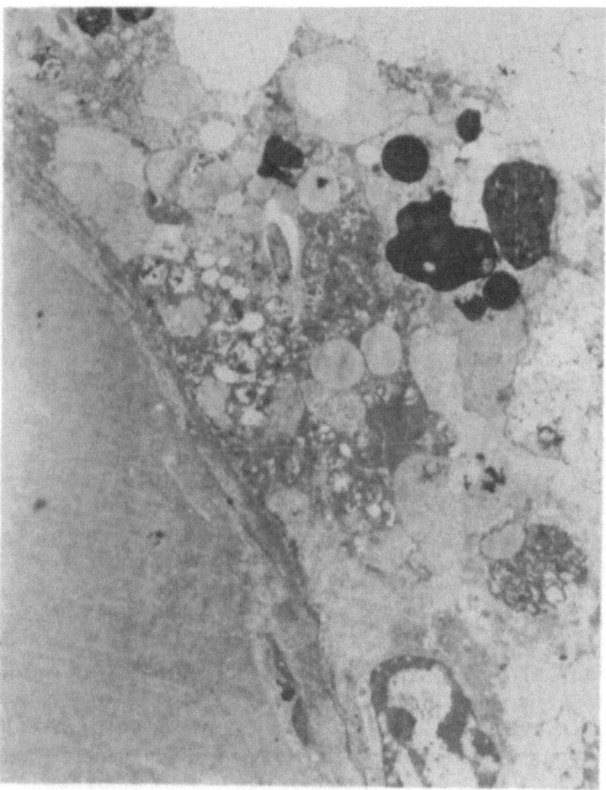

Fig. 2. Electron microscopy. Detail of the tumor. At the junction of the choroid and of the retina, the choriocapillaris disappears, many tumoral cells are dying and there are many pigmented macrophages. In front there is a large serous detachment of the pigmentary epithelium.

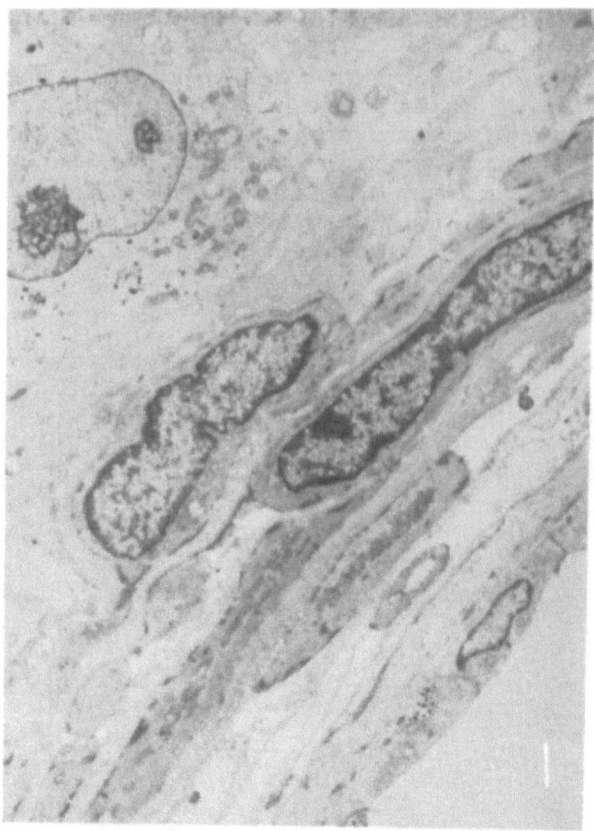

Fig. 3.   Electron microscopy. A tumoral cell reaches the inferior temporal vein which is not invaded. There is only a slight oedema in the middle layers of this one.

EGEBERG, J. & JENSEN, O.A. Malignant melanomas of the human choroid and ciliary body (A comparison of light microscopical and ultrastructural morphology). *Acta path. microbiol. scand.* 80: *519-521* (1972).

ELLIOT, A.J. Recent advances in the diagnosis and management of macular and paramacular tumors. *Canada. J. Ophthal.* 3: *191-201* (1968).

GASS, J.D., SEVER, R.J., SPARKS, D. & GOREN, J. Technique combinée de fondoscopie à la fluorescéine et d'angiographie oculaire. *Arch. Ophthal.* 69: *778-779* (1963).

NORTON, E.W.D. The use of fluorescein in the differential diagnosis of secondary retinal detachments. *Mod. Probl. Ophthal.* Karger édit., Basel. 5: *202-217* (1967).

REESE, A.B., ARCHILA E.A., JONES, I.S. & COOPER, W.C. Necrosis of malignant melanoma of the choroid. *Amer. J. Ophthal.* 69: *91-92* (1970).

Authors' address:
Clinique Ophtalmologique de l'Hôtel-Dieu de Paris
Place de parvis Nôtre-Dame
Paris 75004
France

ON THE SIGNIFICANCE OF THE BRIGHT
DOT-LIKE FLUORESCENCE AT DIFFERENT
MALIGNANT INTRAOCULAR TUMOROUS GROWTH

B. KOVÁCS

(Pécs, Hungary)

This fluorescence angiographic study has been carried out on malignant choroidal melanoma, metastatic choroid carcinoma and retinoblastoma with the main objects in view: What is the most typical staining pattern found in these different malignant tumors? In our series the most frequent pattern of fluorescence was a bright punctate, usually discrete small dot-like spots, which occurred all over the tumor, but more marked at the periphery. They mostly appeared in the arteriovenous phase and tended to become more prominent and numerous during the late venous phase. Then the extension of the dots was permanent and had distinct outlines. The dots persisted for long and in some cases they began to fade half an hour later. This pattern has been described by HILL (1968) and several recent reports have presented this entity as a relatively frequent finding. This phenomenon occurring in different tumors presumably refers to an identical or at least similar pathogenic origin.

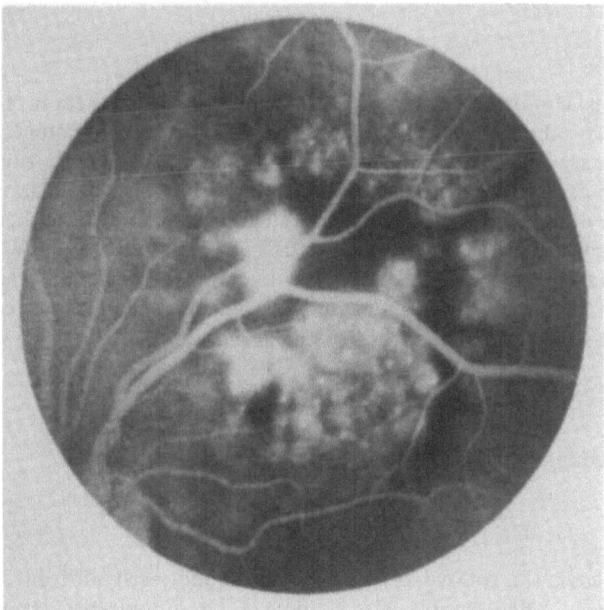

Fig. 1. Flat malignant melanoma. *Case 1*. Fluorescein angiogram, arteriovenous phase.

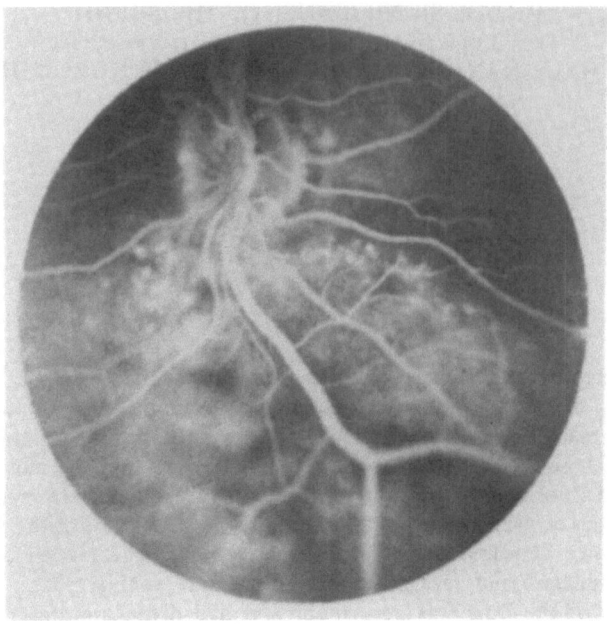

Fig. 2. Highly elevated malignant melanoma, *Case 2*. Fluorescein angiogram, arterio-venous phase.

MATERIAL AND METHOD

This series is comprised of 16 patients who were examined in the Eye Department of the University Medical School of Pécs, and found to have proved primary malignant melanoma in 8 cases, metastatic tumors of choroid in 5 cases and retinoblastoma in 3 cases. Fluorescence angiographic studies were done in all the cases in the standard manner with the Zeiss Jena camera with the Baird Atomic B_4 filter as an exciting filter and KW No. 58 green filter as the barrier. A Fluorescite injection of 5 or 10% was given. Preceding angiography color slides and conventional pictures were taken. The findings were compared with the clinical ones.

RESULTS

The most frequent angiographic findings were as follows:

I. Malignant choroidal melanoma

In all the 8 cases the following patterns were found: early mottling, patchy fluorescence, dot-like spots, late staining. The 'double-circulation' was observed only in two cases.

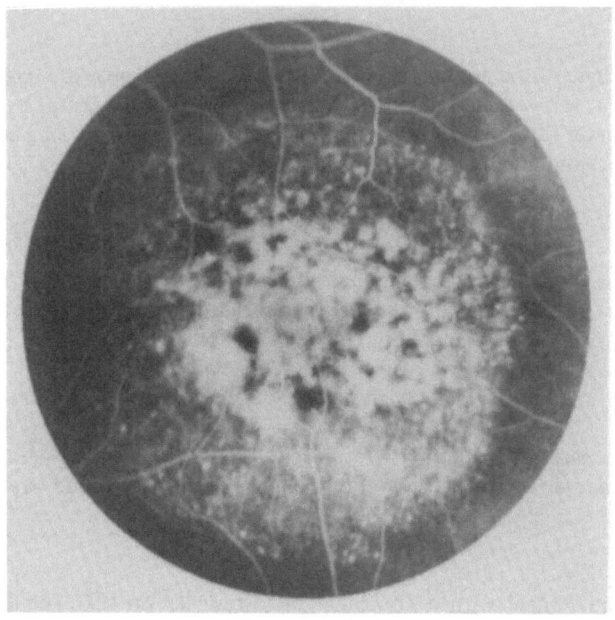

Fig. 3. Choroidal metastasis from bronchial carcinoma, *Case 3*. Fluorescein angiogram, arteriovenous phase.

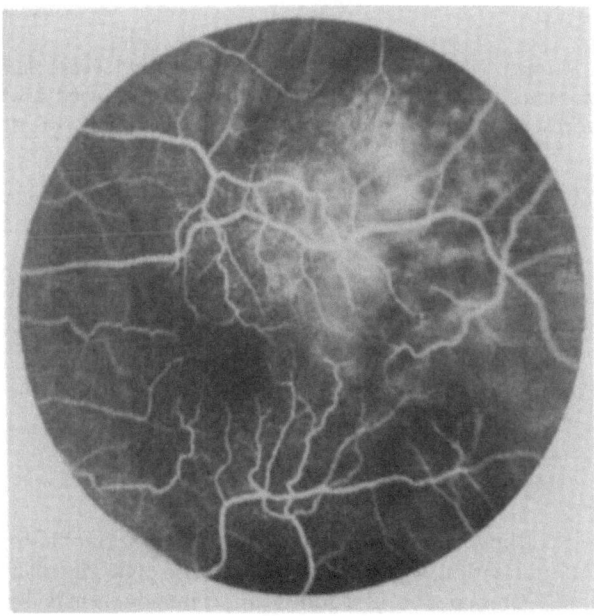

Fig. 4. Choroidal metastasis from breast carcinoma, *Case 4*. Fluorescein angiogram, arteriovenous phase.

275

Case 1.

Flat malignant melanoma in the left eye of a 41-year-old woman. The angiogram showed early mottling and several bright dot-like spots. Six months later the repeated angiography showed an increasing number of these spots and an enlargement of the tumor. Fig. 1.

Case 2.

38-year-old male with a highly elevated tumor in the left eye. The angiogram showed mottled fluorescence and bright dot-like spots in the upper-periferial part of the tumor. Fig. 2.

II. Metastatic choroid carcinoma

In all the cases late staining was present. Three of five cases showed early mottling and dot-like spots. No 'double-circulation' was found at all.

Case 3

44-year-old female with a choroidal metastasis in the left eye as the first clinical manifestation of bronchogenic carcinoma. The angiogram showed prominent patchy fluorescence in the center, and marked, numerous dot-like spots all over the tumor. Fig. 3.

Case 4

67-year-old woman who had radical mastectomy two years earlier, with metastatic carcinoma in the left eye. The angiogram showed a widespread mottled fluorescence and dot-like spots in the periphery of the tumor. Fig. 4.

III. Retinoblastoma

In all of the three cases we observed a very prominent staining, and two of them showed remarkable angiographic feature. At first WETZIG & JEPSON (1966) found that the retinoblastoma exhibited a bright fluorescence. WESSING (1968) reported more detailed observations on the rich vascular supply of the tumor and on the aneurysma-like dilatations of the enlarged vessels.

Case 5

This two-year-old boy was first observed with a large retinoblastoma in the left eye, and enucleation was carried out. In that time the right eye was entirely normal. On occasion of a follow-up examination half a year later, we observed a white tumor in the right macular area. According to the angiography the tumor began to fluoresce during early arteriovenous phase and became more prominent later. There was absence of filling around the tumor. It is of special interest for the present study that punctate dot-like spots appeared in the moderately elevated upper part of the tumor, which became more prominent and numerous as the time passed and they persisted for long. Tortuous, meandering retinal, and a lot of arterio-venous collateral vessels were seen.

DISCUSSION

In all our series the different malignant tumors exhibited a positive fluorescent staining. The pattern of fluorescence showed several kinds of variance, nevertheless the dot-like spots were observed most frequently (81%) and, therefore, were considered the most characteristic feature.

HAYREH (1971) suggested that the punctate fluorescence could represent small localized exudates under the retina or the pigment epithelium. YANKO (1973) believed that they were due to the tumoral vessels filled with dye, running perpendicularly to the tumor's surface. Based on histological findings of melanoma cases they emphasized that the relation of

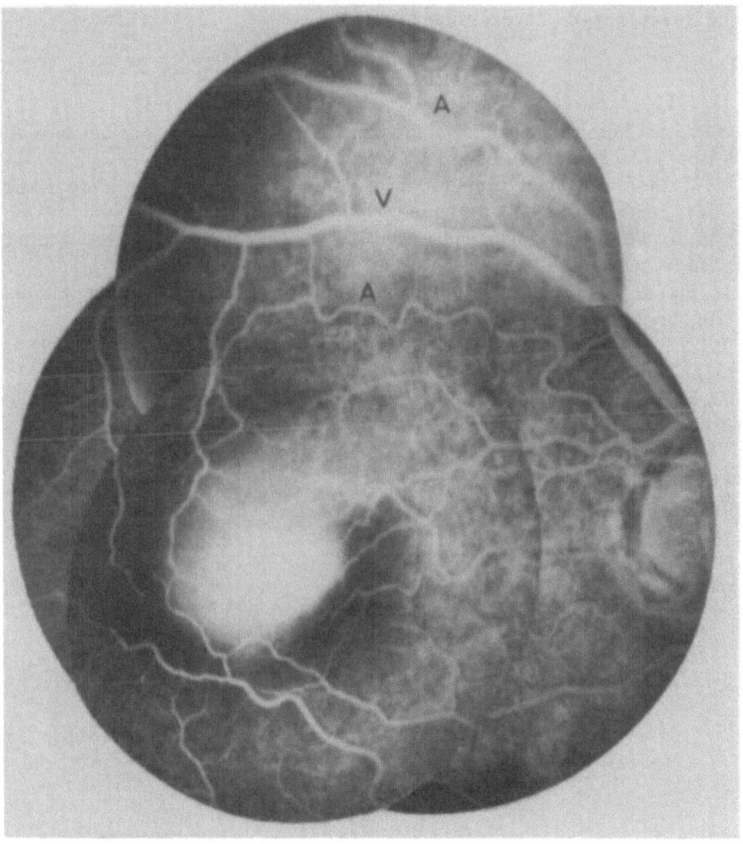

Fig. 5. Retinoblastoma, *Case 5.* with arterio-venous collateral vessels; A = artery, V = vein. Fluorescein angiogram, arteriovenous phase.

punctate fluorescence to retinal pigment epithelium could not be entirely overlooked. Since to the best of our knowledge similar fluorescence pattern has not yet been reported in patients with retinoblastomas, we have paid particular attention to studying our cases angiographically, above all, from the point of view of their vascular alternations. These studies have suggested that these spots may be fluorescent microaneurysms.

This assumption is supported by the following:

1. The filling and staining pattern of the verified microaneurysms are similar to or identical with these dot-like spots.

2. Signs of retinal hypoxia were observed. Retinal hypoxia is accepted as the main etiological factor of microaneurysms.

3. In all cases of retinoblastomas the rapid development (which is also related to the hypoxia) of collateral vessels, may be due to the compression and a vaso-obliterative effect of the quickly expanding tumor.

4. There are histological (WOLTER, 1961) and angiographical (WESSING, 1968) evidences of microaneurysms within retinoblastomas.

Since the different tumors described above showed identical pattern of fluorescence with the retinoblastoma morphologically, it is highly probable that the dot-like spots have similar origin.

REFERENCES

HAYREH, S.S. Choroidal Melanomata. Proc. int. Symp. Fluorescein Angiography, Albi 1969, pp. *115-130* (Karger, Basel 1971).

HILL, D.W. Choroidal tumors, application of fluorescence angiography. *Proc. R. Soc. Med.* 61: *1039-1040* (1968).

WESSING, A. Fluoreszenzangiographie der Retina. Georg Thieme Verlag Stuttgart pp. *140-142* (1968).

WETZIG, P.C. & JEPSON, C.N. Fluorescein photography in the differential diagnosis of retinoblastoma. *Am. J. Ophthal.* 61: *341-343* (1966).

WOLTER, J.R. The Blood Vessels of Retinoblastomas. *Arch. Ophthal.* 66: *545-551* (1961).

YANKO, L. An angiographic and histologic study of the vasculature of choroidal malignant melanoma. *Acta Ophthal. Kbh.* 51: *12-24* (1973).

Author's address:
Department of Ophthalmology
University of Pécs
Ifjuság u. 31
7643 Pécs
Hungary

ANGIOGRAPHIC FOLLOW UP OF CHOROIDAL MELANOMA

K. RUBINSTEIN

(Birmingham, England)

In three situations serial angiography is of essential value for assessment of choroidal melanoma. First, in those cases where the diagnosis is doubtful at the time of first examination, second, as a follow up when the initial pattern is not definitive, and third, as a follow up of conservatively treated tumours.

The assessment of malignancy of a choroidal melanoma is not always easy, even when aided by initial angiography. Simple choroidal naevi give an homogenous, negative (black) clear cut area on fluorogram, similar to that of the haemorrhage. This pattern does not change from early to late stages of the test. The crucial differentiation is between these naevi and the not so dense, dark lesions, small or large, which may show ophthalmoscopically a faint pattern of orange or white specks and are usually called atypical naevi or benign melanoma. Fluorogram shows a mottled pattern, stationary or sometimes even fading away in later stages. These lesions may be observed for years to remain unchanged and yet the fluorescein pattern eventually changes, the original stationary mottling obtained on fluorogram is sharpening and some isolated areas show increasing glow in late stages. (Fig. 1). Ophthalmoscopically one may observe gradual darkening of the lesion but fluorogram change is always much earlier and it signifies a transition from dormancy to active malignant growth.

Several of my cases were followed for up to 15 years vbefore becoming active and then they showed enlargement or an increased elevation or haemorrhagic episodes. Some eyes which were enucleated proved histologically to be malignant, sometimes containing foci of necrosis and consisting of spindle cells with islands of more undifferentiated epitheloid cells, probably represented in fluorograms by insular glowing areas. These lesions respond well to photocoagulation treatment, especially when treated early. They should be designated as melanoma in situ, the terms naevus or benign melanoma are histologically unjustified and clinically misleading, as most of them – if not all – carry a potential of malignancy.

Conservatively treated melanoma requires a careful follow up. The desirable fluorescein angiography pattern after treatment is a completely black, avascular area. This applies to the results of treatment by light coagulation or radiotherapy. (Fig. 2). A repetition of treatment is indicated to the not quite destroyed portions of the tumour which show fluorescein leakage. We have, however, followed up eyes after treatment in which clusters of vessels persisted in the operated areas without any change for over 10 years. These

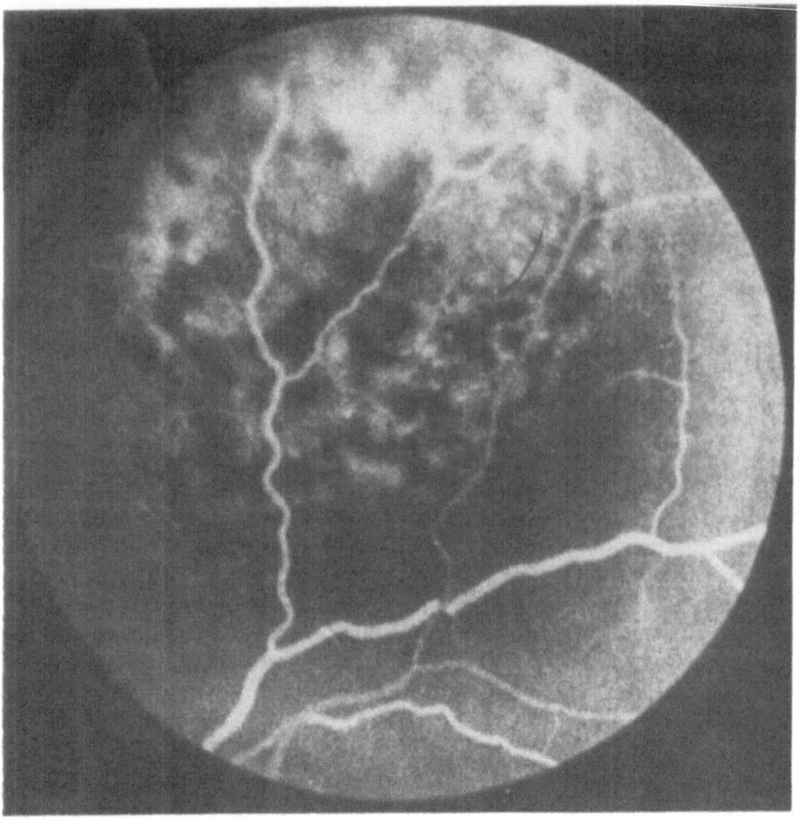

a)

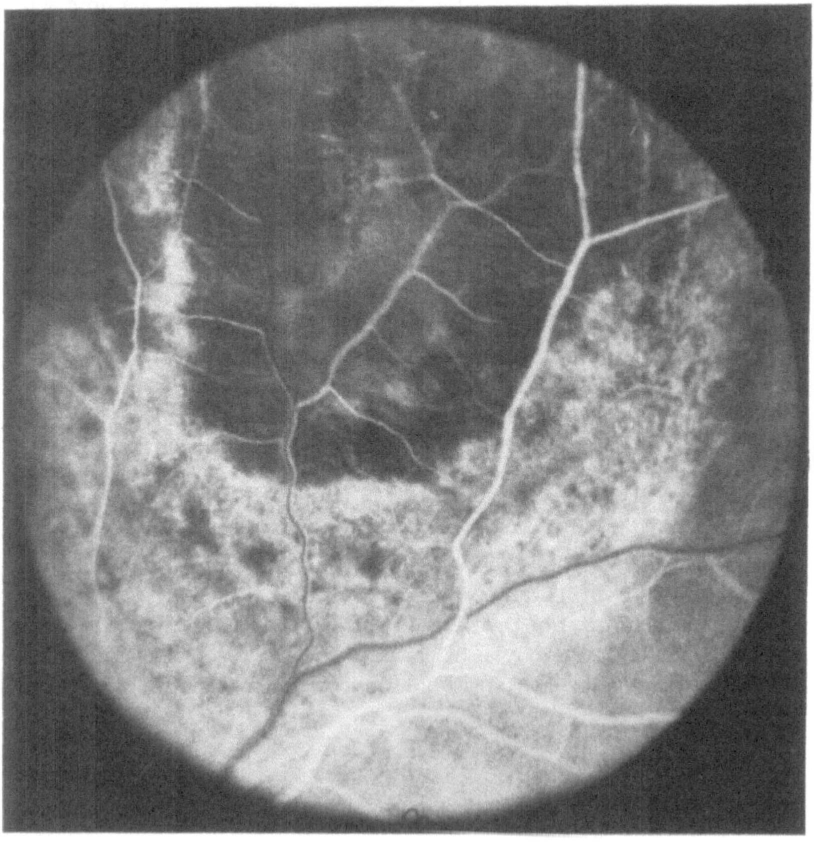

b)

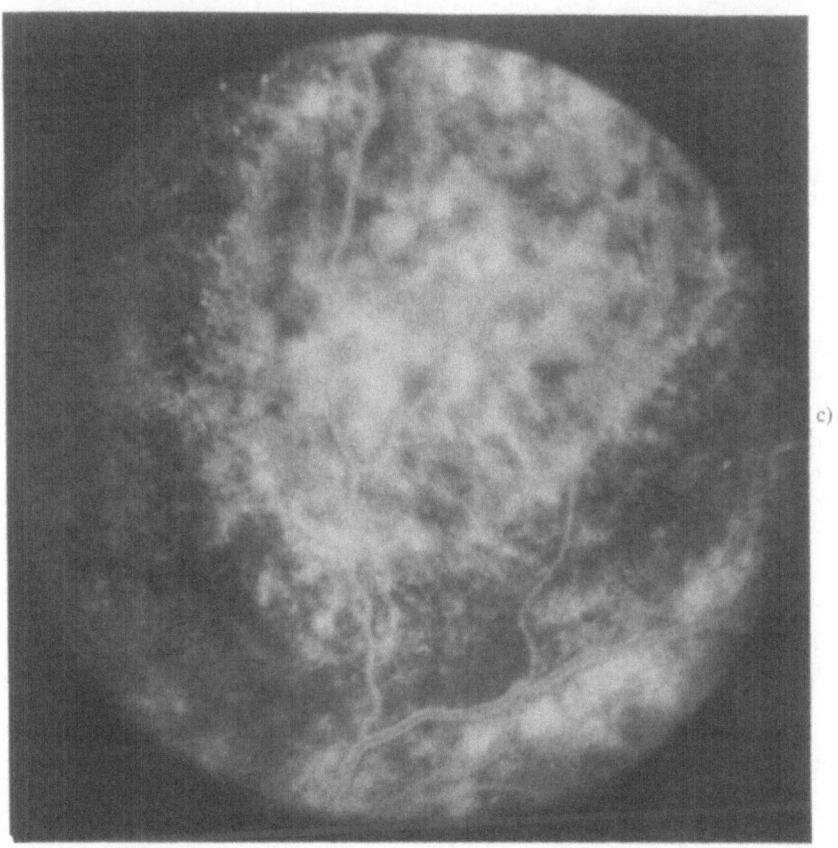

c)

Fig. 1. A female, age 46. a) 1966 angiogram, 9 seconds after injection. The mottled pattern remained unchanged and commenced fading away after 3 minutes; b) 1975 angiogram, 9 seconds after injection; c) 30 seconds after injection showing a typical melanoma pattern, and the glow increasing in intensity in later stages.

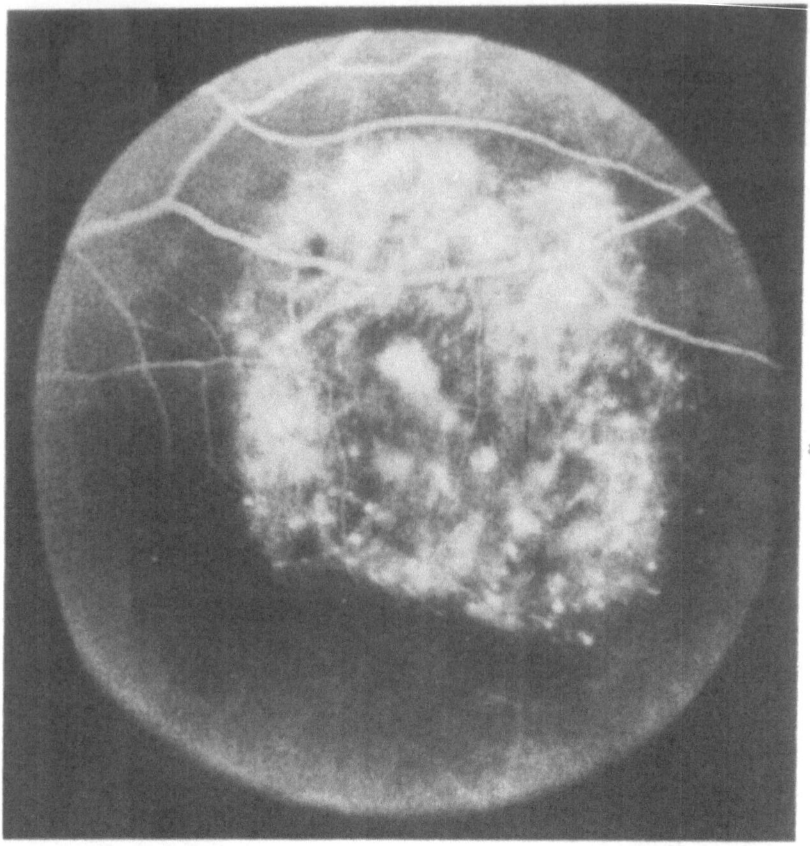

a)

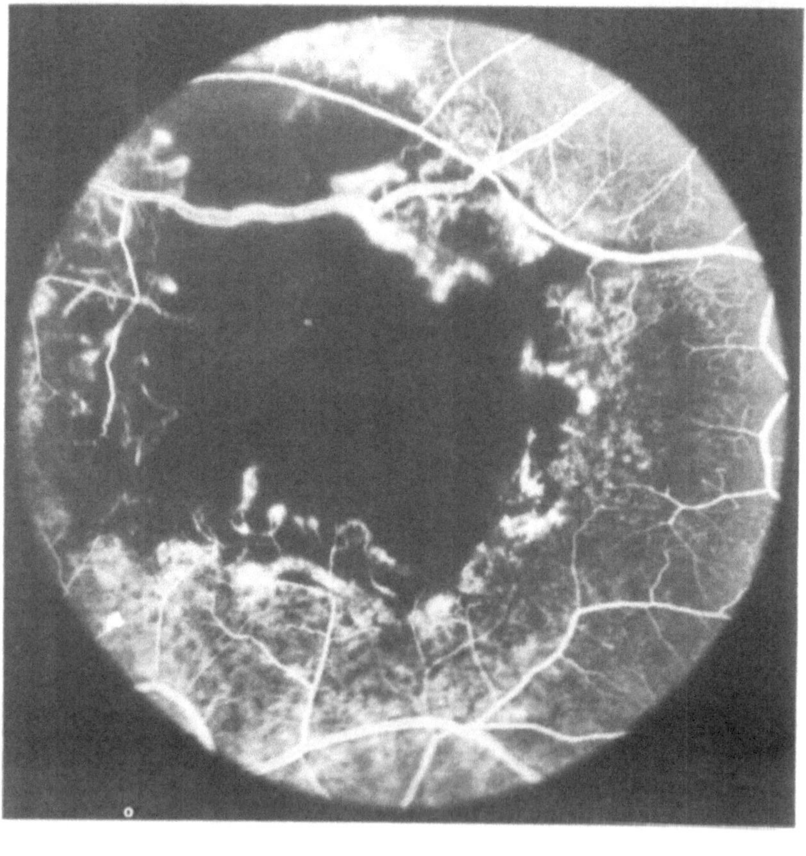

b)

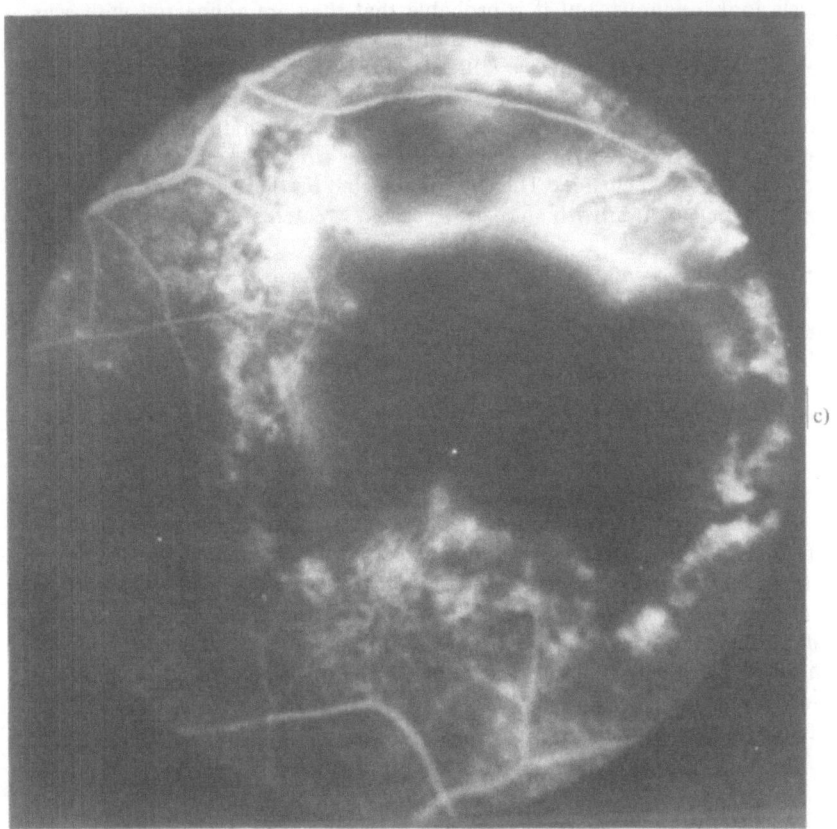

c)

Fig. 2. A male, age 43. a) 1973 angiogram, 20 seconds after injection showing a pattern typical of malignant melanoma; b) 3 years later (1976) angiogram, showing complete destruction of tumour, 8 seconds stage; c) 1 minute stage.

vessels look ominous, but it is probable that they are connected with scar tissue which sometimes stains too, and they seem innocuous. Inspite, however, of this long follow up we still regard these vessels with suspicion. As a rule in cases which showed clinical recurrence, a new irregular pattern of choroidal vessels was seen on fluorograms before ophthalmoscopic signs of new activity. Repeated fluorescein angiograms showed progressive increase in the size of vessel clusters. The eyes enucleated on these grounds proved to contain a malignant growth amongst a scarred, treated area.

Author's address:
10 Pritchatts Road
Edgbaston
Birmingham B15 1QT
Great Britain

DISCUSSION

Dr Norton: I just like to point out the conflict that is facing ophthalmologists to-day. You heard Dr Oosterhuis make the statement that the diagnosis of malignant melanomas means you should take the eye out. On the other hand Dr Rubinstein showed some cases which he has followed for 16 years and he feels confident on the diagnosis and yet the patient must be living otherwise I doubt he could follow them. There is this conflict on how to manage pigmented lesions in the fundus and I wonder if Dr Gass would initiate the discussion.

Dr Gass: There are many problems concerning the management of small melanomas, and we do not have time to discuss all of them. One of the basic problems is: Is our present classification of malignant melanomas accurate? Can we rely on the fact that a spindle-A melanoma is indeed a malignant tumor. All of the evidence available today suggests that a spindle tumor is a benign tumor or is a very, very lowgrade malignancy. That brings us to a second problem: Is the P-32 test really a test of mitotic activity within the tumor? I do not believe that it is. There is no relationship between the degree of positivity of the P-32 test when done in a spindle-A melanoma versus an epitheloid cell melanoma. It would appear, therefore, that the P-32 test cannot differentiate a highly malignant tumor with much mitotic activity from a tumor that is either benign or of low-grade malignancy.

Another problem with the P-32 test is that most of the data available concerning this test has come from study of eyes where the clinician has known ahead of time that he is dealing with a malignant melanoma. Relatively little data is available concerning P-32 testing of lesions that are not melanomas. When the test is negative, the eyes are not removed. We do not know the histology of those lesions with a negative test. In 1955, dermatologists were in hopes that the test would permit an accurate diagnosis of a malignant melanoma prior to removal of a dermal lesion. For a few years, the dermatologic literature contained a number of reports concerning the correlation of P-32 testing and cutaneous lesions. They had the advantage over the ophthalmologist in that they were able to study both suspected benign tumors as well as melanomas. They also were able to excise all of the lesions for histologic study. While they too found a high correlation between a positive P-32 test and a malignant melanoma, they also found a significant incidence of both false positive and false negative tests. For this reason, the dermatologists have abandoned the test. We cannot rely on the P-32 test as being one that distinguishes a malignant melanoma from a non-malignant tumor. It is probable that the P-32 test, when positive, is indicative of the presence of a tumor that is solid and that contains many cells, and that is about all the information that it is providing. I think it is a valuable test, but it is a test that should be used only after the clinician has decided that there is a high probability that the tumor in question is a malignant melanoma and that he is prepared to enucleate the eye. On the operating table, prior to enucleation, a P-32 test should be done. If the P-32 test is positive, then it confirms, but does not prove unequivocally that the tumor is a malignant melanoma. If the test is negative, then it should alert the physician to the possibility and perhaps probability that the tumor in question may not be a malignant melanoma despite its clinical appearance.

Now for some comments concerning the management of patients with small pigmented tumors that are causing no visual disturbance. First of all, the clinician cannot rely on angiography to clearly differentiate a malignant melanoma from a large choroidal nevus. A great variety of staining patterns are seen overlying benign choroidal nevi. While there are some angiographic clues as to the presence of a malignant melanoma, its greatest use is in providing additional photographic information to be used in following the patient for evidence of change. The clinician must however be cautious in interpreting angiographic changes that occur subsequently. Dr Rubinstein showed a nice case of a lesion that on subsequent examination showed no change in size, but showed an apron-shaped area of depigmentation of the pigmentepithelium inferior to the tumor. There was also additional staining on the surface of the tumor. This does not necessarily mean that the tumor in question is a malignant melanoma. It is only showing angiographic evidence that the pigment epithelium is damaged, but such pigment epithelial damage may occur secondary to a nevus as well as a melanoma. The area of depigmentation inferior to the tumor is related to nothing more than prolonged detachment of the retina extending inferior to the tumor. I believe that small slightly elevated pigmented tumors of less that seven disc diameters in size should be observed for evidence of growth, if they show no unequivocal evidence of malignancy such as extension through Bruch's membrane.

Dr Oosterhuis: I agree with Dr Gass that the P-32 test will not give a differentiation between a spindle A, spindle B or epitheloid cell type melanoma; only histologic examination can give this information at the moment. In Holland we have a great experience of the P-32 test because most of the melanoma suspects are referred to our clinic. The P-32 test is related to the number of cells but only to a minor degree in case the number of mitoses is small. Thus, inflammatory lesions like sarcoidosis or prominent non-proliferating lesions such as haemangioma may show an increase of activity of about 30–40%. As P-32 actively participates in the phosphonucleotide metabolism there is a great correlation between the number of mitoses and increase of P-32 test.

A positive test between +60 and +100% is strongly in favour of a malignancy and up till now in all patients with a P-32 of 100% or more, even in very small tumors, the tumors proved to be melanomas on histologic examination. A 100% malignancy was also found in the tumor suspects of 60-100% positive, when the results of fluorescence angiography and perimetry also pointed to malignancy.

Generally in medicine, when a malignancy is established, treatment is started as soon as possible to consider if small melanomas of the choroid are an exception to this rule is beyond the scope of this paper.

Dr Norton: Could I ask you two questions. One of your cases had a negative P-32 test and a year later a positive P-32 test. You took the eye out and it was a haemangioma. So you have one false positive; we have now a whole collection in the United States. Secondly, if you have a small lesion like this, that you thought had a 90% chance of being a malignant melanoma and that it was the patients only eye, what would you do?

Dr Oosterhuis: If it is the patient's only eye, he belongs to the fortunately small number of special cases for which no strict rules for treatment can be given.

Mr Rubinstein: The eye that you saw was enucleated, it was a malignancy. Of the 18 cases, which perhaps you remember I was talking about in Miami 5 years ago, 6 had by now tumours growing from this kind of lesion. What I wanted to say really, is that you talk in terms of morphology, about spindle cells, epitheloid cells etc. If you talk to your dermatologist or to your oncologist, they don't talk about that, they talk about immunity. They have got melanomata of the skin that come and go. It is a normal feature of a melanoma. They now have got sera but when they tried them on people they did not work, but they worked experimentally, and they prohibit the growth of melanomas. And I am sure that the answer here is that they are melanomata that show no growth for years. But if you can treat easily without losing the eye and without losing the sight in the eye, then I veer slowly towards the attitude that obviously enucleation is not the treatment for them. They are flat childishly easy to destroy with light coagulation although I have not been doing this, as you know, for all these years because otherwise I would not have the follow-up and I am delighted whenever my colleagues under whose care these patients are tell me, don't treat this, this is benign, I am happy because I have the patients back. But I come to the point that they really should be treated conservatively with ease and safety and not to have to watch them every year for the next 20 years.

Dr Limon: Je voudrais demander à Mr. Rubinstein si il estime que l'examen angiographique qu'il fait apres ces photocoagulations tumorales forme un critère suffisant pour affirmer que la lésion est détruite. Comme Mr. Oosterhuis a insisté, il y a des propagations à très longue distance et elles peuvent se faire par une mince couche de cellules peu pigmentées parceque ce sont souvent des formes pseudo-épithéliales et je ne crois pas que dans ces cas il y ait une traduction angiographique.

Mr Rubinstein: Cases after conservative treatment are checked with fluorescein, I do not discharge them. The fact that none of them had secondaries is perhaps an answer to the second part of your question. It worries me however when I see photographs like Oosterhuis' showing the extension of the tumour beyond the limits.

Dr Gass: I would like to say just one more thing about the treatment of these small tumors. To me photocoagulation treatment of these small tumors in the back of the eye should be confined to those few patients who develop and maintain a serous detachment overlying a small tumor that cannot be clearly differentiated from a benign choroidal nevus. The treatment should be directed only to the site of the leak overlying the tumor. I think it is unwise, however, to only photocoagulate all of the questionable pigmented choroidal tumors. This reminds me of the dermatologist who years ago decided to cut off, or burn off, all cutaneous moles with the thought that they could prevent patients from developing malignant melanomas. I just think it is a little bit absurd to treat these pigmented choroidal tumors even if they are slightly elevated before you have taken time to watch them. If they are spindle-A tumors or nevi, the patient will probably do quite well following photocoagulation. If it happens that it is a malignant tumor, one which is capable of metastasising, it is very unlike that you will cure the patient with the photocoagulator and as a matter of fact, there is a good possibility that you might disseminate the tumor. At least the statistics that Martin Vogel has presented, and I do not know if anyone would care to comment on them, would suggest that they had a significantly high mortality rate in treating small melanomas with photocoagulation. I think that photocoagulation for a malignant melanoma is something that should never be done unless the patient understands that he is taking a high risk in choosing that form of therapy.

Dr Hayreh: I think it is a matter of philosophy which we are indulging in. The attitude in our department is totally different and we are aware of Dr Gass's views. We feel that if P32 is positive and on angiography and ultrasonography we also find a characteristic pattern of a malignant melanoma, then we are inclined to enucleate the eye in view of the better five year survival results in persons with enucleated eyes. It has been shown that if small tumors are enucleated early, there is a better long term survival rate. And this is the opinion of Dr. Blodi, based on analysis of his material.

NODULAR CHOROIDAL MASSES IN PATIENTS WITH SARCOIDOSIS

WILLIAM S. LESKO, M.D., MORTON H. SEELENFREUND, M.D.
& THOMAS S. MERRILL

(New York, USA)

Two patients referred for fluorescein angiographic studies of choroidal masses are presented. Both patients presented with visual blurring and were found to have elevated choroidal lesions without evidence of other ocular inflammation.

The angiographic changes in these patients and the posterior uveal changes in sarcoidosis are discussed.

MATERIALS AND METHODS

Serial fluorescein angiography was performed using 5ml. of 10% sodium fluorescein and Zeiss retinal camera. Kodachrome II and KodakTri-X pan films were used with standard procedures for photography.

Case 1

A 40 year old black male presented with visual blurring in his right eye. Examination revealed visual acuity of 20/30 O.D. and 20/20 O.S. with a small area of 'edema' inferior to macular in right eye without any other signs of uveitis (Fig. 1).

No therapy was given and the patient presented six weeks later with further visual blurring. Examination now revealed an elevated lesion in the inferior macula area and a new lesion inferior to the disc (Fig. 2). Ultrasonogram revealed a small 'choroidal elevation' (Fig. 3).

He was admitted to the hospital and found to have adenopathy. A biopsy of a supraclavicular lymph node biopsy was compatible with Boeck's Sarcoid. Treatment with Prednisone reduced the size of the lesion and returned the visual acuity to 20/25 (Fig. 4).

Case 2

A 34 year old black female with visual blurring in her left eye was referred to the retinal service at Mt. Sinai Hospital for possible hemangioma of the choroid. Visual acuity was reduced to 20/40 and a large elevated lesion was noted superotemporal to the disc. No other ocular inflammatory changes were noted. A fluorescein study showed extensive late staining of the lesion (Fig. 5).

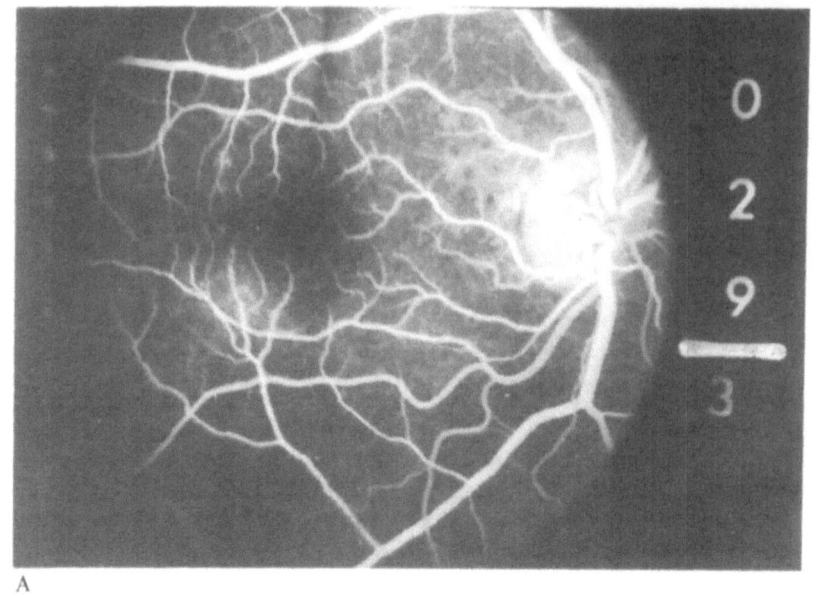

A

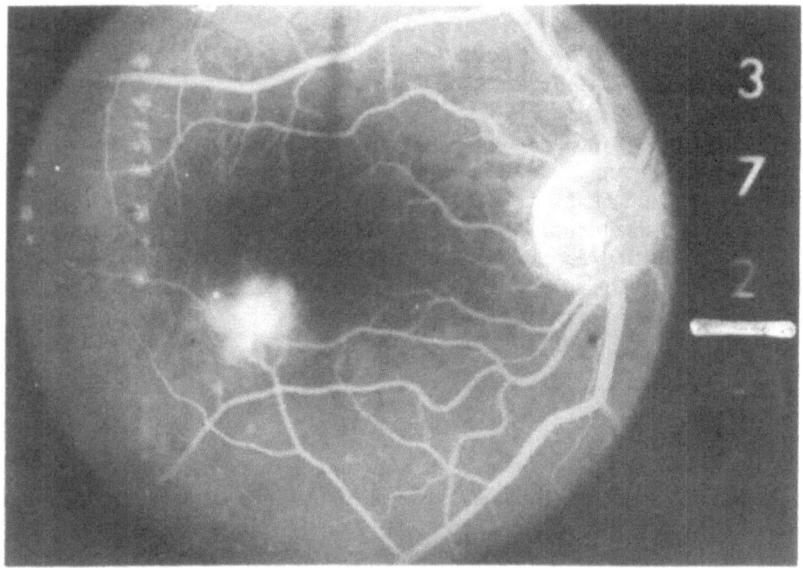

B

Fig. 1. A & B Angiogram taken one week after initial visit.

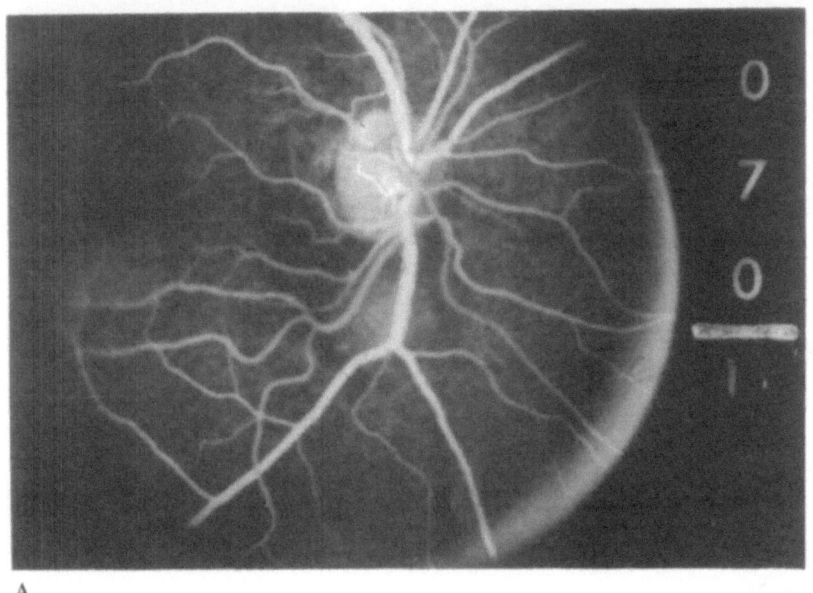

A

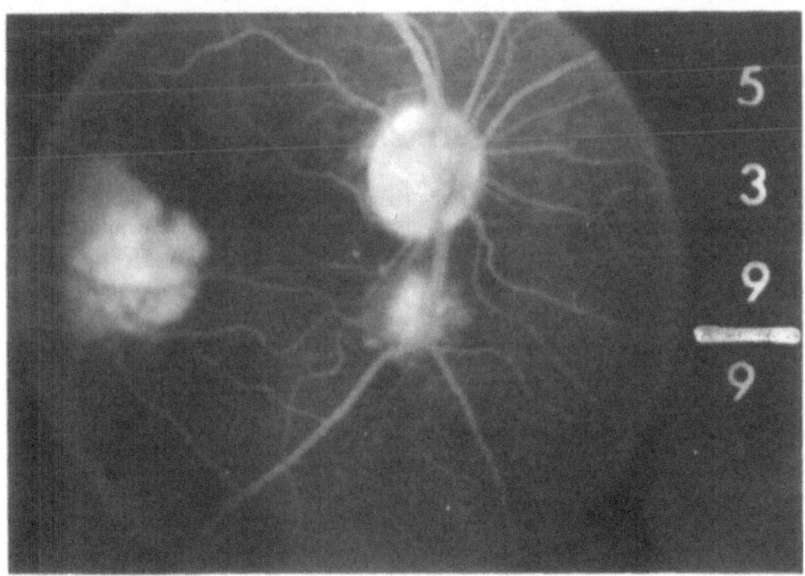

B   Fig. 2. A, B, C Large elevated lesion and satellite area after six weeks.

291

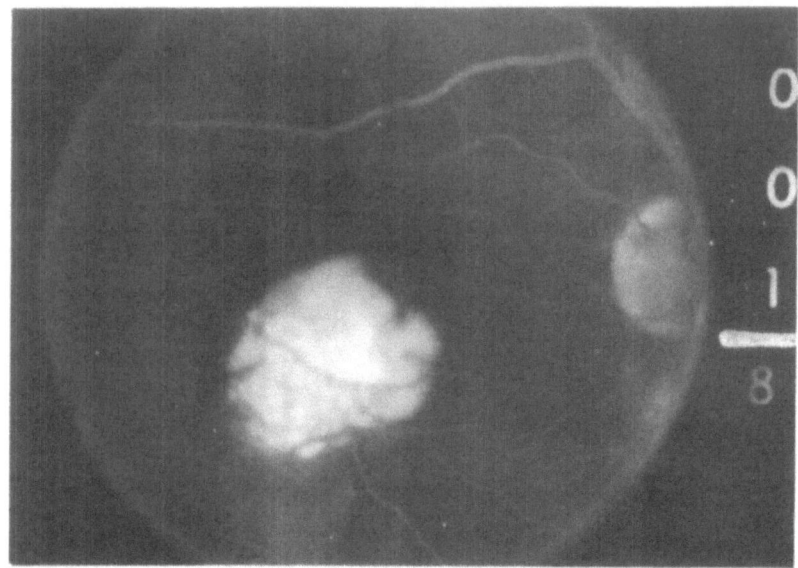

Fig. 2c

A review of her past medical records revealed a biopsy performed 4 years prior because of lymphadenopathy which was compatible with Boeck's Sarcoid. No therapy was given at that time.

After a two month course of Prednisone the lesion flattened and pigmented with return of visual acuity to 20/20 (Fig. 6).

DISCUSSION

Posterior involvement in sarcoid is relatively rare (JAMES, et al., 1964). The classic and common findings include perivascular candle wax dripping, preretinal and intravitreal nodules, and focal retinal exudates (FRANCESCHETTI & BABEL, 1949).

Isolated nodular tumefaction of the posterior pole can present puzzling differential in the absence of other findings. Nodule lesions of the optic disc without other ocular changes have been reported (BURNS, 1976; LATIES & SCHEIE, 1972). Also, nodule changes of the retina associated with 'classic' picture of sarcoid are common.

GASS reported a clinico pathologic correlation (GASS & OLSON, 1973) where nodules were found to be subpigment epithelial granuloma. The cases presented here demonstrate mass-like elevations with associated fluorescein changes. With therapy the clinical improvement was monitored with serial changes in angiography. The lesions flattened and reduced fluorescein stain was demonstrated.

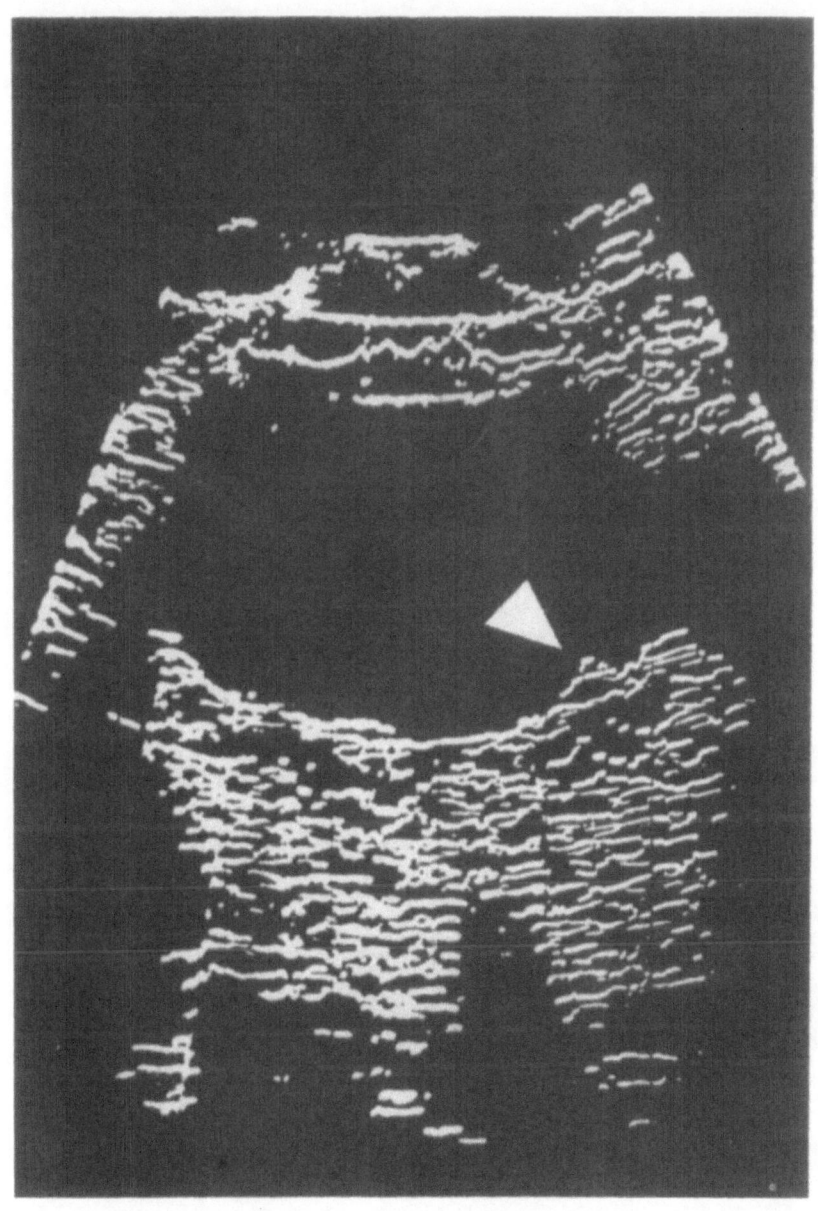

Fig. 3. Ultrasonogram in Case 1.

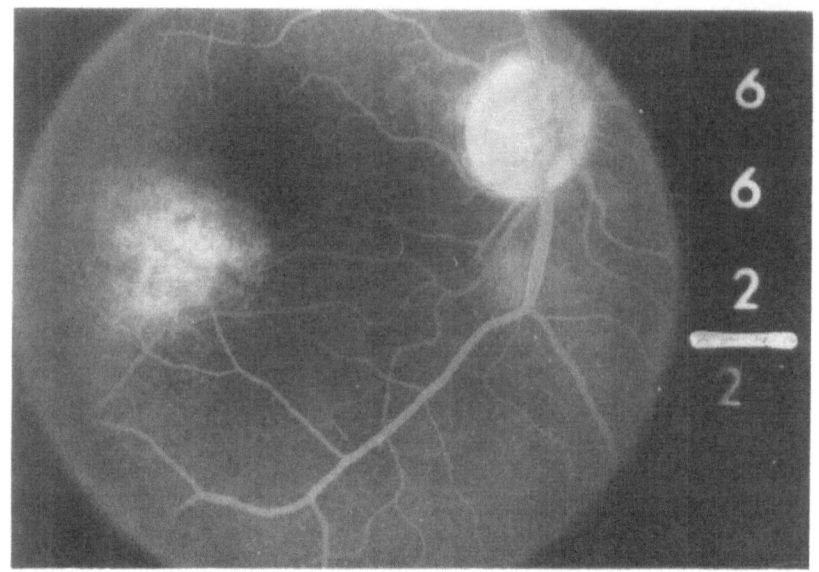

A

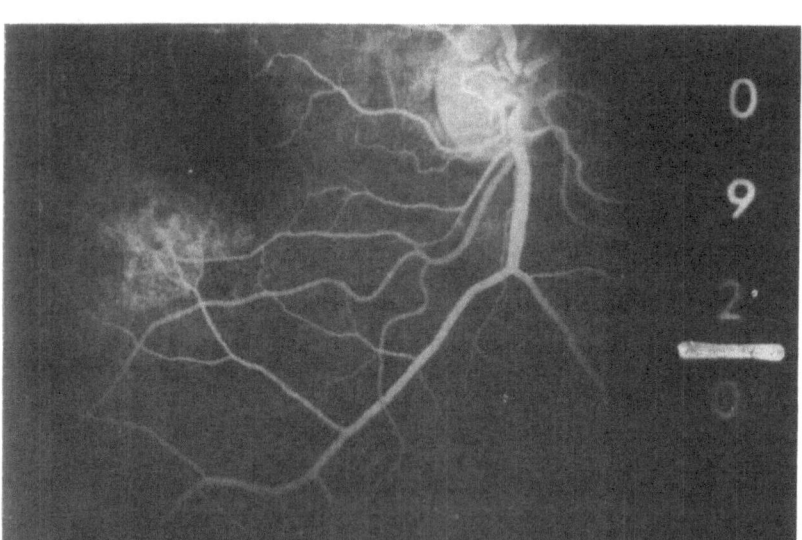

B

Fig. 4.   A & B After treatment with steroid.

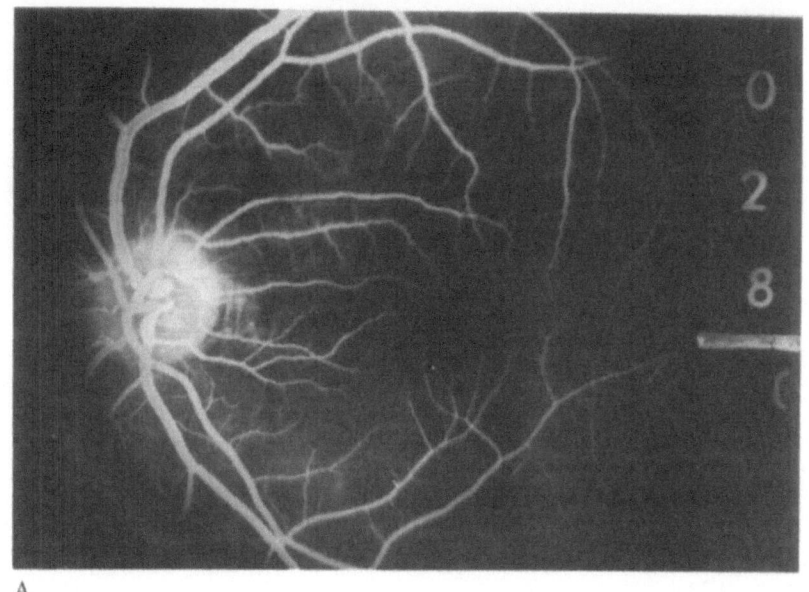

A

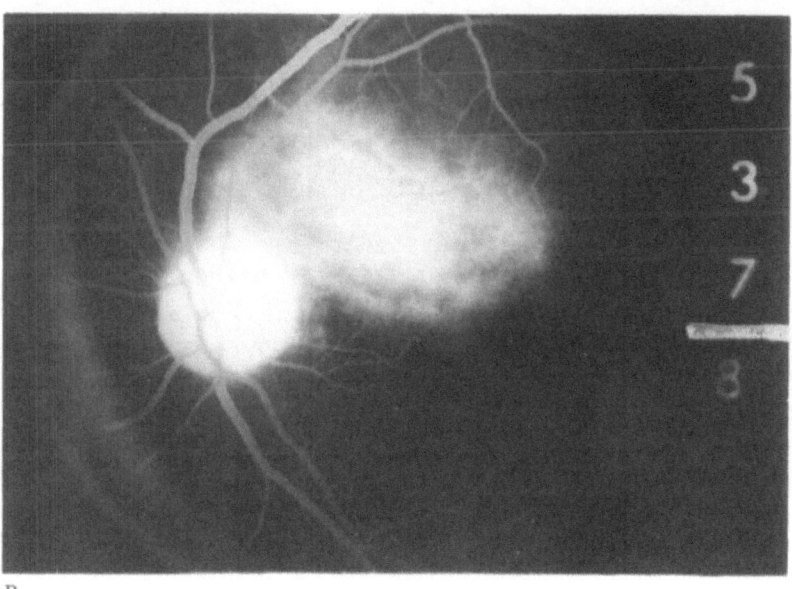

B

Fig. 5. Case 2 A & B Showing late staining of lesion.

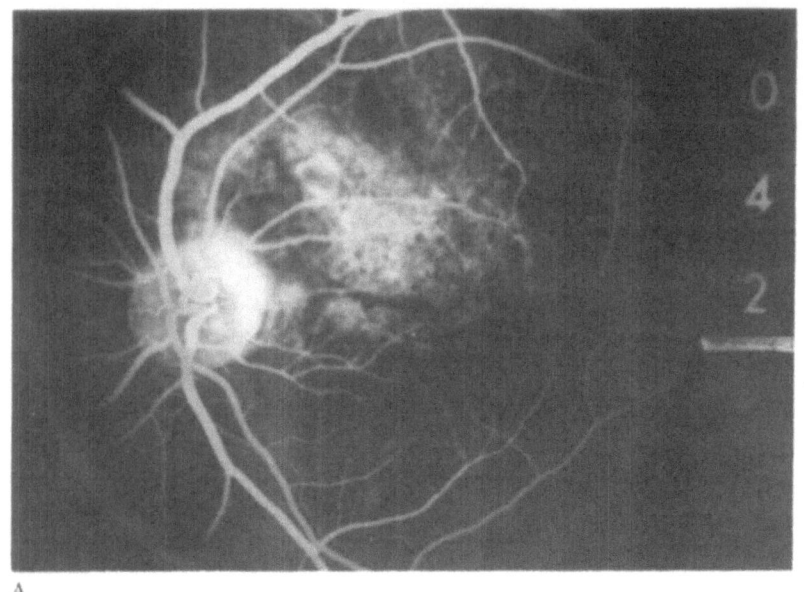

A

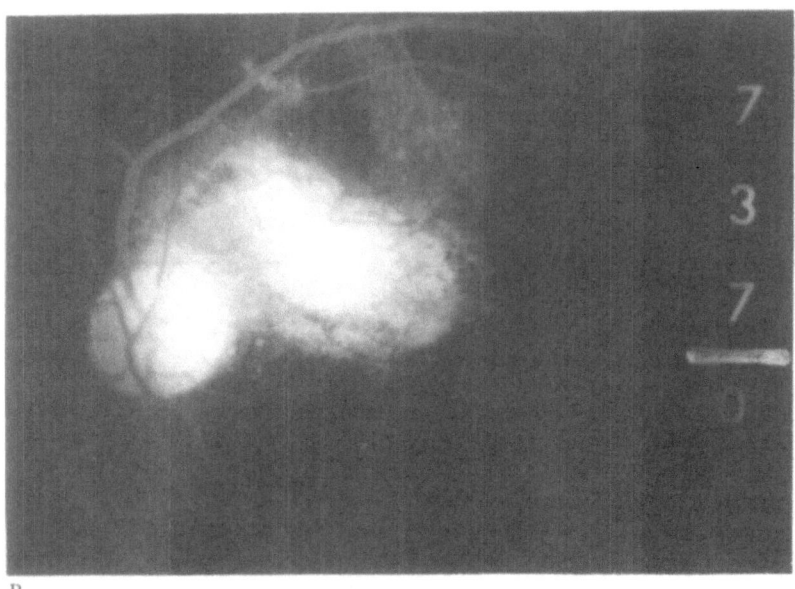

B

Fig. 6. A & B After therapy showing reduced staining and increase in pigmentation.

SUMMARY

Two cases of nodular posterior pole masses are presented. Both cases were found to have systemic sarcoid and no other ocular changes. The changing fluorescein patterns with systemic therapy are reviewed.

REFERENCES

BURNS, C.L. Unusual ocular presentation of sarcoidosis. *Ann. Ophthal.* 7: *69-71* (1976).

FRANCESCHETTI, A. & BABEL, J. La chorio-retinite en 'taches de bougie', manifestation de la maladie de Besnier-Boeck. *Ophthalmologica* 118: *701-710* (1949).

GASS, J.D.M. & OLSON, C.L. Sarcoidosis with optic nerve and retinal involvement. *Trans. Am. Acad. Ophthal. & Otolaryng.* 77: *739* (1973).

JAMES, D.G., ANDERSON, R., LANGLEY, D. et al. Ocular sarcoidosis. *Br. J. Ophthal.* 48: *561* (1964).

LATIES, A.M. & SCHEIE, H.G. Sarcoid granuloma. *Am. J. Ophthal.* 74: *60* (1972).

Authors' address:
Mount Sinai School of Medecine
of the City University of New York
New York, N.Y.
USA

OPTIC DISC AND PERIPAPILLARY CHOROID.
A CINEFLUOROANGIOGRAPHIC STUDY*

J.J. DE LAEY, P.Y. EVANS, T. STRANSKY & F. LENTINI

(Ghent, Belgium/Washington, D.C., USA)

Controversy still enshrouds the hypothesis that the peripapillary choroid contributes significantly to the blood supply of the optic nerve head. The study of optic disc fluorescence and thus vasculature is not an easy one, as the images obtained depend upon several factors. ERNEST & ARCHER (1973) consider 4 components: 1. transillumination of the optic disc from fluorescein in retrobulbar vessels, 2. filling of the primary vasculature of the nerve head from the short posterior ciliary arteries, 3. optic disc venous drainage accompanied by venous drainage from the peripapillary retina and 4. leakage of fluorescein from the peripapillary choroid into the nerve head. The study of optic disc vasculature is thus only possible in the early phases of the fluoroangiography, when the diffusion is not yet important.

METHODS

Normal volunteers and glaucoma patients were studied by cinefluoroangiography. The normal volunteers were aged between 18 and 45, whereas the 3 glaucoma patients were 43, 56 and 70. The methods for cinefluoroangiographic recording have been described in another paper (EVANS et al., 1973).

The choroidal and optic disc fluorescence were first studied by direct frame analysis in 30 normal individuals; some of them were compared several times. A densitometric study was then performed in 11 normals and the 3 glaucoma patients. Using a microdensitometer (Enraf, Nonius) a linear scanning was done on each second frame of the original negative till complete filling and then on each 16 th frame. Different reference points were chosen for scanning at the level of the temporal optic disc and the temporal peripapillary region, avoiding large retinal vessels. In each case the density of the central retinal artery was also followed. The densitometric readings were plotted for each recording, as a percentage of the maximal fluorescence. The results were plotted and the progression coefficient (m) was calculated statistically for the different parts of the curve. This coefficient was used to determine the slopes of the idealized lines for each part of the curve.

---

*   This work was supported in part by a grant from Research to Prevent Blindness.

299

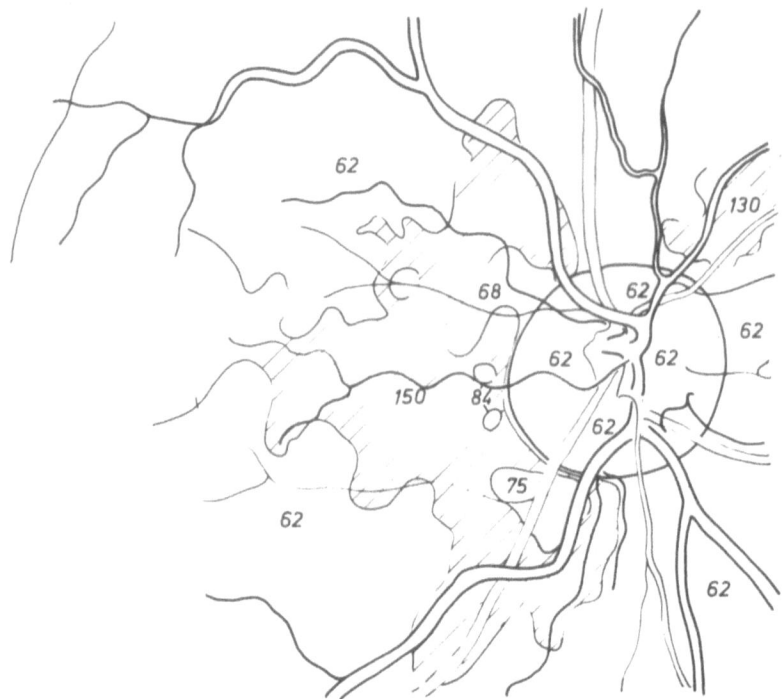

Fig. 1. Direct frame analysis of a cinefluoroangiography in a normal. The numbers refer to the frame from which on diffuse fluorescence was observed.

RESULTS

I. Direct frame analysis

In all of the 30 normal subjects a patchy filling of the choroid with relatively defined areas of choroidal filling delay was observed. In 16 cases such an area extended directly to the disc border without any strip of perfused choroid in between. In 9 cases the area of delayed choroidal filling was in contact with at least one third of the fluorescing optic disc (Fig. 1). These areas were more often situated on the temporal than on the nasal side of the disc. In two cases the areas of delayed perfusion included a segment of optic disc which was adjacent to the delayed choroidal area. In both cases the part of the disc started to fluoresce before the neighboring choriocapillaris (Fig. 2). In the others, however, the segment of the papilla adjacent to the delayed filling area did not differ significantly from the other parts of the disc.

The average filling time of these delayed areas, measured from the first outline of the dark spot to its complete fluorescence, was 2.79 sec. with a range of 0.9–7.65 sec. Two areas which were filled only after 6.9 and 7.65 sec. maintained an increased fluorescence for several seconds.

A common observation was that many of these areas of delayed fluorescence were not homogeneously dark. In some instances choroidal vessels were seen crossing them. Also inside these patches were smaller islands with earlier fluorescence, most often appearing just after the earliest appearance of dye in the choroid.

Direct frame analysis was also performed in 3 cases of glaucoma. No significant differences in the choroidal filling pattern was observed. These three cases were also studied by densitometry and will be discussed below.

II. Densitometric studies

1. Normal eyes

In 7 of the 11 normal cases studied by densitometry, the disc fluorescence started somewhat earlier than the adjacent choriocapillaris. (0.1-1.45 sec.; mean difference 0,5 sec.). In one case the initial moment was the same and in 3 the peripapillary choriocapillaris fluorescence preceded the disc fluorescence (0.05 sec. in two instances, 0,3 sec. in the third case).

In all of the normals a biphasic curve was obtained with a rapid initial rise and a second slower increase towards maximum fluorescence (Fig. 3). The values of the progression factor (m), which determine the angle of the first part of the curve, are given in Table I. In all but 3 cases the progression rate was somewhat more rapid for the first part of the disc curve than for the first part of the choroidal curve. The progression coefficient for the first part of the central retinal artery curve was greater than the progression coefficient for the first part of the optic disc and choroidal curves in all but

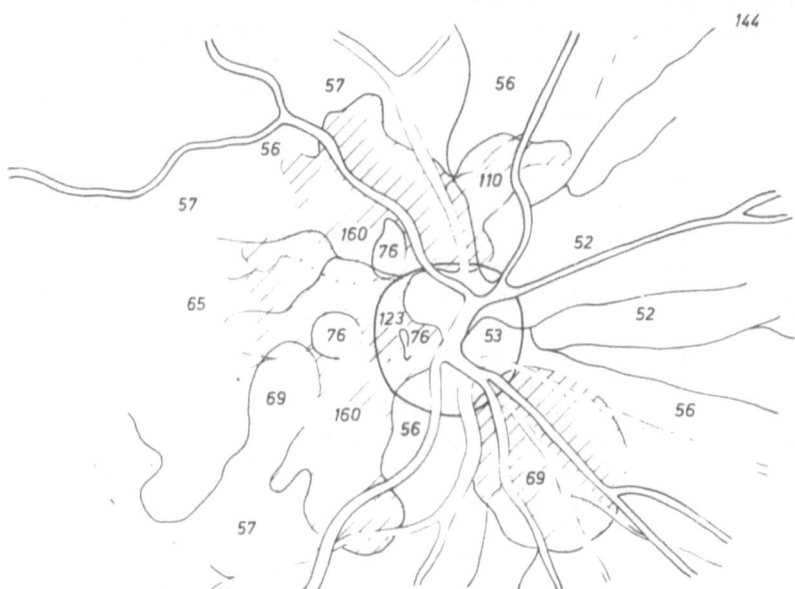

Fig. 2. Direct frame analysis in a normal. Note that the dark area includes partially the temporal segment of the optic disc.

301

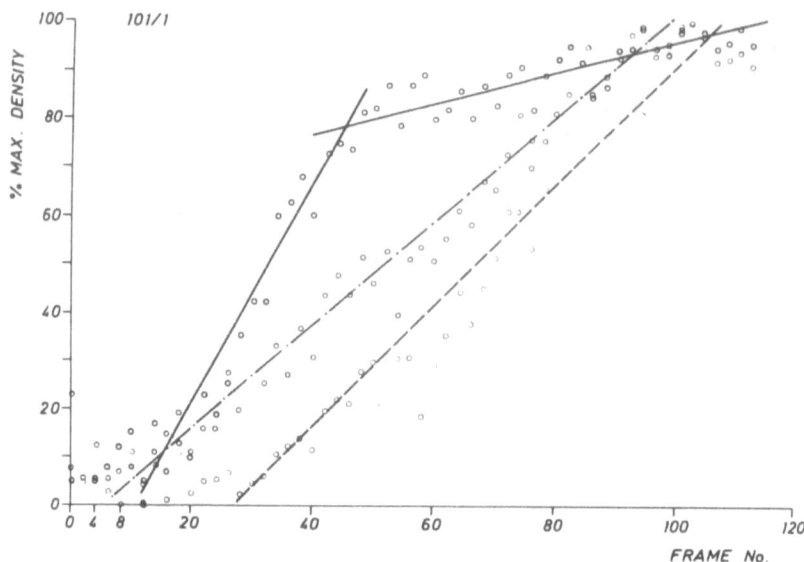

Fig. 3. Densitometry of the temporal optic disc (point-streak line), of the temporal peripapillary region (interrupted line) and of the central retinal artery at the optic disc (continuous line); in a normal.

two instances. However, usually the fluorescent blood appeared later in the central retinal artery than in the optic disc.

The mean of the 11 normals was also calculated and plotted. Here again, as could be expected, a dissociation of the mean optic disc curve and the mean choroidal curve was obtained. Both curves reached their maximum at about the same time (4.4 sec. after the increase began).

Densitometric studies were also performed in 3 glaucoma cases. The oldest patient (70 years old) showed marked disc cupping (C/D ratio 0.8) and a pronounced Bjerrum scotoma. In this case the densitometric readings were done on two different cinefluoroangiographies of the same eye and the results were comparable. In the other cases (ages 43 and 56) the discs were considered within normal limits (C/D ratios of 0.4 and 0.3). In one case with normal discs and fields the optic disc curve preceded the choroidal curve just as in our normal cases. The ocular tension during examination was only slightly increased (25 mm Hg). In the two other glaucoma patients, the choroidal curve was situated to the left of the optic disc curve, with a more rapid increase for the former. It is noteworthy that the tonometry of the eye with still normal disc and reversed densitometric curves was 32 mm Hg at the time of the cinefluoroangiography.

DISCUSSION

Frame-by-frame analysis of normal cinefluoroangiographies already indicates that in a great number of cases there is no direct relationship between the optic disc fluorescence and the filling of the juxtapapillary chor-

302

iocapillaris. This was further confirmed by the densitometric data. One possible objection is that the screening effect of the pigmentepithelium limits the visualization of choroidal fluorescence. This argument is not valid however since similar results were obtained in both lightly as well as darkly pigmented normal patients.

In some cases the great parallelism between the choroidal and disc curves suggests a common vascular origin of both the choriocapillaris and the optic nerve head vasculature. The short post. cil. arteries could well perform this function, and their importance has been stressed by many authors (HAYREH, 1970; ANDERSON, 1970; HENKIND & LEVITZKY, 1970, ERNEST & ARCHER, 1973). In other cases no parallelism was noted; this does not contradict the 'ciliary theory' but indicates that the disc capillaries can fill from multiple feed points (HENKIND & LEVITZKY, 1969).

The densitometric method used did not allow us to estimate the importance of the radial peripapillary capillaries.

The cases of glaucoma were too few to draw general conclusions. Also the fact that 2 patients were older than the normal controls do not allow comparison with them. However, the data obtained in 2 glaucomatous eyes indicates a greater susceptibility of the optic nerve than of the choroid to intraocular hypertension. This was not only observed in the older patient with glaucomatous cupping, but also in the younger patient where the cinefluoroangiography was taken with a tension of 32 mm Hg.

Table I. Values of the progression coefficient for the first part of the densitometric curve of the temporal optic disc, the temporal peripapillary choriocapillaris and the central retinal artery in 11 normal and 3 glaucoma cases.

	Case	Roll No	m1 Temp. Disc	m1 Temp. Chor.	m1 Central Ret. Art.
Normals	1 L.B.	147/2	2,93	2,78	3,76
	2 K.	64/1	3,86	3	4
	3 W.	101/1	2,22	2,5	3,84
	4 M.E.	144/1	5,16	3,86	5
	5 M.I.	29/4	6,02	5,09	5,39
	6 K.S.	139/3	6,12	9,27	12
	7 H.E.	139/2	4,56	4,83	6,2
	8 J.J.	181/2	6,56	2,88	3,02
	9 G.	151/4	6,77	6,67	8,31
	10 D.	15	6,5	4,4	8
	11 H.R.	153/1	3,46	2,26	5,08
Glaucoma	1 J.	151/2	3,49	3,52	4,96
	2 M.L.E.	176/2	2,70	2,95	4,64
	3 A.Z.	101	2,4	2,78	5,30

SUMMARY

Direct frame-by-frame analysis of normal cinefluoroangiographies suggests that in a large number of cases the perfusion of the optic nerve head is independent from the peripapillary choriocappillaris. Densitometric studies on the same material, however, suggest that both may have a common vascular origin. A great deal of variation exists. Our preliminary results in glaucoma confirms a greater susceptibility of the optic nerve head than of the peripapillary choroid to increased intraocular tension.

REFERENCES

ANDERSON, D.R. Vascular supply to the optic nerve of primates. Amer. J. Ophthal. 70: 341-351 (1970).

ERNEST, J.T. & ARCHER, D. Fluorescein angiography of the optic disk. Amer. J. Ophthal. 75: 973-978 (1973).

EVANS, P.Y., SHIMIZU, K., LIMAYE, S., DEGLIN, E. & WRUCK, J. Fluorescein cineangiography of the optic nerve head. Trans. Amer. Acad. Ophthal. Otolaryng. 77: 260-273 (1973).

HAYREH, S.S. Pathogenesis of visual field defects. Role of the ciliary circulation. Brit. J. Ophthal. 54: 289-311 (1970).

HENKIND, P. & LEVITZKY, M. Angioarchitecture of the optic nerve. I. The papilla. Amer. J. Ophthal. 68: 979-986 (1969).

Authors' addresses:
Department of Ophthalmology
University of Ghent
Ghent
Belgium

Department of Ophthalmology
Georgetown University Medical Center
Washington, D.C.
USA

A STUDY OF THE OPTIC DISC FLUORESCENCE
BY PHOTOGRAPHIC SUBTRACTION

DONALD T.T. TJIA , M.D. &
JAN VAN DER WONING, Med. Photogr.

(Amsterdam, The Netherlands)

INTRODUCTION

Subtraction is a well-known technique in radiology. It was first described in 1934 by ZIEDSES DES PLANTES, a Dutch neuroradiologist, who stated the principle of subtraction as follows: 'When there is a difference between two radiographs of the same part of the body, this difference can be cancelled out by covering one radiograph with the diapositive of the other'. Subtraction is now widely used in angiography. The diapositive reversal radiograph or 'mask' must be the exact opposite of the scout radiograph. Usually a mask having about 50% of the density of the negative will produce optimal result.

The aim of subtraction in radiography is the elimination of structure images that otherwise are superimposed over various regions that may be of pathological interest to the radiologist. This is particularly used in the study of vascular arborisation in the skull.

In fluorescein photography the structure of retinal vessel walls in combination with adequate filters produce a very distinct vascular pattern. In the choroid as well as in the optic disc these vascular details are obscured by diffuse fluorescence.

It is our aim to study the optic disc circulation by subtraction of fluorographs of different stages. The study of retinal haemodynamics by means of subtraction of fluorographs has been done before in 1972 by MIKUNI & FUJII. They used the shorter intervals. In step by step subtraction with different time intervals we tried to get an insight of the haemodynamic features, especially of the influx of the optic disc capillary system.

TECHNIQUE

Enlarged 4 x 5 inch transparencies of the optic disc region are made from routine 35 mm fluorescein angiographic negatives using sheet film. Time of exposure of the sheets film is determined by the most dense negative. Care is taken to ensure that all films undergo the same developing procedures which is achieved by an automatic developing machine. The outfit which is at our disposal can be computerized and is capable of developing 8 sheet films in one turn under the same reproducible conditions.

The reversed sheet film series are produced by contactprinting and are also automatically developed. To subtract perfectly it is necessary to have more or less the same projection of the subject and to make the diapositive film or mask of the same contrast as the original negative. This can be achieved with the aid of a density wedge or visually by superimposing the negative by its reversed base film. A patternless grayish picture will result. If so, the separate image of the difference of two serial fluorographs of the same angiogram could only be caused by difference in fluorescence and not by photographic artefacts. In other words it is not only possible to subtract differences in shape, size or position but also in fluorescence.

This means sequential proportional subtraction is possible. In our subtraction technique the preceding fluorograph (base film) will always function as the diapositive or mask. In doing so, white reflections in the print correspond with fluorescence increasing areas.

The mounted film combinations can be printed on film or paper. We print directly on paper.

RESULTS AND DISCUSSION

Our present knowledge in and around the optic nerve head has largely been obtained from post mortem studies using a variety of injection and digestion or tissue classification techniques as described by MICHAELSON (1948), ASHTON (1951), KUWABARA & COGAN (1965), and JOCSON & GRANT (1965), and by x-ray microradiography by FRANÇOIS & NEETENS (1954).

Immense clinical and experimental studies on the circulation of the optic nerve head have been made by HAYREH et al. (HAYREH 1969 a, b. 1970; HAYREH & PERKINS 1968, 1969; HAYREH, REVIE & EDWARDS 1970). Also HENKIND & LEVITZKY (1969) studied the angioarchitecture of the papilla.

Recent articles published by ANDERSON (1969 a, b, c; 1970 a, b) provide an excellent review of light microscopy of the optic nervehead as well as original observations on the ulstrastructure of this region.

Cineangiographic studies by EVANS et al. (1973) expressed the close relationship between the choroidal flush and the dye inflow into the disc capillaries. So, a blood supply of the disc from the choroid was sustained.

ERNEST (1973) stressed the fact that there is no direct relationship between the peripapillary choroid and the optic disc. The choroidal feeders are independent of the vessels which branch to the optic disc.

ANDERSON again (1974) mentioned anastomotic connection to the vessels of the piamater and retina. There has been undue emphasis on the fact that the short posterior ciliary arteries supply the disc, as well as unwarrented assumptions, that responses to the optic disc circulation can be predicted from studies of choroidal circulation.

Our method intends to contribute a study of the optic disc circulation in the normal untouched human eye.

In the interpretation of the different stage subtractions there are 3 possibilities:
1. white reflections indicating an increase in filling;
2. black reflections indicating an emptying phase;
3. gray shades in case of no change in fluorescence.

Fig. 1 shows us subtraction in the first period ($14''/15''$, $15''/16''$). There is a simultaneous and equal change in fluorescence of the optic disc as well as the choroid. So far optic nerve head and choroidal fluorescence go together.

Fig. 2. In subtraction in later stages with greater interval the following can be noted: the optic disc fluorescence decreases much faster than the choroidal fluorescence. In our opinion this can be explained by a difference in structure of the capillaries in the optic disc and the choroid.

Fig. 3 is a subtraction picture of 20″ and 25″. In the recirculation period there is a considerable increase of fluorescence of the optic nerve head sharply outlined to the peripapillary choroid.

Fig. 4 The parent fluorographs show a very distinct fluorescence of a

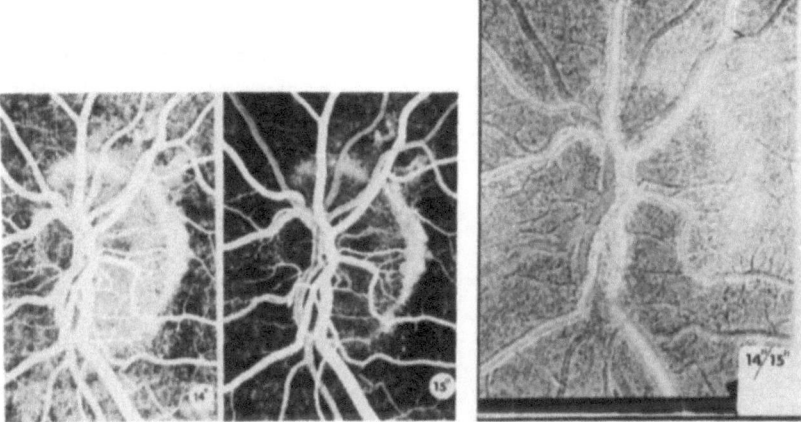

Fig. 1. Parent fluorographs (left) and subtraction (right). See text for explanation.

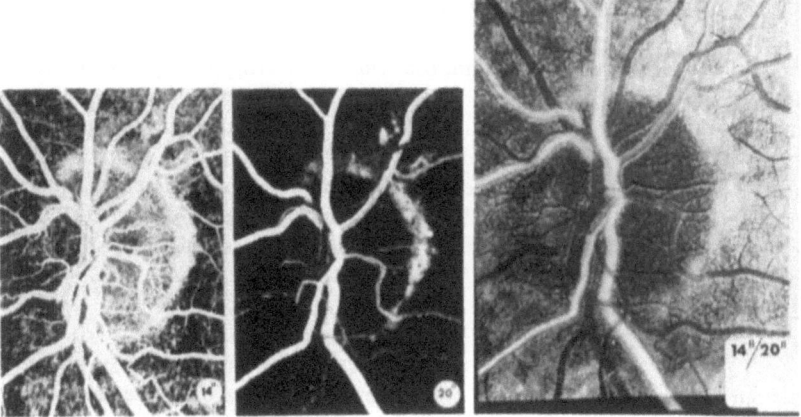

Fig. 2. Parent fluorographs (left) and subtraction (right). See text for explanation.

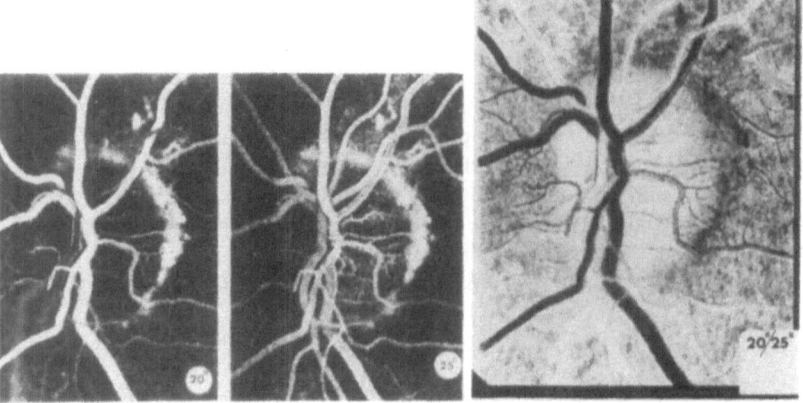

Fig. 3. Parent fluorographs (left) and subtraction (right). See text for explanation.

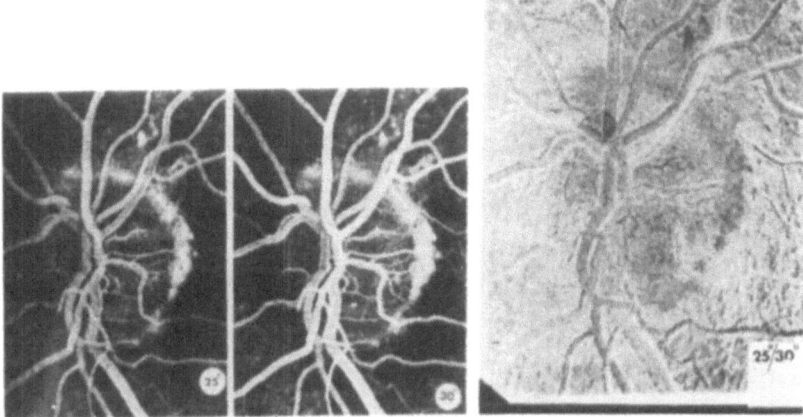

Fig. 4. Parent fluorographs (left) and subtraction (right). See text for explanation.

peripapillary crescent on the temporal side with atrophic pigment epithelium. In the subtracted picture the crescent is dark, which means it is an
emptying phase. The optic disc has a dark centre but there is a lighter haze
in the peripheral part of the disc. This must be explained by a late feeding
of the disc from the border, either out of the deep surrounding peripapillary
tissue (GRAYSON & LATIES 1971), or from the choroid (COHEN 1973),
or both. The source of this late borderline fluorescence of the disc is still
unclear.

CONCLUSION

It is our aim to give a contribution in the problem of the disc vascularisation
by subtracting optic disc fluorographs of different stages with different intervals of time.

In the late arterial and early venous phase we noted equal reflections of optic disc and surrounding tissue. The capillary system of the optic disc and choroid in this stage go together both from posterior cilio-arterial branches. In the later venous phase the disc darkens more than the surrounding choroid. This means that the capillary system of the disc is emptying more rapidly. So this suggests a difference between both capillary systems. The more dynamic proces in the disc vascularisation compared to the choroidal circulation is also evident in the picture of recirculation: The choroid is static, the disc fills up again. This static feature of choroidal filling is an agreement with the consideration of the choroid as a 'cavernous body'. In the late stages refilling of the disc from the border is obvious.

In this preliminary report we only wanted to show the subtraction method as a possible tool to study retinal circulatory dynamics. Yet much work has still to be done, especially in the later phases.

REFERENCES

ANDERSON, D.R. & HOIT, W.F. Ultrastructure of the intraorbital portion of human and monkey optical nerve. *Arch. Ophthalmol.* 82: *506-330* (1969a).

ANDERSON, D.R. & HOYT, W.F. Ultrastructure of human and monkey lamina cribosa. *Arch. Ophthalmol.* 82: *800-814* (1969b).

ANDERSON, D.R. & HOYT, W.F. Ultrastructure of meningeal sheats: normal human and monkey optic nerves. *Arch. Ophthalmol.* 82: *659-674* (1969c).

ANDERSON, D.R. & HOYT, W.F. Ultrastructure of the optic nerve head. *Arch. Ophthalmol.* 83: *63-73* (1970c).

ANDERSON, D.R. & HOYT, W.F. Vascular supply to the optic nerve of primates. *Am. J. Ophthalmol.* 70: *341-350* (1970c).

ASHTON. *Brit. J. Ophthalmol.* 35: *189* (1951)

COHEN, A.I. Is there a potential defect in the blood-retinal barrier at the choroidal level of the optic nerve canal? *Invest. Ophthal.* 12: *513-519* (1973).

ERNEST, J.T. & ARCHER, D. Fluorescein angiography of the optic disk. *Am. J. Ophthal.* 75: *973-978* (1973).

EVANS, P.Y., SHIMIZU, K., LIMAYE, S., DEGLIN, E. & WRUCK, J. Fluorescein cineangiography of the optic nerve head. *Trans. Am. Acad. Ophthal. & Otolaryng.* 77: *260-273* (1973).

FRANÇOIS, J. & NEETENS, A. Vascularization of the optic pathway: I. Lamina cribrosa and optic nerve. *Br. J. Ophthal.* 38: *472-488* (1954).

GRAYSON, M.C. & LATIES, A.M. Ocular localization of sodium fluorescein. Effects of administration in rabbit and monkey. *Arch. Ophthal.* 85: *600-609* (1971).

HAYREH, S.S. & PERKINS, E.S. Clinical and experimental studies on the circulation and optic nerve head. In: Cant, J.S. (ed.), The William Mackenzie Centenary Symposium on the Ocular circulation in health and disease, pp. *71-86.* London, Kimpton (1969a).

HAYREH, S.S. Blood supply of the optic nerve head and its role in optic atrophy, glaucoma and oedema of the optic disc. *Brit. J. Ophthal.* 53: *721-748* (1969b).

HAYREH, S.S. Pathogenesis of visual field defects: role of the ciliary circulation. *Brit. J. Ophthal.* 54: *289-311* (1970).

HAYREH, S.S., REVIE, I.H.S. & EDWARDS, J. Vasogenic origin of visual field defects and optic nerve changes in glaucoma. *Brit. J. Ophthal.* 54: *461-472* (1970).

HENKIND, P. & LEVITZKY, M. Angioarchitecture of the optic nerve. I. The papilla. *Am. J. Ophthal.* 68: *979-996* (1969).

HERDER, B.A. DEN. Personal communication (1976).

JOCSON & GIANT. *Arch. Ophthal.* 73: *707* (1965).

KUWABARA & COGAN. *Arch. Ophthal.* 64: *904* (1960).

MICHAELSON, I.C. & CAMPBELL, A.C.T. The anatomy of the fine retinal vessels. *Trans. Ophthal. Soc. U.K.* 60: *71-112* (1940).

MIKUNI, M. & FUJII, S. Subtraction method in fundus photography. Report 1: Simplified method of subtraction and application to fluorescence fundus photography. *Acta Soc. Ophthal. Jap.* 76: *331-339* (1972).

ZIEDSES DES PLANTES. Subtraktion. Georg Thieme Verlag, Stuttgart (1961).

Authors' address:
Eye Clinic of the
Free University
De Boelelaan 1117
Amsterdam
The Netherlands

IN VIVO MEASUREMENTS OF DIFFUSION OF FLUORESCEIN INTO THE HUMAN OPTIC NERVE TISSUE

I. BEN-SIRA, M. LOEBL, B. SCHWARTZ & C.E. RIVA

(Boston, Massachusetts, USA)

In a previous paper (BEN-SIRA & RIVA, 1975), it was shown that the dilution curve of fluorescein recorded from a retinal artery is practically identical to that of indocyanine green dye (ICG), Fig. 1. This is due to the fact that, normally, neither dye diffuses out of the circulatory system between the site of injection and the retinal vessel. In the event fluorescein does diffuse from the vasculature, into the tissues, between these two loca-

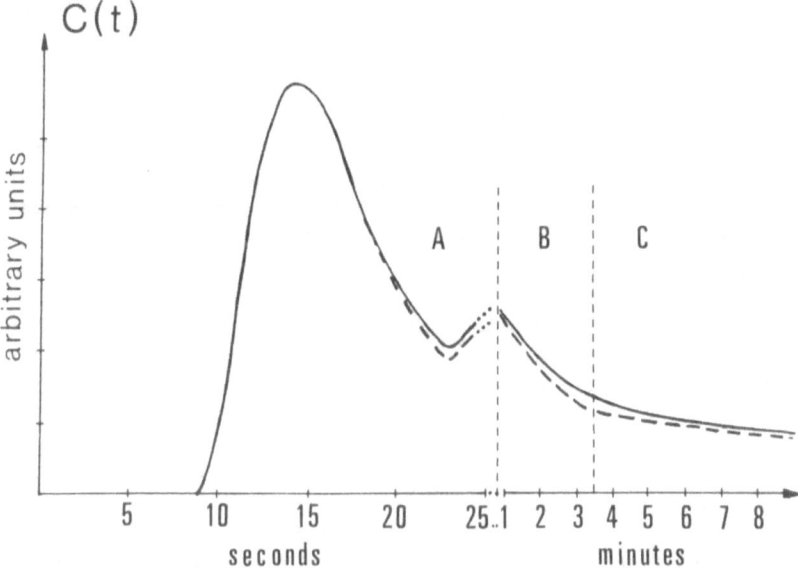

Fig. 1. Dye dilution curves recorded with a fundus reflectometer from a retinal vessel of a normal subject after injection of a mixture of 500 mg fluorescein and 50 mg ICG into the antecubital vein. The vertical scale indicates dye concentration. Compare the fluorescein curve (broken line) to the ICG curve (solid line), and note the three parts: (A) first passage, where both curves are practically identical. (B) fluorescein curve decays slightly faster than ICG curve, because fluorescein is distributed both in the plasma and in extracellular fluid, whereas ICG is only in plasma. (C) ICG curve decays faster than fluorescein curve because ICG is eliminated faster by liver than is fluorescein by kidneys.

311

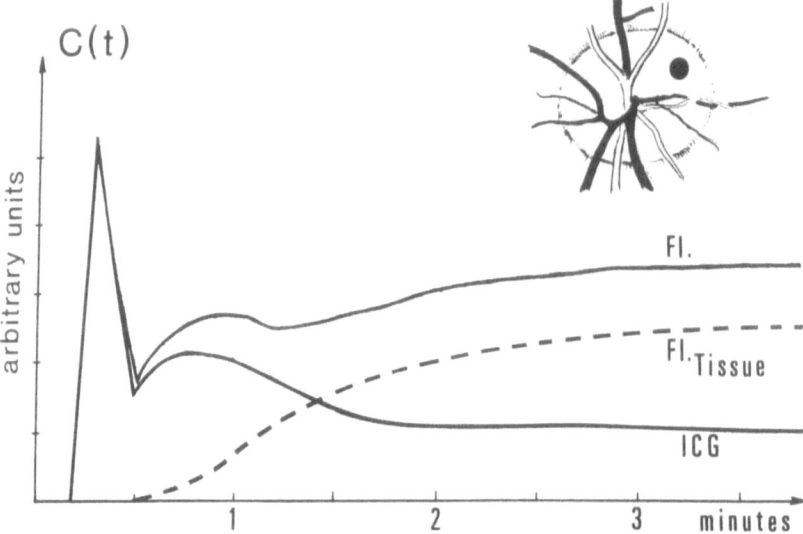

Fig. 2. Dilution curves of fluorescein (Fl) and ICG recorded simultaneously from a spot in the optic disc (black dot in schematic drawing). The amount of dye that has diffused into the optic disc tissue (broken line) was obtained by subtracting the ICG curve from the fluorescein curve.

tions, the dilution curves of both dyes will differ from each other. The difference between the two curves depends upon the time constant of the diffusion process, the ratio between the intravascular volume and the volume of the tissues, the rate of blood flow, and other factors.

Dilution curves of fluorescein and ICG have been recorded from the optic disc tissue in normal human subjects (Fig. 2). Based on these recordings, and applying Goldmann's theory of fluorescein diffusion into the optic nerve (GOLDMANN, 1973), it has been shown that fluorescein does not permeate the capillaries of the optic disc. There is a slow accumulation of fluorescein in the disc — probably dye from the choroid that has entered the optic nerve from the periphery.

This report describes dilution curves of fluorescein and ICG taken from the optic discs of seven patients with ocular hypertension and six patients with glaucoma. These glaucoma patients included: three open angle glaucoma (two of them after a filtering operation); one chronic closure angle glaucoma and two low tension glaucoma (one with diabetes mellitus). All the ocular hypertensive patients had fluorescein curves similar in shape to that of normal subjects. All patients with glaucoma had fluorescein curves similar to the one in Fig. 3, where, during the time of recording (~35 sec.), the fluorescence intensity remains at a constant high level following a sharp initial increase. The bolus-like passage seen with ICG has disappeared.

These results show that in glaucoma patients there is an increased accumulation of fluorescein in the region of the optic disc tissue from which

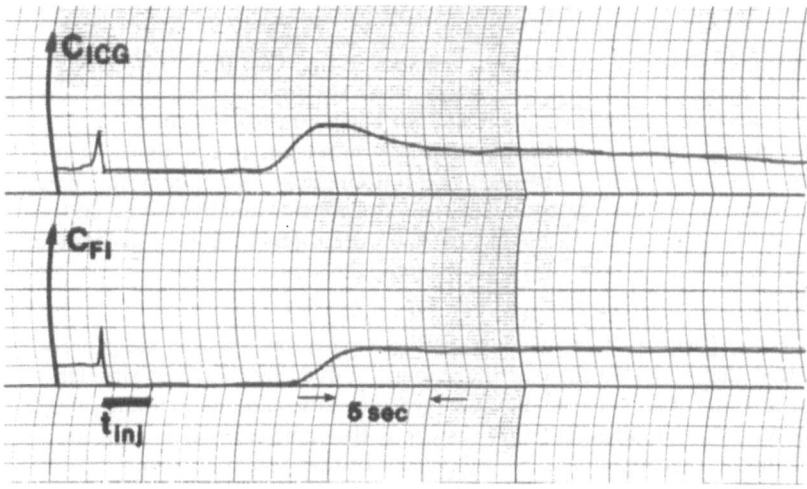

Fig. 3. Representative ICG and fluorescein curves recorded simultaneously from the optic disc of a patient with chronic simple glaucoma. The spikes at the beginning of the recordings signal the start of the injection time ($t_{inj.}$).

fluorescence is detected. We do not yet know whether this indicates changes in the permeability of the disc capillaries or is a manifestation of retrobulbar fluorescence. Further measurements in patients with ocular hypertension are needed in order to establish whether early leakage of fluorescein in the optic disc tissue precedes visual field defect.

ACKNOWLEDGEMENT

This work was supported by Public Health Service grants EY-00227, 1-RO1-EY-01242-01 and 5-RO1-EY-00936-02 from the National Eye Institute, National Institutes of Health and by Research to Prevent Blindness, Inc. — William Friedkin Award.

REFERENCES

BEN-SIRA, I. & RIVA, C.E. Fluorescein diffusion in the optic disc. *Invest. Ophthalmol.* 14: *205-211* (1975).
GOLDMANN, H. Transfer of fluorescein from blood vessels to disc tissue: The theory. *Invest. Ophthalmol.* 12: *475-484* (1973).

Authors' address:
Eye Research Institute
of Retina Foundation
20 Staniford Street
Boston, Mass. 02114
USA

Requests for reprints to:
Editorial Services Unit
Eye Research Institute of Retina Foundation
20 Staniford Street
Boston, Mass. 02114
USA

DISCUSSION

Dr Fonda: I want to make some remarks on the presentation of Dr Riva. I have 3 remarks. The first in general what we measure by dilutioncurve technique is illuminance variation and not concentration variation; moreover the relation between luminance and concentration is not linear. Third: owing to the different diffusibility of fluorescein and indocyanin green surely the non-linear relation between fluorescein concentration and its luminance is different from that of indocyanin green. Taking account of these observations how can you compare the dilution curves for the two dyes?

Dr Riva: I will try to remember the three questions. First, in the paper we showed that when we changed the amount of dye there was a linear relation in the optic disc between fluorescence intensity and the amount of dye injected. Second, when the first passage is the same for both eyes, it means that during this time there is no diffusion of fluorescein into the tissue. All the fluorescein remains in the vascular system. In this case there is still proportionality between intensity and concentration. Only in the case where fluorescein diffuses out, there is no more proportionality between intensity and concentration of fluorescein in the vessels. In the case of glaucoma where there seems to be leakage of dye and, in fact, you are right, I should have put intensity of fluorescence instead of concentration.

CHOROIDAL CIRCULATION IN GLAUCOMA

ARTURO A. ALEZZANDRINI, M.D.

(Buenos Aires, Argentina)

It is not our intention to discuss at this point the techniques of fluoro-angiography of the choroidal vessels. We have referred to this in previous studies (ALEZZANDRINI, 1971; 1972).

As far as the technique which has been used for the fluorangiography of the retina is concerned, we used intravenous injections of 10 cc of 10% fluorescein. We feel that the use of indocyanine green dye (ICG) as a contrasting substance is most interesting, the larger molecule of ICG prevents the penetration to the small vessels of the choriocapillary layer, and therefore the choroidal angiogram is much more detailed. Although we have not had much experience with this dye, in view of that of other authors (FLOWER et al., 1974) we consider that it is extremely helpful.

Our observations are based on the analysis of glaucoma patients at different clinical stages of the disease. These include: (a) full peripapillary choroidal deficit, and (b) vascular disorders of the optic disc.

FULL PERIPAPILLARY CHOROID DEFICIT

In 1951, CRISTIANI suggested that glaucomatous atrophy of the optic disc would result from a deficit in the blood flow of the peripapillary choroid net with resulting ischemia. This was confirmed experimentally in monkeys by HAYREH & PERKINS (1968); here the increase in the intraocular pressure produced ischemia and obliteration of the small peripapillary choroid vessels. The deficit is generally greater in the upper sections of the temporal side; this is made readily evident by an absence in the deep fluorescein and a very suggestive dark shadow in the infrared (Fig. 1).

BLUMENTHAL, GITTER, BEST & GALLIN (1970), by means of controlled angio-fluresceinography with the suction cup, showed in man that as the IOP increases the flow in choroid and retina is reduced, and the circulatory collapse is much greater in the first at lower tension levels than in the second.

ZIMMERMAN, DE VENECIA & HAMASAKI, by increasing the intraocular pressure, experimentally provoked in monkeys excavations and ischemic lesions in the retrolaminar portion of the optic nerve.

ROSEN (1969) angiographically showed a reduction in choroid circulation in two cases of papillary atrophy of unknown etiology. These facts are the ones that took HAYREH (1969) to affirm that '... the choroidal contri-

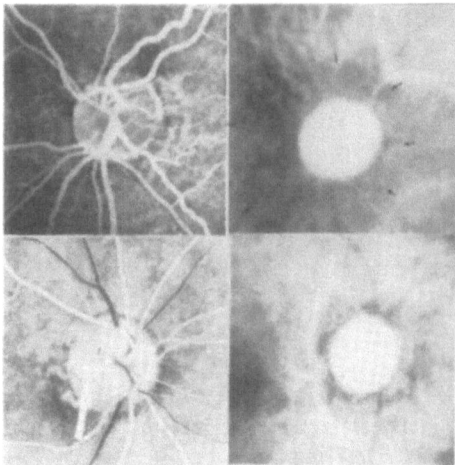

Fig. 1. *Top*: Chronic simple glaucoma. Choroid silence with more marked background fluorescense decrease in the temporal sector. Lesion of the peripapillary pigmentary epithelium due to circulatory deficit. The infrared technique shows a shadow in the shape of a ring surrounding the papilla.
Below: Chronic simple glaucoma with papilla excavation. Abnormal vessels appear on the papilla and in the infrared technique dilatation of the choroid vessels.

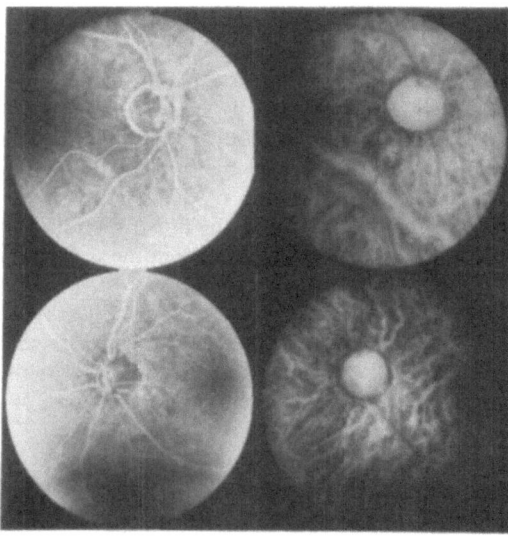

Fig. 2. 2 cases of chronic simple glaucoma with papilla excavation. Dilatation of the choroid vessels with shunt appearance between retinal and choroid vascular systems.

316

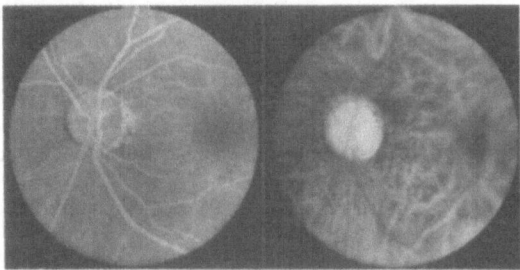

Fig. 3. Chronic simple glaucoma with normal visual field. Normal distribution of choroid vessels is observed.

bution to the blood supply of the optic disc and the peripapillary choroid is most susceptible to obliteration by the elevated intraocular pressure would go a long way towards explaining the pathogenesis of the nerve fibre bundle defects, cupping of the optic disc and cavernous degeneration of the optic nerve in glaucoma ...'.

It is in this way that in glaucoma patients all the peripapillary area is dark, without fluorescense, even in the retinal arterio-venous time (Fig. 1); as the excavation advances with the nasal displacement of the vessels (Fig. 2), this phenomenon tends to disappear and the monochromatic technique − with infrared light − discovers the presence of thick, dilated choroid vessels, which are not visible while the papilla is normal (ALEZZANDRINI & MANZITTI, 1972) (Fig. 3).

INTRADISCAL VASCULARIZATION DISORDER

It is a fact that the vascularization diminishes with the increase of the excavation, physiologically more important at the chorio-capillary level than in the small retinal capillaries. To this respect, RAITA & SARMELLA (1970) add the peripapillary strophy of the pigmentary epithelium as a sign of the alteration of choroidal circulation in glaucoma, especially in young patients.

Our experience (ALEZZANDRINI, 1974) confirms these findings to which abnormal anastomosis between the central artery and the choroidal system are frequently associated (this has not been mentioned to date by other authors), and which would be true shunts by means of which the eye tries to compensate the circumpapillary choroidal ischemia.

SUMMARY

The author's experience in the study of choroidal circulation in patients with chronic simple glaucoma is reported. It is generally possible to observe with the infrared monochromatic light technique that in the early clinical stages of the disease the circulation decreases at the level of the Zinn-Haller's circle. As soon as atrophy of the optic nerve starts, a marked dilatation of the large circumpapillary choroidal vessels can be observed as well as, very frequently, an actual anastomosis between the surface retinal vessel net and the choroid net or probably the posterior ciliary arteries.

REFERENCES

ALEZZANDRINI, A.A. Choroidal circulation studied with infrared fluorescein angiography. *Mod. Probl. Ophthal.* 19: *44-49* (1971).

ALEZZANDRINI, A.A. Choroidal circulation. Scientific Exhibit. IX° Pan-American Ophth. Congr., Houston (1972).

ALEZZANDRINI, A.A. Angiofluoresceinography in glaucoma. *Archivos Oftal. de Bs As.* 49: *269-276* (1974).

ALEZZANDRINI, A.A. & MANZITTI, E. Angiofluoresceinography in congenital glaucoma. *Archivos Oftal. de Bs As.* 47: *347-362* (1972).

BLUMENTHAL, M., GITTER, K.A., BEST, M. & GALIN, M.A. A fluorescein angiography study during induced hypertension in humans. *Am. J. Ophthal.* 69: *39-40* (1970).

CRISTIANI, G. Common pathological basis of the nervous ocular system in chronic glaucoma. *Brit. J. Ophthal.* 35: *11-16* (1951).

FLOWER, R., FINKELSTEIN, D., D'ANNA, S., HOCHHEIMER, B., ORTH, D. & PATZ, A. Simultaneous choroidal and retinal angiography. Scientific Exhibit. Am. Academy of Ophthal. & Otolaryng., Dallas, Texas (1974).

HAYREH, S.S. Blood supply of the optic nerve head and its role in optic atrophy, glaucoma and oedema of the optic disc. *Brit. J. Ophthal.* 11: *721-748* (1969).

HAYREH, S.S. & PERKINS, E.S. Proceedings of a Symposium held at the Royal College of Physicians and Surgeons of Glasgow. Ed. Kimpton, London: *71* (1968).

RAITTA, CH. & SARMELLA, T. Fluorescein angiography of the optic disc and the peripapillary area in chronic glaucoma. *Acta Ophthalm.* 48: *303-308* (1970).

ROSEN, E.S. Fluorescence photography of the eye. Ed. Butterworths, London: *79-82* (1969).

ZIMMERMAN, L.E., DE VENECIA, G. & HAMASAKI, D.I. Pathology of the optic nerve in acute experimental glaucoma. *Invest. Ophth.* 6: *109-112* (1967).

Author's address:
Ayacucho 307
1025 Buenos Aires
Argentina

THE PRECURSORS OF DISCIFORM
MACULAR DEGENERATION

STEPHEN S. FEMAN M.D., &
WICHARD A.J. VAN HEUVEN, M.D.

(Albany, N.Y., USA)

Disciform macular degeneration often causes reduced visual acuity in the older population (KAHN & MOORHEAD, 1973). Statistical surveys indicate that approximately 25% of the older population has some manifestation of this disorder (SORSBY, 1966). The fluorescein angiographic features of disciform macular degeneration are well known (GASS, 1967). Frequently, both eyes are not involved at the same time; one eye may develop a typical macular lesion at some time before the other. Examination of fellow eyes may reveal disorders that are precursors of the disciform lesion. To understand the predisciform lesion, the fellow eye of every disciform macular degeneration patient needs a detailed examination. The angiographic findings in good seeing fellow eyes, when disciform macular degeneration is first noted in the other eye, are described below.

DRUSEN

The histopathologic features of drusen have been reported (FARKAS, 1971). However, the fluorescein angiographic characteristics are less specific. In general, drusen are at the level of the retinal pigment epithelium, remain constant in size during angiography, have their brightness peak within one minute of dye injection, and fade with the choroid.

Lesions of this variety were seen in 100% of the eyes. In 34% of the patients, drusen were the only pathologic features in the fellow eyes. The size, shape and distribution of these lesions prevented accurate analysis. The drusen were too small to measure and too numerous to count. In addition, these lesions had a minimal effect on visual acuity. The average visual acuity of these eyes was 20/30. There were only two such fellow eyes with a best corrected visual acuity less than 20/40 (Fig. 1A + B).

RETINAL PIGMENT EPITHELIAL
DETACHMENTS

Another lesion of the retinal pigment epithelium appears as a large drusen. It has a measurable size and maintains its fluorescence after the choroidal background has faded. This may represent staining of material beneath the retinal pigment epithelium, a variety of retinal pigment epithelial detachment. Other retinal pigment epithelial detachments may be of a greater size.

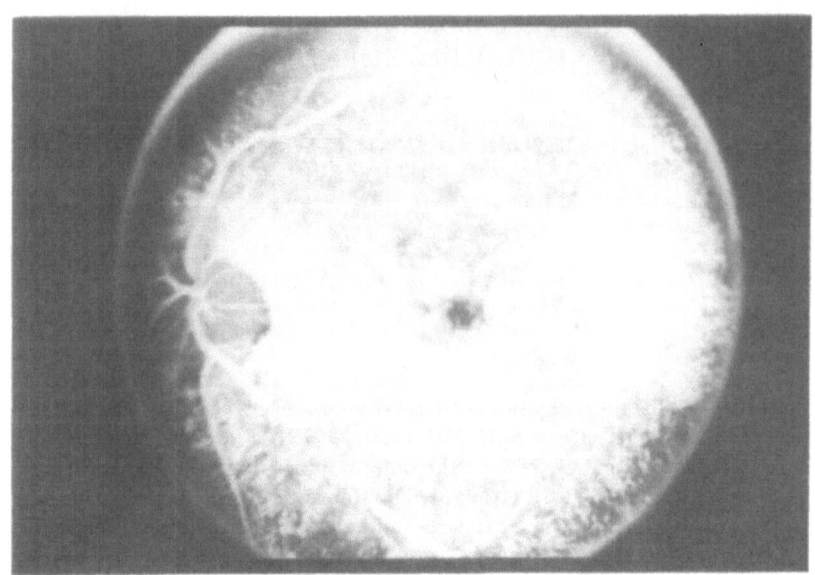

Fig. 1A

EARLY DRUSEN STAGE

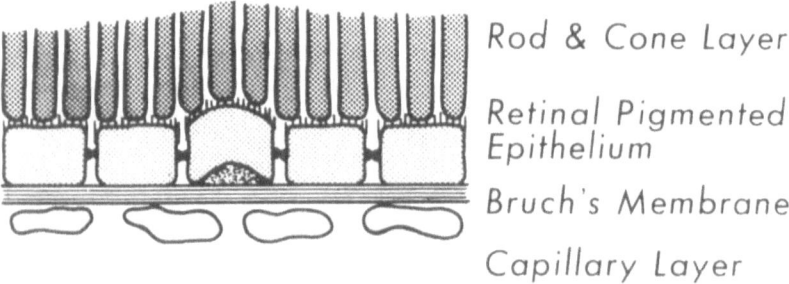

Rod & Cone Layer

Retinal Pigmented
Epithelium

Bruch's Membrane

Capillary Layer

Fig. 1B

The fluorescein characteristics of retinal pigment epithelial detachments are:
1. diffuse filling from the choroid, and 2. distinct borders. Retinal pigment
epithelial detachments and drusen appeared as combined lesions in 50% of
the fellow eyes. The mean visual acuity of these eyes was 20/40; however,
the visual acuity ranged from 20/20 to 20/200 depending on how much
foveal involvement was present (Fig. 2).

320

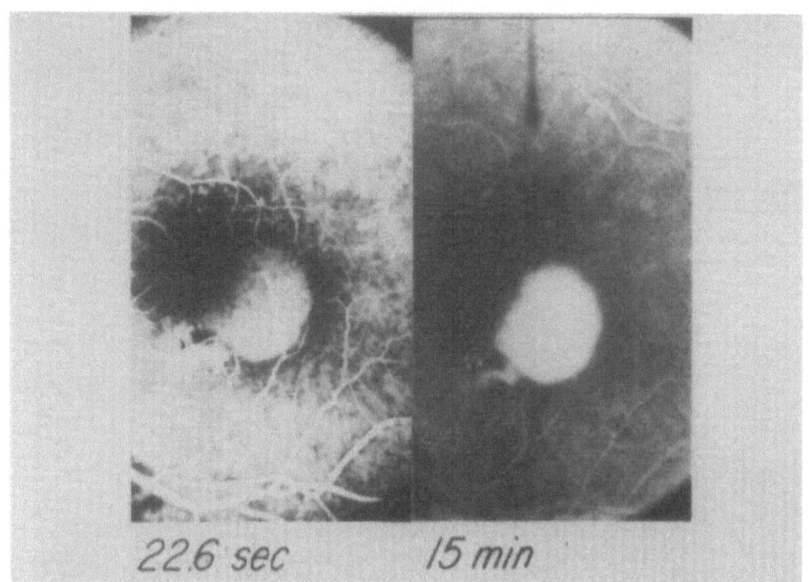

Fig. 2A

RETINAL PIGMENT
EPITHELIAL DETACHMENT

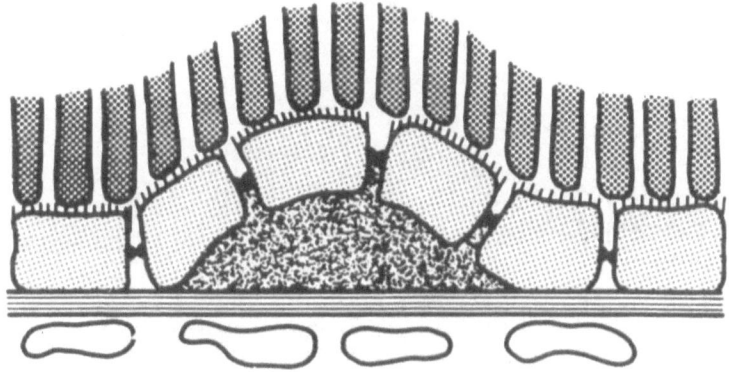

Fig. 2B

**SEROUS NEURO-SENSORY DETACHMENTS
WITH SUBRETINAL NEOVASCULARIZATION**

The fluorescein angiographic characteristic of a serous neurosensory retinal detachment is its indistinct border. That is, fluorescein fills the center of the lesion, but the periphery of the lesion is uncertain. This is because the

321

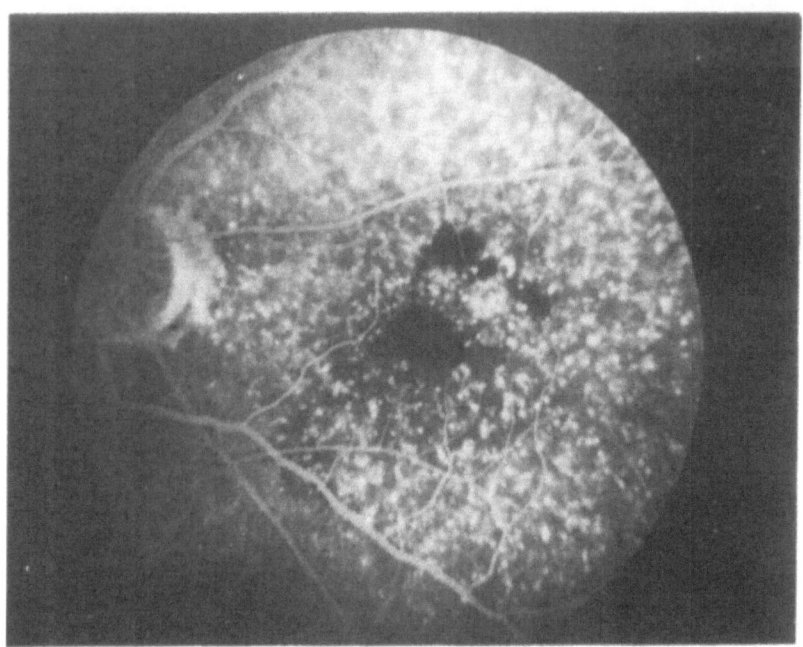

Fig. 3A

SUB-RETINAL HEMORRHAGE

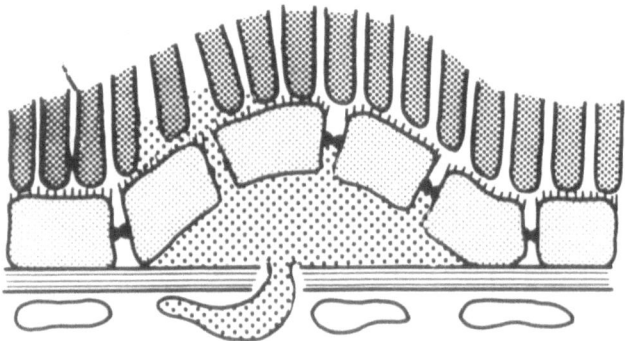

Fig. 3B

margins blend imperceptibly with the adjacent non involved retina. In the present series, this lesion was usually accompanied by a focus of subretinal neovascularization or hemorrhage. In such lesions, the fluorescein appeared to progress from the choroid into the subretinal neovascular tissue and then under and into the neurosensory retina. Frequently, the neovascular tissue

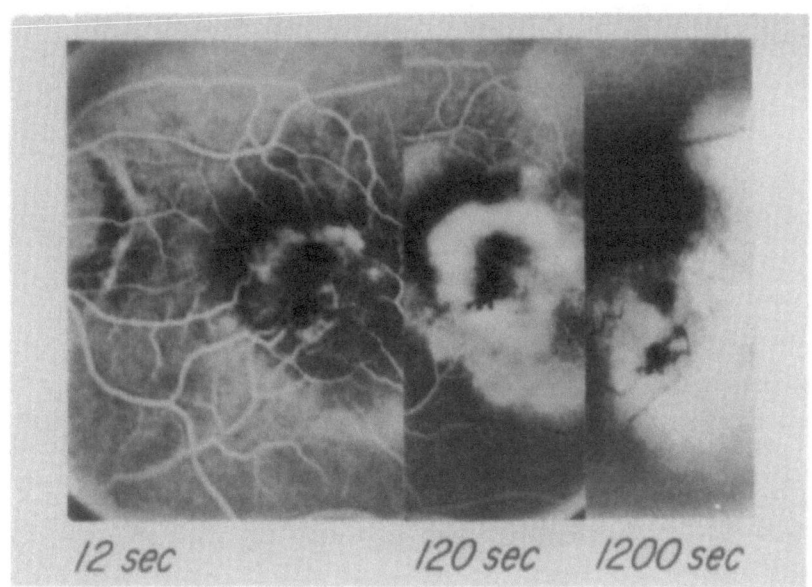

Fig. 3C

SUB-RETINAL
NEOVASCULARIZATION

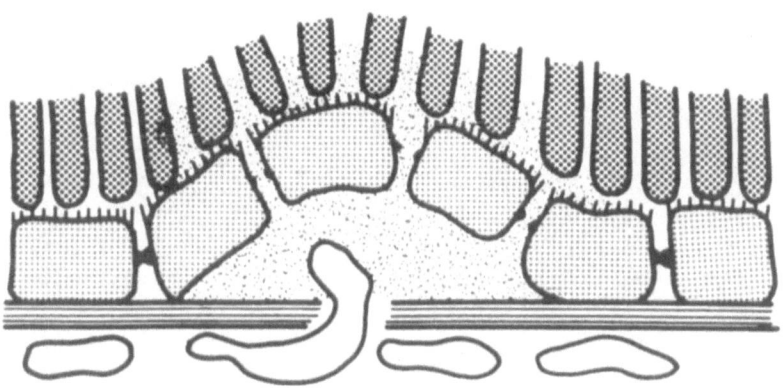

Fig. 3D

was accompanied by a hemorrhage that blocked some aspect of dye transit. For this reason, when subretinal hemorrhage and serous neurosensory detachment is noted without neovascularization, it is assumed that the neovascularization is present but not visible through the overlying hemorrhage (Fig. 3).

323

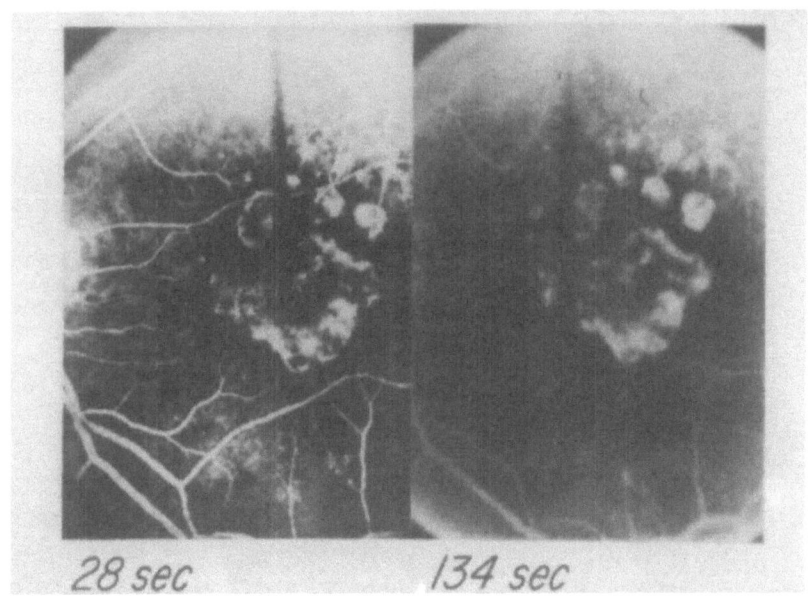

Fig. 4A

ATROPHIC DEGENERATION

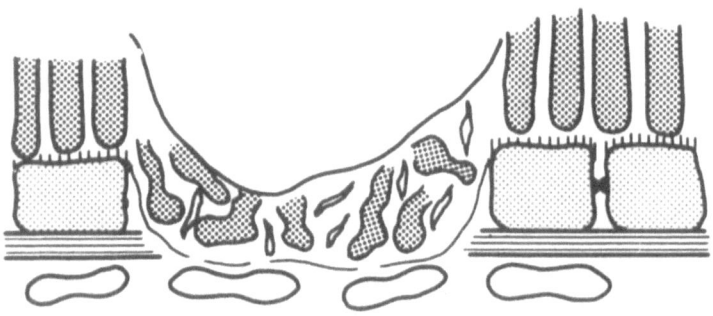

Fig. 4B

In this series of fellow eyes, serous neurosensory detachment with vascularization was present in 14%. The mean visual acuity of such eyes was 20/80. However, in some eyes the visual acuity was as good as 20/40 when the lesion was at a distance from the fovea.

324

ATROPHIC APPEARING RETINAL PIGMENT EPITHELIAL DEGENERATION

In three fellow eyes, large areas of retinal pigment epithelial degeneration were present at the posterior pole. The lesions were extra foveal and had distinct edges. During angiography the lesions filled with fluorescein in the choroidal phase. They remained visible late after venous phase as the scleral fluorescence silhouetted the choroidal vessels. At no time was fluorescein able to leak through these lesions into the neurosensory retina. The visual acuity was 20/100 in each of these eyes (Fig. 4A + B).

SUMMARY

In order to find the cause of disciform macular degeneration it is necessary to study uninvolved eyes. When one eye developes disciform degeneration, the fellow eye may contain the precursor of the disorder. This study demonstrated that 34% of fellow eyes contain only drusen; 50% contain drusen and retinal pigment epithelial detachments; and 13% contain drusen, retinal pigment epithelial detachments, subretinal neovascularization and serous neurosensory edema. The lesion in this 13% is identical to extrafoveal disciform macular degeneration and will probably progress to the typical lesion. Therefore, the lesion that combines drusen and retinal pigment epithelial detachment is the most obvious precursor to disciform degeneration. Therapy to the retinal pigment epithelial detachments may be a means of preventing progressive disciform macular degeneration.

REFERENCES

FARKAS, T.G. Drusen of the retinal pigment epithelium. *Survey of Ophthal.* 16: 75 (1971).

GASS, J.D.M. Pathogenesis of disciform detachment of the neuroepithelium. *Am. J. Ophthal.* 63 (2): *617* (1967).

KAHN, H.A. & MOORHEAD, H.B. Statistics on blindness in the model reporting area of the U.S. Dept. H.E.W. Pub. No. (NIH) 73-427, U.S. Government Printing Office, Washington, D.C. (1973).

SORSBY, A. The incidence and causes of blindness in England and Wales. Her Majesty's Stationery Office, London (1966).

Authors' address:
Retina Offices
Department of Ophthalmology
Albany Medical College
Albany, N.Y. 12208
USA

DISCUSSION

Dr Deutman: Is there anyone who wants to discuss Dr Femans paper? I think it was rather straightforward. The problem is, of course, to know when the people are going to have visual problems, perhaps therefore the perimetric profiles discussed by Dr Greve will be of importance in the future. The problem is, of course, that many patients get a sudden decrease of vision and then it may be to late. Dr Gass, could you comment?

Dr Gass: What needs to be done, I suppose, is to take a group of these patients that have large drusen in the macula and to randomly select one for treatment. It is possible by putting a spot of photocoagulation on each of these drusen to cause it to disappear. The fact that they disappear and that the fundus looks a lot better does not necessarily mean that it is going to help the patient. But I think that it is a study to consider. It has some risks involved because some of these drusen will have new vessels under them and if you treat the drusen in an occasional patient you will precipitate a macular haemorrhage.

Mr Bird: Can I make a comment? We followed 108 patients between 1 and 5 years in whom there was disciform degeneration in one eye and no serous detachment in the other and we found that each year there is a 12% risk for the other eye suffering a disciform lesion. We thought with this low risk that it probably was not reasonable to go ahead and do any kind of prophylactic treatment though I accept that may be wrong. Of these 108 patients we found no correlation between the evolution of the disciform lesion of the second eye and the pigment epithelial changes or the number of drusen or the size of drusen below 800 μ. Those who did not develop disciform lesions had exactly the same features as those who did. There was, however, significant correlation between the development of this disciform lesion in the second eye and large confluent drusen greater than 800 μ. In addition we found a high degree of correlation between the risk of getting a disciform lesion and what we called drusen, lesions in which dye accumulated during fluorescein angiography.

DIFFERENTIAL PERIMETRIC PROFILES
IN DISCIFORM MACULAR DEGENERATION:
STAGES OF DEVELOPMENT

E.L.GREVE, P.J.M. BOS, P.T.V.M. DE JONG & D. BAKKER

(Amsterdam, the Netherlands)

INTRODUCTION AND METHODS

The purpose of this study is to describe the central and paracentral visual function in drusen and disciform macular degeneration and in the stages between these two extremes of the disease. The functional defects will be compared with the fluorescein angiographic findings.

In 1973 GASS described a four year follow-up of 200 patients with drusen. In 49 cases that had only drusen 20% had serious loss of vision during this period. Another 25% lost two lines of the visual acuity chart. In 91 cases in which one eye had disciform macular degeneration and the other eye had drusen, 33% of the cases with drusen had serious loss of vision and another 33% lost two lines of the visual acuity chart. From this study it is clear that a significant number of cases with drusen deteriorate in a period of a few years.

We will try to establish the stages of deterioration of visual function during the proces that leads from drusen to disciform macular degeneration. Such a description might be of value to identify that stage of the disease in which laser coagulation can best be performed. We have obtained data in 20 patients that were studied during the last year. It is not a longitudinal study. The follow-up period is still not long enough to demonstrate significant deterioration in all individual patients. Different stages of development were observed in different patients. This provides a working hypothesis for the natural history of visual function of the disease in the individual patient.

All patients were examined by means of differential central single stimulus static perimetry. By differential perimetry we mean that perimetry was performed at two levels of adaption. In this case the levels were photopic (3 cd.m^{-2}) and mesopic (0.003 cd.m^{-2}). Comparing the intensity of defects under photopic and mesopic circumstances provided valuable information. The intensity of mesopic and photopic defects will be expressed as an M/P ratio. If the M/P ratio is 1.0 this means that the intensity of the photopic and mesopic defects is equal. If the M/P ratio is larger than 1 this indicates that the mesopic intensity is greater than the photopic intensity. The meridians of static perimetry were selected on the basis of ophthalmoscopy and fluorescein angiography.

Scotopic campimetry has been described by FRANÇOIS & VERRIEST (1956). It is not suitable for clinical purposes.

Kinetic mesopic campimetry has been advocated by JAYLE (1958) who concluded that this method is superior to photopic kinetic campimetry. For

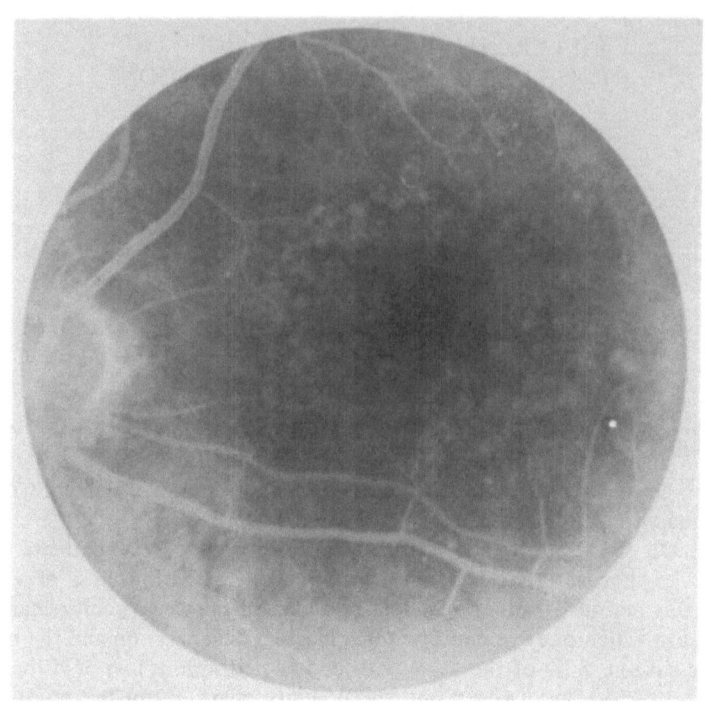

Fig. 1. F.F.A. of case 1.: drusen

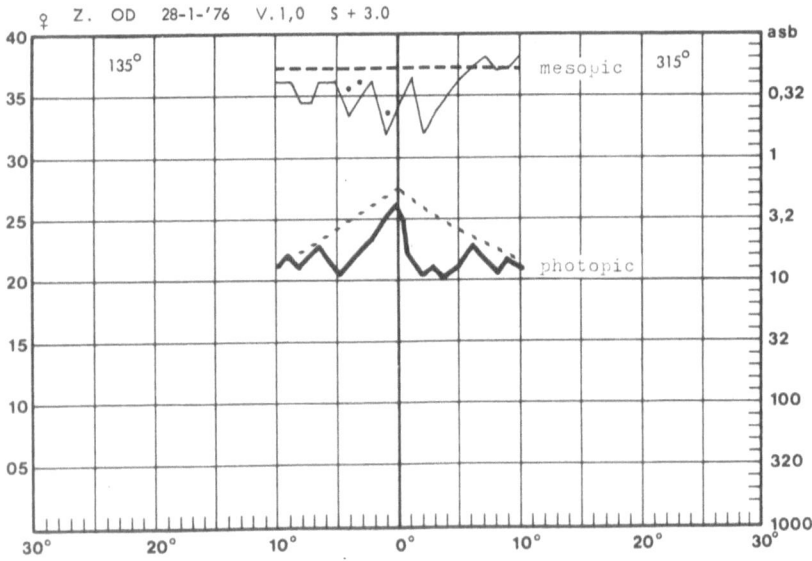

Fig. 2. D.S.P. (Differential Static Perimetry) of case 1.: relative paracentral defects with good central sensitivity. M/P ratio is 1.

328

reasons explained elsewhere static perimetry is to be prefered for visual field examinations that aim at comparing mesopic and photopic results (GREVE, 1973).

The results will be illustrated on the basis of 4 case-reports.

CASE REPORTS

Because of the limited space available only the F.F.A. photographs and perimetric profiles are shown.

Case 1

Woman of 68 years who has a visual acuity of 1.0 in the right eye and of 0.25 in the left eye. The right eye has drusen and the left eye a late stage of disciform macular degeneration. Both the fundus and the fluorescein angiography show a classic picture of drusen (Fig. 1.). The differential static perimetry shows relative paracentral defects where central sensitivity is still quite good. The M/P ratio is 1. (Fig. 2).

Case 2

Woman of 67 years. Visual acuity in the right eye is 0.9 and in the left eye 1.0. The left eye shows only drusen, some of them confluent (Fig. 3). The differential static perimetry shows an increase of the paracentral defects and here it is the mesopic intensity that increases more than the photopic intensity so the M/P ratio is larger than 1. (Fig. 4). The right eye of this patient shows large confluent drusen and a local retinal pigment epithelial (R.P.E.) detachment (Fig. 5). One wonders if there is also some sub-foveal fluid or foveal oedema. Fluorescein angiography shows the R.P.E. detachment. Differential static perimetry shows a paracentral defect with a mesopic intensity that is greater than the photopic intensity and a central defect (Fig. 6). Again there was an M/P ratio greater than 1. The difference between this left eye and the right eye is that central sensitivity is affected in the right eye.

Case 3

A man of 68 years with visual acuity in the right eye of 0.5 and in the left eye of 1.0. The right eye shows drusen and R.P.E. detachment with extension of fluid under the fovea. Fluorescein angiography shows the pigment epithelial detachment but no leakage (Fig. 7). The left eye has only drusen. The differential static perimetry of the right eye shows paracentral and central defects with an M/P ratio that is larger than 1. (Fig. 8). In this case the central defect is deeper than in case 3 (right eye).

Case 4

A man of 60 years old with disciform haemorrhagic exsudative macular degeneration. Fluorescein angiographic shows the typical picture with leakage (Fig. 9). Differential static perimetry shows a large central and paracentral defect with a M/P ratio of more than 1. (Fig. 10).

329

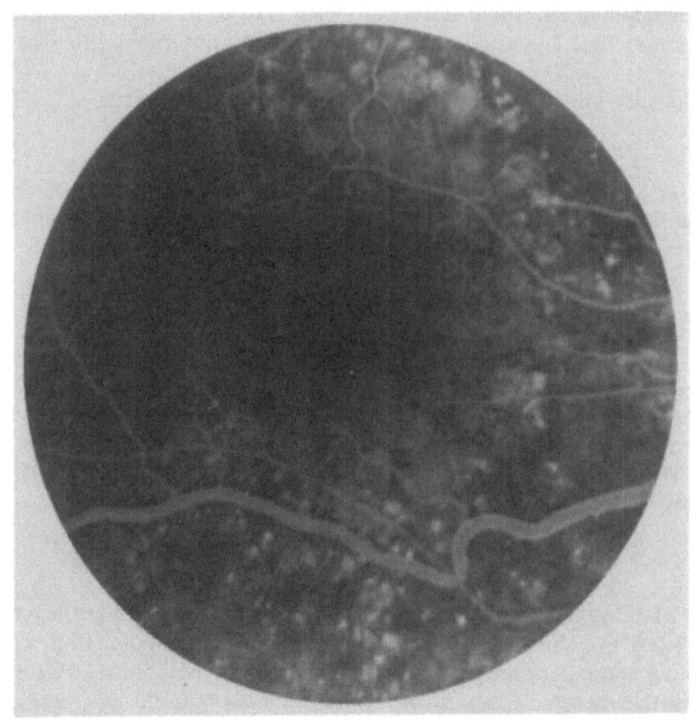

Fig. 3. F.F.A. of case 2 (left eye): drusen

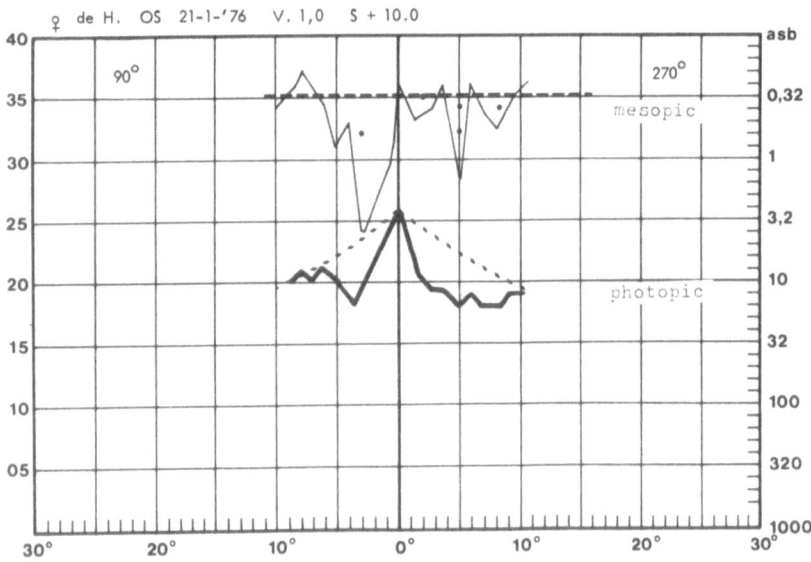

Fig. 4. D.S.P. of case 2 (left eye): paracentral defect with intensity greater than in case 1. and increase of M/P ratio in the defect.

330

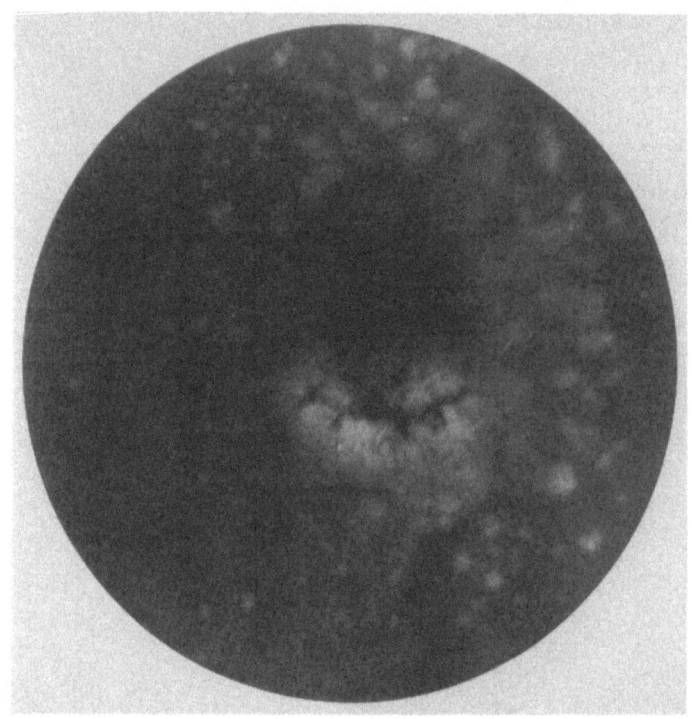

Fig. 5. F.F.A. of case 2. (right eye): drusen and small R.P.E. detachment.

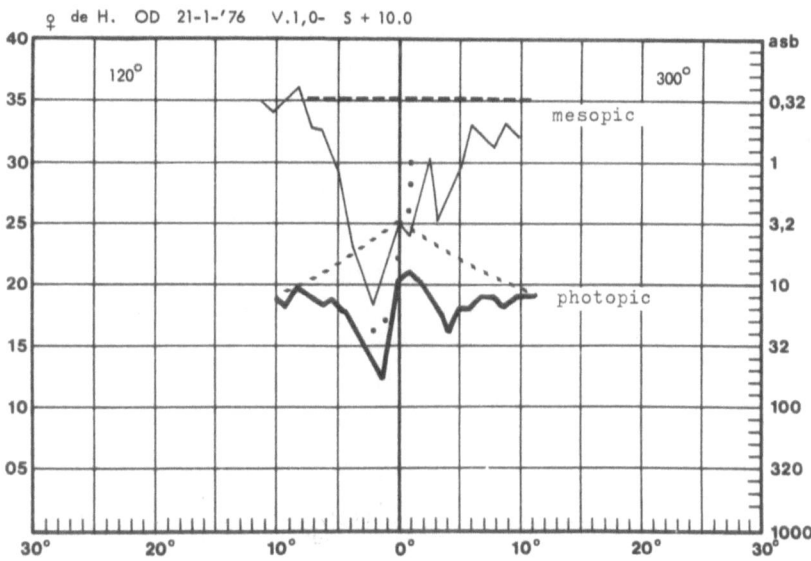

Fig. 6. D.S.P. of case 2 (right eye): paracentral defect of intensity greater than in case 2 (left eye) and in addition the appearance of a central defect with an M/P ratio greater than 1.

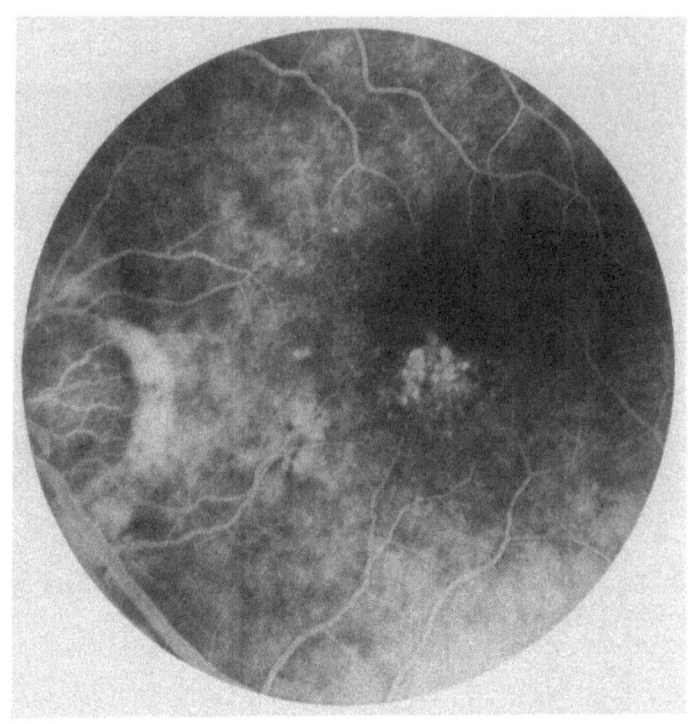

Fig. 7. F.F.A. of case 3: R.P.E. detachment; no leakage.

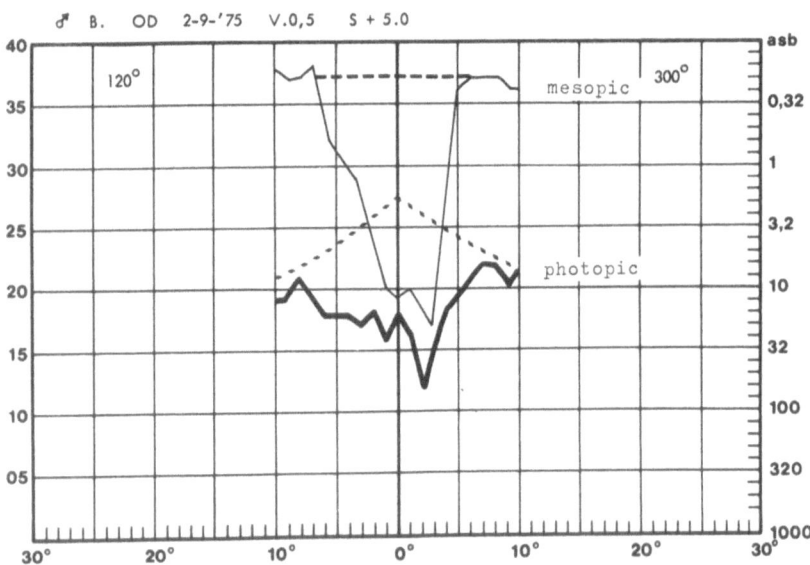

Fig. 8. D.S.P. of case 3: Paracentral defect as in case 2 (right eye) and a central defect with an intensity that is greater than the intensity of the central defect of case 2. M/P ratio greater than 1.

DISCUSSION

The case reports shown here demonstrate the typical configuration of defects as measured by central static perimetry. The different stages of the development of the desease have been grouped from I to IV. The group II has been subdivided in a group IIa and IIb. The stages are based on the configuration of the defect and the behavior of the mesopic/photopic ratio. An overview of the stages is given in Table I. Again it is emphasized that these stages are a working hypothesis. Certainly not all defects in disciform macular degeneration develop in the way described here. For practical purposes however the described cases are the most interesting because only cases with paracentral detachment of the retinal pigment epithelium (R.P.E.) are available for treatment. In group I and IIa the fundus and fluorescein angiographic findings are described as drusen. In group I there are relative paracentral defects and the mesopic/photopic ratio is 1.0 (case I).

In group II a deeper paracentral defect develops and the mesopic/photopic ratio increases. From this study and from earlier work an central serous choriopathy (GREVE et al. 1972, 1973, 1976), we have concluded that the increase of the mesopic/photopic ratio means that there is fluid either under the retinal pigment epithelium or under the retinal neuro-epithelium. In the case of stage IIa ·it is impossible to prove that there is fluid under the confluent drusen but it is highly probable (case 2 left eye). The clinical difference between stages I and stages IIa is in the size of the drusen. Stage IIa is close to a small retinal pigment epithelium detachment.

In stage IIb the fundus shows a hazy appearance of the fovea suggesting that foveal edema is present (case 2, right eye). The difference between IIa and IIb is that in addition to the paracentral defect now there is also a central defect with an increasing central mesopic/photopic ratio. The transition from stage IIa to IIb is an important one because it indicates that the localized parafoveal sub R.P.E. fluid of stage IIa has extended under the fovea. In stage IIa we only deal with a paracentral defect that in principle is available for treatment. Visual acuity in stage IIb is still quite good. On fluorescein angiography no leakage could be shown. In stage III there is a clear R.P.E. detachment with foveal oedema and there is a marked increase of the relative central defect which corresponds with the foveal oedema (case 3). On fluorescein angiography again there is no leakage. In fact the stages I, II and III are the most interesting of this study, because they are the early stages of development of disciform macular degeneration. Stage IV is already a relatively late stage with a deep central and paracentral defect (case 4).

An extremely useful and new finding from our study is that the mesopic/photopic ratio indicates the presence of fluid or call it oedema. We use this routinely if we are in doubt whether there is foveal oedema or not. As shown in Table I, fluorescein angiography in the early stages indicates the retinal pigment epithelium detachment but not the foveal oedema.

Careful biomicroscopy of the fundus may indicate the foveal oedema. Differential static perimetry is a highly sensitive and objective means of detecting foveal oedema and a welcome confirmation of biomicroscopy

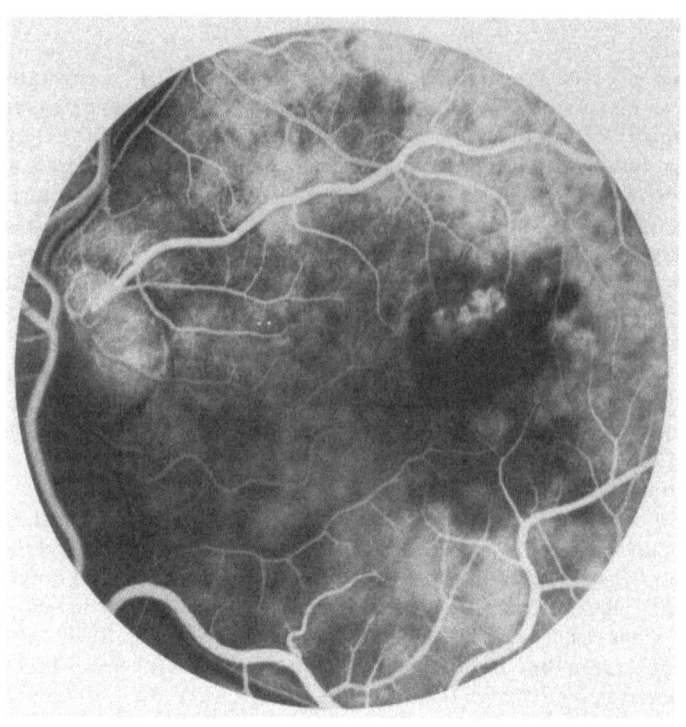

Fig. 9.   F.F.A. of case 4: disciform macular degeneration with leakage.

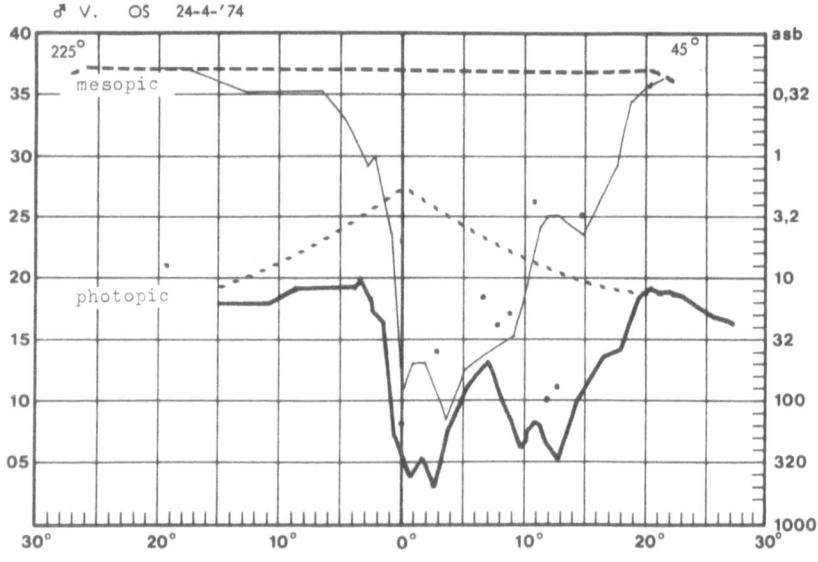

Fig. 10.   D.S.P. of case 4: large central and paracentral defect.

	I	II A	II B	III	IV
FUNDUS	DRUSEN	DRUSEN	R.P.E. DETACH. + ? SUBFOVEAL FLUID ?	R.P.E. DETACH. + SUBFOVEAL FLUID	DISCIFORM MACULAR DEGENERATION
F F A	DRUSEN	DRUSEN	R.P.E. DETACH. NO LEAKAGE	R.P.E. DETACH. NO LEAKAGE	D.M.D. LEAKAGE
V F					
	SLIGHT PARACENTRAL DEFECTS	DEEPENING PARACENTRAL DEFECT M>P	BEGINNING DETERIORATION OF CENTRAL SENS M>P	FURTHER DETERIORATION OF CENTRAL SENS M>P	DEEP CENTRAL DEFECT LATE STAGE
M/P RATIO	1.0	1.2 – 1.5	1.8	1.5	1.2
V A	1.0	1.0	0.75 – 1.0	0.5	< 0.5

findings. We feel that differential static perimetry is a better indicator of the severity of the disease than fluorescein angiography. Both diagnostic methods should go hand in hand in the early stages of disciform macular degeneration. Also differential static eprimetry showed severe defects when visual aquity was still good. The reason for this is that the para-foveal retina is affected in an earlier stage than the fovea itself.

Now a few remarks about therapy. BIRD stated in 1974 that until a method is devised of indentifying eyes at high risk it is likely that prophylactic laser coagulation of senile choroidal macular degeneration will remain in abeyance. Bird's series of laser coagulation in avascular disciform macular degeneration suggested that laser coagulation can improve visual acuity, at least temporarely. If one looks at the stages of development of disciform macular degeneration as indicated by differential static perimetry one is tempted to suggest that stage IIb might be the stage were laser coagulation could prevent further deterioration of central sensitivity. We have not yet started laser coagulation in that stage because we want to extend our follow-up period, but we hope to be able to use differential static perimetry as a prognostic index in the early stages of development of disciform macular degeneration.

SUMMARY

The purpose of this study is to describe the central and paracentral visual function in drusen and in disciform macular degeneration and in the stages between these two extremes of the disease. The functional defects will be compared with the fluorescein angiographic findings. Function is measured by means of central single stimulus static perimetry at a mesopic and photopic level of adaptation.

The results show:
1. A typical configuration of defects in the different stages of drusen and disciform lesions. The transition to the stage with foveal oedema is indicated very well by differential static perimetry.
2. A greater intensity of defects at mesopic levels of adaptation than at photopic levels of adapation in the case of sub-retinal or sub R.P.E. fluid.
3. Differential static perimetry is better indicator of the severity of the disease than fluorescein angiography.
4. Differential static perimetry showed severe paracentral defects when visual acuity was still good.
5. A stage of development of the disease where profilactic laser coagulation might be practised is suggested.

REFERENCES

BIRD, A.C. Recent advances in the treatment of senile disciforme macular degeneration by photocoagulation. *Brit. J. Ophthal.* 58: *367* (1974).

GASS, J.D.M. Drusen and disciform macular detachment and degeneration. *Arch. Ophthal.* 90: *206* (1973).

FRANÇOIS, J. & G. VERRIEST. Conclusions des études sur le champ visuel central scotopique au moyen de tests de Livingston. *Ann. Oculist* 189: *605-620* (1956).

GREVE, E.L. Single and multiple stimulus static perimetry in glaucoma; the two phases of visual field examination. *Docum. Ophthal.* 136: *1-355* (1973).

GREVE, E.L., P.J.M. BOS, R. MESKER & M. LEDEBOER. Static perimetry and fluorescein angiography in central serous choriopathy. Pres. at the Meeting of the N.O.G. (Dutch Ophthalmological Society) (1972).

GREVE, E.L., W.M. VERDUIN & M. LEDEBOER. The two-colour threshold in static perimetry. Read at the sec. Int. Symp. on Recent advanges in colour vision deficiencies.; Edinburgh (1973). *Mod. Prob. Ophthal.* 13: *113-118* (1974).

GREVE, E.L., P.J.M. BOS., P.T.V.M. DE JONG & D. BAKKER. Central static perimetry in maculopathies. Pres. at the Meeting of the N.O.G. (Dutch Ophthalmological Society) (1976).

JAYLE, G.E. & L. AUBERT. Le Camp visuel mésopique en pathologie oculaire. Actualités Latines d'Ophthalmologie. Masson, Paris, *50-115* (1958).

Authors' address:
Eye Clinic of the University of Amsterdam
Wilhelmina Gasthuis
1e Helmersstraat 104
Amsterdam
The Netherlands

DISCUSSION

x: I would like to ask Dr Greve whether he has used his perimetric profiles in other diseases with macular oedema especially in central serous retinopathy. I am asking him this question because recently we found that if an adaptometric curve is plotted in patients with quite typical central serous retinopathy, you get a very distinct and marked scotopic defect which is peripheral to the macular oedema and this somehow could correlate with his results.

Dr Greve: In fact, in 1972 we started this project on central serous choroidopathy and it was then we found that the mesopic defects were much deeper. There were two defects: one of the pigment epithelial detachment and one of the neuro epithelial detachment. The defect of the neuro epithelial detachment correspond exactly to the perimetric defect. Why we have not done scotopic perimetry is because it is a very difficult method of measuring visual function. You are coming to problems of adaptation, problems of fixation and all that. I think mesopic perimetry provides as much information as does the scotopic perimetry. We have carried out examinations in a lot of other macular diseases which have been reported recently to the Dutch Ophthalmological Society and, for instance, dry senile macular degeneration does not have this mesopic-photopic ratio, the recently described neuro-epitheliopathy of Bos and Deutman does not have this mesopic-photopic ratio, so we really feel that it is a very good tool for finding out if there is oedema or not.

FLUORANGIOGRAPHIC STUDY OF CHORIORETINAL LESIONS IN HIGH MYOPIA

N. STANGOS, P. TRAIANIDIS, A. PAPOULIS, J. KAMBOUROGLOU & K. PSILAS

(Thessaloniki/Greece)

It is worth pointing out that little data is available concerning fluoroangiography of high myopia. This led us to work on the findings of fluorescein angiography in axial high myopia.

As in almost every subject, fluorescein angiography provides data for a pathogenetic study and on the other hand, information useful in the assessment of the influences of therapy.

MATERIAL AND TECHNIQUE USED

For the fluoroangiography we used the Topcon TRC-F$_3$ fundus camera which allows us to take 3 photographs per second. In this way, we have

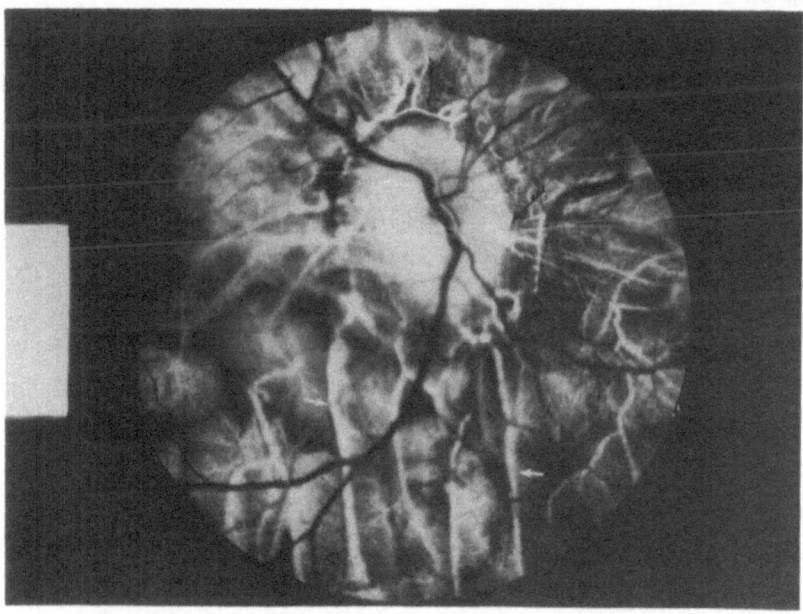

Fig. 1. Albinotic fundus in high myopia: choroidal phase. Proximal peripapillary annular vascularisation (Zinn-Haller ring-arrows). Radially arranged choroidal vessels starting from the disc area (white arrows).

been able to study effectively choroidal filling. We used ampoules of sodium fluorescein 10%. Our material includes the examination of 40 patients with high axial myopia of greater than -8d. and aged between 16 and 75. In all these patients, the abnormal length of the axis of the globe was verified using ultrasound biometry.

FINDINGS AND CONCLUSIONS

A detailed description of fluoroangiographic findings in high myopia will be published in one of our future papers. Circumstances allow us only to mention our general conclusions.

Because the angiographic recording refers to the posterior pole, our study deals with peripapillary and macular changes. Angiographic studies of high myopia allow good recording of choroidal circulation because most myopic fundi are pale (Fig. 1) and in many segments there is atrophy of the pigment epithelium especially in peripapillary regions (Fig. 2).

A. Peripapillary changes

The study of peripapillary choroidal circulation led to the following findings:

a. In cases of myopic crescent the peripapillary choroid is partially shown in the crescentic area (Fig. 3). It has a plexus-like appearance and in a few cases cilioretinal branches arising from this plexus can be easily seen (Fig. 4).

b. When atrophy or a peripapillary staphyloma exists:

1. In one-third of cases the peripapillary choroidal vasculature is complete (Fig. 1), while in the remainder of cases it appears incomplete with irregular

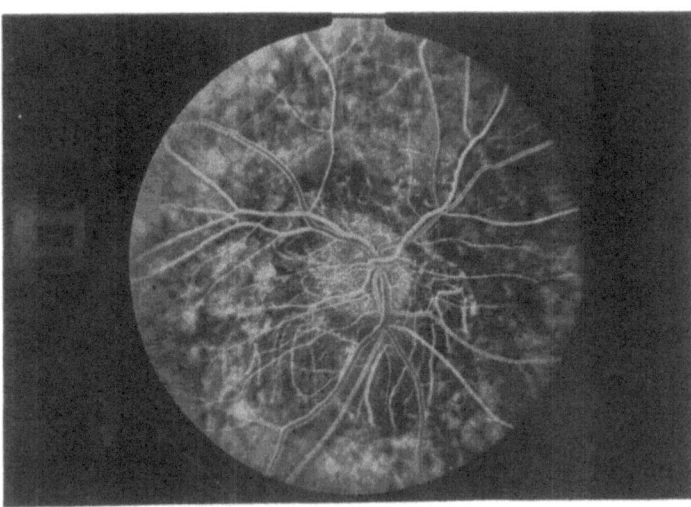

Fig. 2. Peripapillary atrophy of the pigment epithelium in high myopia.

340

filling (Fig. 5). Analysis of the relationship between choroidal filling and pigment epithelial changes has not yet been undertaken.

2. In some cases a second wider vascular ring appears with incomplete or complete vascular filling in the venous phase and is probably venous in origin (Fig. 6). Thus, this indicates that the peripapillary choroidal circulation consists of a series of concentric circles (AMALRIC, 1969).

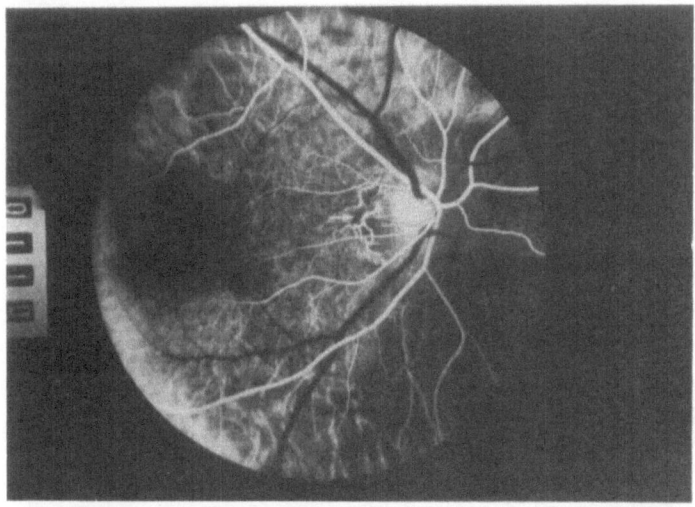

Fig. 3. Myopic crescent. Partially shown peripapillary choroidal annular vascularisation (arrow-arterial phase).

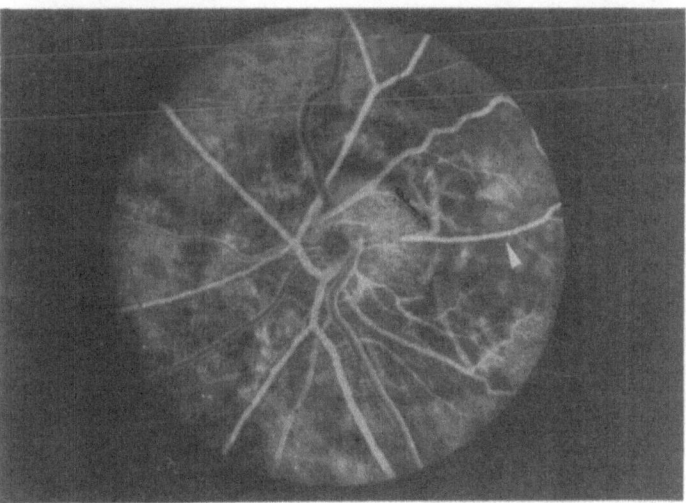

Fig. 4. Emergence of cilioretinal branch stemming from the peripapillary choroidal vascular plexus (arrows).

3. In addition we found radially arranged choroidal vessels starting from the disc (Fig. 1) and other vessels emerging from points in the periphery (Fig. 5). These vessels form a dense choroidal peripapillary framework.

4. Capillary fluorescence gradually disappears from the myopic crescent and myopic cone (Fig. 5). In the late venous phase hyperfluorescence appears at the margin of the atrophic ring (Fig. 5). In the late phases occasional areas of fluorescein leakage occur.

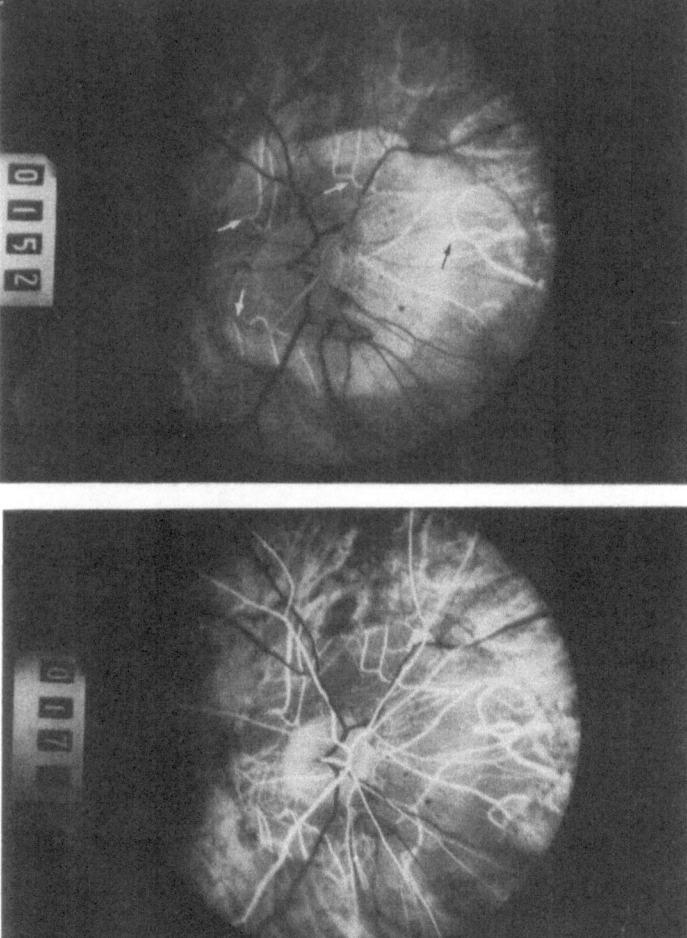

Fig. 5. Choroidal phase: peripapillary emergence of choroidal branches in the area of an atrophic ring in high myopia (white arrows). A more peripheral emerging branch is shown by the black arrow.

b. Early arterial phase. The choroidal peri apillary vascularisation becomes more rich.

342

5. The appearance of peripapillary choroidal vessels becomes less common in ratio to the age of the patient.

6. However, it is possible to have intense peripapillary sclerosis with good central visual acuity if the macular changes are mild (Fig. 5).

7. The peripapillary choroidal vessels remain fluorescent during the late venous phase. In two cases we found ruptures of Bruch's membrane simu-

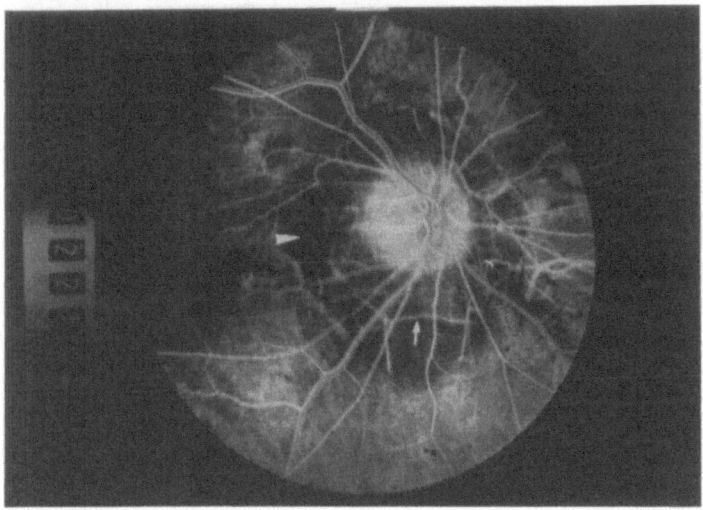

Fig. 6. Larger ring-shape peripapillary choroidal vascularisation (arrow). The atrophic ring lacks choroidal capillaries.

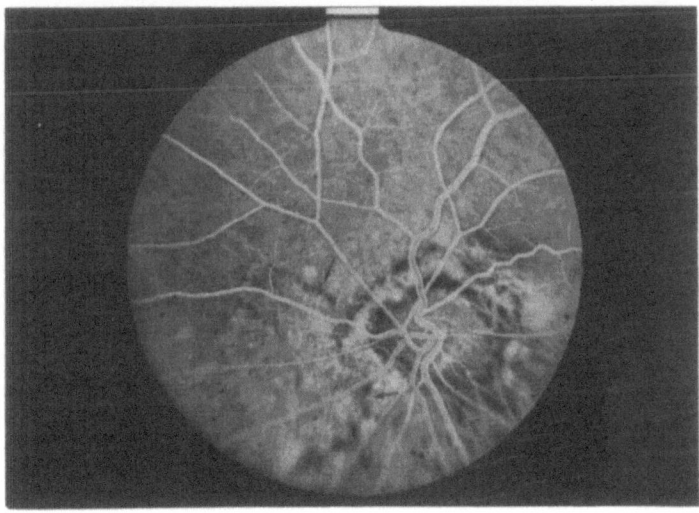

Fig. 7. High myopia. The arrows indicate radial ruptures of Bruch's membrane.

343

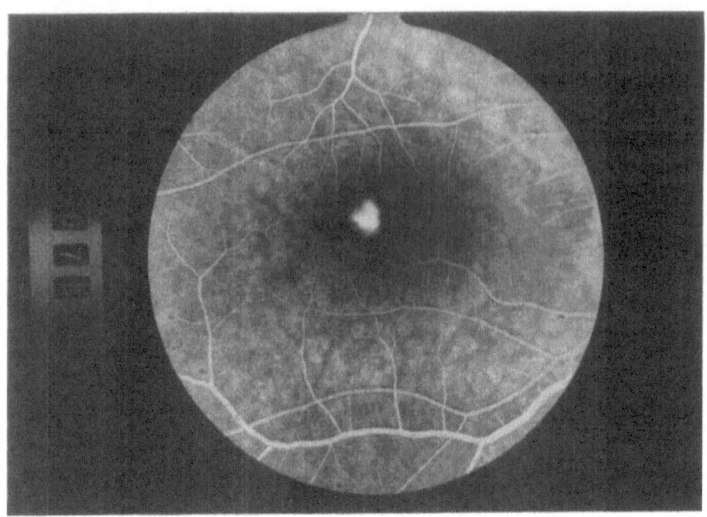

Fig. 8. Intense diffusion of dye in macular area. The other eye shows a Förster-Fuchs spot.

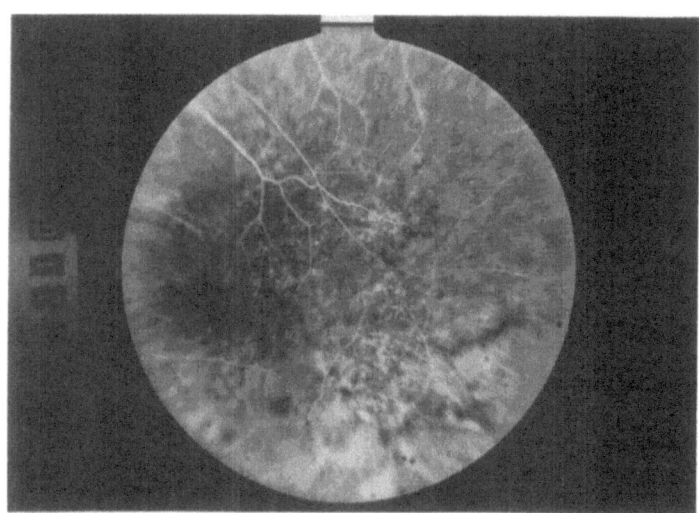

Fig. 9. Macular dry degenerative lesions in high myopia.

lating early angioid streaks radiating from the peripapillary area (Fig. 7). In these cases extensive degenerative changes were found in the macular area.

B. The fluoroangiographic study of the macular area

In high myopia shown according to the severity of the individual case:
1. Pigment epithelial changes with good vision.
2. Late dye leakage and subretinal new vessels, representing an early stage of a Förster-Fuchs spot (Fig. 8), or associated with a preexisting Förster-Fuchs spot (Fig. 9). This leakage may be some distance from the foveola and angiography is helpful in guiding laser treatment (WESSING, 1972; P. FRANÇOIS et al., 1975; GASS 1973).
3. Finally, fluoangiography helps in the true depiction of dry lesions in the macular area (Fig. 9) which according to the severity of the case are thas classified between the simple disturbance of the pigment epithelium and extended choroidal atrophy accompanied by necrosis most vascular elements (P. FRANÇOIS et al., 1975).

REFERENCES

AMALRIC, P. Circulation choroidienne. In: P. Amalric (ed.). Fluorescein angiography. Proceedings of the International Symposium on Fluorescein Angiography: *192-203*. Karger (1971).

BLATT, N. Augenhintergrund Veränderungen bei hochgradige Myopie. *Klin. Mbl. Augenheilk.* 146: *391-411* (1965).

FRANÇOIS, P., D'HOINE, G. & TURUT, P. La macula de l'oeil myope. *Confér. Lyon d'Ophtal.* 126 *(1975)*.

GASS, J.D.M. Choroidal neovascular membranes, their visualization and treatment. *Trans. Am. Acad. Ophthal. & Otolaryng.* 77: *310-320* (1973).

WESSING, A.M.D. Photocoagulation guided by fluorescein angiography. In: Shimizu, K. (ed.). Fluorescein angiography. Proceedings of the International Symposium on Fluorescein Angiography (ISFA), Tokyo 1972: *410-415*. Igaku Shoin Ltd, Tokyo (1974).

Keywords:
fluorangiography
high myopia
peripapillary circulation
choroidal circulation

Authors' address:
University Eye Clinic
Thessaloniki
Greece

JUVENILE JUXTAPAPILLARY HEMORRHAGIC CHOROIDITIS

SURESH R. LIMAYE, M.D. VERNON G. WONG, M.D.
& JEAN-J. DE LAEY, M.D.

(Washington, D.C., USA)

Lesions adjacent to the optic nerve head have always been of great interest to ophthalmologists; the etiology has remained obscure. A hemorrhagic exudative lesion involving choroid and retina adjacent to the optic disc has been described in presumed ocular histoplasmosis (SCHLAEGEL & KENNEY, 1966), a disease once thought to occur exclusively in the U.S.A. However, this entity appears to affect on the other side of the Atlantic (BRAUNSTEIN et al., 1974). A typical macular disciform lesion in presumed ocular histoplasmosis is common, but its counterpart near the disc is rare and may be difficult to categorize in the absence of peripheral punched-out chorio-retinal scars. The following two cases will illustrate this point.

A nineteen year old Caucasian female was examined on August 24, 1973, for symptoms of metamorphopsia. In 1969, she was hospitalized with the diagnosis of right optic neuritis, at another institution. The neurological

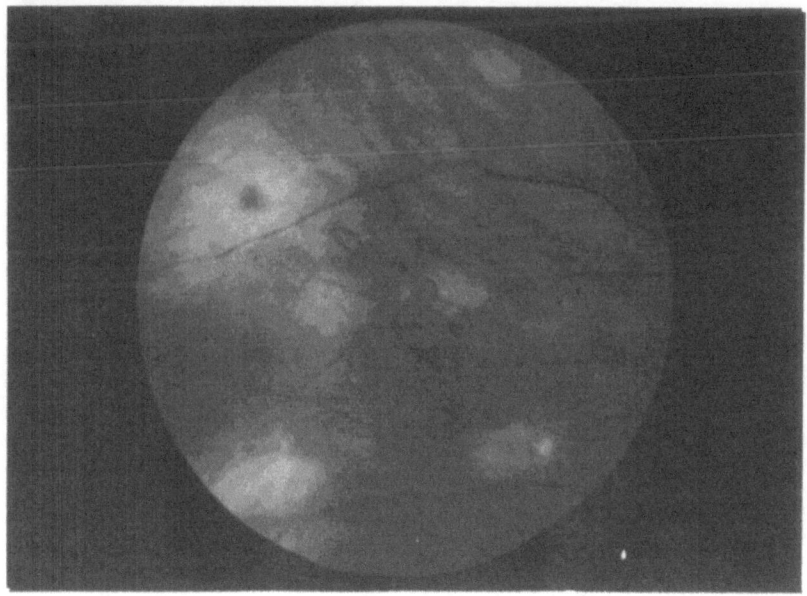

Fig. 1. *Case 1*, 'Histo-spots' in mid periphery.

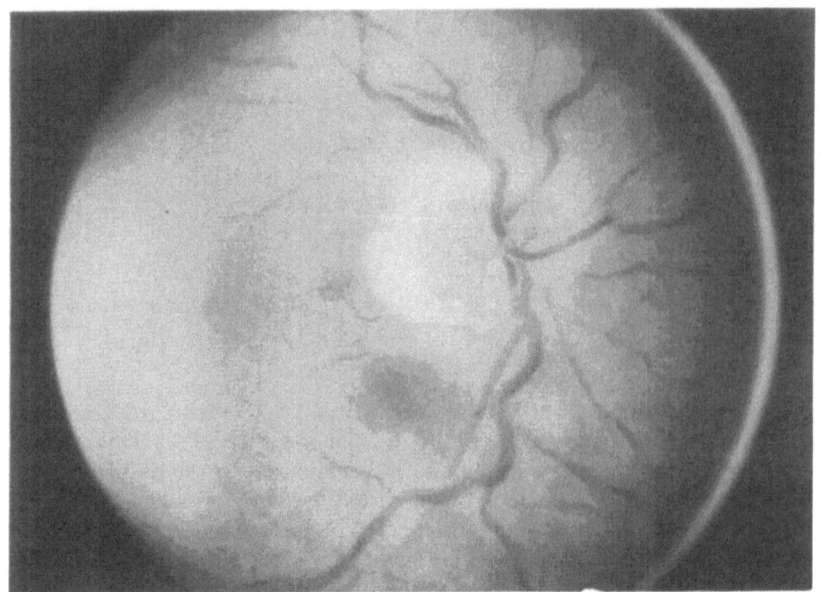

Fig. 2. *Case 1*, Fundus photo taken 4 years earlier (courtesy of Hospital Center, Washington, D.C.)

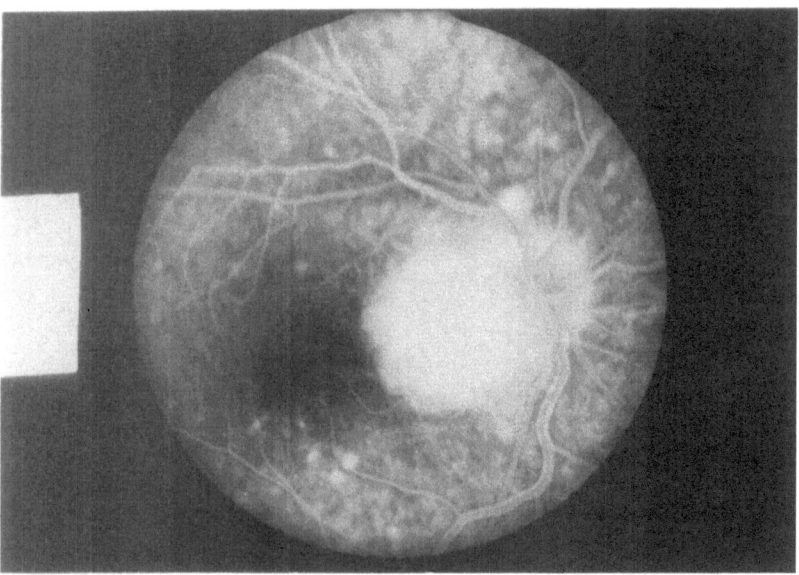

Fig. 3. *Case 1*, Late A. V. phase showing hyperfluorescein of juxtapapillary tissue and small round lesions.

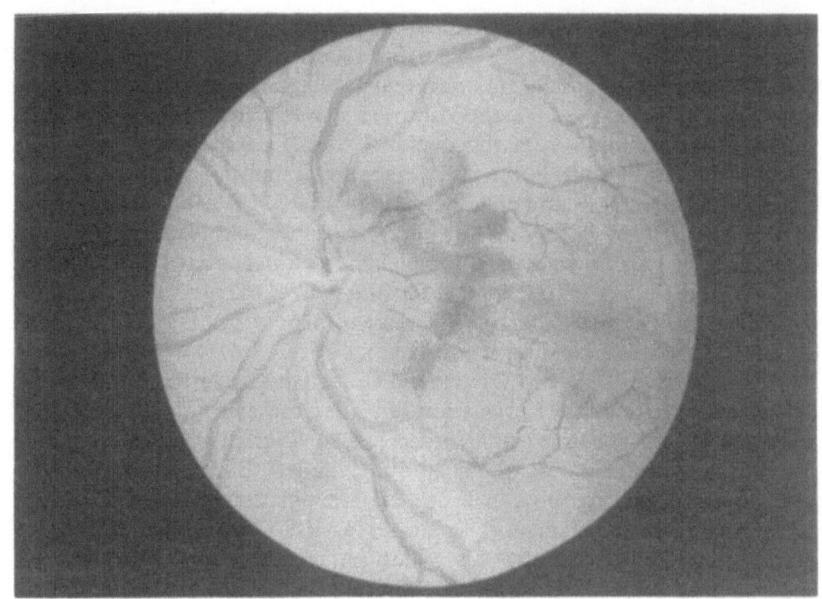

Fig. 4. *Case 2*, Juxtapapillary hemorrhagic lesions with retinal folds.

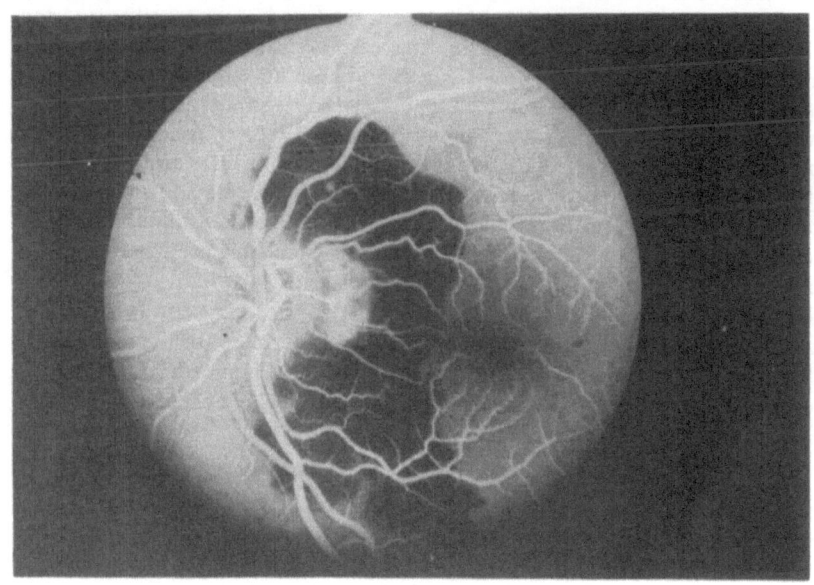

Fig. 5. *Case 2*, Subretinal leakage surrounded by subretinal hemorrhage.

work-up was reported as negative. Her visual acuity was 20/25 in the right eye and 20/20 in the left eye. There was a Marcus Gunn pupil on the right side. Slit-lamp examination did not reveal inflammatory cells in the anterior segment. The fundus examination showed a triangular, elevated subretinal whitish scar extending from the temporal border of the optic disc to the macula. There were folds in the overlying internal limiting membrane. Several 'histo-spots' were seen in the mid-periphery (Fig. 1). The left fundus also showed 'histo-spots' in the mid-periphery. A fundus photo of the right eye taken four years earlier showed a hemorrhage which eventually absorbed (Fig. 2). The fluorescein angiogram illustrates dye leakage with staining of the triangular scar area and hyper-fluorescent 'histo-spots' (Fig. 3). Serological test for histoplasmosis was reported as negative.

A second case is that of a 24 year old Caucasian female who was referred on February 11, 1975, for evaluation of an hemorrhagic lesion near the left optic disc. She had noticed sudden decrease in vision of this eye. Her visual acuity was 20/20 in the right and 20/50 in the left. Both anterior chamber and vitreous failed to show evidence of inflammation. There was a large subretinal hemorrhage adjacent to the optic disc (Fig. 4). The rest of the examination was normal and 'histo-spots' were not seen. The hemorrhage had increased over a few days, but eventually it became partially resolved. The fluorescein angiogram demonstrated subretinal fibrovascular leakage adjacent to the disc margin (Fig. 5). The histoplasmic skin test was purposely avoided and the serological test for histoplasmosis was reported negative.

DISCUSSION

An acute onset of nodular optic neuritis leading to typical peripapillary atrophy in presumed ocular histoplasmosis has been recently reported (HUSTED & SHOCK, 1975). Our first case appears to be similar to the above report; presenting as optic neuritis and later developing into peripapillary scarring and 'histo-spots'. In contrast, the second patent had only hemorrhagic exudative lesion near the optic disc with conspicuous absence of 'histo-spots'. The triad of peripheral punched-out chorioretinal lesions, peripapillary scar and hemorrhage disciform of the macula may not be present in every case of presumed ocular histoplasmosis. Similar cases of juxtapapillary hemorrhagic lesions have been seen in Europe. There seems to be a tendency to overdiagnose ocular histoplasmosis (SCHLAEGEL, 1975). Whether we are misdiagnosing this condition or not remains to be seen. For the ophthalmologist, fluorescein angiography is of value for the differential diagnosis of subretinal fibrovascular tissue causing hemorrhagic exudative lesions and lesions such as drusen of the optic disc which cause hemorrhages in adjacent retina.

REFERENCES

BRODRICK, J.D. Drusen of the disc and retinal hemorrhages. *Brit. J. Ophthal.* 57: *229-306* (1973).
BRAUNSTEIN, A., ROSEN, A. & BIRD, C. The ocular histoplasmosis syndrome in United Kingdom. *Brit. J. Ophthal.* 58: *893-898* (1974).

HUSTED, R.C. & SHOCK, J.P. Acute presumed histoplasmosis of optic nerve head. *Brit. J. Ophthal.* 59: *409-412* (1975).

SCHLAEGEL, T.F., JR. & KENNEY, D. Changes around the optic nerve head in presumed ocular histoplasmosis. *Am. J. Ophthal.* 62: *454-458* (1966).

SCHLAEGEL, T.F. JR. Ocular Histoplasmosis. Internation. Ophthalmology Clinic. Little, Brown & Comp., Boston 15(3): *3* (1975).

Authors' address:
Georgetown University Medical Center
Washington, D.C.
USA

DISCUSSION

Dr Deutman: The cases of Dr Limaye really look very much like histoplasmosis; however, you have to be careful that they are not drusen of the disc giving rise to subretinal new vessels but I am sure they were not there. Dr Henkind, would you like to comment? You have such a beautiful display outside on drusen of the disc and disciform macular degeneration.

Dr Henkind: When the first Albi conference was held in 1969 the entity of disc drusen and associated hemorrhages and particularly those beneath the pigment epithelium and retina was unknown. The first papers seemed only to appear from Chezchoslovakia and the United States in that year. I do not know if Dr Limaye's cases do or do not have disc drusen. To aid in the diagnosis, one should do ultrasounds. We used B- scan, but Don Gass says A-scan would even be better. We do not know whether the drusen have to be calcified in order to give the echo. I think myself the best way to look at these patients is not to look at these patients if they are young but look at their family. We have been impressed that, with one exception that I remember now, all these patients with disc drusen and associated hemorrhages had family members, father, mother, sister or brother with disc drusen. I have one child in particular whom I first saw at age 3 1/2 who had no obvious drusen at that age. Five years later she has very obvious drusen and I suspect that you can have relatively normal discs until later in life. The thing that impressed me in Dr Limaye's cases was the last case. There is no visible physiological pit and that is typical for disc drusen. The cases we have seen of disc drusen had flat discs and abnormal vascular patterns on the disc and to me that is almost typical for disc drusen. If you see the absence of a physiological cup and a crowded disc that is a very good sign, at least in our hands of disc drusen. I do not know if the cases of Dr Limaye do or do not have that, but it is not an uncommon entity.

Dr Norton: I would just hasten to add that it really was a known entity before 1969. Dr Reese had it described in the first edition of his book on tumors.

Dr Henkind: You are talking about his mistaken diagnosis of tuberous sclerosis.

Dr Norton: No, I am talking about hemorrhagic lesions associated with drusen of the nerve head and I saw patients myself in the fifties.

Dr Henkind: Oh yes, Dr Reese mentions that but we are not talking about the same lesions. Dr Reese mentions the hemorrhages which are peripapillar and above the disc: these have been known for years but the subretinal hamorrhage, the first bona fide case I have been able to find is Ostradovic, I think, in the Polish literature and, of course, Sanders from St. Louis was the first to report this in this country. But when he mentioned his case apparently at the AOS, 12 other cases were reported by other members. I am sure it has been seen before and generally missed.

MORPHOLOGY OF THE PIGMENT EPITHELIUM

L. MISSOTTEN

(Louvain, Belgium)

As an introduction to this morning session on the pathology of the pigment epithelium, a review of some well known facts on its normal morphology and function could be helpfull.

The retina is a part of the central nervous tissue inserted into the eye, a piece of neuro-ectoderm surrounded by mesodermal tissues such as the choroid and the vitreous body. The intercellular milieu of nervous tissue differs from that in mesodermal tissues, and, for that reason, it has to be separated from the surrounding tissues.

The pigment epithelium (P.E.) provides the barrier towards the choroid. It is a monolayer of hexagonal cells. Electron microscopy (E.M.) demonstrates how well they fit together. Surrounding each cell a terminal bar complex forms a tight bond with each neighbour. A perpendicular section of this complex shows the zonula adhaerens, providing the mechanical adhesion between cells and the zonula occludens, restricting diffusion between the cells through the intercellular cleft.

The nature of this barrier to diffusion has been explored in many ways; let us mention two of them. SHIOSE (1973) demonstrated by histochemical means that peroxidase diffuses freely in the chorio-capillary layer and Bruchs membrane, filling the basal infoldings of the pigment epithelial cells and diffusing in the intercellular spaces between the P.E. cells up to the zonula occludens but never beyond.

LASANSKY & DE FISCH (1966) have demonstrated the barrier to diffusion in another way. After preparing a P.E. in vitro, they detect a potential difference of 10 to 20 millivolt accross this layer. In this way not only an active transport mechanism for ions is demonstrated but also the fact that the terminal bars restrict the back diffusion of these ions in such a way that a potential difference may be build up.

Together these experiments demonstrate that the terminal bar system is impermeable to proteins, to ions and, as is well known, to substances such as fluorescein.

The basal surface of the P.E. has numerous infoldings of the plasma membrane, best seen in a flat section, with mitochondria in the cytoplasma adjacent to this area. A similar configuration: basal infoldings + mitochondria is seen in all epithelia concerned with active transport such as the renal tubulus or the epithelium of the ciliary body. This suggests an active transport function for the P.E. The direction of the transport may be different for different substances but there are good reasons to suppose that the bulk of fluid transport is toward the choriocapillaries in order to suck the retina in close contact with the apical area of the P.E.

At the apical surface each photoreceptor of the retina is surrounded partially by expansions of the P.E. cell. This area of close association is the site of numerous and intense interactions and we would like to mention three of them.

The tips of the photoreceptors break off and are ingested by the pigment epithelial cells. This has been shown by YOUNG & BOK (1969). It is a rather slow proces, requiring weeks for complete digestion of a rod.

Another interaction has been demonstrated by DOWLING (1960). When dark adapted rats are put in a bright environment the retinene disappears from the photoreceptors and is stored as vitamin A in the pigment epithelium. During dark adaptation the reverse proces occurs: vitamin A disappears from the P.E. and is incorporated as retinene in the visual cells of the retina. This exchange is complete in about half an hour; another interaction investigated by STEINBERG et al. (1970) requires only seconds. An intracellular electrode in a P.E. cell records a hyperpolarisation when a flash of light strikes the retina. The potential is generated by the apical membrane as is shown by the fact that its polarity is reversed in the C wave of the ERG. This potential may be due to a light sensitivity of the pigment epithelium; more likely however it is the result of an interaction with the photoreceptors of the retina.

A last word about the pigment that shields the photoreceptors from extraneous light. GABEL et al. (1973) have shown that its transmission is very low for short wave lengths: only approx 10% for blue and 25% for green light. This high absorption results in an attenuation by a factor of about 20 times of the fluorescence of the choroid during fluorescence angiography.

These measurements also explain why the shifting of the blue exiting wavelength from 500 to 525 nanometers gives better fluorograms of the choroidal circulation, as has been shown by Delori at this symposium. For longer wavelengths the pigment epithelium is almost perfectly transparent.

REFERENCES

DOWLING, J.E. Chemistry of visual adaptation in the rat. *Nature* 188: *114* (1960).

GABEL, V.P., BIRNGRUBER, R., HILLENKAMP, F., WALLOW, I.H.L. & SCHMOLKE, W. Uber die Lichtabsorption am Augenhintergrund. *Ber. Deutsche Ophthal. Gesellschaft.* 73: *362-367* (1973).

LASANSKY, A. & De FISCH, F.W. Potential, current, and ionic fluxes across the isolated retinal pigment epithelium and choroid. *J. Gen. Physiol.* 49: *913-924* (1966).

SHIOSE, Y. In Electron Microscopic Atlas in Ophthal. Ed. Yamada E. and Shikano S. Georg Thieme, Stuttgart 1973.

STEINBERG, R.H., SCHMIDT, R. & BROWN, K.T. Intra cellular responses to light from cat pigment epithelium: Origin of the electroretinogram c-wave. *Nature* 227: *728-730* (1970).

YOUNG, R.W. & BOK, D. Participation of the retinal pigment epithelium in the rod outer segment renewal process. *J. Cell. Biol.* 42: *392-403* (1969).

Author's address:

St. Raphaël Hospital, Department of Ophthalmology

Capucijnenvoer 35

3000 Louvain, Belgium

354

BRUCH'S MEMBRANE

STEPHEN J. RYAN, M.D.

(Los Angeles, USA)

Bruch's membrane has been the subject of extensive investigation, particularly as to its structure because of its importance in the pathogenesis of macular degenerations. WOLFRUM (1908) described the collagenous layer and the elastica of Bruch's membrane as well as the lamina vitrea as a glassy membrane. This classic description was somewhat forgotten in subsequent reports until the classic series of papers by HOGAN et al. (1971). Indeed, the ultrastructural studies by HOGAN provide the basis for much of this review of Bruch's membrane. HOGAN has preferred to describe the ultrastructure of Bruch's membrane in terms of five layers, bounded by the basement membrane of the retinal pigment epithelium (RPE) on its inner side and the basement membrane of the choriocapillaris on its outer side (HOGAN, 1967; HOGAN & ALVARADO, 1967; HOGAN et al., 1971; HOGAN & WOOD, 1973). Between these basement membranes are the inner collagenous zone and outer collagenous zone, which are separated by the elastica layer.

The basement membrane of the retinal pigment epithelium is 0.3 millimicra thick (HOGAN et al., 1971). Its fine filaments join the retinal pigment epithelial cell basement membrane to the adjacent collagen (HOGAN et al., 1971; HOGAN, 1967). The inner collagenous zone is 1.5 millimicra thick. The elastica does not lend itself to a measurement of thickness because it is a meshwork with gaps and holes through which collagen passes, maintaining continuity between the inner collagenous zone and outer collagenous zone. The outer collagenous zone is approximately 0.7 millimicra thick. Again, it has a similar collagen structure to that of the inner collagenous zone. The basement membranes of the choriocapillaris is approximately 0.14 millimicra thick. In the intercapillary region between the channels of the choriocapillaris, there is less ground substance and the collagen seems more dense than that in the outer collagenous zone (HOGAN, 1967; HOGAN et al., 1971).

It should be noted that there are those who prefer to think of the ultrastructure of Bruch's membrane in terms of two distinct layers: The basement membrane of the RPE and all external to that as being another layer of collagen related and derived material. FINE and others point out that the intercapillary region has a collagen layer which is continuous with the collagen of Bruch's membrane (FINE, 1973).

The function of Bruch's membrane is not known with certainty. It does, however, have a similar appearance to that membrane separating the pulmonary capillaries from adjacent air sacs. The mechanism of transport from the choriocapillaris to the pigment epithelium would seem to be via direct diffusion. There are no indications of active transport.

The major interest in Bruch's membrane is related to its role in the pathogenesis of macular degenerative processes. It does show the most prominent and frequently the earliest aging changes of all the retinal and choroidal layers. It is the opinion of HOGAN that the inner collagenous layer shows the first aging changes with subsequent changes in the elastica and outer collagenous layer and then in the intercapillary region (HOGAN, 1967). The question as to whether these changes are secondary to the function of the retinal pigment epithelium or choriocapillaris or actually related to the collagen and ground substance of the tissue of Bruch's membrane itself remains unanswered. The relation to the changes in the macular retina is also unknown.

With aging, there is an increased PAS positivity of this abnormal material in the collagenous zone. There is vesicular, granular, and filamentous material on the inner collagenous layer, which extends to the outer collagenous layer as well as altered collagen fibers. The elastic zone in aging demonstrates an increased basophilia which correlates with a moth-eaten appearance and increased density around a central core and then deposits of needle-like crystals on electron microscopy. The basophilic change precedes drusen formation which consists of deposits of amorphous granular material with round or oval globules of varying size. The drusenoid or colloid material can accumulate in the inner collagenous layer. Other drusenoid material is finaly fibrillar. In the intercapillary region, there is vesicular material and clumps of wide spacing fibers, long and osmophilic fibers, and dark granular ground substance.

In considering Bruch's membrane, the crucial consideration in where does aging end and disease begin. The thickening and hyalinization of Bruch's membrane correlates with an increased amount of collagen as well as change in its character. This substance also produces the intercapillary thickening. Basophilia is associated with calcific deposition. Drusenoid material can be seen within the RPE or deposited in Bruch's membrane, presumably by the RPE. Electron microscopy demonstrates an amorphous granular material with lipid globules and calcium crystals. This material may interfere with the exchange of metabolites or breakdown products between the choriocapillaris and ultimately the receptors.

The crucial question then remains as to the interrelation of the retina, the retinal pigment epithelium, Bruch's membrane, and the choriocapillaris. In these degenerative processes, the retina can show degeneration with loss of receptors and gliosis. The retinal pigment epithelium can demonstrate degeneration, migration, drusen formation with lipoidal degeneration, and proliferation with metaplasia to fibroblastic activity as well as phagocytic transformation. In the subretinal pigment epithelial region, these can be drusen, lipid accumulation or exudation, new vessel formation, and fibroblastic proliferation. Bruch's membrane can demonstrate granular transformation, thickening and hyalinization, intercapillary thickening, fibrillary degeneration, basophilia, calcification, fracture, and hemorrhage. There can also be the production of abnormal basement membrane by the pigment epithelium accumulating in the sub-RPE and RPE zones (KENYON, 1974). The choriocapillaris can show hemorrhage, atrophy, and obliteration.

In a discussion of colloid material, SARKS noted that there can be coarse granules with fat, calcium, and mucopolysaccharides (SARKS, 1973). KLEIN felt that this might be related to the inner cuticular portion of Bruch's membrane (KLEIN, 1951). HOGAN emphasized the lipoidal degeneration of retinal pigment epithelium (HOGAN, 1967; HOGAN & ALVARADO, 1967; HOGAN & WOOD, 1973). GASS felt that there was an eosinophilic layer of portein exudate derived from the choriocapillaris (GASS, 1967). FARKAS et al. (1971) felt that this colloid was secondary to degeneration of the RPE by release of lysosomal enzymes. SARKS demonstrated this material to be PAS positive and to vary with different stains (SARKS, 1973), and again we would support that a number of previous suggestions as to the importance of this may be seen. There can be some discrepancy with fluorescein angiography since new vessels may not be seen despite their presence demonstrated histologically. Neovascularization of the periphery and peripapillary area, on the other hand, is not of pathogenetic significance (SARKS, 1973).

The case that we have demonstrated clealy shows that abnormal basement membrane material can be seen as one of the causes of increased thickening of Bruch's membrane; specifically that associated with the retinal pigment epithelium and the inner collagenous layer (KENYON, 1974).

The importance of Bruch's membrane rests with its crucial function as a membrane between the source of nutrition, the choriocapillaris, and the pigment epithelium modifier of this nutrition for the sensory retina. The great interchange between these metabolically active areas requires the modification of the pigment epithelium and the diffusion of these substances across Bruch's membrane. The crucial question as to whether these aging changes in Bruch's membrane are secondary to changes in the pigment epithelium or choriocapillaris cannot be answered at present and remains a subject for speculation.

REFERENCES

FARKAS, T.G., SYLVESTER, V. ARCHER, D. The ultrastructure of drusen. *Am. J. Ophthalmol.* 71: *1196* (1971).

FINE, B.S. Personal communication (1973).

GASS, J.D.N. Pathogenesis of disciform detachment of the neuroepithelium. I. General concepts and classification. *Am. J. Ophthalmol.* 63: *579* (1967).

HOGAN, M.J. Bruch's membrane and disease of the macula. *Trans. Ophthalmol. Soc. United Kingdom* 87: *113* (1967).

HOGAN, M.J. & ALVARADO, J. Studies on the human macula. IV. Aging changes in Bruch's membrane. *Arch. Ophthalmol.* 77: *410* (1967).

HOGAN, M.J., ALVARADO, J.A. & WEDDELL, J.E. Histology of the human eye. Philadelphia, W.B. Saunders Company (1971).

HOGAN, M.J. & WOOD, I. The retinal pigment epithelium. *Trans. Pac. Coast Oto-Ophthalmol. Soc.* 54: *11* (1973).

KENYON, K.R. Personal communication (1974).

KLEIN, B.A. Macular lesions of vascular origin. *Am. J. Ophthalmol.* 34: *449* (1951).

SARKS, S.H. New vessel formation beneath the retinal pigment epithelium in senile eyes. *Brit. J. Ophthalmol.* 57: *951* (1973).

WOLFRUM, M. Contributions to the anatomy and histology of the choroid in man and higher animals. *Graefe's Arch. Ophthalmol.* 65: *307* (1908).

Author's address:
Department of Ophthalmology
University of Southern California
Estelle Doheny Eye Foundation
Los Angeles, California
USA

DISCUSSION

Dr Henkind: I should like to ask Don Gass: on the basis of his studies, what does he think drusen are? There seems to be a lot of confusion to what drusen really are.

Dr Gass: Well, I think that the case Dr Ryan showed presents changes that are different from most cases of drusen. Most drusen, the discrete lesions that we see in the back of the eye, are composed of material lying beneath the basement membrane. The basement membrane is normal, or when I say normal, with the light microscope it appears to be normal. The case that Dr Ryan showed, clearly indicated that there was an excessive amount of basement membrane material. You noticed that it had a very fine nodular appearance that was very diffuse in the back of the eye. So, it suggests that there may be more than one type of drusen. I do not think anybody knows where drusen come from. There has been a debate on that going on for years and we have not solved it yet.

Dr Ryan: I would like to ask Don: in light of your case of drusen with the six breaks and sites of separate subretinal neovascularization, if you care to amplify on your comment regarding a study of treating drusen. Do you worry that in treating drusen in eyes with such good vision, there might be occult neovascularization, which might be stimulated to hemorrhage and a rapid downhill course for that macula?

Dr Gass: It is a worry if you decide to treat these patients. Not only if you are going to do a study of patients, with nothing but drusen, but it also points out that if you treat patients for pigment epithelial detachment or a neovascular membrane, if you place therapy on these drusen, you may occasionally get hemorrhages. It is of interest that that eye which had six breaks under a drusen in one area, had no other breaks of Bruch's membrane in the entire macular area, and the eye which had a detachment had no breaks in Bruch's membrane.

CORRELATION OF FLUORESCEIN
ANGIOGRAPHY AND HISTOPATHOLOGY

J. DONALD M. GASS, M.D.

(Miami, Florida)

This report concerns the correlation of biomicroscopic, fluorescein angiographic, and histopathologic findings in four patients who had diseases affecting the retinal pigment epithelium.

CASE 1

This 56-year-old man was followed at regular intervals because of loss of central vision in both eyes secondary to the presumed ocular histoplasmosis syndrome (POHS). Figure 1 demonstrates two of the multiple atrophic, punched-out appearing choroidal lesions present in both eyes. These lesions showed evidence of fluorescence during the early, as well as the late stages of angiography. Figure 2 reveals the histopathologic findings of one of the atrophic lesions depicted in Figure 1. There was focal loss of the choroidal tissue including Bruch's membrane, retinal pigment epithelium, and the

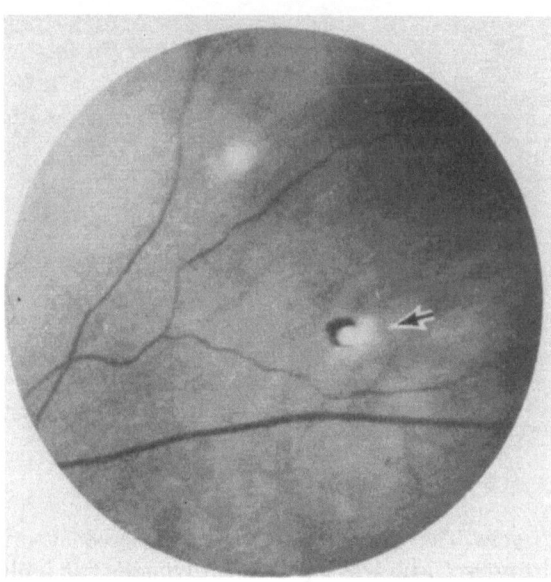

Fig. 1. *(Case 1)* See Fig. 2 for histopathology of lesion indicated by arrow.

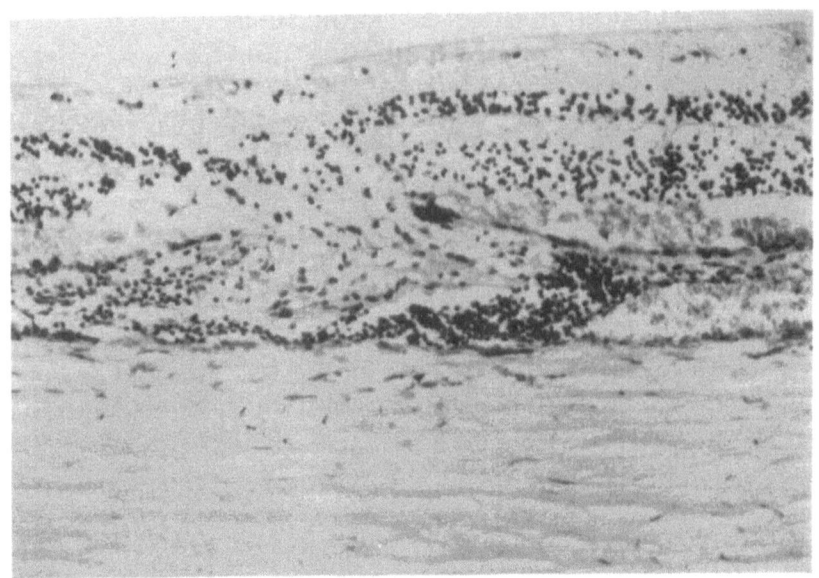

Fig. 2 *(Case 1)* Histopathology of lesion shown in Fig. 1.

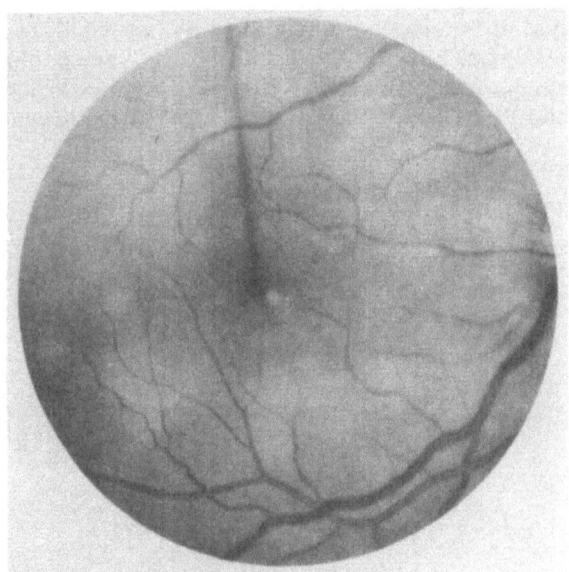

Fig. 3. *(Case 2)* A. Right macula.

outer retinal layers. The choroidal defect was replaced by retinal tissue, presumably atrocytes. There was a prominent lymphocytic infiltration surrounding the base of the lesion. There was proliferation of the pigment epithelium at the margin of the lesion. Similar findings were present in each

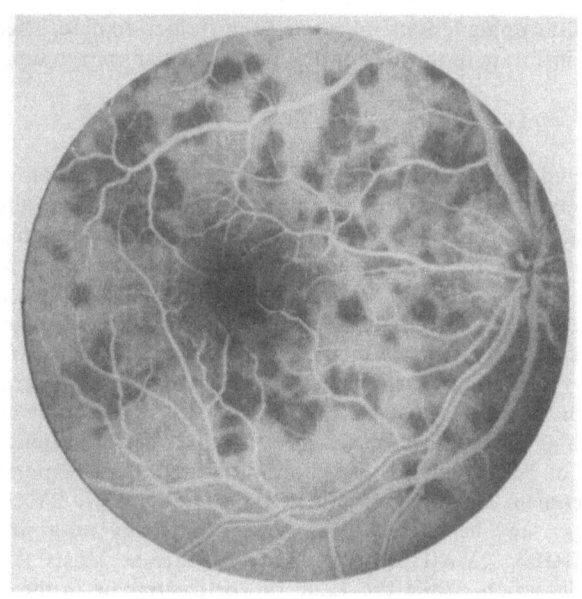

Fig. 3. (*Case 2*) B. Early angiogram

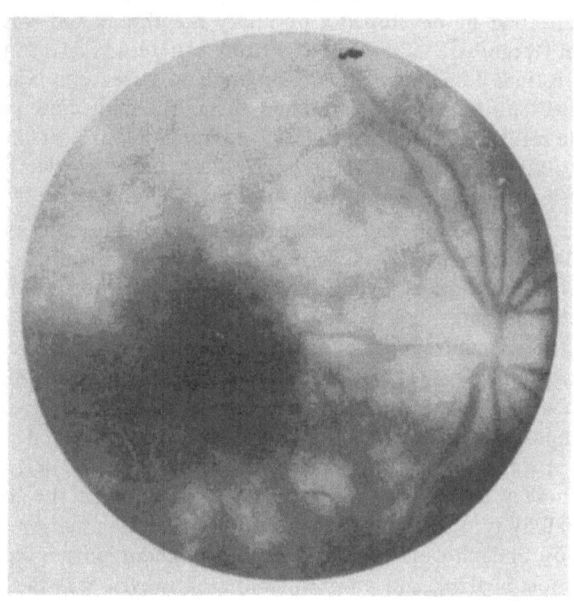

Fig. 3. (*Case 2*) C. Late angiogram

of three focal atrophic lesions that have been studied to date. There was no lymphocytic infiltrate in the area of disciform macular scars in both eyes.

Comment

The unexpected findings in this patient were: 1) the presence of retinal glial cells that are ophthalmoscopically transparent, filling the focal defect in the choroid, and, 2) the prominent lymphocytic infiltrate surrounding the base of the peripheral lesions, that clinically appeared to be inactive atrophic scars. These findings may be important in explaining: 1) the changes in pigmentation and size that have been observed to occur in some of these peripheral lesions over a long period of time (GASS & WILKINSON, 1972), as well as, 2) the initial development of serous exudation, choroidal neo-vascularization and subretinal bleeding at the site of the focal scars when they are located in the macular area. The findings are in keeping with the observations of focal lymphocytic choroiditis underlying hemorrhagic dis-ciform detachment of patients with POHS (GASS, 1967, RYAN, 1975). These findings may be related to an antigen antibody reaction first sug-gested by WOODS & WAHLEN (1959) taking place at the site of previous histoplasma infection. While the value of corticosteroids in these patients has been debated, these findings suggest that there is some rationale to their use in the early treatment of macular detachment in this disease.

CASE 2

Posterior Sympathetic Ophthalmia. This 34-year-old man sustained a pene-trating corneoscleral laceration in his left eye in September, 1975. Fol-lowing surgical repair he developed a pupillary membrane and was referred to the BPEI in December, 1975, for vitrectomy. There was ultrasonographic evidence of a retinal detachment in the left eye. A vitrectomy via the pars plana was done. The retina was reattached during the immediate postopera-tive course. He returned in February, 1975, complaining of spots in his right eye. His acuity was 20/20. The left eye was blind and atrophic. There was minimal injection of the conjunctiva in both eyes. There were a few inflam-matory cells in the vitreous and anterior chamber of the right eye. There was a heavy flare in the anterior chamber of the left eye. Figure 3, A, B, and C, demonstrates the clinical and fluorescein angiographic findings in the right eye. Multiple, small, slightly elevated, creamy-white, mottled lesions at the level of the pigment epithelium and choroid were scattered in the posterior pole of the eye. There was no subretinal fluid. The lesions were discretely nonfluorescent during the initial phases of angiography, and they gradually stained in a diffuse manner during the later phases. The clinical diagnosis of posterior sympathetic uveitis was made. The left eye was enucleated. There was minimal lymphocytic infiltration in the iris. There was diffuse, patchy lymphocytic and granulomatous inflammation involving the ciliary body and choroid. Giant cells and pigment phagocytosis were present. The most striking and unusual finding, however, was the presence of multiple focal areas of choriocapillaris obliteration by inflammatory cells and an overlying mound of epithelioid cells lying between the intact Bruch's membrane and the focally elevated and thinned pigment epithelium (Dalen-Fuchs nodules) (Fig. 4). Special stains for fungi and acid fast bacilli were negative. The patient received systemic corticosteroid therapy and within several weeks the lesions had resolved leaving only faint alterations in the pigment epithelium posteriorly.

Comment

This patient demonstrated clinical evidence in the right eye and histopathologic evidence in the left eye of sympathetic ophthalmia that was confined largely to the posterior uveal tract. The ophthalmoscopic and angiographic findings in the right eye suggested that the fundus lesions were caused by partial obstruction of the choriocapillaris and focal invasion of the choroid and subpigment epithelial space by epithelioid cells similar to those seen histologically in the left eye. The clinical and angiographic pictures were somewhat similar to that seen in acute posterior multifocal placoid pigment epitheliopathy (GASS, 1968). Unlike this disease, however, they were slightly raised, their surface showed a slightly mottled appearance, and they rapidly resolved without leaving significant pigmentary changes in the pigment epithelium.

CASE 3

This 71-year-old man with bilateral macular drusen recovered normal vision after a sercus detachment of the macula in his left eye. Histopathologic

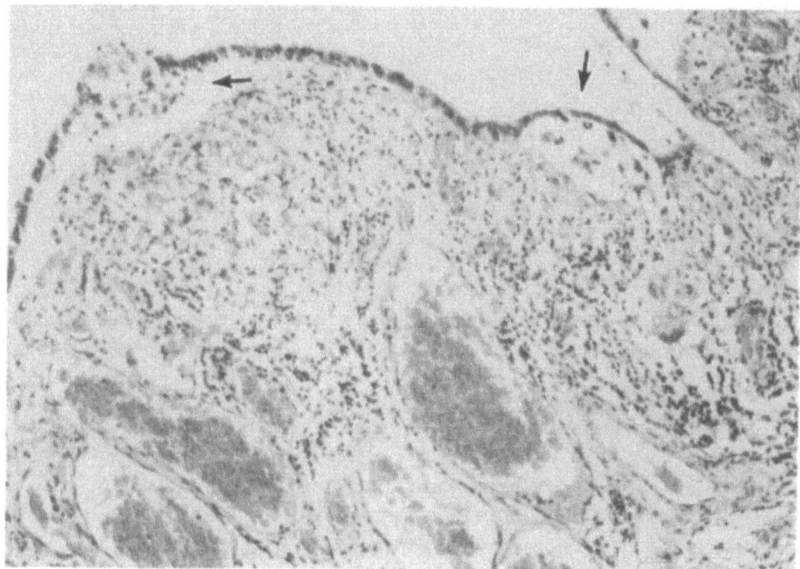

Fig. 4. (*Case 2*) Histopathologic findings in the posterior choroid of the left eye. Note mound of epithelioid cells (arrows) between the thinned pigment epithelium and Bruch's membrane overlying an area of closure of the choriocapillaris.

examination revealed hyperplasia of the pigment epithelium, but no evidence of a break in Bruch's membrane at the site of fluorescein leakage. At the site of a single drusen in the opposite macula that was otherwise normal, there were six small breaks in Bruch's membrane and a choroidal neovascular tuft extending through each break into the drusen.

CASE 4

The previously reported biomicroscopic, angiographic, and histopathologic findings in a woman with a peculiar adult form of vitelliform foveal dystrophy were presented (GASS, 1974).

REFERENCES

GASS, J.D.M. Pathogenesis of disciform detachment of the neuroepithelium. V. Disciform macular degeneration secondary to focal choroiditis. *Am. J. Ophthalmol.* 63: *661-687* (1967).

GASS, J.D.M. Acute posteror multifocal placoid pigment epitheliopathy. *Arch. Ophthalmol.* 80: *177-185* (1968).

GASS, J.D.M. A clinicopathologic study of a peculiar foveomacular dystrophy. *Tr. Am. Ophthalmol. Soc.* 72: *139-156* (1974).

GASS, J.D.M. & WILKINSON, C.P. Follow-up study of presumed ocular histoplasmosis. *Tr. Am. Acad. Ophthalmol. & Otolaryngol.* 76: *672-694* (1972).

RYAN, S.J. Histopathological correlates of presumed ocular histoplasmosis, In: Ocular Histoplasmosis, Proceeding of the Ocular Histoplasmosis Symposium, Ed. T.F. Schlaegel, Jr., M.D., Boston, Little, Brown and Company, 15: *125-137* (1975).

WOODS, A.C. & WAHLEN, H.E. The probable role of benign histoplasmosis in the etiology of granulomatous uveitis. *Tr. Am. Ophthalmol. Soc.* 57: *318* (1959).

Author's address:
Department of Ophthalmology
University of Miami School of Medicine
1638 N.W. 10th Avenue
Miami, Florida 33152
USA

DISCUSSION

Dr Henkınd: I should like to ask Don Gass: on the basis of his studies, what does he think drusen are? There seems to be a lot of confusion to what drusen really are.

Dr Gass: Well, I think that the case Dr Ryan showed presents changes that are different from most cases of drusen. Most drusen, the discrete lesions that we see in the back of the eye, are composed of material lying beneath the basement membrane. The basement membrane is normal, or when I say normal, with the light microscope it appears to be normal. The case that Dr Ryan showed, clearly indicated that there was an excessive amount of basement membrane material. You noticed that it had a very fine nodular appearance that was very diffuse in the back of the eye. So, it suggests that there may be more than one type of drusen. I do not think anybody knows where drusen come from. There has been a debate on that going on for years and we have not solved it yet.

Dr Ryan: I would like to ask Don: in light of your case of drusen with the six breaks and sites of separate subretinal neovascularization, if you care to amplify on your comment regarding a study of treating drusen. Do you worry that in treating drusen in eyes with such good vision, there might be occult neovascularization, which might be stimulated to hemorrhage and a rapid downhill course for that macula?

Dr Gass: It is a worry if you decide to treat these patients. Not only if you are going to do a study of patients, with nothing but drusen, but it also points out that if you treat patients for pigment epithelial detachment or a neovascular membrane, if you place therapy on these drusen, you may occasionally get hemorrhages. It is of interest that that eye which had six breaks under a drusen in one area, had no other breaks of Bruch's membrane in the entire macular area, and the eye which had a detachment had no breaks in Bruch's membrane.

DISEASES AFFECTING THE PIGMENT EPITHELIUM

A.C. BIRD & A.M. HAMILTON

(London, England)

Diseases causing swelling and subsequent atrophy of the pigment epithelium and choriocapillaris taken many forms, and attempts have been made to identify distinct clinical entities within this group of diseases on the basis of their morphological and behavioural characteristics. These include Harada's disease (SHIMIZU, 1973), placoid pigment epitheliopathy (GASS, 1968), geographical (or serpiginous) choroidopathy (HAMILTON & BIRD, 1974) and acute retinal pigment epitheliitis (KRILL & DEUTMAN, 1972).

HARADA'S DISEASE

This presents with bilateral retinal detachments at the posterior pole under which focal pigment epithelial disease can be identified. Fluorescein angiography shows obstruction of the background choroidal fluorescence during the initial transit of dye, subsequent accumulation of dye within the areas of focal pigment epithelial disease and finally leakage of dye into the sub-retinal space. The detachment often enlarges, causing total or subtotal retinal detachment. Spontaneous resolution of the disease occurs after weeks or months, leaving multifocal pigment epithelial changes manifested by loss of pigment in the pigment epithelium and hyperpigmentation. The ocular disease resolves rapidly when treated with steroids but will recur if the steroids are withdrawn too early. This disease is associated with uveitis of variable severity which may become severe (Vogt-Koyanagi syndrome).

Aural symptoms, depigmentation of the iris, skin, eye lashes, eyebrows, or other hair, occurs in a minority of cases. No cause is known of this disease.

ACUTE POSTERIOR MULTIFOCAL PLACOID PIGMENT EPITHELIOPATHY (APMPPE)

This is characterised by acute visual loss and in the fundus there are multi-focal yellow-white placoid lesions at the level of the pigment epithelium. Rapid resolution of these lesions occurs with permanent alteration of the pigment epithelium and minimal damage to the adjacent choroid or retina. Significant visual improvement occurs during recovery which may be complete.

Uveitis is not a prominent feature of this disease and there is no associated detachment of the retina.

367

The cause of APMPPE has yet to be established but virus infections (GASS, 1968; RYAN & MAUMENEE, 1972; ANNESLEY, TOMER & SHIELDS, 1973; FITZPATRICK & ROBERTSON, 1973) and tuberculosis and erythema nodosum (VAN BUSKIRK, LESSELL & FRIEDMAN, 1971) have been reported as associated diseases. Recently adenovirus type 5 infection has been identified in a patient with APMPPE (AZAR, GOHD, WALTMAN & GITTER, 1975).

'PLACOID PIGMENT EPITHELIAL DISEASE' AND RETINAL DETACHMENT

Two patients were described with acute multifocal pigment epithelial disease associated with posterior retinal detachment in the early phase of the disease (BIRD & HAMILTON, 1972). These patients had pigment epithelial disease and the detachment stimulating Harada's disease, but the detachment resolved spontaneously within a few days with recovery of vision. The pigment epithelial lesions and the rapid recovery were similar to APMPPE although the scarring was often less marked than might have been expected. During the recovery phase slow filling of the choriocapillaris was recorded which was identical to that reported by VAN BUSKIRK et al. (1971). This observation suggested that the choriocapillaris was the initial site of the disease and that the pigment epithelial lesion represented local infarction.

It was commented by us that both patients had received penicillin during the period immediately preceding disease. We have subsequently recorded fourteen further cases with similar disease and of these six had received a penicillin derivative immediately prior to the onset of symptoms (four had received ampicillin). One patient had previously suffered a skin rash which was attributed to penicillin sensitivity. It is conceivable that the disease suffered by these patients represents an immune complex disease affecting the choriocapillaris in response to an allergen which in some patients was penicillin. In the other patients the allergen has not been identified as yet, and we are proposing during the next weeks to investigate these patients further.

GEORGRAPHICAL (OR SERPIGINOUS) CHOROIDOPATHY

This disease is characterised by recurrent subacute multifocal pigment epithelial disease which usually affects both eyes (HAMILTON & BIRD, 1974). During the early phase the pigment epithelial lesion appears grey or yellow, and swollen, without overlying retinal detachment. The lesion evolves over a period of months during which time it becomes well defined, grey and flat, followed by atrophy of the pigment epithelium and underlying choriocapillaris. During the evolution of the lesion there is no change in its shape or size. The disease appears to progress over several years, during which time further pigment epithelial lesions occur. This disease is accompanied by relatively little vitreous or anterior chamber signs of inflammation. Juxtapapillary lesions occur early in the disease and new lesions are frequently but not invariably contiguous with the pre-existing lesion. The cause of this disease is unknown.

ACUTE RETINAL PIGMENT EPITHELIITIS

This disease has an acute onset and visual symptoms may be mild. The typical lesion is near the macula and consists of a greyish swollen area of pigment epithelium. Resolution occurs over a few weeks, during which time the pigment epithelium becomes grey and is surrounded by a pale yellow halo-like zone. Fluorescein angiography in the acute stage may show some blocking of the background choroidal fluorescence and after resolution there is usually hyperfluorescence corresponding with the surrounding halo, but it is often remarkably subtle (KRILL & DEUTMAN, 1972). The involvement is usually bilateral although the second eye may be affected weeks after the first. The cause of this disease is unknown.

COMMENTS

It is important to characterise these conditions as carefully as possible so that distinct disease entities can be recognised. Such a classification is valuable in order to identify the prognosis of each disease. Equally a search for the cause of these diseases is unlikely to be successful without such a subdivision; surveys of a group of patients with more than one disease are unlikely to reveal significant aetiological factors.

It is quite likely that the clinical conditions now classified as APMPPE, and geographic choroidopathy may include more than one disease entity. It is equally possible that a single aetiologic agent may produce a variable clinical picture. This is illustrated by onchocerciasis in which a single disease may produce disease varying from localised mild irregular loss of pigment in the pigment epithelium to widespread atrophy of retina, pigment epithelium and choroid (BIRD, ANDERSON & FUGLSANG, 1976). Such a consideration, whilst important, should not deter efforts to subdivide fundus diseases into distinct clinical entities since it is possible to amalgamate certain groups into a single disease category when aetiologic factors have been identified.

REFERENCES

ANNESLEY, W.H., TOMER, T.D. & SHIELDS, J.A. *Amer. J. Ophthalmol.* 76: *511* (1973).
AZAR, P., GOHD, R.S., WALTMAN, D. & GITTER, K.A. *Amer. J. Ophthalmol.* 80: *1003* (1975).
BIRD, A.C., ANDERSON, J. & FUGLSANG, H. *Brit. J. Ophthalmol.* 60: 2 (1976).
BIRD A.C. & HAMILTON, A.M. *Brit. J. Ophthalmol.* 56: *881* (1972).
FITZPATRICK, P.J. & ROBERTSON, D.M. *Arch. Ophthalmol.* 89: *373* (1973).
GASS, J.D.M. *Arch. Ophthalmol.* 80: *177* (1968).
HAMILTON, A.M. & BIRD, A.C. *Brit. J. Ophthalmol.* 58: *784* (1974).
KRILL, A.E. & DEUTMAN, A.F. *Amer. J. Ophthalmol.* 74: *193* (1972).
RYAN, S.J. & MAUMENEE, A.E. *Amer. J. Ophthalmol.* 74: *1066* (1972).
SHIMIZU, K. *Trans. Amer. Acad. Ophthalmol. & Otolaryng.* 77: *281* (1973).
VAN BUSKIRK, E.M., LESSELL, S. & FRIEDMAN, E. *Arch. Op halmol.* 85: *369* (1971).

Authors' address:
Moorfields Eye Hospital
City Road
London EC1V 2PD

ACUTE MULTIFOCAL POSTERIOR PLACOID PIGMENT EPITHELIOPATHY AND ARGON LASER PHOTOCOAGULATION. AN ANGIOGRAPHIC COMPARISON

J.A. BERNARD, J. DUREUIL, G. COSCAS, A. GAUDRIC & J. HAUT

(Paris, France)

The angiographic syndrom of the Acute Multifocal Posterior Placoid Pigment Epitheliopathy (AMPPPE) depends on the age of the lesions.

1. At the acute stage, the lesions are marked by a blocked fluorescence, which lasts about one hundred seconds. This blockage has also been interpreted as a filling defect, as a real choroidal silence (BONNIN); i.e. the absence of perfusion of the choriocapillaris. At the end of the second minute, the plaques disappear, and the choroidal pattern seems rather uniform. This aspect may be the result of the physiological diffusion out of the choroidal vessels, or, for HAYREH the result of a backward veinous circulation in the choriocapillaris. On the very late angiograms, the plaques

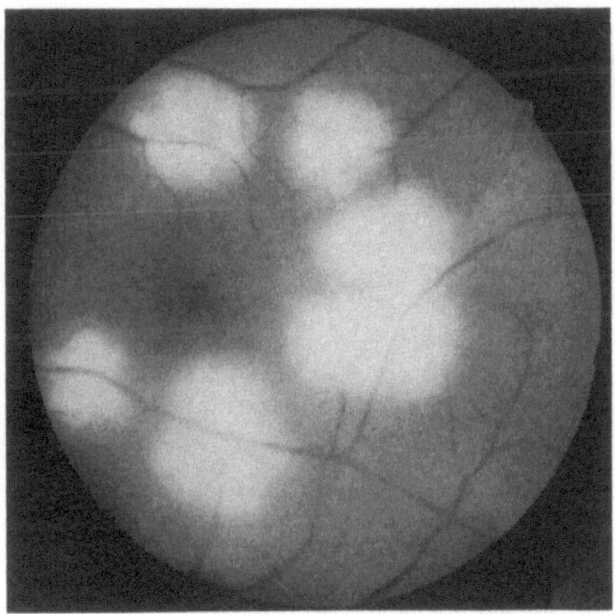

Fig. 1. Red free picture of Laser coagulation, experimentally made on the retina before enucleation.

371

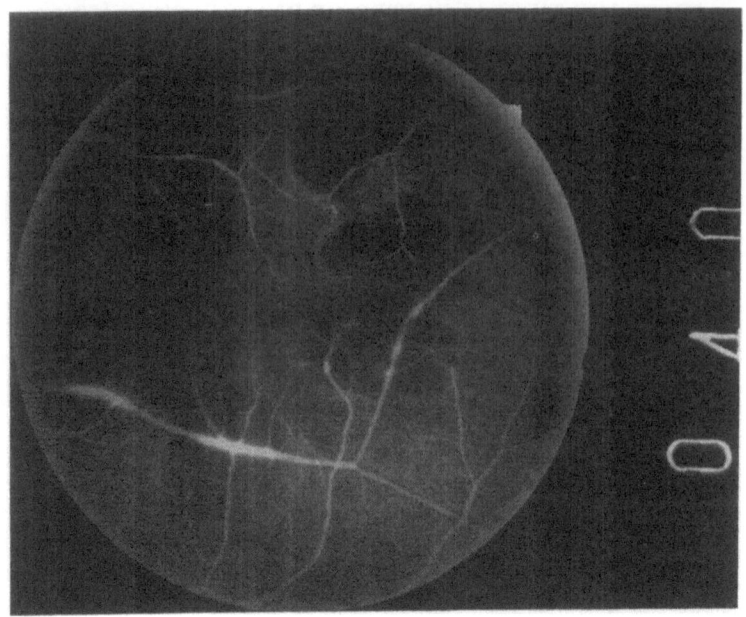

Fig. 2. 40 seconds after the fluorescein injection, there is a 'blockage' of fluorescence on the photocoagulated areas.

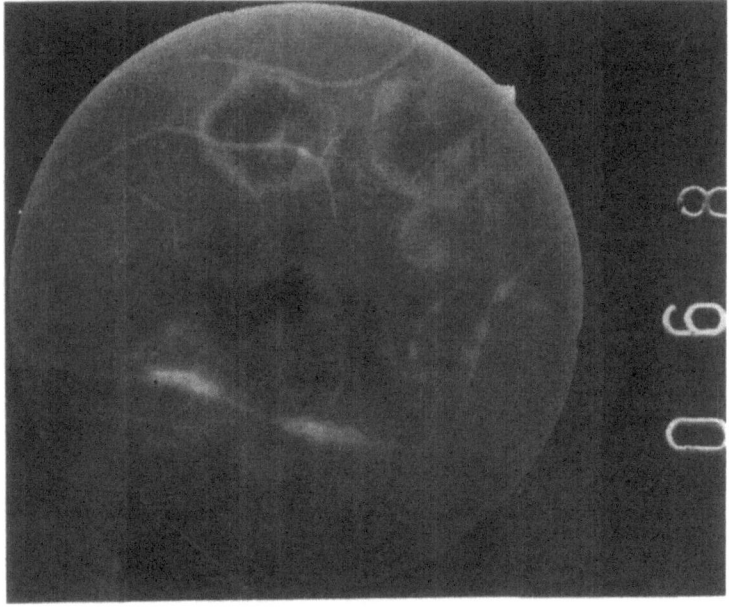

Fig. 3. These areas begin to stain after 70 seconds.

372

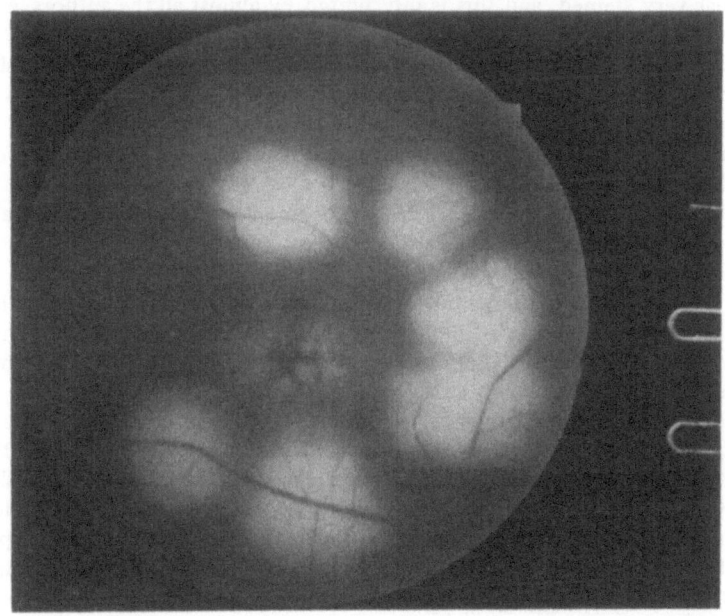

Fig. 4. Heavy staining after 30 minutes. Note the cystoid edema due to the malignant melanoma of the choroid (Fig. 5).

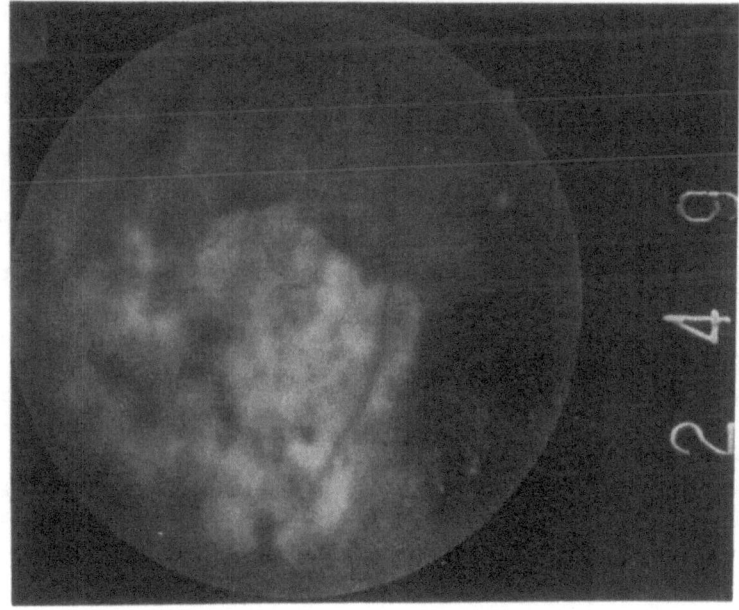

Fig. 5. The late angiogram of the malignant melanoma.

appear very stained, and this is interpreted by almost all the authors, as the consequence of the tissular lesion.

2. At the sequellae stage, the AMPPPE scars are only marked by a slight central pigment clumping with a typical polycyclical hyperfluorescent boarder. This is interpreted as the diffusion of the dye out of the choriocapillaris, under the pigmentary epithelium, which is destroyed on a larger area.

The explanation of the AMPPPE syndrome is not clearly demonstrated, as no one has any histological data.

Some authors (J. FRANÇOIS, J.J. DE LAEY, M. BONNET) think that this disorder is the consequence of a 'choriocapillaritis'. As a matter of fact, this theory explains a great part of the clinical, angiographic and sometimes biological symptoms of this disease, and also is in good correlation with HAYREH's experiments on monkeys.

But other experimental occlusions of the choriocapillaris, made by STERN & ERNEST (1974), with latex microspheres, and the study of some cases of Disseminated Intravascular Coagulopathy (D.I.C.), show a different pattern of the angiogram, where the lesions appear fluorescent without any delay as it is in the AMPPPE. This aspect is typical of the Elschnig spot, which was histologically described in 1904. Neither does AMALRIC's triangular syndrom show any lesions comparable to the AMPPPE.

Consequently to these considerations, one must keep the first hypothesis, made by D. GASS, in 1968, when he described the first cases, emphasizing the important role of the pigmentary epithelium.

As everyone knows, the Argon Laser photocoagulation brings a maximal damage to the pigmentary epithelium. This is well demonstrated on the experimental histological datas.

As a matter of fact, the photocoagulation lesions and the AMPPPE ones have, after 2 or 3 weeks of evolution, the same aspect of a central pigmentation and a hyperfluorescent borderline.

On a 53 year old woman, who had a malignant melanoma of the left eye (Fig. 5), we performed before enucleation 6 'plaques' of one to one and a half disc-size, around the macula (Fig. 1), which was not detached but only involved by a cystoid edema.

The angiogram of these coagulations appears very comparable with the AMPPPE one:
— blocked fluorescence (or non-filling effect?), during about 100 seconds (Fig. 2).
— coloration of the plaques beginning on the boarder of the lesions (Fig. 3).
— heavy tissular staining on the late angiograms (Fig. 4).
— besides these points, the involvement of the wall of a vein crossing a plaque is also very comparable to the one we demonstrated in a clinical case (Fig. 2).

CONCLUSIONS

AMPPPE lesions and photocoagulation lesions are angiographically very alike. As the histological datas demonstrate the proeminent involvement of the pigmentary epithelium in the Laser coagulations, we have to think that epitheliopathy remains a very good definition of this very peculiar disorder of the ocular fundus.

Authors' address:
J.A. Bernard
1, rue Scheffer
75016 Paris
France

VARIOUS PRESENTATIONS OF PIGMENT EPITHELIOPATHIES AND CHORIOCAPILLAROPATHIES

ABDEL–LATIF SIAM, F.R.C.S. Ed.

(Cairo, Egypt)

Since the first report made by GASS (1969) of acute posterior multifocal placoid pigment epitheliopathy (APMPPE) many other reports appeared in the literature with similar and additional features. AMALRIC & BONNIN (1969), MAUMENEE (1970), DEUTMAN (1972) and ANNESLEY (1973), described almost identical cases. VAN BUSKIRK (1971) and DEUTMAN (1972) found erythema nodosum in two of the cases. KIRKHAM (1972) reported on similar cases associated with retinal vasculitis and papillitis. BIRD & HAMILTON (1974) presented cases with bilateral serous detachment of the retina. SAVINE et al. (1974) stressed the protean manifestations of such a disease which was associated in their cases with uveitis, papillitis episcleritis, macular mottling and serous detachment of the retina. DEUTMAN (1974) reported a case associated with an increased white blood count in the spinal fluid. SIAM (1975) found macular oedema & macular star in two typical cases. He wondered about the fluorographic evidence of capillary 'ischaemia' and the extensive retinal pigment epithelial affection in the whole inschaemic territory.

All the above reports appeared to be of the same category as those initially described by GASS (1968), since they were all characterised by isolated, flat, rapidly resolving lesions with a characteristic fluorographic pattern.

KRILL & DEUTMAN (1972) and DEUTMAN (1974) reported on cases under the name of acute retinal pigment epitheliitis. They thought they were dealing with a different disease process of unknown aetiology on the basis of a different clinical picture, a different clinical course and a specific fluorographic pattern. DEUTMAN (1974) pointed out the similarity of such cases to chronic central serous choroidapathy but indicated the fluorographic difference from the recent cases. He stated that in acute pigment epitheliitis low acuity occurs without fluorescein leakage, whereas in recent central serous choriodopathy leakage in nearly always present. They thought of a possible subclinical virus inflammation, involving only the macular pigment epithelium. FREIDMAN (1975) described similar cases with two additional features, bilaterality and recurrence followed by complete resolution.

SIAM (1975) described peculiar cases with a peculiar fluorographic pattern & associated with severe macular involvement in the form of considerable macular oedema. The lesions were followed by scarring of the retina

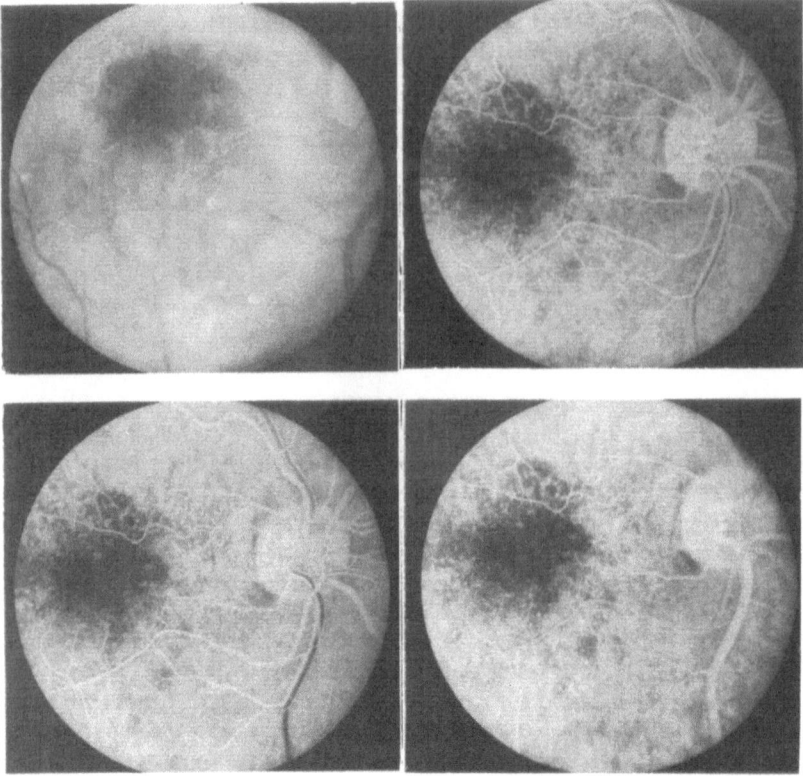

Fig. 1. *Case 1*: a) Fluorographic appearance when first seen with innumerable dot-leakage.

and choroid in the focus affected. He could not fit his cases in the groups of diseases so far reported.

We report here on yet other cases of unknown nature presenting with an acute onset of generalised retinal oedema hiding the choroidal pattern, mainly at the posterior pole including papillary and macular oedema and associated with severe and widespread choriocapillary and pigment epithelial reaction and leading to severe visual failure. They had a fairly rapid course and ended in severe and extensive choriocapillary retinal pigment epithelial damage (Fig. 1a, b and c). The cases did not appear to be favourably altered by intensive steroid therapy.

We wonder in this context about the widespread, bizzare and dissimilar reaction of the retinal pigment epithelium and choriocapillaris and the great difference in the visual affection in cases of Vogt-Koyanagi-Harada syndrome.

Another group of reports concerns an apparently different class of diseases of a possible inflammatory or degenerative nature & running a much more sluggish course. Such reports include: serpiginous choroiditis described by LANTIKANINEN & ERKKILÄ (1974), geographical choroidopathy by

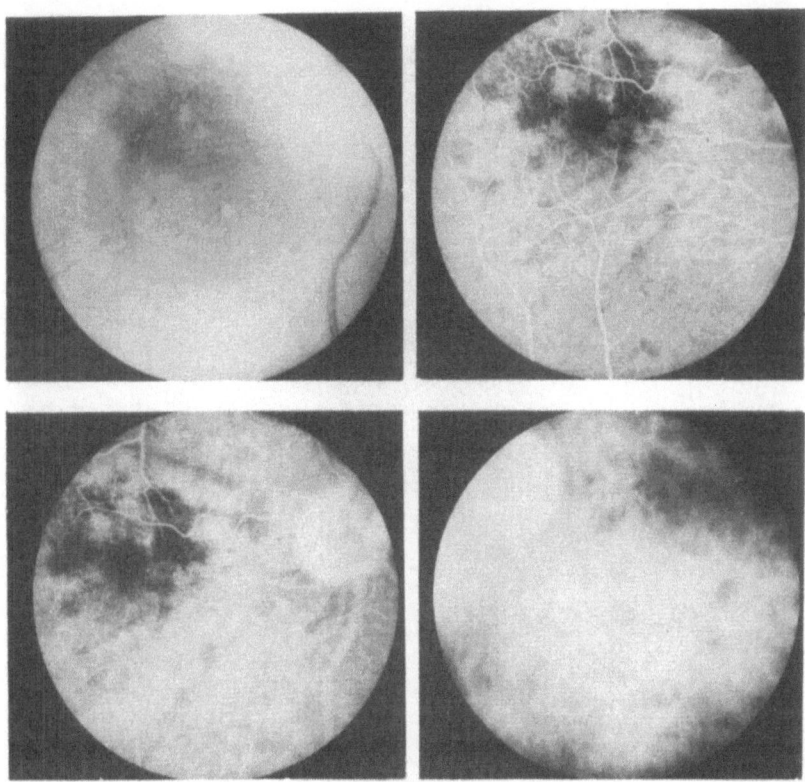

b) Appearance three weeks later with generalised 'choriocapillaritis' & disc oedema.

HAMILTON & BIRD (1974) and geographical helicoid peripapillary choroidopathy by SCHATZ et al. (1974). Although the example we present here
(Fig. 2) appears to belong to this group, it ran a prolonged course and had a
quite different effect on vision on the two sides. Vision was reduced to
counting fingers in the eye first affected, while the second eye (Fig. 2b) sim-
ilarly diseased two years later, retained 6/6 vision. Its course did not seem to be
affected with steroids or immunosuppressive drugs. This eye appears to have
retained a surviving island of the choriocapillaris in the macular area. The
extensive choriocapillary & retinal pigment atrophy following the disease is
evident in Fig. 2.

DISCUSSION

Since the classic description of GASS (1968) of the so-called acute posterior
multifocal placoid pigment eptheliopathy many disease forms have been
described and various clinical pictures reported. From the protean nature of
reports made under the same disease entity and the various names given to
what appeared to be the same disease and the controversy about the

379

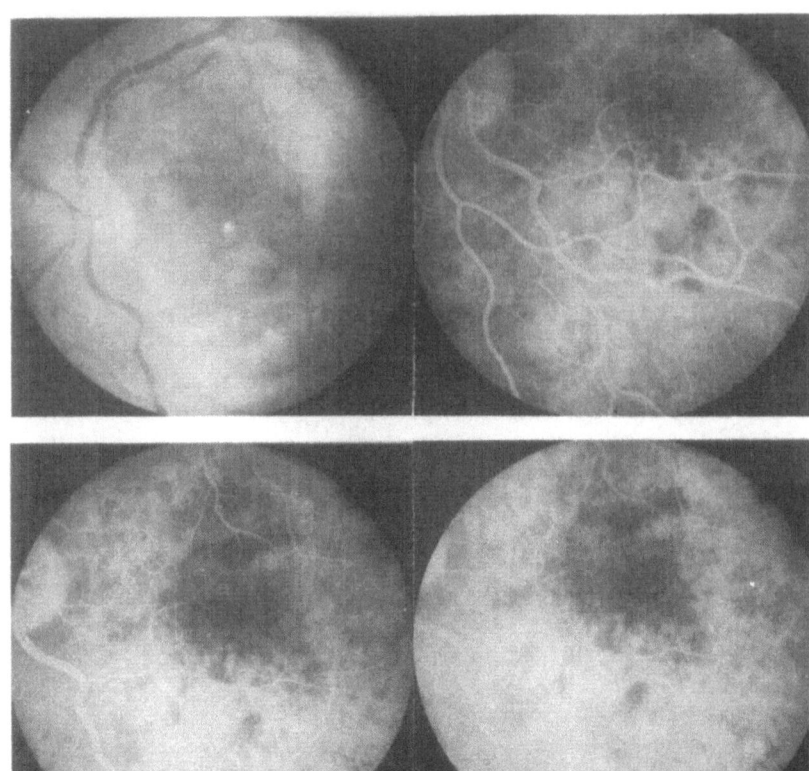

c) Left eye of same case.

anatomical site of primary affection, it soon became obvious that we are probably dealing with a new group of diseases not yet identified. It is also possible that we are dealing with various presentations of the same disease affecting primarily one or more layers. The close anatomic and physiologic intimacy of the choriocapillaris, Bruch's membrane and the retinal pigment epithelium has been pointed out by BABEL (1971) so that it is difficult to envisage affection of one layer without involvement of the other. There is difference of opinion, however, about the primary site of disease. GASS (1968) believed that the disease he described was a primary retinal pigment affection, but did not exclude however, the possibility of a rapidly resolving inflammatory process in the choriocapillaris involving the pigment epithelium. DEUTMAN (1972) thought that placoid epitheliopathy may be caused by an allergie inflammatory reaction of the choriocapillaris and that the disease was probably an acute multifocal choriocapillaritis. The responce to steroids, however, has been poor, KIRKHAM & FFYTCHE (1972), DEMAILLY (1975). SIAM (1975) thought that the acute inflammation takes place primarily in the choriocapillaris with secondary affection of the

380

pigment epithelium. Various intensities of the same disease can involve more or less of one or more layers, leading to various clinical pictures. In the severe cases he presented (1975) the deeper layers of the choroid were evidently affected leading to deep focal chorio-retinal sears. He brought fluorographic evidence of delayed filling of the choriocapillaries probably due to spasm leading to inschaemia and contributing to the inflammatory degenerative process. Choriocapillary 'ischaemia' appeared to be an important factor in the causation and location of the placoid foci, SIAM (1975). BIRD & HAMILTON (1972) thought that in the acute stage of the disease, reduced blood flow in the choroidal capillaries causes focal swelling of the retinal pigment epithelium due to focal ischaemia. The chorio-retinal barrier is vulnerable to many injurious factors, ischaemic, inflammatory or toxic. Thus affected, it allows toxins and fluids to pass into the neuroepithelium leading to oedema or detachment. Depending on the capillary bed affected, and the severity of the reaction, various clinical pictures can result. If the peripapillary choriocapillaris is affected 'papillitis' may become part of the clinical picture, whereas if the macular choriocapillary region is in-

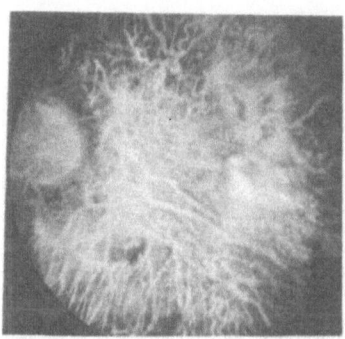

Left eye of Fig. 2

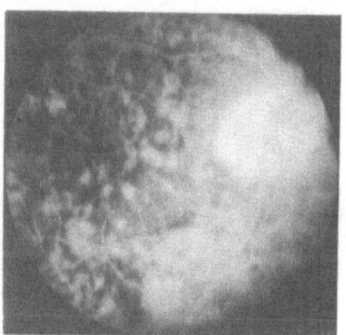

Fig. 1   Case 2 (4 weeks later)

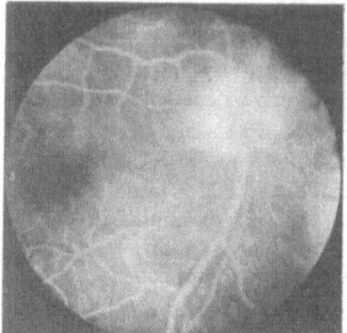

Fig. 1   Case 2 (at onset)

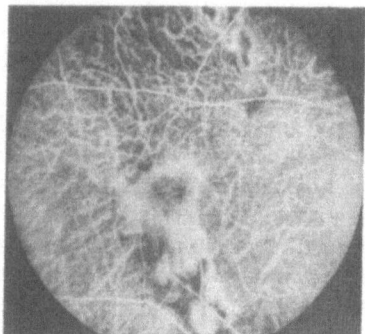

Right eye of Fig. 2

Fig. 2.   A case of bilateral subacute geographic choriodopathy followed by generalised choriocapillary & pigment epithelial atrophy, still retaining good visual acuity on the right side.

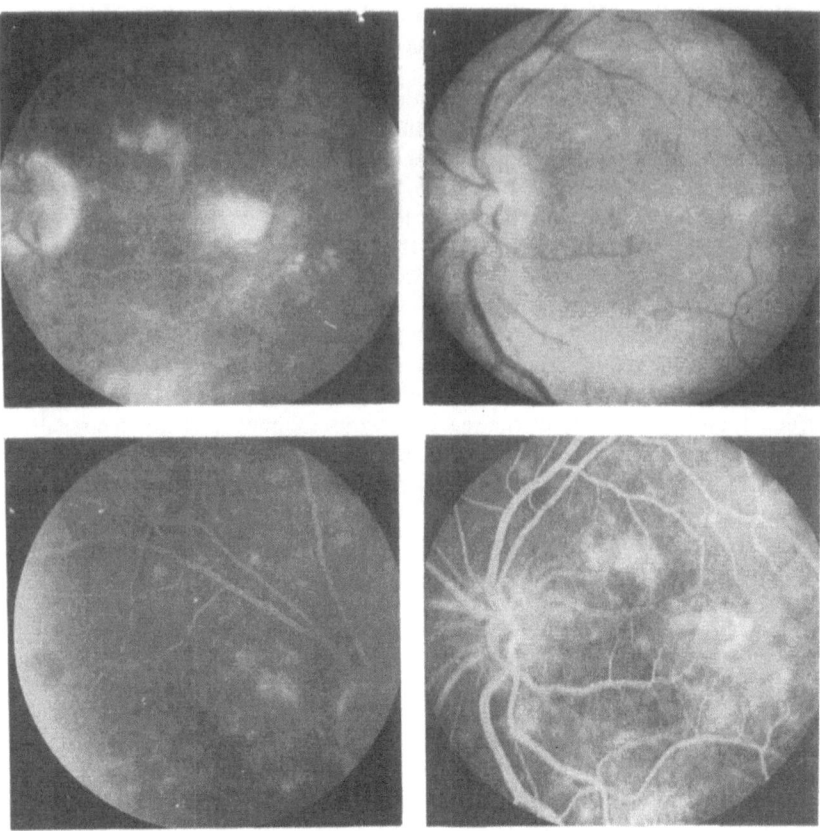

Fig. 3. Left eye of a bilateral widespread focal choriocapillaritis with left central visual failure & failing to improve 6 months later.

volved macular oedema or even central serous detachment can occur. The same disease can cause a vasculitis. A generalised choriocapillary and retinal pigment epithelial reaction can occur with extensive oedema and severe retinal pigment alterations, associated with more or less visual deterioration, as exemplified by two obscure case we present here as well as by cases of Vogt-Koyanagi-Harada's syndrome. An abiotrophic retinal pigment epithelium can react markedly to nocuous factors by extensive inflammatory and degenerative phenomena. Conversely an infectuous mechanism might be a stimulus to subsequent abiotrophic change, SCHATZ et al. (1974). A heriditary basis for choroidopathy has been suggested by KRILL & ARCHER (1971).

CASE PRESENTATIONS

We present here the following eight examples to illustrate the protean & varied manifestions of either or several diseases, not yet well recognised.

Two cases of the so-called acute posterior multifocal placoid pigment epitheliopathy of GASS (1968) one with bilateral macular oedema which resolved completely in a few weeks' time, and one with a macular exudate in the form of a macular star which again resolved with subsidence of the disease which remained unilateral.

One case of widespread bilateral focal choriocapillary affection with macular involvement of a peculiar from associated on one side with severe visual loss (Fig. 3).

One case of deep 'choriocapillary' infiltration with recurrent macular oedema together with retinal vasculitis. Good visual acuity was, however, preserved after several attacks of choriocapillaritis.

One case presenting with bilateral severe focal 'choriocapillaritis' of unknown nature leading to macular scarring & severe visual deterioration.

Two obscure cases of acute diffuse choriocapillary & pigment epithelial reaction with generalised retinal oedema & followed by severe generalised pigment epithelial degeneration & migration and associated with focal choriocapillary atrophy, Fig. 1 (Case 1 & Case 2).

One patient with subacute progressive apparently serpiginous choriocapillaritis and pigment epitheliitis of a peculiar inflammatory and/or degenerative type, followed by generalised retinal pigment and choriocapillary atrophy on one side, associated with loss of central vision. The other eye followed, two years later, but ran a different course with preservation of central vision, although the macular area was involved and inspite of the generalised pigment epithelial and choriocapillary atrophy, except a perhaps for a surviving island of choriocapillaris in the macular area. (Fig. 2).

None of the above cases appeared to respond favourably to steroid therapy.

REFERENCES

AMALRIC, B. & BONNIN, P. Angiographie fluorescéinique. *Bull. Ophthal. Fr.* Numéro spécial (1969).

ANNESLEY, W.H., TOMER, T.L. & SHIELDS, J.A. *Amer. J. Ophthal.* 76: *511* (1973).

BABEL, J. Proc. Int. Symp. Fluorescein Angiography. Albi, 1969: *216.* Karger, Basel (1971).

BIRD, A.C. & HAMILTON, A.M. *Brit. J. Ophthal.* 56: *881* (1972).

DEMAILLY, PH. & BERNARD, J.A. In: Oeil et cortisone. Masson et Cie. Soc. Fr. d'Ophthalmologie, p. *321* (1975).

DEUTMAN A.F., OOSTERHUIS, J.A., BOEN-TAN, T.N. & AAN DE KERK, A.I. *Brit. J. Ophthal.* 56: *863* (1972).

DEUTMAN, A.F. *Amer. J. Ophthal.* 78: *571* (1974).

FRIEDMAN, M.W. *Amer. J. Ophthal.* 79: *567* (1975).

GASS, J.D.M. *Arch. Ophthal.* (Chicago) 80: *177* (1968).

KIRKHAM, T.H., FFYTCHE, T.J. & SANDERS, M.D. *Arch. Ophthal.* (Chicago) 56: *875* (1972).

KRILL, A.E. & ARCHER, D. *Amer. J. Ophthal.* 72: *562* (1971).

KRILL, A.E. & DEUTMAN, A.F. *Amer. J. Ophthal.* 74: *193* (1972).

LAÄTIKAINEN, L. & ERKKILÄ, H. *Brit. J. Ophthal.* 58: *777* (1974).

MAUMENEE, A.E. *Amer. J. Ophthal.* 69: *1* (1970).

SAVINO, P.J., WEINBERG, R.J., YASSIN, J.G. & PILKERTON, A.R. *Amer. J. Ophthal.* 77: *659* (1974).

SCHATZ H., HAUMENEE, A.E. & PATZ A. *Trans. Amer. Acad. Ophthal. & Otolaryng.* 78: *747* (1974).

SIAM, A.-L. Proc. 8th Panhellenic Ophthal. Congr. Ioannina, 1975, p. *556* (1975).

VAN BUSKIRK, E.M., LESSEL, S. & FRIEDMAN E. *Arch. Ophthal.* (Chicago) 85: *369* (1971).

Author's address:
Opthalmology Department
Ein Shams University
Cairo
Egypt

INFLAMMATIONS OF THE CHOROID

KOICHI SHIMIZU, KEIICHI YOKOCHI & YOSHIHARU KOBAYASHI

(Maebashi, Japan)

In the past clinical studies on inflammations of the uveal tract, a lot of attention seems to have been paid to focal choroiditis entities caused by identifiable specific organisms. In the present paper, I am going to mainly discuss diffuse exudative choroiditis of still unknown etiology and particularly the disease of Harada. Incidentally, the diseases of Harada and Behcet comprise the two most frequent uveitis entities in present Japan.

The disease of Harada is characterized by its acute onset, bilaterality and occasional signs of meningeal irritation. The ocular manifestation invariably appears as serous detachment of the sensory retina starting in the posterior fundus. Signs of anterior uveitis and skin manifestations are later clinical signs of the disease.

In our previous reports (SHIKANO & SHIMIZU, 1968; SHIMIZU, 1973) we have proved that the retinal detachment is due to multifocal serous leakage from the choroid into the subretinal space. There are three types of

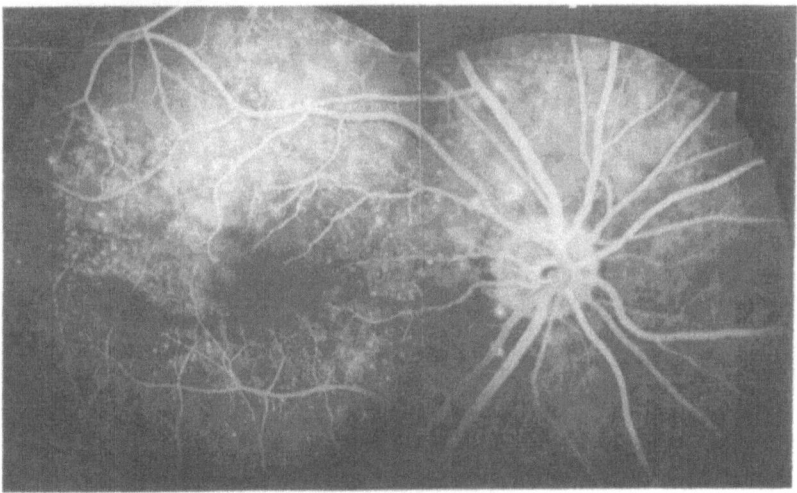

Fig. 1. Harada's disease, ca.80 seconds after injection. Numerous dots of fluorescein are disseminated over the papillomacular and surrounding areas. The dots are either stationary or enlarging in size.

leakage of dye. It may start as numerous discrete fluorescent dots which gradually enlarge like so many inkblots. This type is more common in milder forms of the disease. In severer and acuter type of the disease,

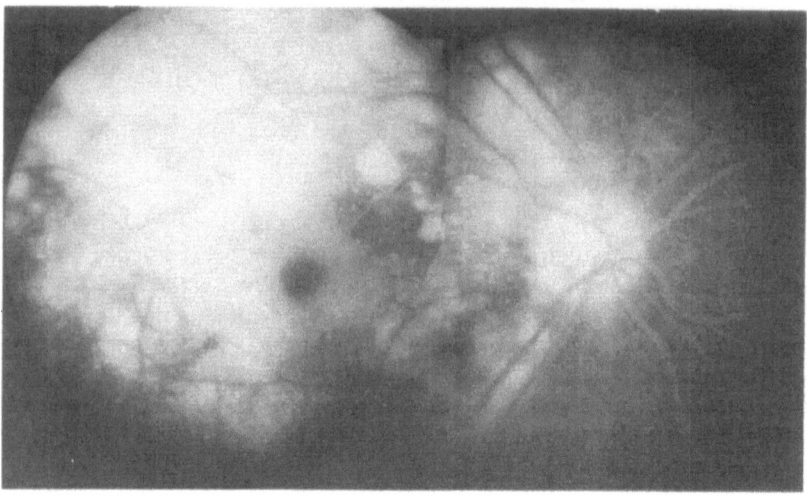

Fig. 2. Same as above, 16 minutes after injection. Fluorescein has accumulated behind the detached neuro- and pigment epithelium. Dots of fluorescein are still discernible. The optic disc shows hyperfluorescence.

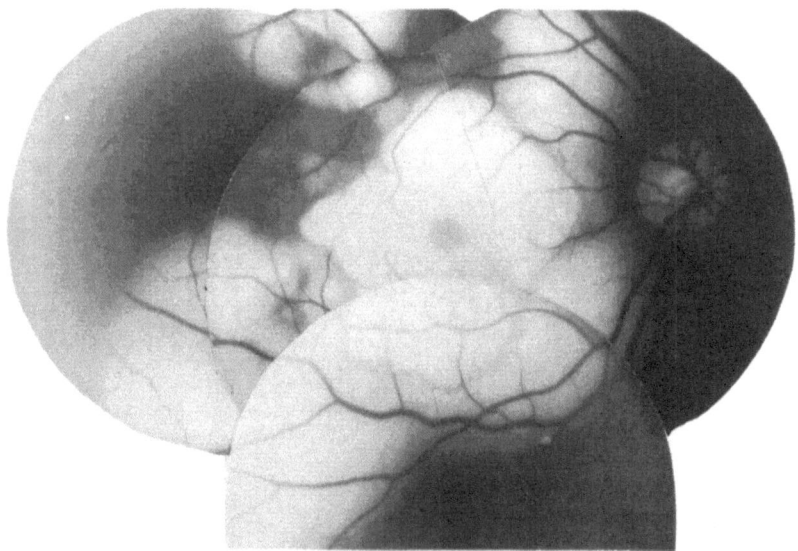

Fig. 3. Same as above, 2 hours after injection. Dye pooling behind the pigment epithelium is obvious. The peripheral fundus is unaffected.

386

fluorescein angiography reveals numerous areas of choroidal hypofluorescence. In later angiograms, these hypofluorescent areas begin to show patchy hyperfluorescene indicating leakage of dye. After a few days have passed since the onset of the disease, fluorescent angiography reveals numerous dots of fluorescence which are discrete and which do not show increase in size even in the late angiogram. This last feature seems to indicate the presence of invasion of epitheloid cells into the retinal pigment epithelium (Fig. 1).

The late angiograms in the early stage of Harada's disease regularly shows accumulation of dye behind the detached neuroepithelium and the pigment epithelium. The detachment of the pigment epithelium is most manifest when the fundus is observed several minutes or even hours after injection of dye (Fig. 3 & 4). The dye pooling behind the detached pigment epithelium looks like cobblestones of various sizes. The macular area regularly forms one unit of a few millimeters in diameter surrounded by a well-defined nonfluorescent borderline.

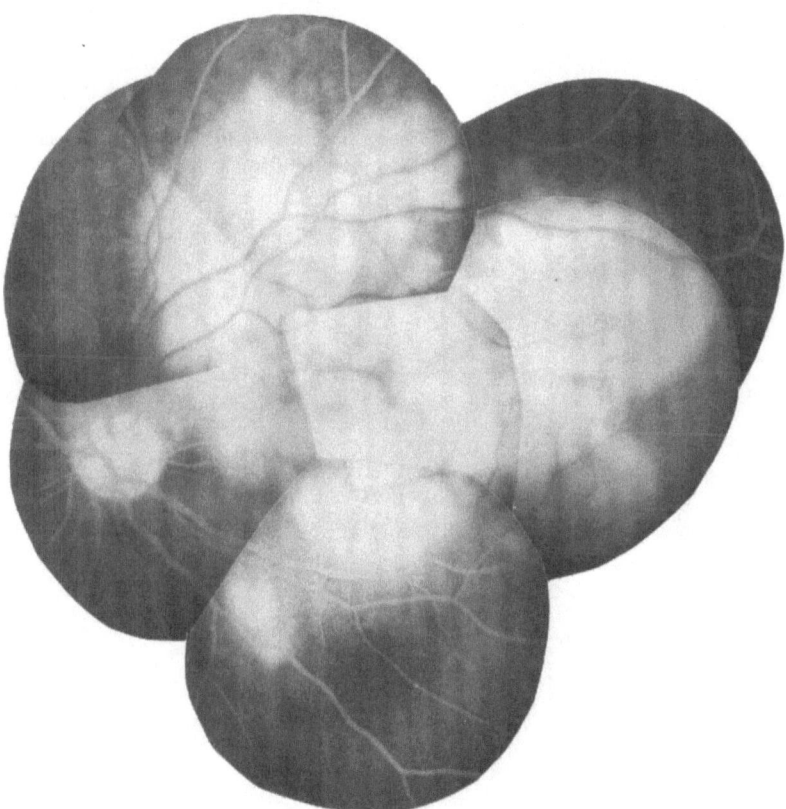

Fig. 4. Harada's disease (fulminant type), 22 minutes after injection. Multiple areas of hyperfluorescence correspond to dye pooling behind the detached pigment epithelium. The macular area has formed one unit with the dark fovea in its center. The affected fundus area is sharply demarcated from the neighboring uninvolved fundus.

The detachment of the neuro- and pigmentepithelium is confined to the posterior fundus areas in the early stage of the disease. The neighboring peripheral fundus is remarkably free from abnormal findings (Fig. 3 & 4).

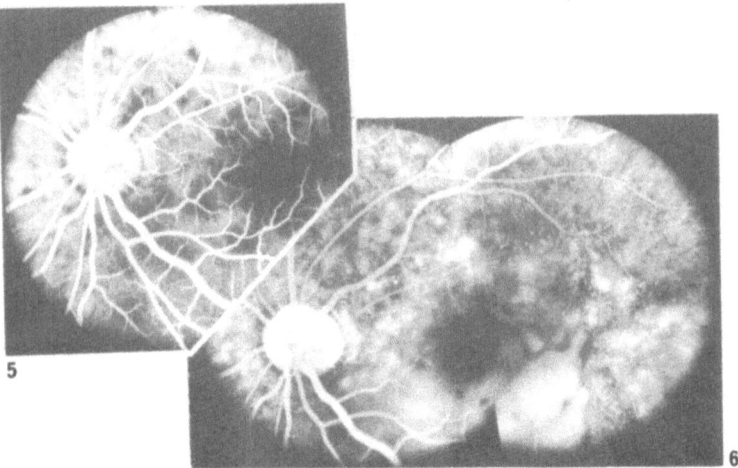

Fig. 5. Sympathetic ophthalmia, 15 seconds after injection. Numerous nonfluorescent patches indicate delayed onset of choriocapillaris perfusion.
Fig. 6. Same as above, 2 minutes after injection.

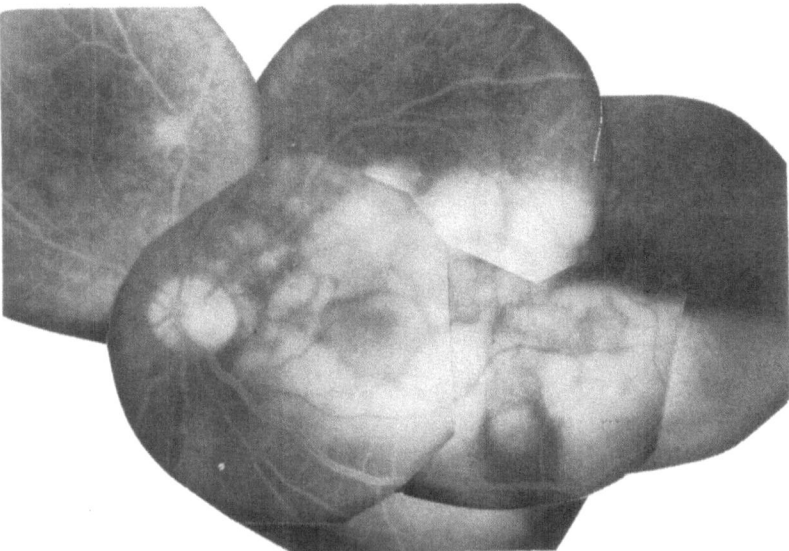

Fig. 7. Sympathetic ophthalmia, 25 minutes after injection. Areas of pooled dye behind the pigment epithelium are arranged like cobblestone in the posterior fundus. The peripheral fundus is virtually unaffected. The initially nonfluorescent patches now present faint hyperfluorescence.

388

Also, the retinal vessels are virtually unaffected except slight engorgement and tortuosity secondary to uneven retinal surface. Hyperfluorescence of optic disc vessels is a regular feature and usually persists several months after other inflammatory signs have subsided.

It has been often claimed (SHIMIZU, 1973) that there exists a close similarity between the fundus manifestations of the disease of Harada and sympathetic ophthalmia. I shall present a typical, untreated case of sympathetic ophthalmia with fluorescein angiographic features that are indistinguishable from those of Harada's disease.

The patient, a 26-year-old female (K.N., 74-1883), suffered from traumatic rupture of the cornea with prolapsus of the iris which remained untreated for 6 weeks. Sympathetic ophthalmia developed and the patient came to us 5 days after onset. The sympathized eye showed multiple retinal detachment in the posterior fundus and looked almost identical to Harada's disease. Fluorescein angiography showed multiple areas of initial nonfluorescence (Fig. 5) and patchy hyperfluorescence in the later angiogram (Fig. 6). The after-phase angiogram, taken 25 minutes after dye injection, showed multiple areas of dye-pooling behind the detached pigment epithelium. The abnormal findings were confined to the posterior fundus areas leaving the neighboring fundus areas practically unaffected.

The disease of Harada and sympathetic ophthalmia thus seem to share almost identical fluorescein angiographic features in common. The occasional presence of multiple hypofluorescence might lead one to assume that these two diseases might fall into the same group as the acute posterior multifocal placoid pigmentepitheliopathy (APMPPE). While it is true that the latter condition is also characterized by its bilaterality, initial nonfluorescence and multiple hyperfluorescence in later angiograms and also by involvement of the optic disc, the similarity ends there. In APMPPE, multifocal degeneration of the pigment epithelium is the rule after the acute phase has burned out. In the disease of Harada and sympathetic ophthalmia, diffuse depigmentation of the choroid is the usual event after cure of the disease but focal punched-out choroidal degeneration is infrequently observed. Also, Dalen-Fuchs nodules in Harada are dissimilar to what we see after cure of APMPPE.

The disease of Behcet and sarcoidosis also belong to the category of diffuse choroiditis similar to Harada. Though it is dangerous to oversimplify the mode of fundus involvement of Behcet's disease because of its polymorphic nature, it is safe to state that the latter usually affects the retinal vessels inducing generalized hyperpermeability of vessel wall. The pigment epithelium seems to be not seriously affected as in the case of Harada.

I shall close my introductory paper on inflammation of the choroid with a few words over the presumed ocular histoplasmosis. It is almost certain that histoplasmosis is either not endemic or only thinly disseminated in Japan. Still, we have occasionally seen cases with so-called ocular histoplasmosis showing macular neovascularization, peripapillar and peripheral choroidal atrophy. Histoplasmin skin test was only occasionally positive. This is a fit subject of geographic ophthalmology and a lot of effort will be needed to clarify the nature of this disease entity.

REFERENCES

SHIKANO, S. & SHIMIZU, K. Atlas of fluorescence fundus angiography. p. *125-135*. Igaku-Shoin, Tokyo, and W.B. Saunders, Philadelphia (1968).

SHIMIZU, K. Fluorescein microangiography of the ocular fundus. p. *91-99*. Igaku-Shoin, Tokyo, and Williams & Wilkins, Baltimore (1973).

SHIMIZU, K. Harada's, Behcet's, Vogt-Koyanagi syndromes – are they clinical entities? *Trans. Amer. Acad. Ophth. Otolaryng.* 77: *OP281-290* (1973).

Authors' address:
Department of Ophthalmology
Gunma University School of Medicine
3-39-15 Showamachi
Maebashi
371 Japan

DISCUSSION

Dr von Winning: I was impressed, in the pictures of Dr Shimizu, by the early occurrence of a dark spot in the macula in the cases of Harada's disease. I wondered how this could be explained. The retinal vessels did not seem to show gross changes and perhaps this intracellular swelling of the retina could not be explained by subretinal and still less by subpigmente-pithelial exudation. I should want to ask Dr Shimizu if this is a constant early finding in Harada's disease and how its occurrence is explained.

Dr Shimizu: I just showed you a few typical instances of Harada's disease. I have experienced over 80 cases of Harada's disease and I can say that almost every early case of Harada looks like the picture I showed you, on colour photographs and in fluorescein angiograms. The dark spot in the macula can be explained by assuming the presence of a filter-like structure right in the central fovea and within the neuroepithelium. The background fluorescence from the pooled dye behind the detached pigment epithelium will be effectively blocked by this filter-like structure. You are quite right in pointing out that the retinal vessels are not involved in Harada except, I should say, the optic disc vessels. The macular dark spot is, therefore, of entirely different nature from what you see in cases of cystoid macular edema.

Dr Siam: I would like to ask Dr Shimizu whether, in the 80 cases of Harada's disease he mentioned, he did come accross the complete syndrome of Vogt-Koyanagi-Harada as I have shown in the two cases with similar fluorographic patterns.

Dr Shimizu: The difficulty in definition between Harada's and Vogt-Koyanagi's syndrome lies in the fact that Dr Harada wrote only in Japanese and Dr Koyanagi wrote only in German. Another difficulty is that Harada's disease and also sympathetic uveitis seem to be coming less and less severe these days. They used to follow a much more severe course 30 or 40 years ago so that the whole disease picture is changing. Among my 80-odd cases, I think I didn't see more than 3 which would fit into the concept of Vogt-Koyanagi with massive anterior segment involvement and poliosis and every-thing. Harada is a moderate form of Vogt-Koyanagi.

FLUORESCEIN ANGIOGRAPHY IN UVEAL EFFUSION

H. PAULMANN & K. HEIMANN

(Cologne, W. Germany)

The uveal effusion syndrome of SCHEPENS & BROCKHURST was first described in 1963 based on their observations of 17 patients. Its clinical features are as follows: annular choroidal detachment combined with non-rhegmatogenous retinal detachment, typical shifting of the subretinal fluid according to gravity and posture, minimal or no signs of uveitis. Predilected

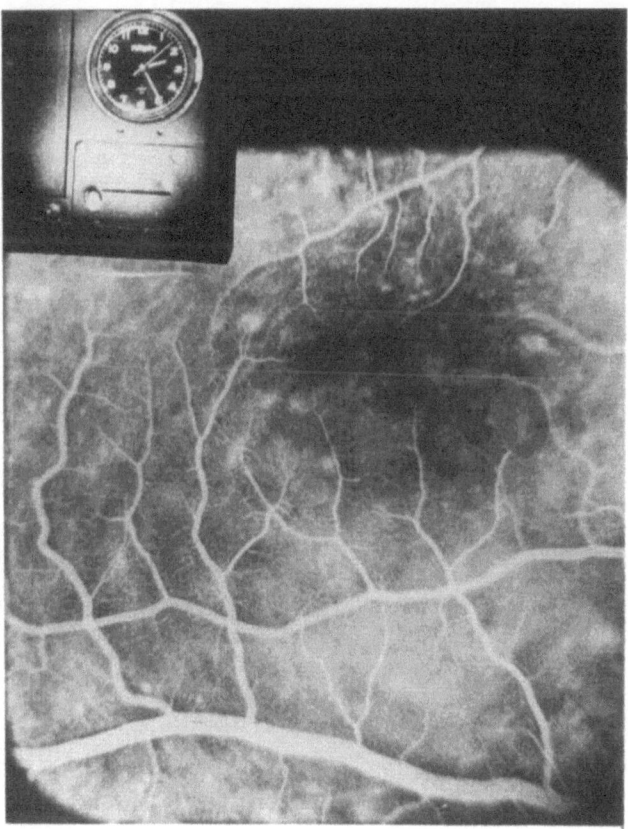

Fig. 1. *Case 1*. Multiple tiny leakages of dye in the early venous phase. Staining of subretinal fluid.

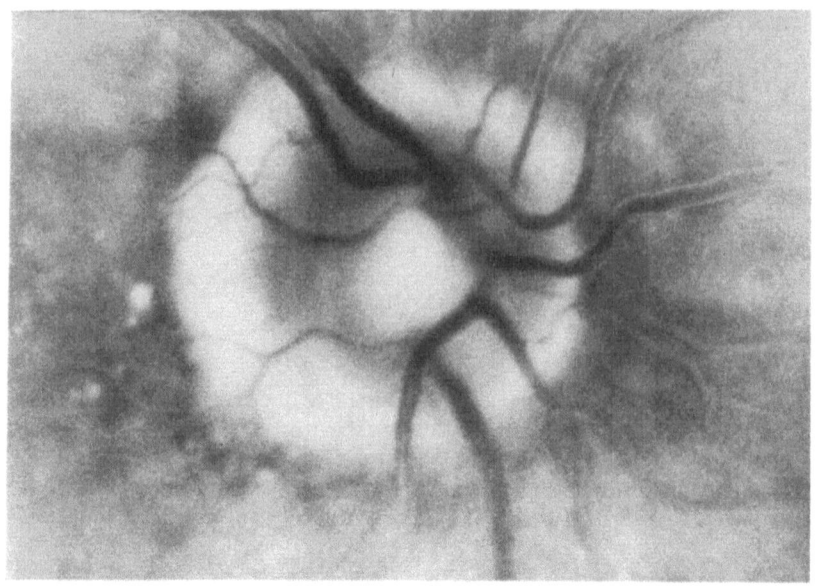

Fig. 2. *Case 1*. Fluorescein ring of the disc without capillary abnormalities in the late phase.

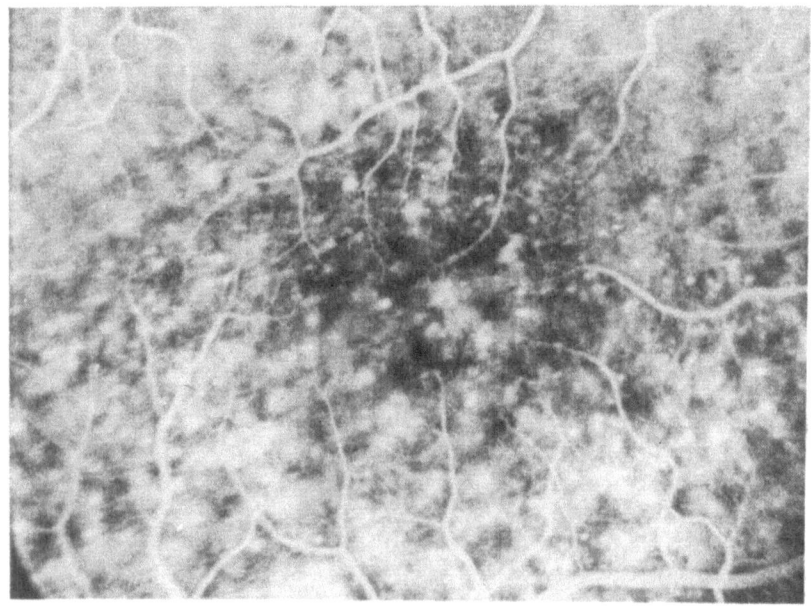

Fig. 3. *Case 1*. Multiple granula-like spots without confluence in the venous stage.

392

are middle-aged men. In 1974 we saw three patients with uveal effusions. Because of the rare descriptions in literature, we want to demonstrate our fluorescein angiographic findings.

CASE 1

A 57-year-old man was seen for the first time at Univ. Eye Clinic Cologne in 1974. Vision was reduced to 0.3 on his right eye, nulla lux on his left eye caused by retinal detachment unsuccessfully operated on five years ago. Ophthalmoloscopically we found an almost complete choroidal detachment of nearly 360° with a flat central serous retinal detachment.

Fluorescein angiography showed normal transit of dye (Fig. 1). During the arterial phase, there was a soft mottling of the posterior pole. In the venous stage multiple tiny leakages of dye arose within the retinal detachment with confluence in the late phase after ten minutes. During the early phase appeared a ring of fluorescein around the disc, which remained sharply marked through all the stages, differing much from the angiographic picture of an oedematous nervehead. No capillary abnormalities were to be

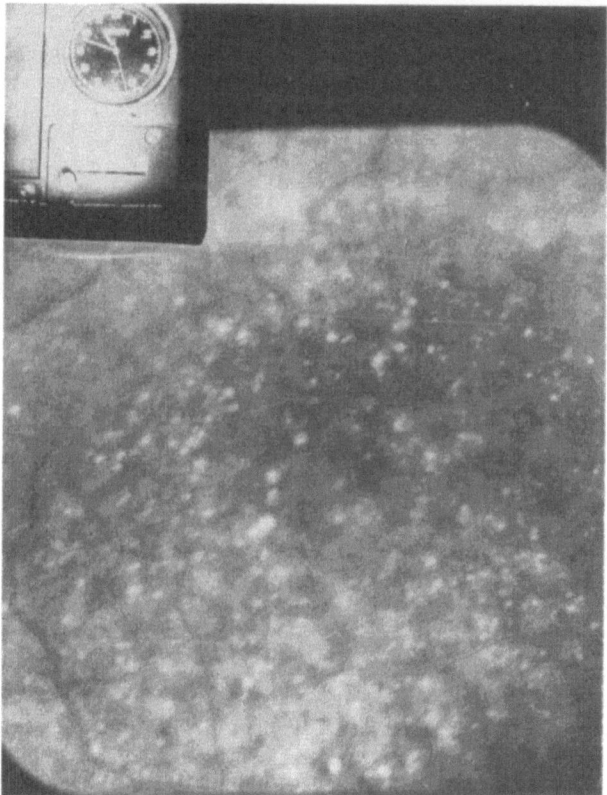

Fig. 4. *Case 1*. Drusen-like spots still containing dye in the latest phases.

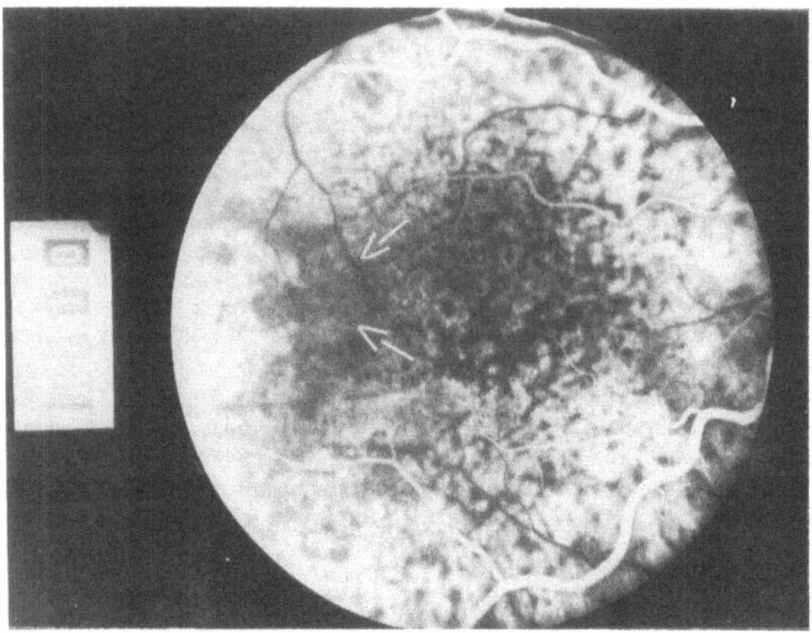

Fig. 5. *Case 2*. Pigmentproliferations besides small areas of depigmentation in the late arterial phase. Still absence of background fluorescence (arrow).

seen on or around the disc (Fig. 2). Treatment with steroids and Rheoma-krodex brought complete reattachment of both the retina and choroid.

In this stage, fluorescein angiography revealed a dense mottling during the arterial phase; in the venous phase multiple fine granula-like spots appeared with a good visible demarcation, some drusen-like spots still containing dye could be seen even in the latest phases (Fig. 3, 4).

CASE 2

A 25-year-old woman complained of marked loss of sight of the right eye, which she had for two weeks. Another transient decrease of vision had occurred twelve months before but vision had returned without treatment six weeks later. Examination by slitlamp microscopy revealed no inflammatory signs. Ophthalmoloscopically there was a ballooning retinal detachment with a tumor-like choroidal detachment of nearly 360°. In the upper part of the retina, there were pepper and salt-like patches, some suggestive of scars. Right visual acuity was 0.4.

Fluorescein angiography revealed pigmentproliferations besides small areas of depigmentation. There was confluence of dye and staining of the subretinal fluid in the lower part of the fundus (Fig. 5, 6). Under treatment with steroids and Rheomakrodex choroidal and retinal detachment were resolved within three weeks after the first examination. In this stage, angiography offered little further changes: tiny window-like defects of the RPE next to granular hyperpigmentations were scattered throughout the retina (Fig. 7).

The patient was seen subsequently at two to three month intervals, but fluorescein angiography did not change much, except for a slight recovery of the macular shadow, where the drusen seemed to disappear partly. Both patients had a spontanous recurrence of choroidal and retinal detachment, accompanied by starfold macular changes similar to beginning macular edema.

Fluorescein angiography revealed no central leakage of dye, but an increase in mottled appearance with prolonged fluorescein in the underlying choroid (Fig. 8). Shifting of subretinal fluid could be demonstrated easily because of the height of the retinal detachment. But no loss of dye appeared, neither through vessels nor in the subretinal fluid of the detached area (Fig. 9).

Because the symptoms and the course of the disease of our third patient

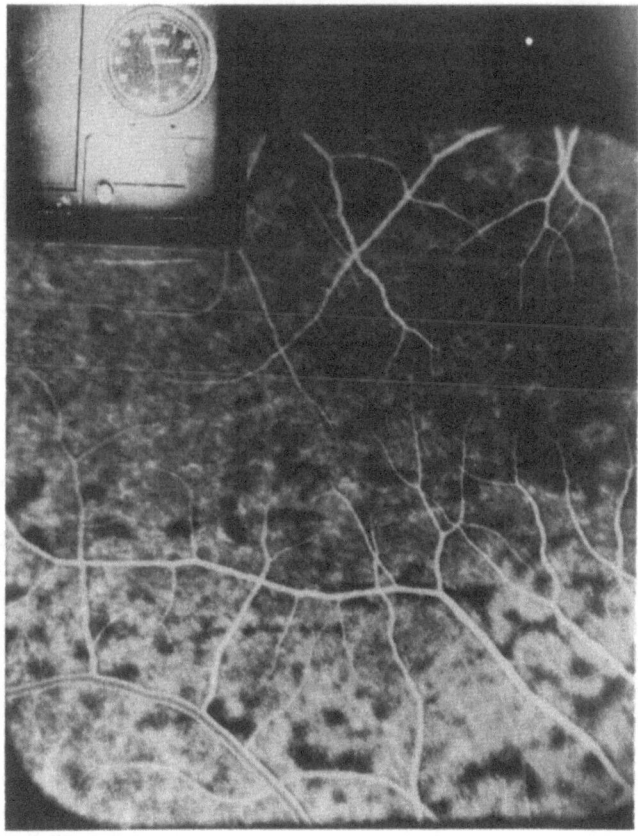

Fig. 6. *Case 2* Multifocal lesions in and around the macula with minimal confluence in the venous stage.

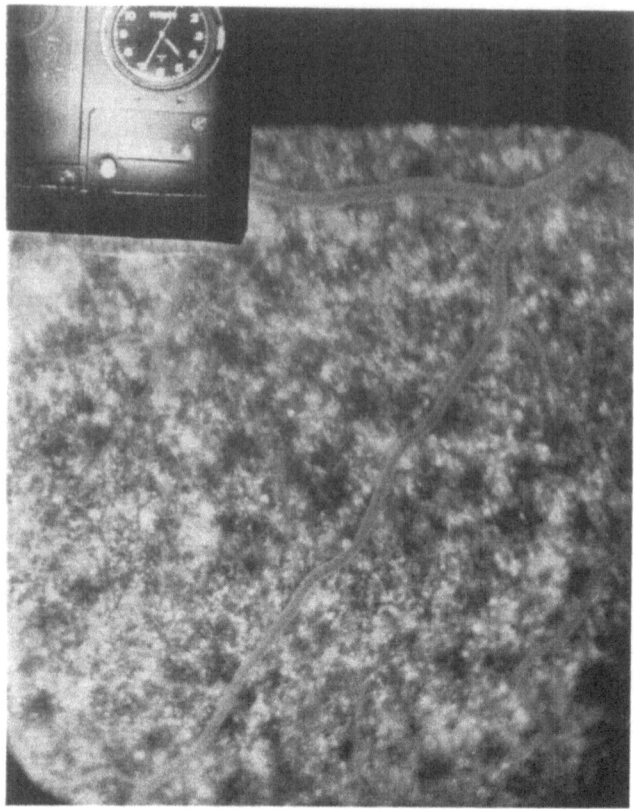

Fig. 7. *Case 2.* Window-like defects of the RPE next to granular hyperpigmentations throughout the retina in the late venous stage.

are so mimilar to that of our demonstrated cases, an explanation will be spared for sake of economy (Table 1).

ROSEN first described fluorescein angiographic changes in uveal effusion with findings similar to ours. Contrary to the observations made by SCHEPENS, DAVIES observed a more heterogenous group with similar symptoms but non dominating bilateral manifestation. According to the descriptions of SCHEPENS, ROSEN and others the clinical feature of uveal effusion is variable. Presumably our demonstrated cases seem to be the early stage of this disease, whose cause is yet unknown. Efficiency of steroids and Rheomacrodex seem to indicate an immunological process with underlying vasculopathy. This hypothesis is supported by histological findings of ROSEN who found signs of an exsudative sclerouveitis with infiltration of plasma cells, eosinophils and lymphocyts. In our opinion this shifting sub-retinal fluid only stands for the monotonous reaction of the choroid caused by different agents. The reaction of the RPE is not quite clear, because on the RPE no serious damages can be observed and as reported by ROSEN, no gross abnormality in enucleated eyes can be demonstrated. Recovery enters with minimal loss of visual acuity, accompanied by pigmentary changes, ressembling a pepper and salt fundus. As DUKE-ELDER and SCHEPENS point out, pigmentary alteration seems to be the result of a long standing choroidal detachment only. It would thus appear, that this kind of epitheliopathy can be regarded as a benign pigmentary disturbance.

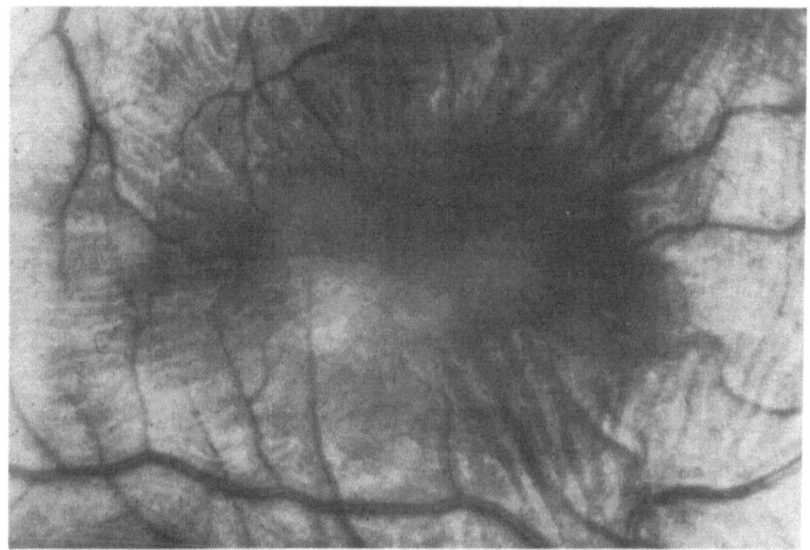

Fig. 8. *Case 1.* Starfold macular changes.

OCULAR FINDINGS (3cases)

serous retinal detachment			
with choroidal detachment	unilat.	case	1+2
	bilat.	case	3
edematous disc.		case	1+2
mild uveitis ant.		case	3
ECG/ERG reduc.		case	1-3
perimetry - scotoma		case	1-3

Table 1. Summary of ocular findings.

| | Visual Acuity | | Duration |
	Initial	Final	
1. F.D. ♂ 58 yr.	OS 0.3	0.6	3 months (1 recurrence)
2. A.L. ♀ 25 yr.	OD 0.4	0.9	2 months (2 recurrences)
3. M.H. ♀ 70 yr.	OD 0.05 OS 0.05	0.6 0.4	∅

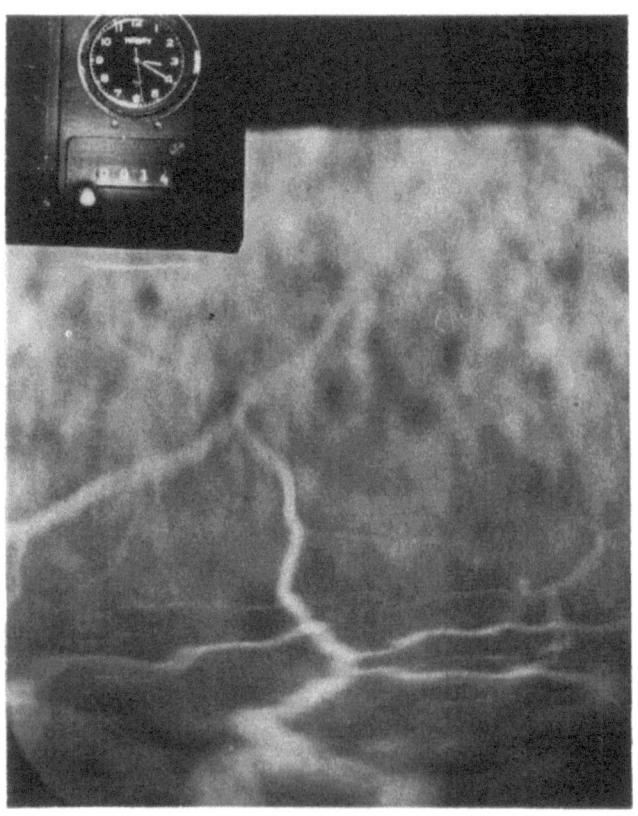

Fig. 9. *Case 2.* Serous retinal detachment without any demarcation line. No loss of dye in the detached area.

398

REFERENCES

SCHEPENS, C.L. & BROCKHURST, R.J. Uveal effusion. *Arch. Ophthal.* 70: *189-201* (1963).

BROCKHURST, R.J. et al. Uveal effusion. II. Report of a case with analysis of sub-retinal fluid. *Arch. Ophthal.* 90: *399-401* (1973).

DAVIES, E.W.G. et al. Annual serous detachment of the choroid. *Trans. Ophthalm. Soc. U.K.* 93: *145-159* (1973).

ROSEN, E. et al. Uveal effusions. *Amer. J. Ophthal.* 65: *509-518* (1968).

DUKE-ELDER, S. System of ophthalmology. Vol. 9, Diseases of the uveal tract, p. *939*. Kimpton, London (1966).

Authors' address:
Universitäts-Augenklinik
Joseph-Stelzmannstrasse 9
5 Cologne 41
West Germany

ANGIOGRAPHIE FLUORESCEINIQUE DU FOND D'OEIL AU COURS D'UNE OPHTHALMIE SYMPATHIQUE

P. BEC, J.L. ARNE, J.P. AUBRY & V. PHILIPPOT

(Toulouse, France)

L'ophtalmie sympathique réalise généralement une atteinte diffuse de l'uvée antérieure et postérieure, gênant l'examen précis du fond d'oeil, ce qui explique la rareté des publications sur ce sujet (GUILLAUMAT 1973).

Nous avons pu observer à différents stades de son évolution, une ophtalmie sympathique originale par son étiologie et dont les manifestations se sont essentiellement localisées à l'uvée postérieure permettant différents examens angiographiques.

HISTOIRE CLINIQUE

Une malade de 34 ans avait présenté depuis l'âge de 4 ans plusieurs poussées de kératite herpétique au niveau de l'oeil gauche qui avaient laissé une importante opacité de la cornée. En 1973, est pratiquée une première kératoplastie lamellaire. Elle est suivie d'une opacification du greffon et d'une hypertonie nécessitant une intervention fistulisante.

En novembre 1974, la malade est revue avec un desmétocèle. Une kératoplastie perforante est pratiquée et au cours de l'ouverture de la chambre antérieure, on note l'existence d'une importante synéchie iridocornéenne qui doit être clivée.

Les suites opératoires immédiates sont satisfaisantes mais 41 jours après l'intervention, la malade se plaint d'une chute d'acuité visuelle de l'oeil droit et est réhospitalisée immédiatement le lendemain du début des troubles.

A l'examen du côté opéré, l'acuité visuelle est réduite à la perception lumineuse; le greffon est légèrement opaque avec de gros plis de la Descemet.

Du côté droit, on note des signes d'uvéites: tyndall de l'humeur aqueuse, précipités rétro-cornéens, léger trouble du vitré laissant toutefois percevoir un important oedème rétinien du pôle postérieur.

Un bilan complet est pratiqué:
— formule numération: normale.
— les différents séro-diagnostics sont négatifs.
— le bilan virologique montre une faible fixation du complément d'antigène herpétique, une absence de virus en culture de tissu.
— le bilan immunologique est pratiqué: le test de transformation blastique à l'uvée est faiblement positif. Différentes recherches d'anticorps par fluorescence sont pratiquées et reviennent négatives.

— la ponction lombaire ramène un liquide clair normo-tendu avec une élévation importante des lymphocytes: 47 lymphocytes par mm 3.

Nous avons conclu à une Ophtalmie Sympathique probablement liée à une manipulation opératoire de la synéchie irido-cornéenne. Un traitement médical est d'abord institué, fait d'immuno-dépresseurs, d'A.C.T.H., et d'antibiotiques. Devant l'insuffisance de ce traitement, l'énucléation de l'oeil gauche est pratiquée avec un résultat très favorable, puisque l'acuité de l'oeil droit remontait rapidement à 9/10e tandis que le fond d'oeil se nettoyait avec un remaniement pigmentaire et un pli rétinien maculaire.

EXAMEN ANATOMO–PATHOLOGIQUE

L'examen anatomo-pathologique est très caractéristique: l'altération pathologique essentielle est constituée par un épaississement et une infiltration granulomateuse de tout le tractus uvéal: choroïde, corps ciliaire, iris. Cette infiltration est constituée en majorité par des cellules lymphocytaires, mais elle comprend également des cellules épithélioïdes et des cellules géantes. Ces dernières formations se rencontrent dans toutes les parties de l'uvée et ne s'accompagnent d'aucune caséification.

Par ailleurs, on trouve plusieurs formations nodulaires constituées par des cellules épithélioïdes et des lymphocytes au niveau de l'épithélium pigmentaire.

La rétine est décollée mais elle ne présente aucun signe d'atteinte inflammatoire, sauf en de rares endroits, autour des vaisseaux. Des foyers de cellules lymphocytaires et épithélioïdes se rendontrent au niveau de la sclérotique.

Il faut noter encore:
— la cicatrice de kératoplastie avec un greffon de structure normale non vascularisé.
— l'aspect normal du cristallin.
— enfin, l'iris ne figure pas en entier sur la coupe: une partie est absente, ce qui reste esten situation de synéchie antérieure au niveau de la rétine irienne.

En conclusion, il s'agit donc de lésions très évocatrices d'Ophtalmie Sympathique avec:
— infiltration granulomateuse uvéale faite de cellules lymphoïdes, épithélioïdes et de cellules géantes.
— nodules de DAHLEN-FUCHS sur l'épithélium pigmentaire.

BILAN ANGIOGRAPHIQUE

Différents examens angiographies de l'oeil droit ont été pratiqués au cours de l'évolution de la maladie.

1. *Le 1er se situe le jour de la réhospitalisation* de la malade, le lendemain du début des troubles, pour chute de l'acuité visuelle de l'oeil droit.

Dès les temps très précoces apparaît une diffusion du colorant sous forme de halos respectant la macula. La fluorescence de ces lésions va augmenter aux temps artério-veineux, prédominant toujours au centre.

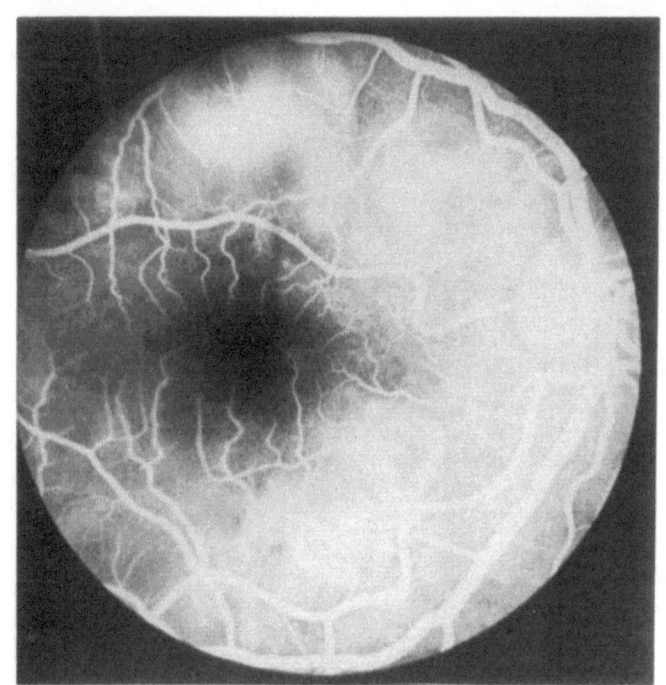

Fig. 1

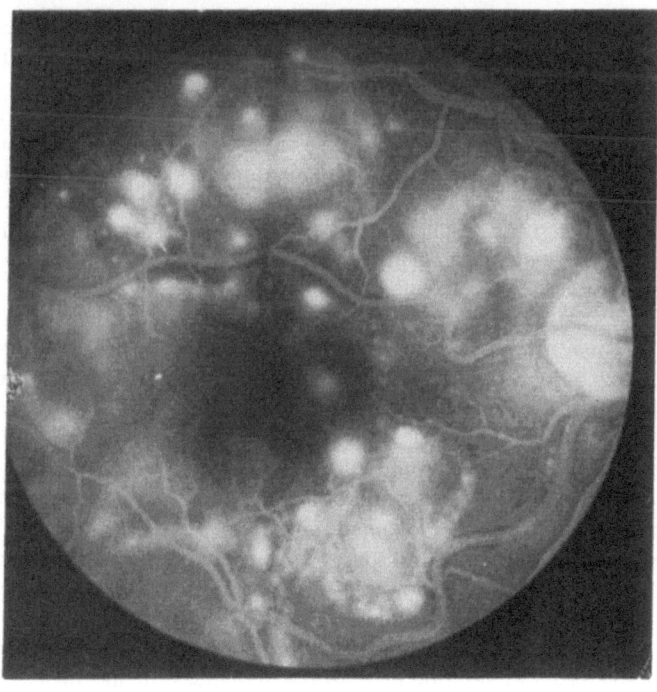

Fig. 2

403

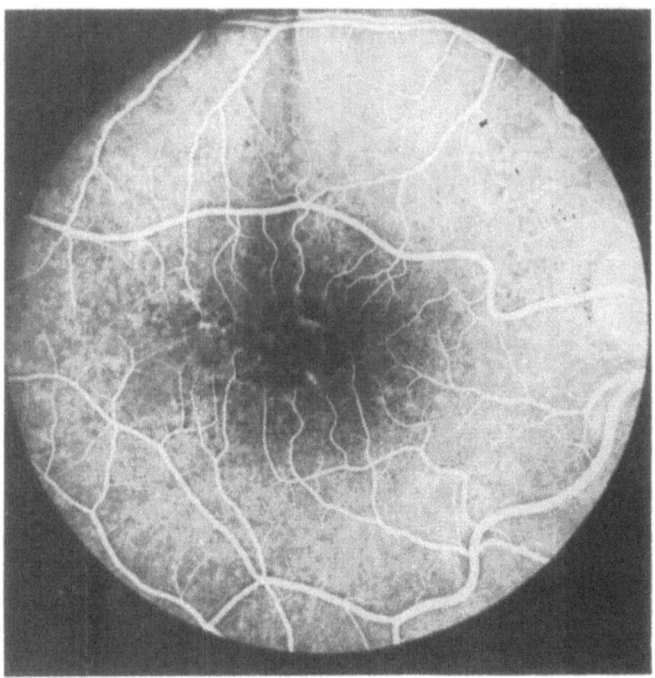

Fig. 3

Lors des temps veineux apparaissent de nouveaux points de diffusion qui présentent des caractères différents des premières lésions notées aux temps artériels. Elles sont limitées, arrondies, intensément fluorescentes de façon homogène. Elles se surajoutent aux premières diffusions en halo, (Fig. 1).

Aux temps veineux tardifs les lésions vont atteindre la zone de la macula et leur diffusion va progressivement augmenter en intensité et en surface pour couvrir bientôt toute l'aire maculaire (Fig. 2). Elles prennent alors un aspect de dégénérescence maculaire sénile exsudative et leur apparition plus tardive qu'en périphérie tient probablement à l'épaisseur de l'épithélium pigmentaire dans la région maculaire.

Aux temps très tardifs, les vaisseaux rétiniens sont parfaitement visibles, se détachant en sombre sur le fond fluorescent: celui-ci est maintenant formé de plages fluorescentes pratiquemment confluentes, occupant tout le pôle postérieur.

2. *Un mois après*, l'examen ophtalmoscopique montre un oedème papillaire avec des hémorragies sus-papillaires et l'apparition d'un pli maculaire. L'angiographie s'est considérablement modifiée: les diffusions précédemment constatées ont totalement disparu. Trois éléments sont frappants:

Lors des temps précoces, le pôle postérieur apparaît comme strictement normal et aucune altération pigmentaire n'est visible.

Aux temps tardifs apparaît un oedème de la papille très accentué avec dilatation veineuse et altération des parois vasculaires et hémorragies temporales supérieures.

La macula présente un pli radiaire certainement rétinien qui est imprégné et qui semble épouser la convexité des deux plis plus profonds, sans doute choroidiens, partant de la macula vers la région temporale et ne semblant pas diffuser le colorant lors du temps tardif.

3. *Trois semaines plus tard*, l'oedème papillaire est en regression nette et il existe peu de diffusion; les veines reprennent peu à peu un aspect normal. Les hémorragies temporales supérieures ont nettement diminué et il n'en persiste que dans le secteur sus-maculaire.

Alors que le pôle postérieur est normal, apparaissent surtout dans le secteur temporo-maculaire, des altérations pigmentaires de type sec, dont la fluorescence prédomine en périphérie.

4. *15 jours plus tard*, le pôle postérieur apparaît cicatriciel, avec des amas pigmentaires. A l'angiographie, les lésions précédentes ont pris un aspect cicatriciel; de fins vaisseaux choroidiens, sclérosés qui semblent exclues de toute circulation, entourent les zones muettes au niveau de l'épithélium pigmentaire. La lésion maculaire un aspect en trèfle (Fig. 3).

On retrouve au niveau de la macula la cicatrice du pli rétinien fluorescente traduisant des altérations majeunes de l'épithélium pigmentaire à ce niveau; les plis choroïdiens ont disparu.

5. *Trois mois plus tard*, l'aspect ophtalmoscopique est totalement cicatriciel. A l'angiographie, les temps précoces révèlent toujours quelques aspects de retard circulatoire physiologique. Les altérations pigmentaires de la macula se retrouvent identiques.

DISCUSSION

1. On est donc frappé par le contraste entre cet aspect absolument cicatriciel au bout de trois mois, s'opposant à l'image très spectaculaire de la première angiographie qui a immédiatement précédé l'énucléation. Il est notamment étonnant de voir l'opposition entre la densité des signes de la première angiographie et la cicatrice que laisse l'affection, excepté dans la région maculaire qui apparaissait très touchée.

2. Plusieurs images angiographiques nous ont posé des problèmes d'interprétation pathogénique que nous n'avons pas pu totalement résoudre.

Lors de la première angiographie, il semble coexister des lésions de type décollement séreux de l'épithélium pigmentaire correspondant aux tâches fluorescentes bien limitées et une imprégnation de l'épithélium pigmentaire luimême par la fluorescéine réalisant ces halos de fluorescence croissante. Des phénomènes cicatriciels se localiseront essentiellement à l'endroit où l'épithélium pigmentaire est plus épais, dans la région maculaire.

Nous n'avons pas su rattacher à son origine et interpréter le pli rétinien maculaire, connaissant l'intégrité habituelle de la rétine lors des Ophthalmies Sympathiques.

BIBLIOGRAPHIE

GUILLAUMAT, L., SELIGMAN, M., MARX, P., LANGLOIS, J. & IRIS, L. Ophtalmie
sympathique de caractère inhabituel: traitement par les immunodépresseurs. *Bull.
Soc. Ophtal. France* 73, 3 (1973).

Adresse d'auteurs:
Service d'Ophtalmologie
Hôpital Purpan
3105 Toulouse
France

406

LESIONS CHORIO-EPITHELIALES INITIALES DANS L'ONCHOCERCOSE OCULAIRE

P. METGE*, M. CHOVET** & E. LOREAL***

(Marseille, France)

Des angiographies systématiques du fond d'oeil ont été réalisées sur 64 sujets onchocerquiens confirmés (116 yeux), à Bamako (Mali), et 20 yeux (10 malades) ont pu être contrôlés après une évolution de 27 mois. Une présentation a déjà été faite (METGE et al., 1974; METGE & CHOVET, 1975) des divers types de lésions constatées. Nous exposons ici les lésions élémentaires des atteintes chorio-épithéliales, leur localisation élective et certains aspects évolutifs.

MALADES ET METHODES

Tous les sujets examinés étaient de race noire et leur age compris entre 18 et 68 ans (age moyen 36 ans).

Le diagnostic d'onchocercose était affirmé dans tous les cas par un critère parasitologique: SNIPP quantitatif ou présence de microfilaires dans la chambre antérieure.

L'examen ophtalmologique comportait la mesure de l'acuité visuelle, de la pression oculaire, un examen biomicroscopique du segment antérieur, du vitré et du fond d'oeil, des rétinographies couleur, anérytres et en fluorescence (Angiographe Topcon).

RESULTATS

Sur 116 yeux examinés, 85 présentaient des lésions d'onchocercose dont 73 étaient des atteintes du segment postérieur associées (51 cas) ou non (22 cas) à des lésions antérieures.

Les lésions postérieures chorio-épithéliales étaient 46 fois discrètes et localisées, 27 fois généralisées; les unes et les autres étaient associées à une atteinte papillaire ou vasculaire rétinienne (44 fois).

Lésions élémentaires

Ce sont des lésions chorioépithéliales rencontrées constamment à un stade d'atteinte discrète. Il s'agit soit d'un foyer isolé d'atrophie épithéliale 'en ilot', 'en placard', soit de taches plus fines, groupées en secteur, parfois l'association de ces deux formes.

*CHU Hotel Dieu   **Hôpital A. Lavéran   ***IOTA
Place Daviel   13013 Marseille   Bamako
13002 Marseille   France   Mali
France

1. Placard

Dans sa forme la plus discrète, c'est un 'îlot' arrondi ou 'placode' de 1/5 à 1/3 de diamètre papillaire; souvent isolé, il peut passer inaperçu à l'ophthalmoscopie: petite zone de rétine un peu plus pâle, de coloration grisâtre ou gris orangé. Il nous a souvent été révélé par l'angiographie: il s'illumine en effet précocement dès le temps de remplissage choroïdien: petite plaque finement granitée, nettement définie, invariable en surface, sans hyperfluorescence tardive, elle apparait comme un effet fenêtre de l'épithélium pigmentaire (fig. 1).

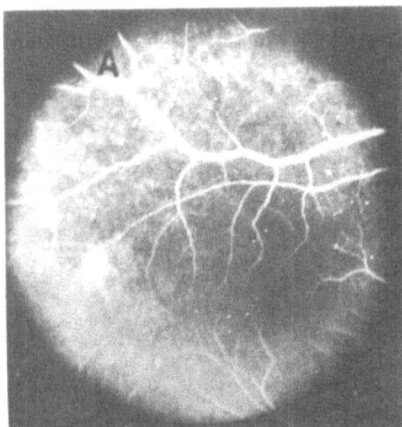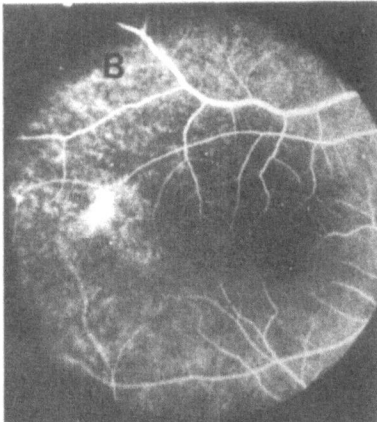

Fig. 1. *Observation 39:* Placode temporale. A. Novembre 1973, femme de 42 ans, A.V.O.D.: 0,7 papille, macula vaisseaux normaux. Petit îlot d'hyperfluorescence paracentral externe.
B. Janvier 1976, A.V.O.D.: 0,4, léger élargissement du foyer.

Sa localisation élective et quasi constante est paramaculaire externe sur le méridien horizontal à 2 ou 3 diamètres papillaires du point fovéolaire. On peut la retrouver aussi du côté nasal au voisinage de la papille.

Un 'placard' plus large de 1 à 2 diamètres papillaires, arrondi à bords nets semble succéder .à l'îlot précédent par élargissement ou coalescence de foyers atrophiques voisins; il a, en effet, la même topographie élective temporale externe. Des mottes pigmentées alternent à sa surface avec des taches et un liseré achromes. Ce placard plus large est entouré d'une couronne d'éléments 'tachetés' (fig. 2 et 3).

2. Foyers 'tachetés'

Les foyers 'tachetés' sont constitués par le groupement, en secteur limité, de fins éléments, de quelques dizaines de microns, d'atrophie épithéliale de teinte claire.

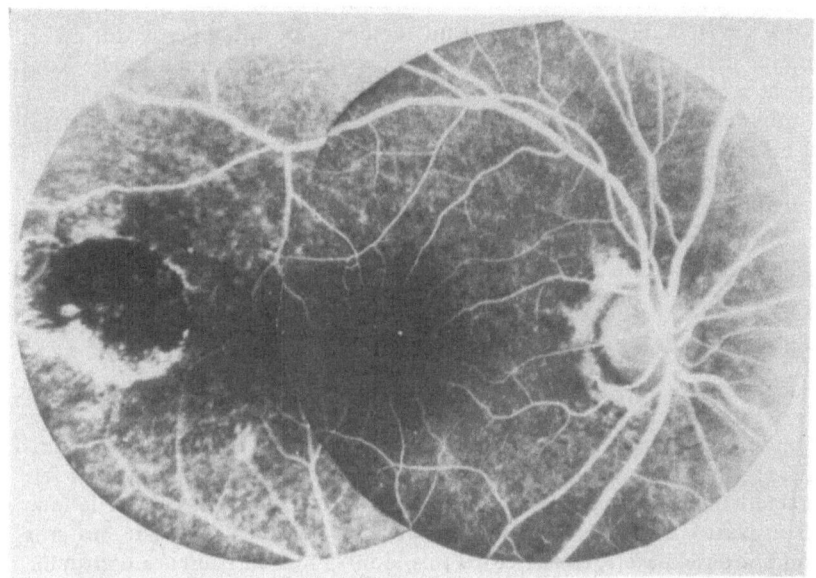

Fig. 2. *Observation 30:* Placard temporal externe.
Homme de 35 ans, SNIPP ++, A.V.O.D. 2/10, Papille décolorée, artères rétrécies et engainées. Placard temporal pigmenté à bordure achrome. Croissant péripapillaire.

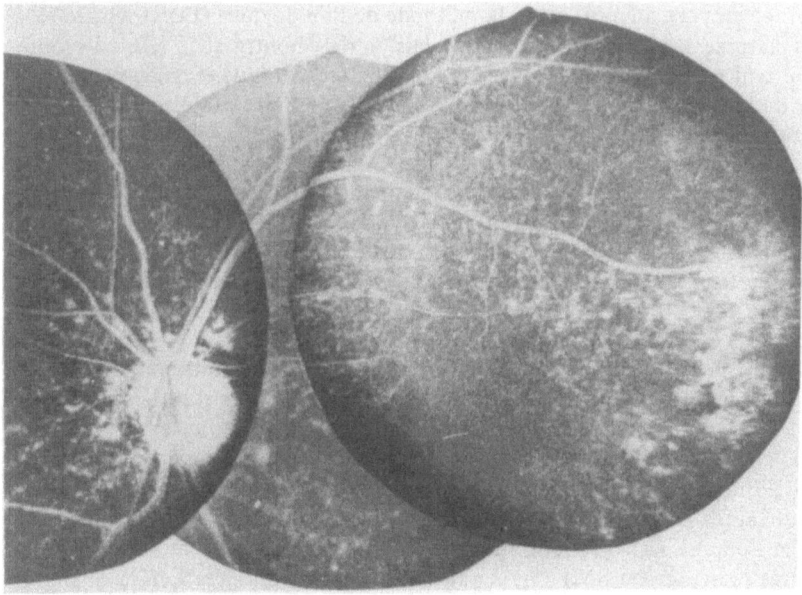

Fig. 3. *Observation 54:* Foyer temporal externe. Homme de 24 ans, A.V.O.G. 10/10, T.O. 12, placard et pommelé temporal externe, petit foyer juxta-papillaire.

409

Un foyer juxta-papillaire nasal ou temporal en îlot, en croissant ou en anneau, paraît être par sa fréquence la deuxième localisation isolée. Nous l'avons rencontré 9 fois chez des sujets dont l'age moyen était 41 ans.

Pommelé annulaire para-central: En couronne plus ou moins complète, ou en croissant autour de la macula avec une prédominance toujours temporale. Cette lésion déjà plus étendue se projette en regard de l'arc des vaisseaux temporeaux. Nous l'avons rencontrée 13 fois sur 73 cas.

Foyer temporo-maculaire: il apparait comme une extension sur la macula, du placard ou du pommelé temporal, nous l'avons rencontré 3 fois comme seule atteinte chorio-épithéliale.

Association

Ces lésions chorio-épithéliales localisées ont été trouvées associées à des atteintes papillaires: 10 fois à une atrophie optique, à bords nets, sans excavation; 4 fois à un oedème papillaire discret cliniquement, mais tout à fait caractéristique en angiographie, avec, 2 fois, une diffusion colorée le long des vaisseaux rétiniens. L'association avec un engainement blanc des gros troncs artériels a été constatée 19 fois, dont 5 fois en l'absence d'atrophie optique.

Evolution

Vingt fonds d'yeux, chez 10 sujets, ont eu un examen de contrôle avec angiographie en janvier 76, 27 mois après le premier examen. Il s'agissait de malades traités par la Di-éthyl-carbamazine à faible dose (50 mg par semaine), et en permanence, selon la méthode de l'un de nous (LOREAL, 1973).

Quatorze fonds d'yeux, chez 8 sujets, n'ont montré acun signe d'évolution tant sur le plan fonctionnel, qu'ophthalmoscopique et angiographique. Les lésions présentées étaient variables, allant de l'atteinte discrète aux formes terminales.

Six globes, chez 4 sujets, ont évolué. Deux concernaient une forme terminale (chorio-rétinite de Ridley). Deux sont présentés ici en illustration: il ságit d'une forme de début à placode temporale isolée qui s'est légèrement élargie (obs. 39, fig. 1), les lésions de l'autre oeil ne variant pas. L'autre cas est une forme temporo-annulaire bipolaire dont les foyers se sont discrètement agrandis (obs. 40, fig. 5). Enfin, sur 2 yeux, les lésions épithéliales n'ont pas varié alors que les papilles se décoloraient.

Trop peu de sujets ont été controlés pour que l'on puisse expliquer les raisons de ces évolutions différentes. Cependant, une raison thérapeutique pourrait être retenue: Les 8 patients (14 yeux) chez lesquels nous n'avons pas trouvé d'évolution en angiographie étaient parasitologiquement blanchis (SNIPP quantitatif négativé, absence de microfilaires dans la chambre antérieure après massage).

A l'opposé les sujets qui ont montré une évolution de leur lésion se sont averés présenter un SNIPP hyper-positif et des microfilaires dans la chambre antérieure. On peut penser que ces derniers sujets ont eu un traitement insuffisant.

Ces éléments et leur groupement ont des aspects variables: L'aspect le plus fréquent est le type 'pommelé' (LAGRAULET, 1969; MONJUSIAU et al., 1965) constitué de fines taches irrégulières donnant à l'ensemble un aspect rugueux, granité ou en 'mie de pain'. On peut appeler ces lésions le 'pommelé en secteur'.

En angiographie, l'augmentation du contraste donne à ces atteintes atrophiques uns aspect brillant, poreux, en pierre ponce, nettement défini et invariable (fig. 4).

Les autres types de lésions tachetées en secteur sont plus rares (8 fois sur 73 atteintes): à éléments ponctués, ronds, réguliers, de même aspect atrophique, clair évoquent des microdrüses ou un aspect de 'ponctuée albescente' ou encore un aspect plus grossièrement mais régulièrement moucheté.

Topographie

Un élément essentiel est la localisation particulière de ces lésions limitées:

Le foyer temporal externe para-maculaire, en îlot, placard ou pommelé est la localisation quasi-constante. Cette zone est, en effet, toujours interessée dans les formes étendues ou généralisées (27 cas), elle participe 45 fois sur 46 aux atteintes localisées; elle apparait enfin comme unique lésion chorioépithéliale dans 21 fundus.

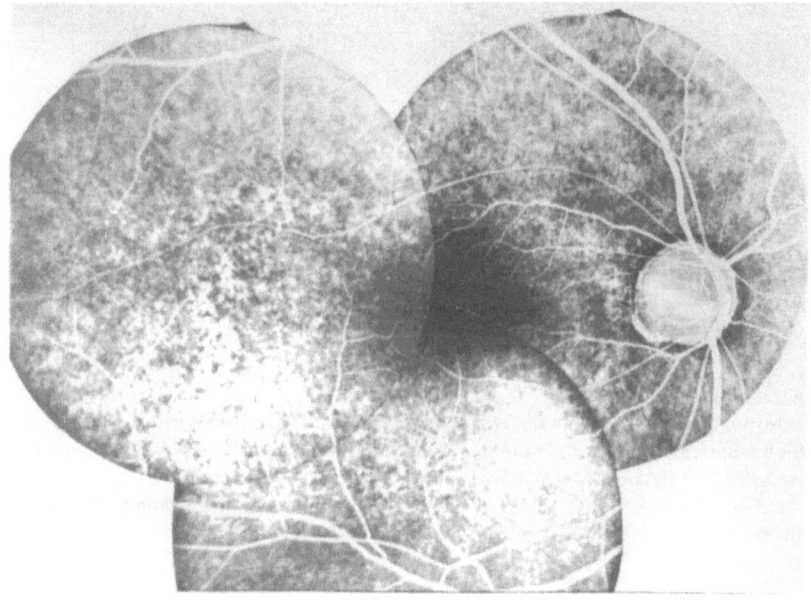

Fig. 4. *Observation 58·* Homme de 40 ans. Novembre 1973, A.V.O.D. 0,9, T.O.: 14. Microfilaires dans la chambre antérieure et sur la cristalloide postérieure. Pommelé paracentral à prédominance temporale. Papille décolorée. Janvier 1976. A.V. 0,4, T.O.: 14;5 microfilaires sur la cristalloide postérieure. Angio: pommelé et atrophie optique identique à précédemment.

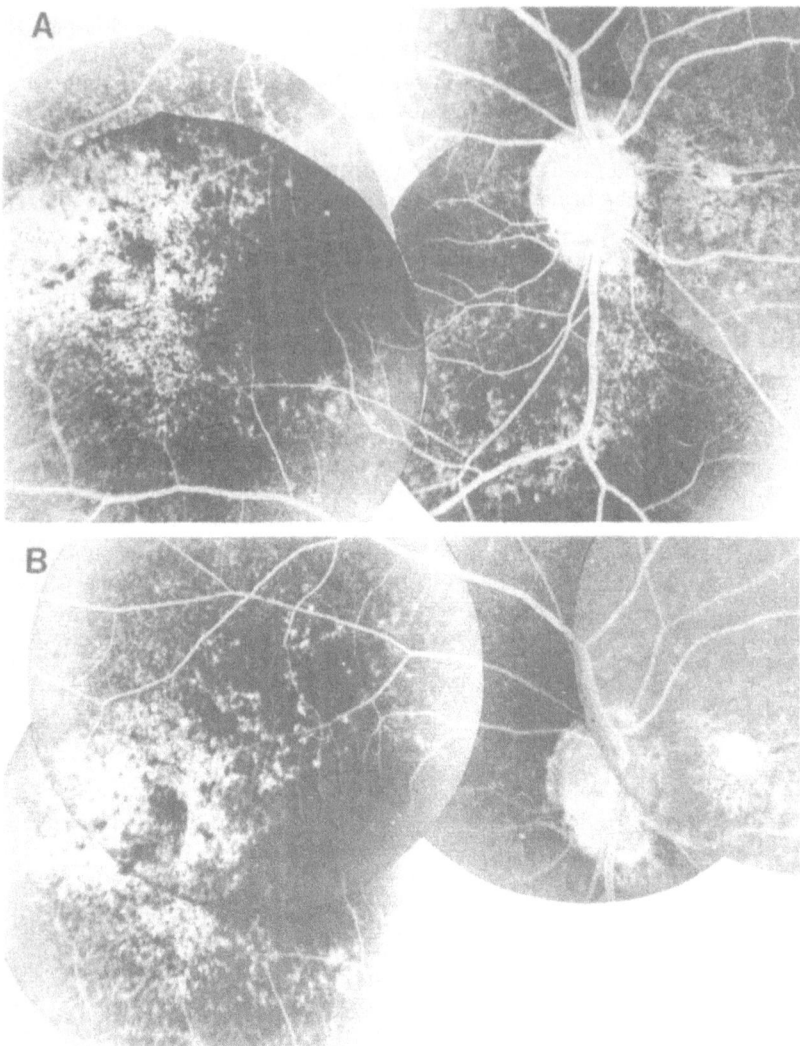

Fig. 5. *Observation 40:*
A. Novembre 1973, homme de 37 ans, A.V.O.D. 0,8. Microfilaires dans la cornée, la chambre antérieure et le vitré antérieur. Fluo: pommelé annulaire bipolaire avec placode temporale et nasale parapapillaire. Papille normale.
B. Janvier 1976, A.V. 0,4, papille décolorée, plus sombre en angiographie. Elargissement du placard temporal et nasal sans modification du pommelé.

COMMENTAIRES

Ces lésions limitées peuvent apparaitre comme des lésions initiales, sans que l'on puisse exclure comme modes de début une atteinte d.emblée plus généralisée.
   La localisation paramaculaire externe est rencontrée de façon constante,

soit isolée (21 cas sur 73), soit associée à une atteinte para-centrale plus ou moins annulaire, ou à des formes plus extensives. Il faut noter aussi la relative fréquence de la localisation péri-papillaire. Cette topographie a été retrouvée par d'autres auteurs, notamment BUDDEN (1973) et BIRD et al. (1976).

Ces lésions ont des corrélations anatomiques, elles correspondent aux orifices de pénétration des vaisseaux ciliaires postérieurs, particulièrement à celui de l'artère ciliaire longue postéro-externe. Les coupes histopathologiques de NEUMANN & GUNDERS (1973) ont montré la présence constante de microfilaires mortes le long de la gaine de ce vaisseau. On peut donc penser qu'il existe un rapport direct entre les voies de pénétration des microfilaires, la libération possible de toxines microfilariennes et le lieu d'élection des lésions initiales.

Par ailleurs, ont sait que dans l'onchocercose cutanée, la migration pigmentaire à un stade tardif est un phénomène habituel. On rencontre chez les vieux onchocerquiens des vitiligos importants, souvent contemporains des lésions chorio-rétiennes. Cette similitude dans la dystrophie pigmentaire du derme et du tapetum pourrait procéder du même mécanisme: soit allergie directe à l'antigène microfilarien, déterminant une chorio-capillarite, soit indirectement par épithéliopathie libératrice de pigment modifié et allergie secondaire de la choriorétine à ce pigment.

RESUME

Des angiographies systématiques réalisées sur 64 onchocerquiens confirmés (116 yeux) au Mali, et un contrôle de 20 yeux 27 mois après, donnent une appréciation de la morphologie, de la topographie et de l'évolution possible des lésions chorio-épithéliales. Un aspect d'atrophie progressive de l'épithélium pigmentaire et de la chorio-capillaire est constant. Il n'y a pas de symptome d'inflammation aigüe ou d'oedème ischémique.

La principale lésion initiale est située dans la région paramaculaire externe. Lésion chorio-épithéliale isolée dans 29% des cas, elle apparait comme un petit îlot atrophique ou un triangle pommelé. Elle peut être au premier plan mais associée (33%) à des lésions atrophiques péri-papillaires ou périmaculaires en croissant ou en couronne.

Cette topographie particulière correspond aux points de pénétration trans-sclérale des vaisseaux ciliaires postérieurs et particulièrement de la ciliaire longue postéro externe.

La pathogénie proposée pourrait être une vascularite allergique à l'antigène micro-filarien, puis secondairement une auto-immunité au pigment modifié.

SUMMARY

Systematic angiography performed on 64 confirmed onchocerquian (116 fundus) at Bamako (Mali), and a 27 month follow-up study on 10 cases, gave an appreciation of morphology, topography and possible evolution of chorioepithelial lesions. An aspect of progressive atrophy of pigment epithelium and choriocapillary, then of large choroidal vessels, is constant. There is no symptom of acute inflammation or ischemic oedema, no leakage. The chief initial lesion begins in paramacular outer region. Isolated chorioepithelial lesion in 29% of cases, it seems like a little atrophic islet, or a mottled triangle. It may be preeminent but connected (33%) with atrophic perimacular or peripapillary crescent or crown. The spread lesions concern 37% of cases. This external paramacular localization corresponds to the point of transcleral penetration of external posterior long ciliary artery, chief microfilarian biological cul de sac of posterior pole.

Ten patients (20 eyes) have been checked after 27 months, only six eyes have suffered a light neighbourhood evolution, which is perhaps linked with treatment.

The proposed pathogenesis would be allergic vascularitis to microfilarian antigen, then a secondary auto-immunity to the changed pigment.

BIBLIOGRAPHIE

BIRD, A.C., ANDERSON, J. & FUGLSANG, H. Morphology of posterior segment lesions of the eye in patients with onchocerciasis. *Brit. J. Ophthal.* 60: *2-20* (1976).

BUDDEN, F.H. Corresp. *Amer. J. Ophthal.* 76: *1027-1028* (1973).

LAGRAULET, J. Parasitoses oculaires: onchocercose. *Clin. Ophtal.* 5: *189-200* (1969).

LOREAL, E. Etat actuel du traitement et de la prophylaxie de l'onchocercose. Document interne, O.C.C.G.E., I.O.T.A. 73 (III) (1973).

METGE, P., CHOVET, M., CAZENAVE, P. & LOREAL, E. Lésions choriorétiniennes localisées dans l'onchocercose. *Méd. Trop.* 34-5: *625-632* (1974).

METGE, P. & CHOVET, M. Angiographie du fond d'oeil dans l'onchocercose. *Bul. Mém. Soc. Fr. Ophtal.* Masson-Paris: *67-74* (1975).

MONJUSIAU, A.G., LAGRAULET, J., D'HAUSSY, R. & GOCKEL, C.W. Aspects ophtalmologiques de l'onchocercose au Guatémala et en Afrique Occidentale. *Bull. Org. Mond. Santé* 32: *339-355* (1965).

NEUMAN, E. & GUNDERS, A.E. Pathogenesis of the posterior segment lesion of ocular onchocerciasis. *Amer. J. Ophthal.* 75 (1): *82-89* (1973).

Mots clefs:

Onchocercose
Chorio-épithéliopathie
Angiographie

Adresse des Auteurs:
22, rue Bel Air
13006 Marseille
France

DOMINANT MACULAR DYSTROPHIES: CYSTOID MACULAR EDEMA AND BUTTERFLY DYSTROPHY

AUGUST F. DEUTMAN, M.D.

(Nijmegen, The Netherlands)

Since 1967 I have been interested in the study of hereditary macular dystrophies (DEUTMAN, 1971). Much has changed since the quotation of DUKE-ELDER (1967): 'The many different clinical pictures described as heredomacular dystrophies probably represent phenotypical manifestations of a fundamentally single dystrophic process and not a number of autonomous lesions'.

Today, we know that there are many different hereditary dystrophies of the macula. To study macular dystrophies adequately, it is of paramount importance to do the whole battery of retinal function tests, such as visual acuity, visual fields, photopic and scotopic electroretinography, electrooculography, dark adaptation studies and colour vision studies. Furthermore it is needless to say that fluorescein angiography is necessary to line out the anatomic lesions more precisely.

During the last two years we have seen in our department 5 different pedigrees with a quite unusual condition, characterized by cystoid macular edema in most younger individuals and atrophic macular dystrophy in most of the older individuals. Personally I studied 3 of these pedigrees, in which the inheritance pattern of the macular dystrophy appeared to be autosomal dominant (Fig. 1). Some of the features of this dystrophy were presented already at the Macular Workshop in Bath (April 1974), at the American Academy Meeting (Dallas 1975) and at the Dedication of the new Bascom Palmer Eye Institute in Miami (January 1976).

This dominant type of cystoid macular edema is furthermore characterized by moderate decrease in visual acuity during the cystoid edema stage (Fig. 2, 3, 4) and poor acuity of around 0.1 during the atrophic stage (Fig. 5, 6), moderate to high hyperopia, often in combination with astigmatism, strabismus and whitish punctate opacities in the vitreous body. All capillaries in the posterior pole may be dilated and this phenomenon is most obvious around the fovea and the disk. The retinal arteries and veins and peripheries are grossly normal.

The electroretinogram (ERG) is also normal, but the electro-oculogram (EOG) is in most cases definitely subnormal.

Colour vision shows a blue-yellow defect in the early stages of the disease process due to the macular edema and a red-green defect with decreased red sensitivity later on, indicating receptor damage. There appears to be a diffuse disturbance of the retinal pigment epithelium, combined with a prob-

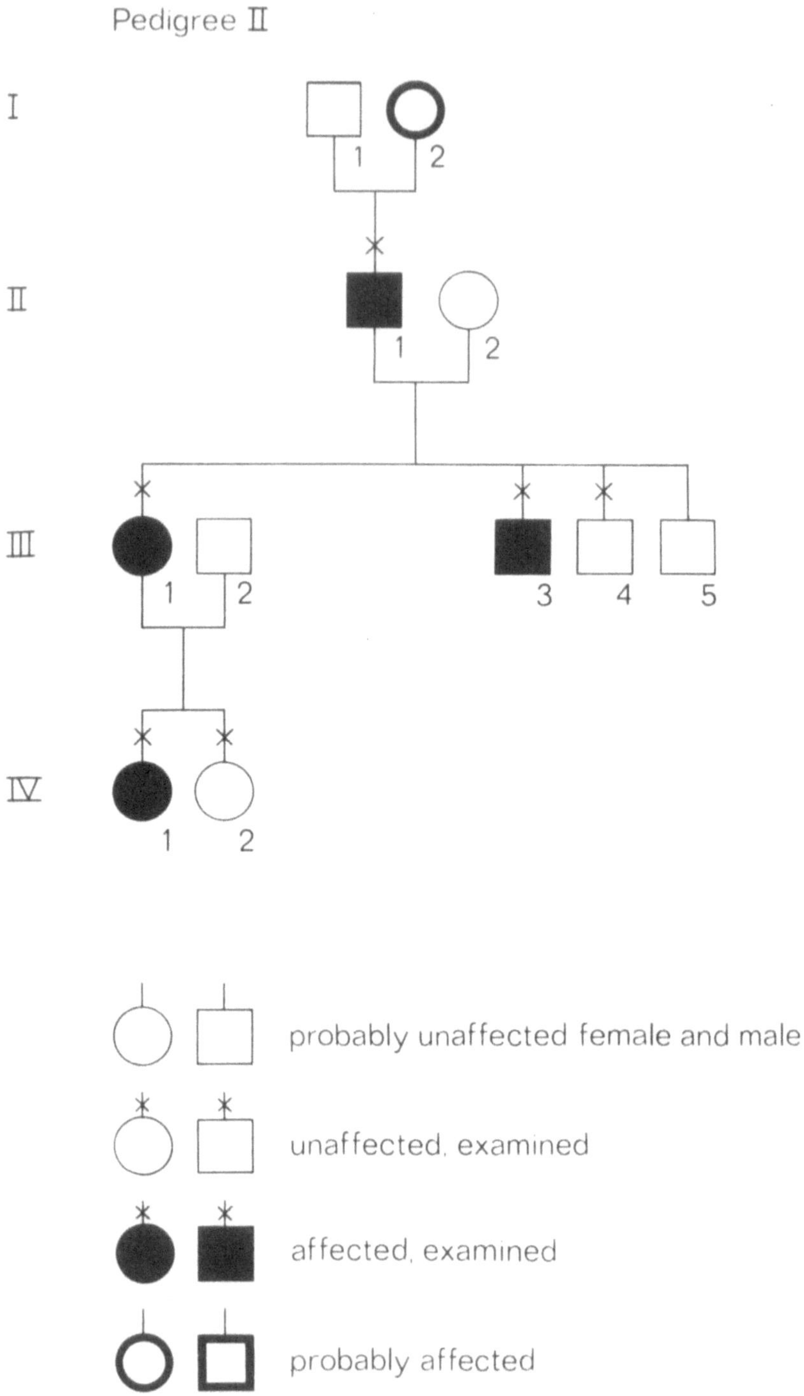
Pedigree II
I
II
III
IV
probably unaffected female and male
unaffected, examined
affected, examined
probably affected

Fig. 1. Pedigree of family with cystoid macular edema, dominantly inherited.

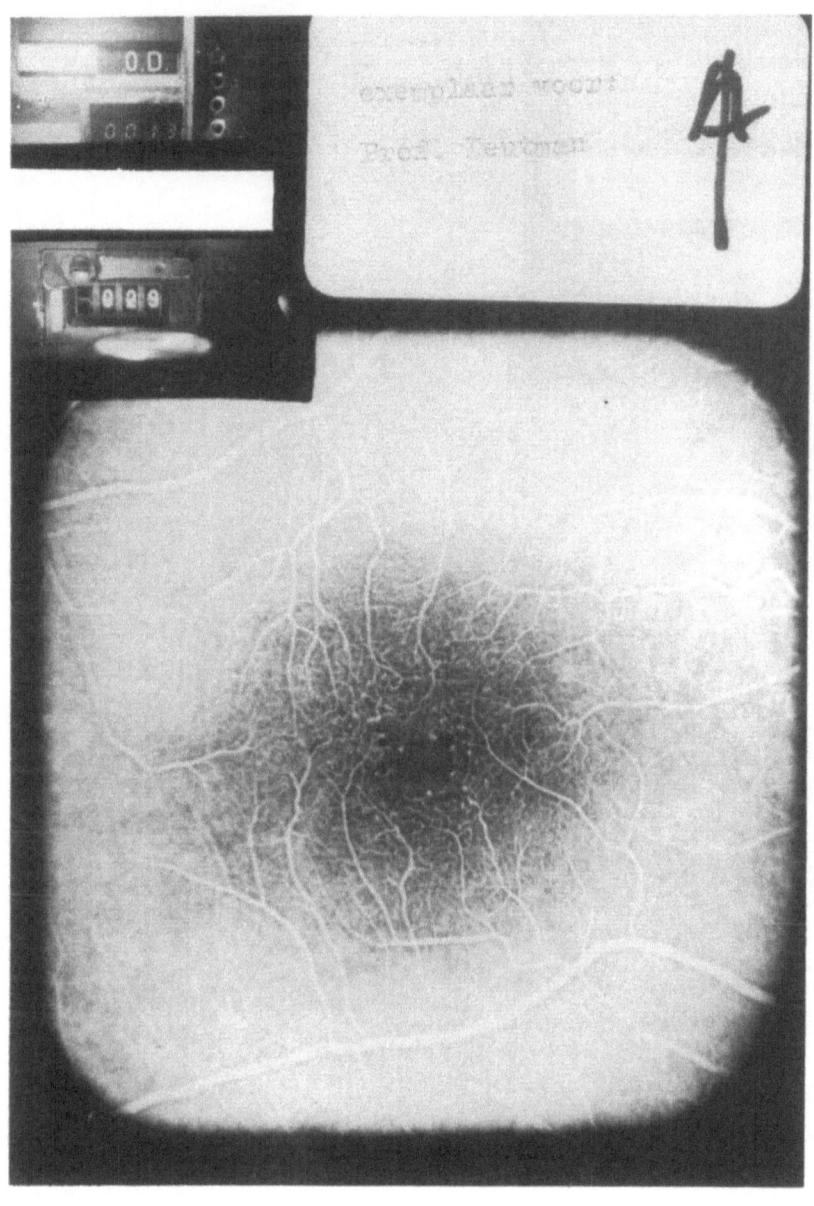

Fig. 2 abcd. Cystoid macular edema, dominantly inherited in a 10-year old girl. Note the dilated and leaking perimacular capillaries.

417

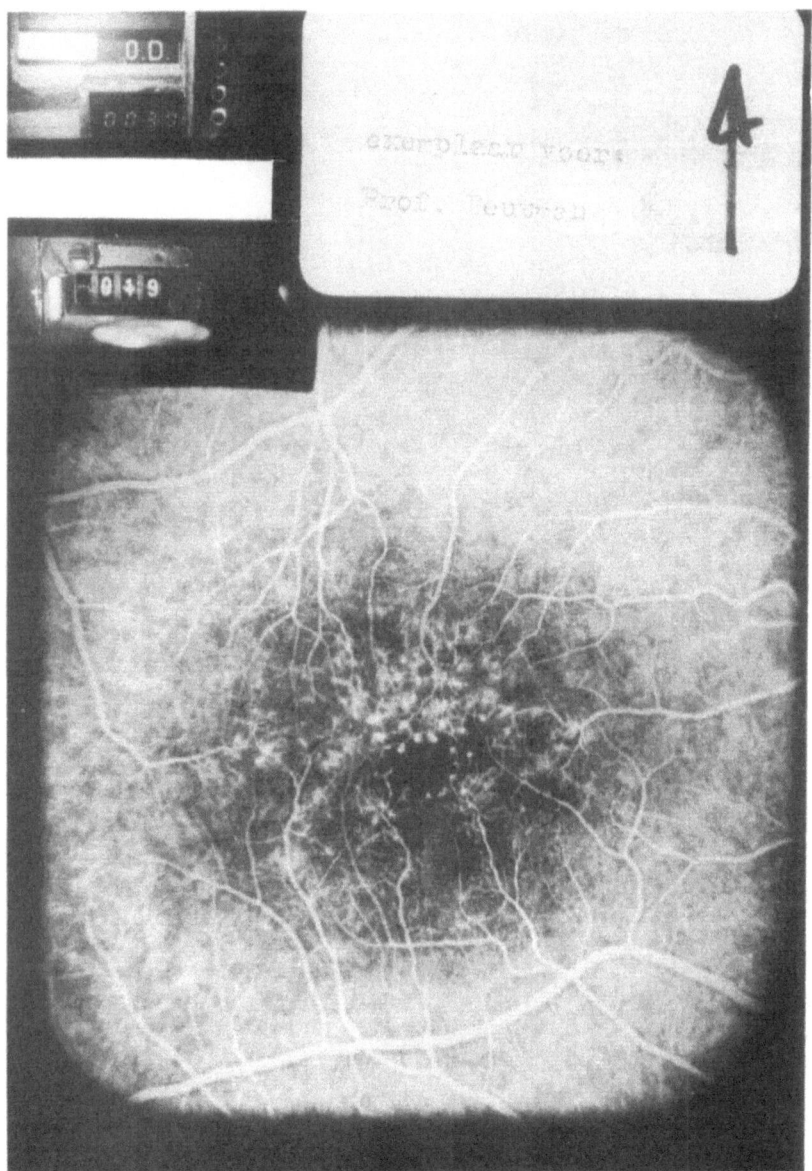

Fig. 2B.

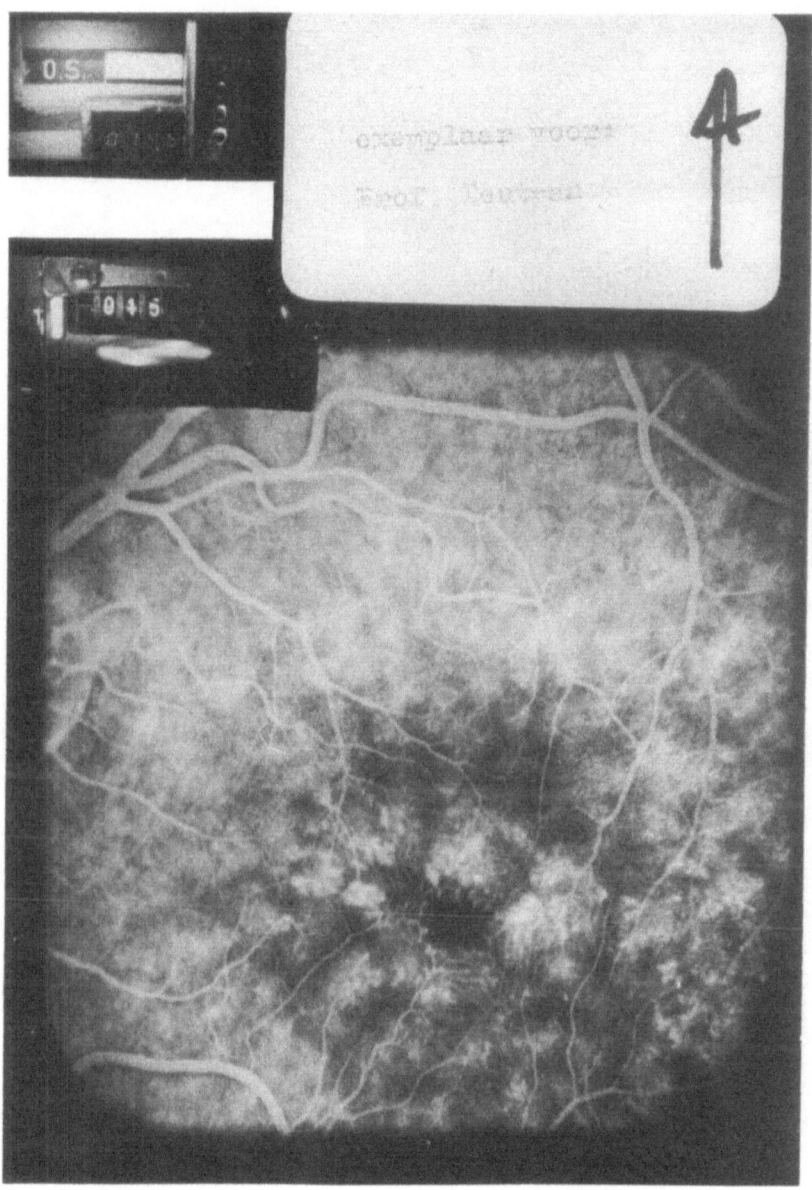

Fig. 2C.

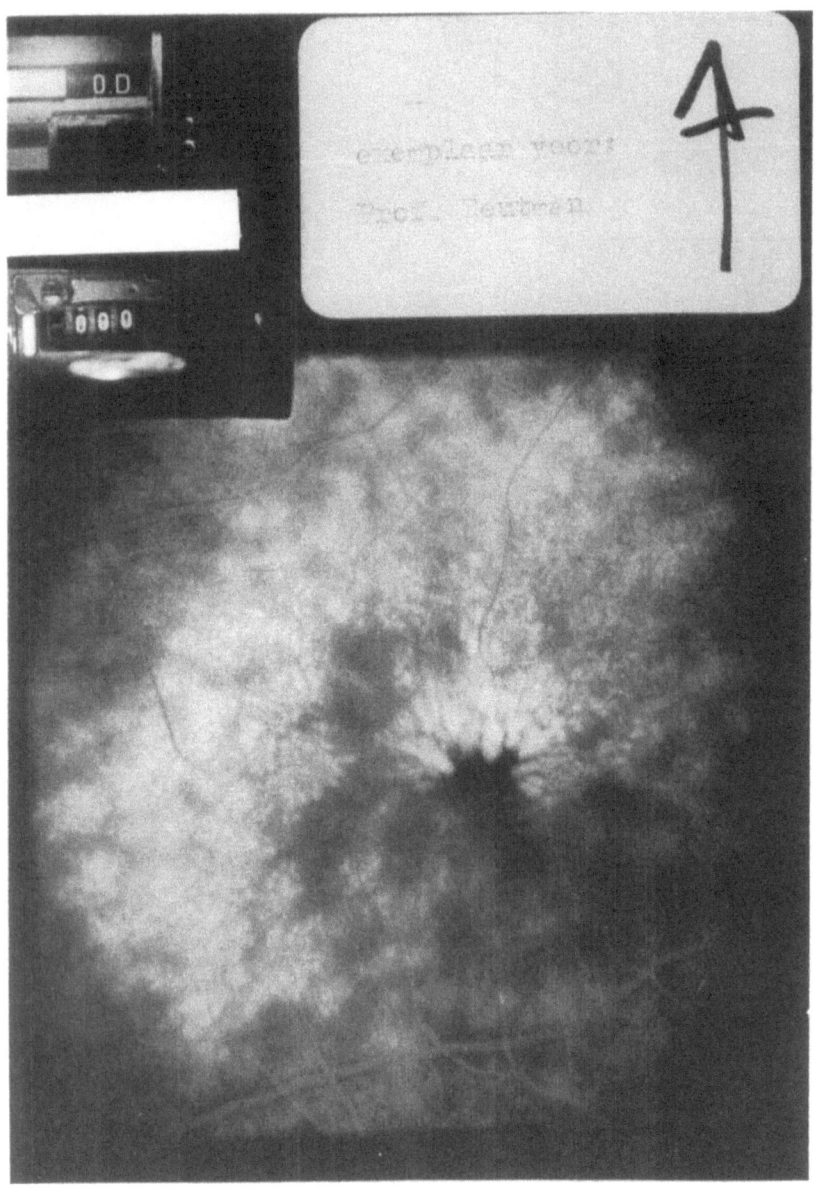

Fig. 2D.

ably secondary type of retinal capillary dilation with leakage. This is well known and has often been noticed in the cystoid macular edema of retinitis pigmentosa (FFYTCHE, 1972), but it is not too common in hereditary macular dystophies.

Like the autosomal dominant vitelliform dystrophy (Best) (DEUTMAN, 1969) and the dominant butterfly dystrophy (DEUTMAN et al., 1970) we have here the rare occasion of a macular dystrophy with a subnormal EOG and a normal ERG.

Other clear dominant macular dystrophies are dominant drusen (DEUT-MAN & JANSEN, 1970), central choroidal dystrophy (SORSBY & CRICK, 1953), pseudo-inflammatory dystrophy (SORSBY et al., 1949), cone dystrophy (KRILL & DEUTMAN, 1972; KRILL et al., 1973) and benign concentric annular macular dystrophy (DEUTMAN, 1974). HAMPTON LEFLER et al. (1971) presented a few years ago another clearly separate type of dominant macular dystrophy with a very polymorphous picture, showing drusen in some and a roundish atrophic reaction in others.

Subretinal neovascularisation may also occur in that condition and this has also been seen in patients with vitelliform dystrophy.

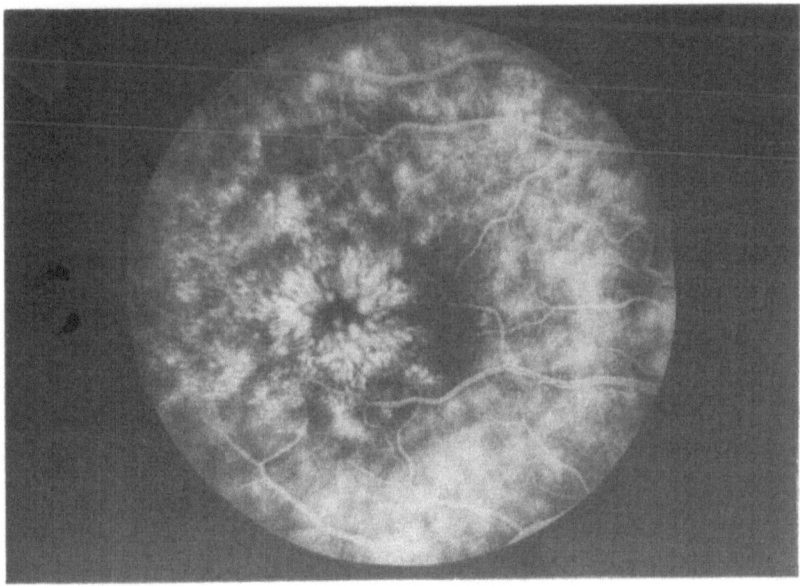

Fig. 3. Cystoid macular edema with autosomal dominant inheritance pattern. Right macula of IV-1 in pedigree depicted in Fig. 1. Note there is also leakage of capillaries around the macular area.

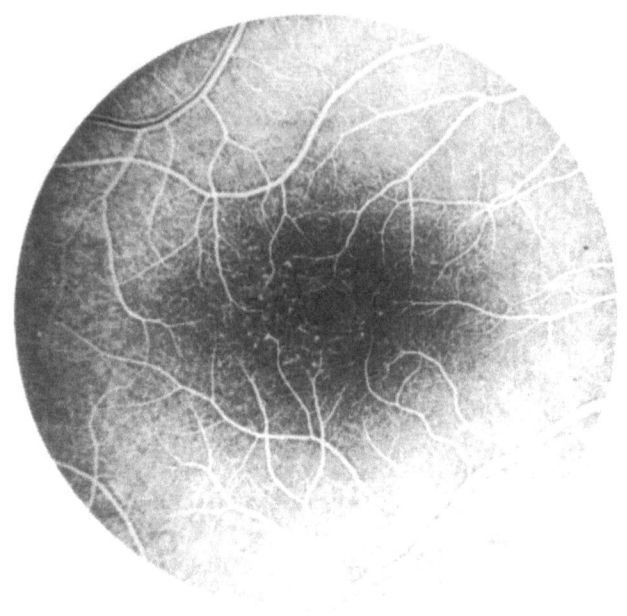

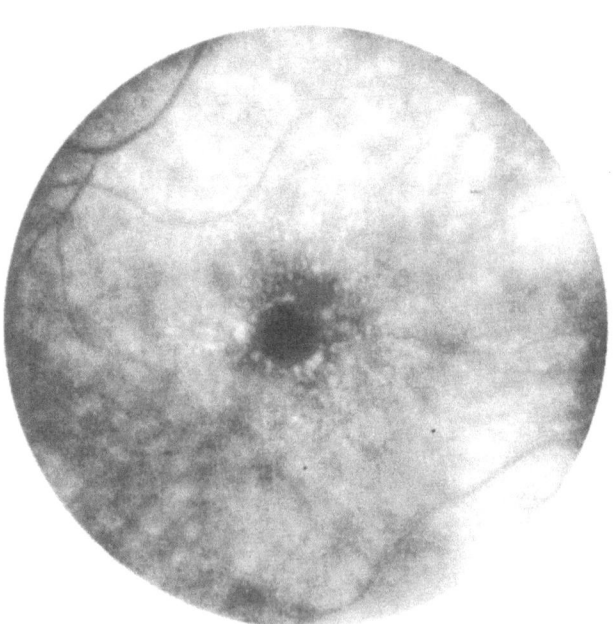

Fig. 4 ab. Another young girl, 9 years of age with a mild type of autosomal dominant macular edema with a subnormal electro-oculogram (EOG).

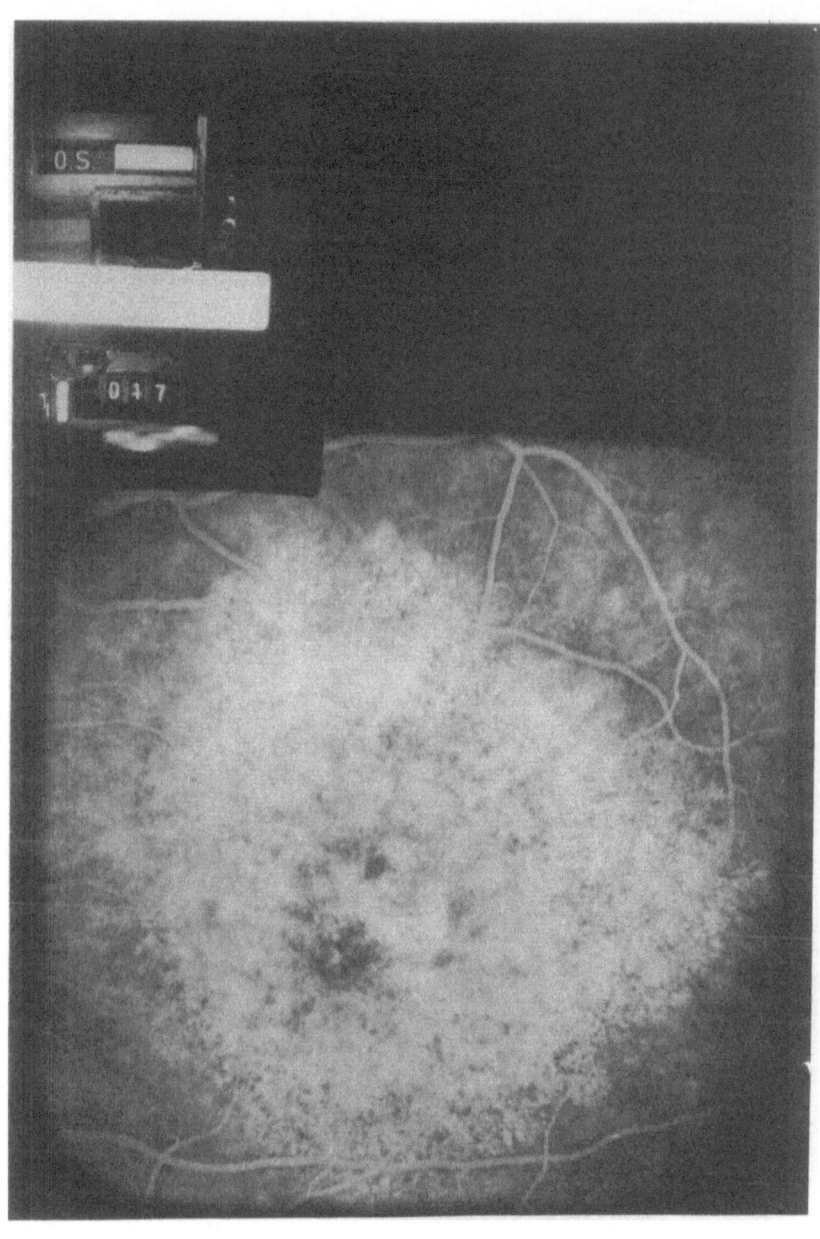

Fig. 5. Atrophic macular lesion in mother of patient whose macula is depicted in Fig. 2.

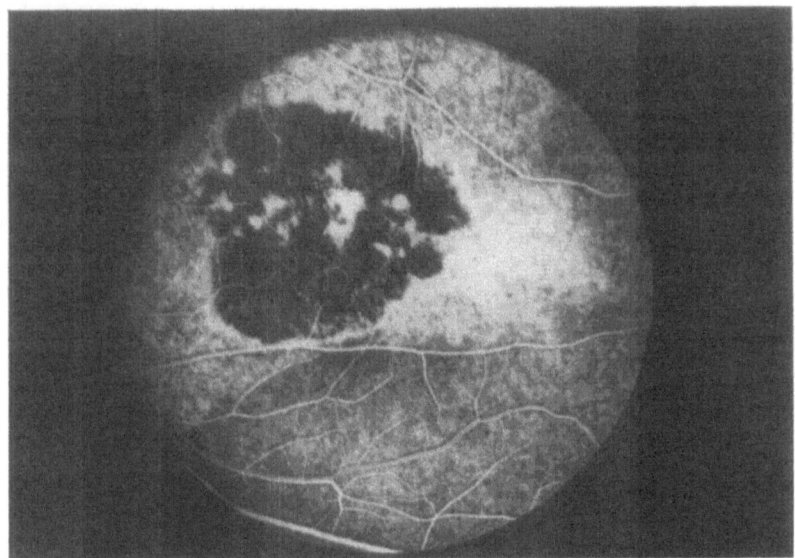

Fig. 6. Atrophic macular lesion with dilated choroidal capillaries in maternal uncle of the patient whose right macula is depicted in Fig. 3 (patient III-3 in the pedigree (Fig. 1)).

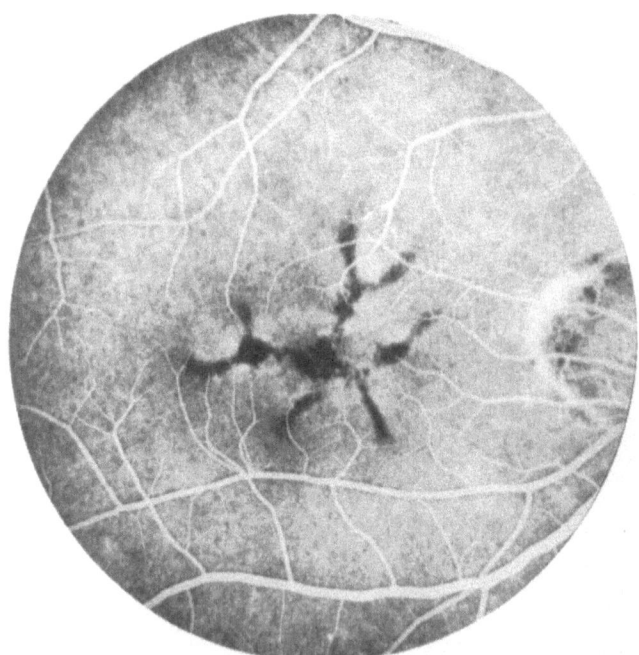

Fig. 7 abc. Butterfly dystrophy and retinal peripheral lesions in a 46-year-old patient with butterflyshaped macular pigment dystrophy. In 8 years time the macular lesions have clearly increased in size.

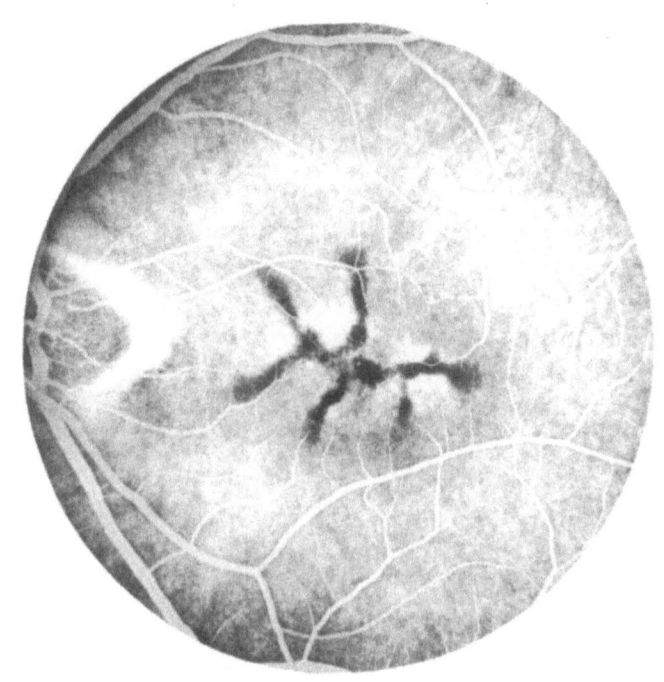

b)

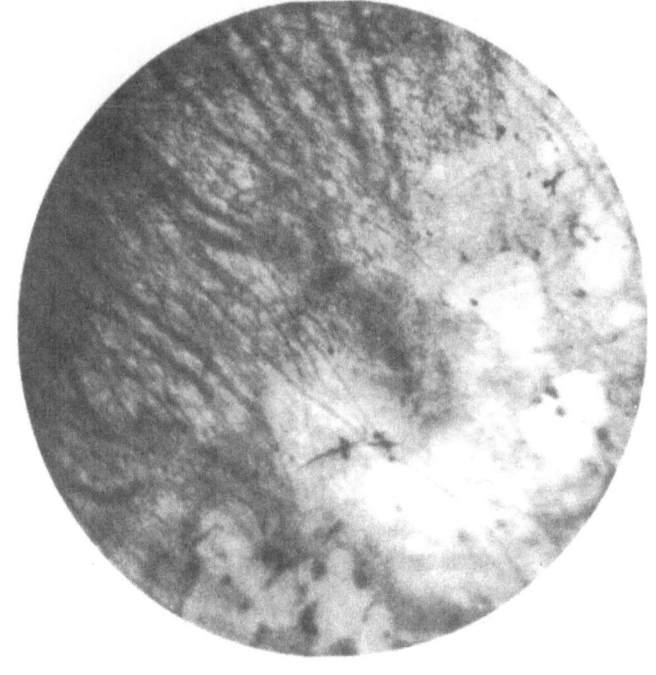

c)

425

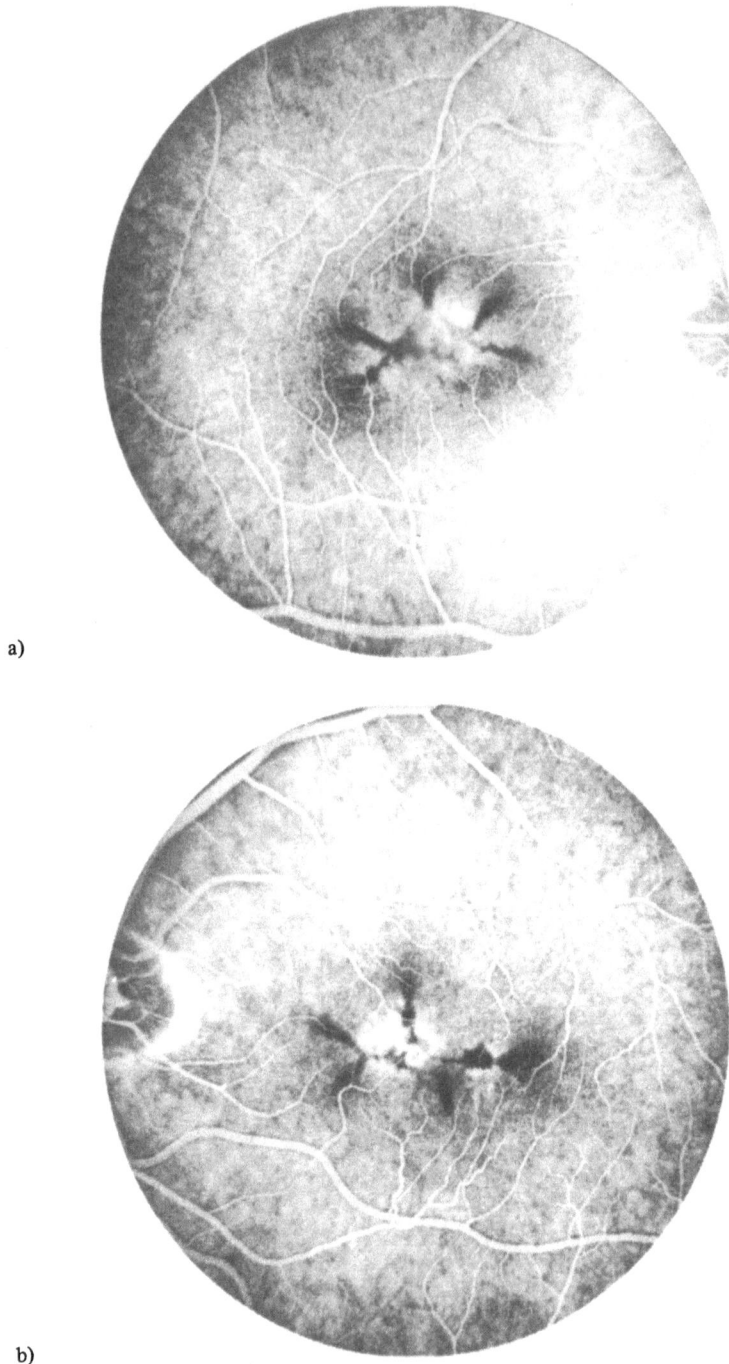

a)

b)

Fig. 8 abc. Butterfly macular dystrophy in a 51-year old man, also showing peripheral lesions.

426

I also had the opportunity to perform a follow-up study in most of the patients with butterflyshaped pigment dystrophy we examined originally in 1969 (DEUTMAN et al., 1970).

The pigmented macular lesions appeared to have extended in most patients towards the perifoveal area. Many reticular and spiderlike pigmented structures now could be seen in the retinal mid- and far periphery (Fig. 7, 8, 9). In the original study there were only a few peripheral retinal changes.

The retinal functions, though, had not changed considerably since the first study and the visual acuity was still 1.0 or only slightly less. The ERG was still normal, whereas the EOG was subnormal in most patients. Colour vision was only slightly affected.

Butterfly-shaped pigment dystrophy of the macula appears to be a very specific disorder, located at the level of the retinal pigment epithelium as is also indicated by the subnormal EOG.

Occasionally a sporadic case may be seen with butterfly like pigmentary lesions. Differenterial diagnosis has to be made with reticular pigmentary lesions secondary to drusen, angioid streaks and serous detachment of the retinal pigment epithelium. In myotonic dystrophy (Steinert) there may also be a macular lesion at the level of the retinal pigment epithelium resembling butterfly dystrophy (DEUTMAN, 1974).

The follow-up study indicated that it is possible that the macroreticular dystrophy described by MESKER et al. (1970) is the same disease process as butterfly dystrophy.

I will not be surprised if in the future more basically different macular dystrophies will be presented.

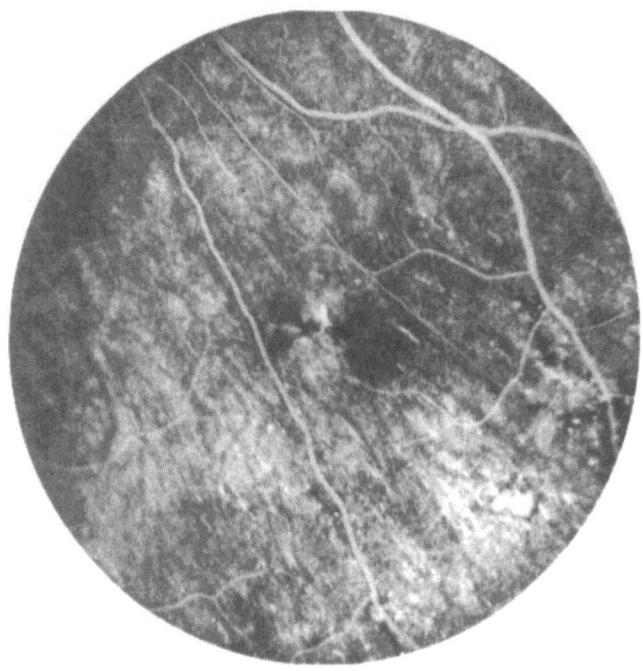

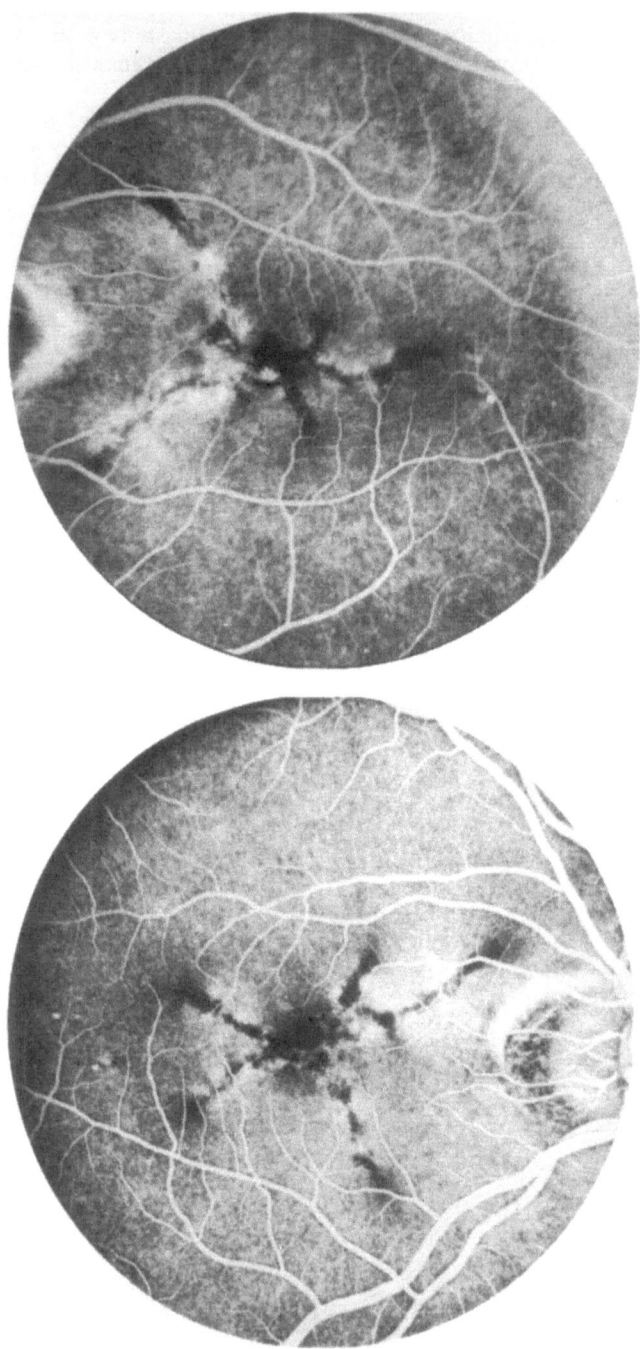

Fig. 9. The 50 -year old brother of the patient whose maculae are depicted in Fig. 7 and Fig. 8, showing diffuse peripheral reticular pigmentations and increased macular changes compared to 1969.

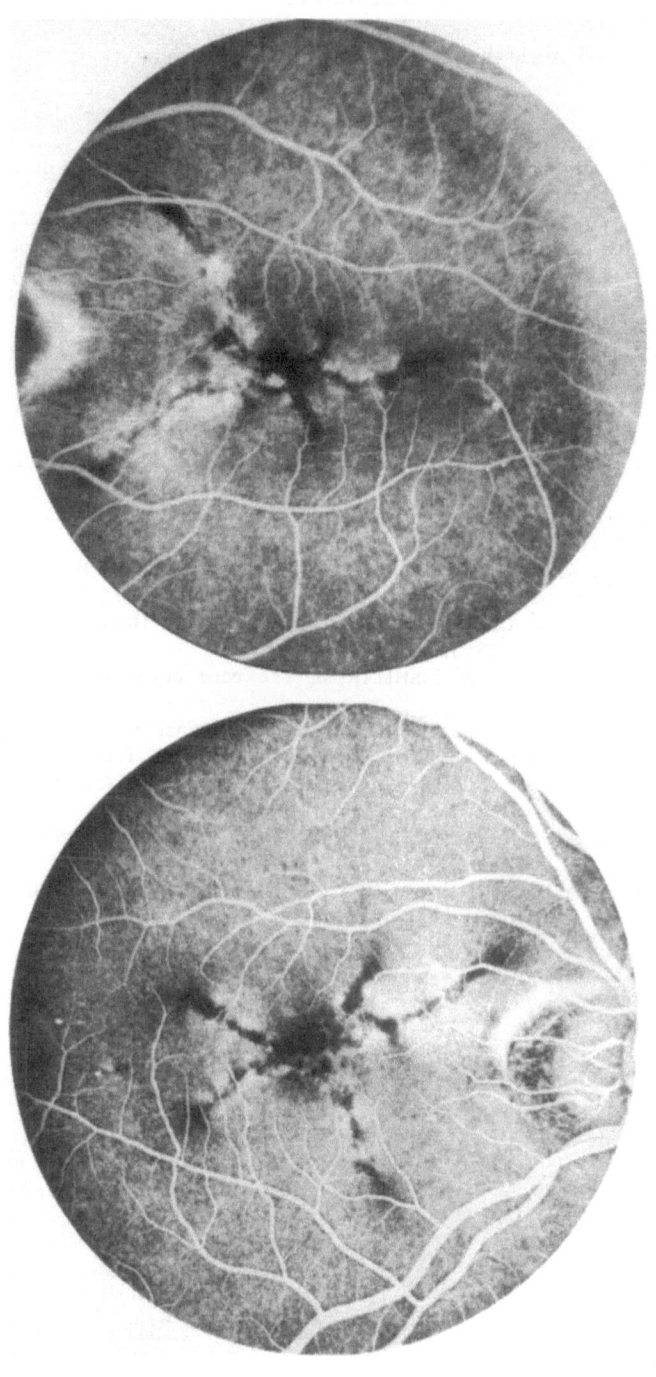

ACKNOWLEDGEMENTS

Mr. A.L. Aan de Kerk made the photographs.

REFERENCES

DEUTMAN, A.F. Electro-oculography in families with vitelliform dystrophy of the fovea. *Arch. Ophthalmol.* 81: *304* (1969).

DEUTMAN, A.F., VAN BLOMMESTEIN, J.D.A., HENKES, H.E., WAARDEN-BURG, P.J. & SOLLEVELD-VAN DRIEST, E. Butterfly-shaped pigment dystrophy of the fovea. *Arch. Ophthalmol.* 83: *558* (1970).

DEUTMAN, A.F. & JANSEN, L.M.A.A. Dominantly inherited drusen of Bruch's membrane. *Brit. J. Ophthal.* 54: *373* (1970).

DEUTMAN, A.F. Benign concentric annular macular dystrophy. *Amer. J. Opthalmol.* 78: *384* (1974).

DEUTMAN, A.F. The Craig Lecture 1974. Genetically determined retinal and choroidal disease. *Trans. Ophthal. Soc. U.K.* 94: *1014-1032* (1974).

DUKE-ELDER, SIR, S. System of Ophthalmology, Vol. X. Disease of the retina, p. *630*. Kimpton, London (1967).

FFYTCHE, T.J. Cystoid maculopathy in retinitis pigmentosa. *Trans. Ophthal. Soc. U.K.* 92: *265-283* (1972).

HAMPTON LEFLER, W., WADSWORTH, J.A.C. & SIDBURY, J.B., JR Hereditary macular degeneration and aminoaciduria. *Amer. J. Ophthalmol.* 71: *224* (1971).

KRILL, A.E. & DEUTMAN, A.F. Dominant macular degenerations. The cone dystrophies. *Amer. J. Ophthalmol.* 73: *352* (1972).

KRILL, A.E., DEUTMAN, A.F. & FISHMAN, M. The cone degenerations. *Doc. Ophthalmol.* 35: *1* (1973).

MESKER, R.P., OOSTERHUIS, J.A. & DELLEMAN, J.W. A retinal lesion resembling Sjögrens's dystrophia reticularis lammae pigmentosae retinae. Perspectives in ophthalmology, vol. 2, ed. J.E. Winkelman & R.A. Crone, pp. *40-45*, Excerpta Medica, Amsterdam (1970).

SORSBY, A. & CRICK, R.R. Central areolar choroidal sclerosis. *Brit. J. Ophthalmol.* 37: *129* (1953).

SORSBY, A., JOLL MASON, M.E. & GARDENER, N. A fundus dystrophy with unusual features. *Brit. J. Ophthalmol.* 33: *67* (1949).

Author's address:
University Eye Clinic
Philips van Leydenlaan 15
Nijmegen
The Netherlands

SECTOR RETINITIS PIGMENTOSA WITH CHRONIC DISC EDEMA

LOUISE A. COPE, M.D., VAN W. TEETERS, M.D.,
ROBERT P. BORDA, PH.D., & JOHN A. MCCRARY, III, M.D.

(Houston, USA)

INTRODUCTION

A familial syndrome is described which, to our knowledge, has not been previously reported. The entity is transmitted by the dominant mode of inheritance. It is characterized by an annular distribution of pigment, which predominates in the nasal and inferonasal retinal quadrants, and chronic edema of the optic nerve, progressing to optic atrophy. Edema of the optic nerve in any variant of retinitis pigmentosa (RP) has not been reported. We believe that the incidence of five cases in this family makes a unique syndrome. Because two of the members have been inadvertently studied for evidence of intracranial pathology, it was deemed necessary to report this family in the ophthalmic literature.

REPORT OF CASES

Case III-2, a 14-year old white male (Fig. 1), was thought to have bilateral papilledema and pigmentary retinopathy on routine fundus examination eight years ago. He was hospitalized for a neurosurgical work-up, which was

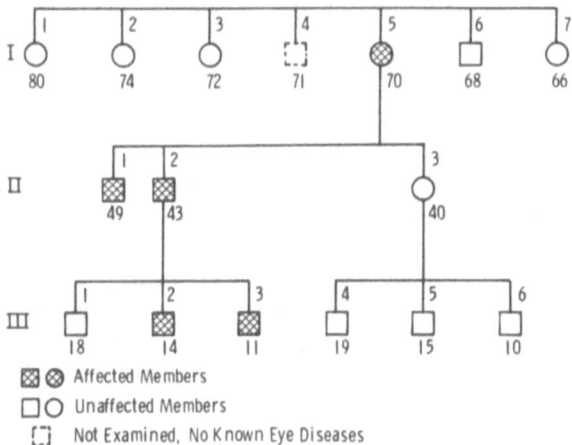

Fig. 1. Family tree, illustrating involvement of sector RP with disc edema in three generations.

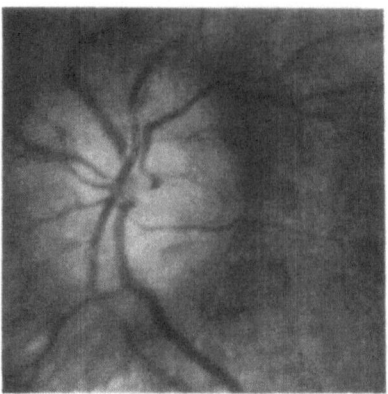

Fig. 2. Left eye of Case III-2

negative. He was discharged with a presumptive diagnosis of pseudotumor cerebri and followed as an outpatient.

The vision in both eyes without correction was 20/20. The positive slitlamp findings were a prominent Schwalbe's line, nasally and temporally, and numerous cellular-like particles, clumped especially in the posterior area of the vitreous. Both optic nerves were yellowish-pink and elevated (Fig. 2). There was a peripapillary rim of subretinal fluid. In the periphery, pigment clumping was apparent over 360 degrees. This degeneration extended posterior to the equator in the nasal and inferonasal quadrants. Fluorescein angiography showed marked leakage from the disc; this appearance had not changed over an eight-year period (Fig. 3). Angiography also showed marked vascular sclerosis and pigment epithelial atrophy in the involved periphery.

Case I-5, a 72-year old white female, began to gradually lose vision in both eyes fifteen years ago. She was felt to have RP and bilateral papilledema, and was hospitalized. The neurosurgical work-up was negative, and she was discharged with no definite diagnosis. The visual loss gradually continued over the years. Vision in the right eye was hand motion at four feet, and in the left eye, hand motion at one foot. Pertinent slit-lamp findings were a striking prominence of Schwalbe's line for 360 degrees and moderate numbers of cells in the vitreous, with predominance posteriorly. There was also syneresis, consistent with her age. Both discs were grayish-white and atrophic. There was severe chorioretinal atrophy in the periphery, with bone spicule formation extending to the disc from the nasal quadrant. There was no leakage of dye from the disc on angiography.

The other involved family members showed a similar type of pigmentary retinopathy and elevated, edematous discs. All but one had a prominent Schwalbe's line. They had no ocular complaints, and their vision was generally good. Angiography of the discs showed profuse leakage in the young and only moderate leakage in the older members (Fig. 4). The visual-field examinations showed both peripheral loss, corresponding to the approximate area of chorioretinal degeneration, and nerve-fiber-bundle defects, consistent with optic-nerve disease. The ERG showed normal photopic but abnormal scotopic responses (i.e., b-wave suppression following dark adaptation). The EOG was normal in all except the oldest member. The involved members were hospitalized for a complete medical evaluation. The only abnormality found was an elevated serum vitamin A level and a depressed serum carotene. A combination of conductive and labyrinthine deafness was found in all members tested.

COMMENT

The pattern of pigment dispersion seen in this family is consistent with sector retinitis pigmentosa. The dominant mode of inheritance and a propensity for involvement of the inferonasal quadrants are typical of sector RP (KÜPER, 1960). A complete annular involvement in the periphery has been described (BIETTI, 1937), and progression of the disease with age has also been reported (MANFREDINI, 1966). The subnormal scotopic ERG seen in this family is also consistent with sector RP, in which the ERG is never extinguished but decreases in amplitude as the retinal degeneration

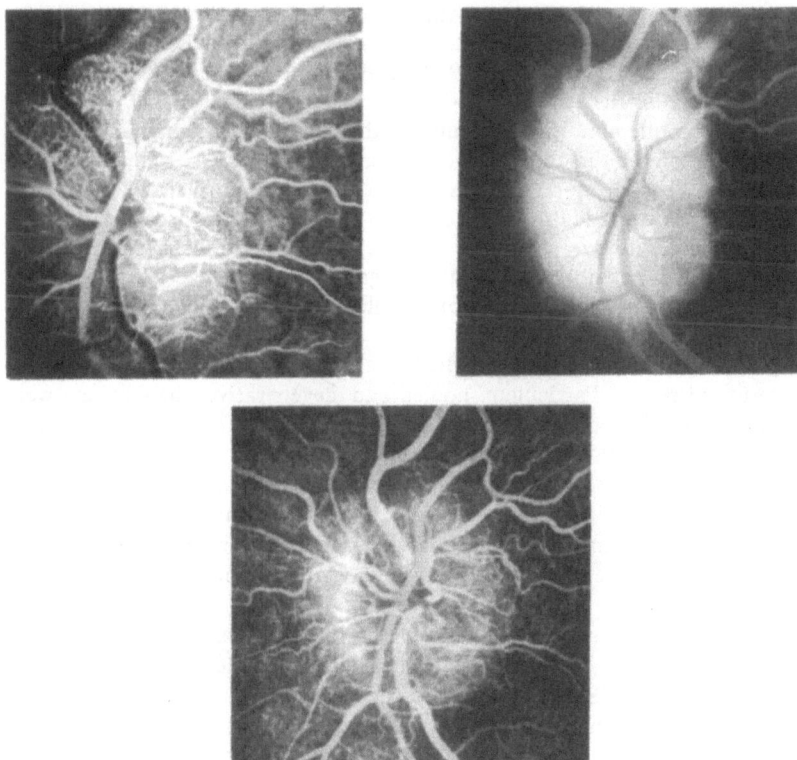

Fig. 3. (a) Early and late angiograms of Case III-2. (b) Early angiogram of Case III-2, eight years ago.

433

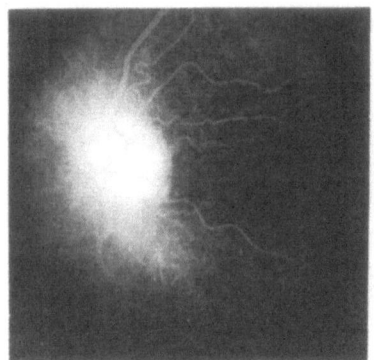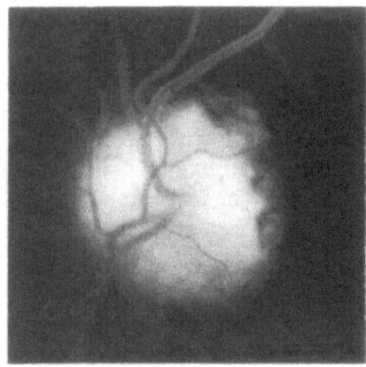

Fig. 4.   (a) Late angiogram of Case III-3. (b) Late angiogram of Case II-2.

progresses (HOMMER, 1959; KÜPER, 1960). The EOG has been reported to be abnormal in sector RP (BOTERMANS, 1972) but was found to be normal in all members of this family except the oldest.

To our knowledge, conductive deafness in combination with labyrinthine deafness has not been reported with sector RP. It is well known that labyrinthine deafness is often associated with classical RP in the recessive form (FRANCESCHETTI & KLEIN, 1954), and otosclerosis has been reported in cases of dominant RP (FRANCESCHETTI & FRANCOIS, 1974).

The metabolic abnormality found in this family (the high vitamin A and low carotene levels) is unusual. According to CAMPBELL et al. (1964) and SHEARER (1964), most patients with RP have subnormal levels of vitamin A and carotenoids in the blood. MIYATA (1964) and KRACHMER (1966) found, however, that the average vitamin A level in the blood of patients with RP is not significantly different from normal. To our knowledge, high vitamin A and low carotene values have not been reported in any variant of RP.

Three of five family members had small, uniformly sized particles in the posterior vitreous. Particulate bodies and degenerative changes are well known in RP (ELSCHNIG, 1904; PRUETT, 1975). Degeneration usually begins with fine, colories particles, seen throughout the vitreous, progressing in time to a collapse of the posterior vitreous, with a great reduction in volume, leaving behind a coarse matrix of interconnecting fibers. This family is different in that the cellular-like particles were concentrated posteriorly in the vitreous body, and there were no rope-like degenerative changes.

There are changes in the optic nerves in this family suggestive of drusen. Hyaline bodies of the disc have three etiological classifications (FRANCOIS & VERRIEST, 1958): (1) idiopathic cases occurring in otherwise normal eyes, with an irregularly dominant mode of transmission; (2) those associated with heredo-degenerative diseases, especially pigmentary retinopathy; and (3) those associated with acquired diseases of the globe and optic nerve, especially optic neuritis, papilledema, optic atrophy, glaucoma, and chorioretinitis. Drusen are known to cause visual-field loss and optic atrophy

(FRANCOIS & VERRIEST, 1958; KAMIN, 1973). Drusen near the disc surface have been repeatedly shown to autofluoresce; however, deeply buried drusen do not (KELLEY, 1974). The discs of three of the family members have an ophthalmoscopic appearance that is compatible with drusen. The drusen of the disc in one person (Case II-2) did autofluoresce. The visual fields demonstrating optic-nerve involvement are also compatible with nerve-fiber-bundle defects caused by drusen. Although the discs in this family have the ophthalmoscopic appearance of drusen, angiography confirms the presence of edema by leakage into the peripillary subretinal space. In drusen alone, there is no leakage of dye onto the retina (SANDERS & FFYTCHE, 1967). The general leakage of fluorescein from the disc capillaries covers any uptake of dye from the drusen themselves. The combination of chronic edema and drusen in this family appears to lead to optic atrophy, as in Case I-5. The remaining family members will have to be followed to determine their ultimate visual function.

In conclusion, these family members represent a unique hereditary disorder, characterized by hearing loss of labyrinthine and conductive type, a prominent Schwalbe's line, cellular-like particles in the vitreous, fundus changes compatible with sector RP, and chronic edema of the optic nerve which appears to progress to optic atrophy.

ACKNOWLEDGMENTS

Many thanks to Marilyn Ekeroot for expert secretarial assistance and to Ditte Jacobsen and Johnny Justice for their excellent photographs.

REFERENCES

BIETTI, G. *Bull. Ocul.* 16: *159-1244* (1937).
BOTERMANS, C.H.G. Handbook of Clinical Neurology, Vol. 13: Neuroretinal Degenerations (P.J. Vinken & G.W. Bruyn, Eds.). American Elsevier, New York, pp. *179-182* (1972).
CAMPBELL, D.A., HARRISON, R. & TONKS, E.L. *Exp. Eye Res.* 3: *412-426* (1964).
ELSCHNIG, A. *Klin. Monatsbl. Augenheilkd.* 42: *429-525* (1904).
FRANCESCHETTI, A. & FRANCOIS, J. Chorioretinal Heredodegenerations. Charles C Thomas, Springfield, Ill., p. *878* (1974).
FRANCESCHETTI, A. & KLEIN, D. *J. Genet. Hum.* 3: *175-183* (1954).
FRANCOIS, J. & VERRIEST, G. *Ophthalmologica* 136: *289* (1958).
HOMMER, K. *Graefes Arch. Ophthalmol.* 161: *16-26* (1959).
KAMIN, D.F. *Arch. Ophthalmol.* 89: *359-362* (1973).
KELLEY, J. *Arch. Ophthalmol.* 92: *263-264* (1974).
KRACHMER, J.H. *Arch. Ophthalmol.* 75: *661-664* (1966).
KÜPER, J. *Klin. Monatsbl. Augenheilkd.* 136: *97-102* (1960).
MANFREDINI, U. *Ann. Ottal.* 42: *669-678* (1966).
MIYATA, M. *Acta Soc. Ophthalmol. Jap.* 68: *1666-1675* (1974).
PRUETT, R.C. *Arch. Ophthalmol.* 93: *603-668* (1975).
SANDERS, M.D. & FFYTCHE, T.J. *Trans. Ophthalmol. Soc. U.K.* 87: *457* (1967).
SHEARER, A.C.J. *Exp. Eye Res.* 3: *427-438* (1964).

Authors' address:
3803 University Boulevard
Houston, Texas 77005
USA

DISCUSSION

Dr Brégeat: Je voudrais poser une question à Mme Cope à propos de sa communication sur la rétinite pigmentaire avec oedème papillaire chronique. Ne pense-t-elle pas qu'il s'agit plutôt de faux oedème papillaire avec druses? Alors le cas n'est pas rare comme elle a eu l'air de le penser et si sur certaines angiographies on n'a pas vu de druses apparaître c'est qu'il s'agissait sans doute, au stade infra-druses, de névroglies immatures de la papille. Dans la famille on voit apparaître des druses et même les scotomes triangulaires qu'elle nous a montré sont en faveur de druses. Le petit oedème que l'on a trouvé autour de la papille serait un oedème réactionnel, car les druses qui évoluent donnent un peu d'oedème et même parfois des hémorragies. Je crois qu'il faudrait dire avec faux oedème papillaire et alors le cas est assez fréquent, car les druses accompagnent très fréquemment les rétinites pigmentaires.

Dr Cope: I mentioned in my presentation that there is a high association of drusen with retinitis pigmentosa. But I have demonstrated unequivocal evidence of edema of the disc in this family. I showed an eleven year old male without ophthalmoscopic evidence of drusen who had marked leakage of fluorescein from the disc and into the retina. There are some discs which I presented in which drusen are probably present; for example, the forty-three year old male. I feel that chronic edema, of a still unknown etiology, is the primary process occurring in these discs and that the drusen are a secondary phenomenon. Dr François has described drusen secondary to optic neuritis, glaucoma and papilledema.

Dr Henkind: I do not think that drusen occur secondarily but that is neither here nor there. In a non selected series of cases done by Dr Friedman of our institution, drusen were found 17 times on 700 consecutive autopsies ... There is no evidence that drusen occur secondarily to papilledema. In our own group I think we have seen leakage from disc capillaries, which would make sense because there are vascular abnormalities in drusen. Even more than that it is peculiar that in your chronic papilledema, if that is what it is, there is no sheathing of the vessels, which is a very common finding. Further more, none of your cases showed any physiological cupping and this again is typical of drusen. If you use ultrasound you might pick up the drusen, in your cases. You may have a new entity, but I think, it is drusen you are dealing with.

Dr Cope: There was sheathing of the vessels in some of the discs I showed, especially in the forty-three year old and seventy year old family members. At any rate, true edema of the nervehead with leakage into the retina has not been reported in association with either drusen of the disc or retinitis pigmentosa. We need to observe more cases of these entities and watch them closely.

Mr Rubinstein: Dr Cope, you convinced at least one person, that is me, that you showed pictures of papilledema.

Dr Gass: I like to say that she convinced two people. She convinced me too. I also think that the patient may have drusen but the interesting thing is that the question has been raised whether indeed not all drusen may at depart be an extracellular deposit related to a vascular anomaly of the disc and what you are showing may just be a severe form of that abnormal permeability. The angiogram certainly demonstrated a marked dilatation of capillaries and marked staining in the retina, and whether this is caused by drusen or not I do not know. It is a very interesting case and quite different from the usual cases of drusen in a young child mistaken for increased intracranial pressure.

Mr Rubinstein: What you did not convince me about is: was it a case of retinitis pigmentosa?

Dr Cope: They were cases of sector retinitis pigmentosa. I come to this conclusion because of the sectorial predominance of the pigmentation inferonasally, because of the good vision despite marked pigment changes in all members except the oldest (who had poor vision from optic atrophy), and because of the subnormal ERG's. I believe this family represents a unique syndrome of sectorial retinitis pigmentosa with chronic disc edema.

LEAKAGE FROM RETINAL CAPILLARIES
IN HEREDITARY DYSTROPHIES

J.G.A. NOTTING & A.F. DEUTMAN

(Nijmegen, The Netherlands)

Fluorescence angiography (fluography) is of great help to establish the amount and extent of retinal pigment epithelium disturbance and choriocapillaris atrophy in various hereditary dystrophies (DEUTMAN, 1971). The retinal circulation in these cases has not been reported to show abnormal-

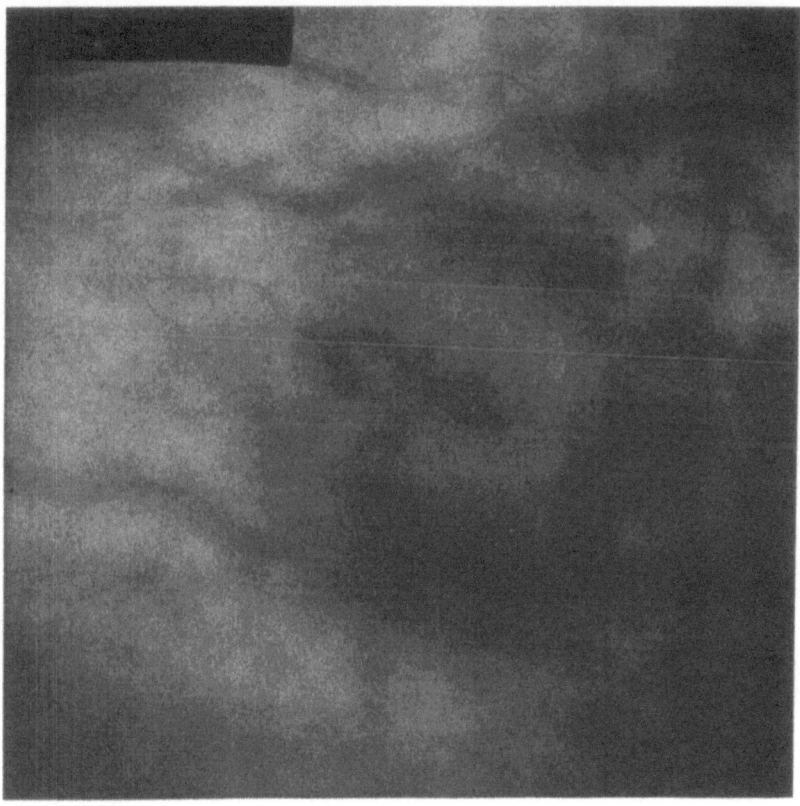

Fig. 1. Retinitis pigmentosa. Male aged 20. Late phase fluography showing cystoid macular edema.

ities, except in *retinitis pigmentosa* where retinal capillary dilatation and cystoid macular edema (CME) have been described by several authors (HYVÄRINEN, 1971; FFYTCHE, 1972; FRANÇOIS et al., 1972; METGE et al., 1974) (see Fig. 1).

In the past few years we examined in our clinic a number of patients with other hereditary dystrophies wherein involvement of the retinal microcirculation could be demonstrated fluographically.

In many cases of *Stargardt's disease* (atrophic macular dystrophy with fundus flavimaculatus) a generalized dilatation of the capillaries in the posterior pole can be seen (Fig. 2). In no instance, however, could we find any late dye leakage from these dilated vessels. In our opinion there is a real dilatation of the capillaries and not only an increased visibility due to the enhanced contrast (reduced background fluorescence).

Several cases of *X-linked juvenile retinoschizis* showed discrete or

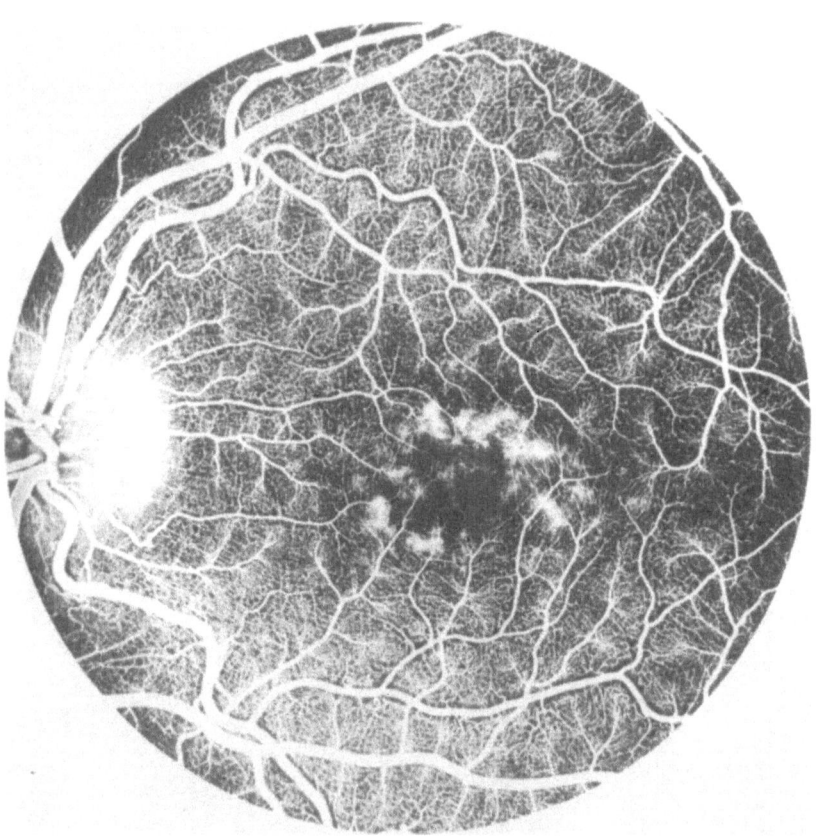

Fig. 2. Stargardt's disease (fundus flavimaculatus). Female aged 22. Extreme generalized capillary dilatation in the posterior pole. Late dye leakage does not occur from these capillaries.

marked pigment epithelium defects as well as dilatation and rarification of the retinal capillaries in the macular area (Fig. 3a). We observed no leakage from these vessels. In one of our cases however, there was late dye diffusion from small veins and dilated capillaries in a peripheral area surrounded by chorioretinal scars (Fig. 3b). We assume that this vasculopathy represents activity of the disease process in the periphery.

In a pedigree with *progressive cone (rod) dystrophy* we saw a girl aged 8 years, showing pigment epithelium defects in the macular area and dilated retinal capillaries in the posterior pole (Fig. 4a) as in fundus flavimaculatus. Her brother aged 17 years, had already progressed to the stage of an extensive atrophic macular lesion with extinguished E.R.G. Fluography in this case revealed a considerable capillary dilatation around the borders of the lesion, with late dye leakage (Fig. 4b, c) whereas no leakage in the central atrophic area could be seen. It is tempting to assume that during the pro-

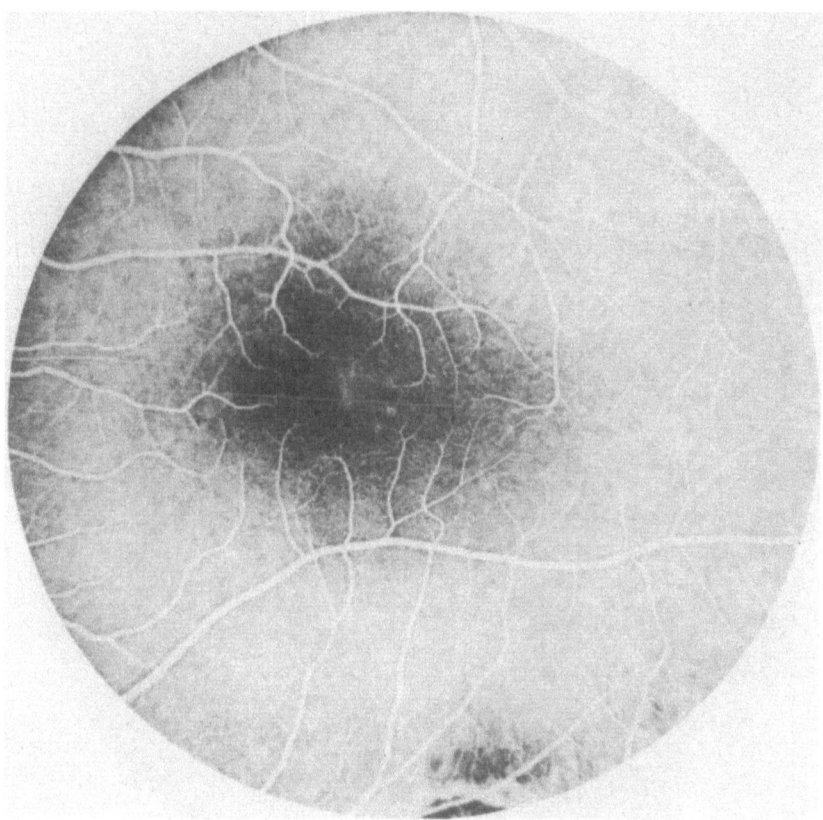

Fig. 3. X-linked retinoschizis. Male aged 16. Note subtle pigment epithelium defects in the fovea and dilatation and rarification of the retinal capillaries in the macular area (a). In the periphery there is an area of retinal vasculopathy with dye leakage from the vessel walls surrounded by chorioretinal scars (b).

gression of the lesion towards the periphery (toxic?) damage of the retinal capillaries takes place in the border zone before the retina becomes completely atrophic.

Retinal capillary dilatation and dye diffusion in a pattern of cystoid macular edema can be seen very clearly in patients with *dominant cystoid macular dystrophy* (D.C.M.D.) (Fig. 5) as described by DEUTMAN (1976), DEUTMAN et al. (1976) and NOTTING & PINCKERS (1976). The outstanding features of this disease are: pigmentary disturbance, cystoid macular edema, cells and opacities in the vitreous and (axial) hypermetropia. The ERG is normal, whereas the EOG is disturbed in the majority of patients. Colour vision shows an acquired type I R-G defectiveness to differing degrees (PINCKERS et al., 1976). Up to this moment we have obtained fluographic documentation of this disease in 18 patients (from 5 different pedigrees). In D.C.M.D. the affection of the inner retinal

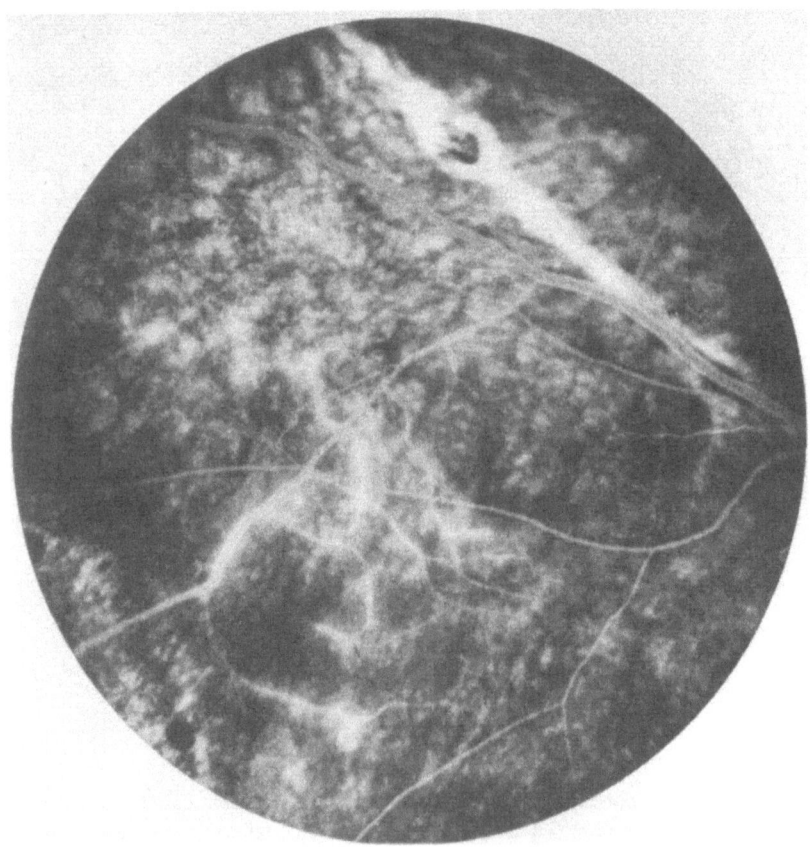

Fig. 3B.

layers is very obvious, but it occurs in combination with a clear disturbance at the level of the pigment epithelium and the question remains open, whether the disease process finds its origin in the outer retinal layers, analogous to other retinal dystrophies.

The vitreal changes might be explained by a continuous slow extravasation of humoral (and probably also corpuscular) blood elements from the retinal capillaries into the vitreous. Possibly the cells in the vitreous have the same origin as in retinitis pigmentosa where they can be observed in most cases. Though progression in D.C.M.D. is very slow generally, a number of patients − all over 30 years of age in our material − have developed a central atrophic lesion, comparable to our cases with progressive cone-rod dystrophy. In these cases we could also demonstrate capillary dilatation and dye leakage in a cystoid pattern around the border of the atrophic area.

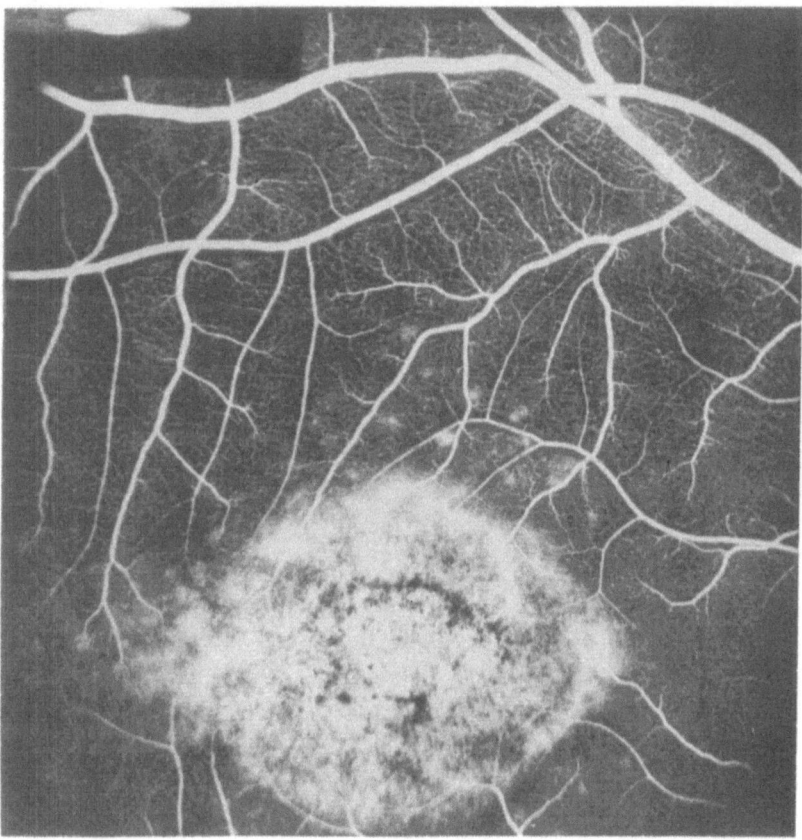

Fig. 4. Progressive cone-rod dystrophy. Female aged 8. There is a rhomboid macular lesion with pigment-epithelium defects and granular hyper pigmentations. Note the retinal capillary dilatation in the posterior pole (a). Her brother aged 17 shows a large atrophic lesion in the posterior pole; the ERG is extinguished. Fluography shows dilated retinal capillaries in the borderzone (b) with late dye leakage (c).

Summarizing, there is ample evidence of retinal capillary involvement in hereditary retinal dystrophies ranging from simple capillary dilatation as in X-linked retinoschizis and fundus flavimaculatus to a full blown picture of cystoid macular edema as in retinitis pigmentosa and D.C.M.D. Further elucidation of the mechanisms by which these phenomena are produced is needed as it could be a help for better classification and understanding of the retinal dystrophies.

REFERENCES

DEUTMAN, A.F. The hereditary dystrophies of the posterior pole of the eye. Thesis, Van Gorcum, Assen, The Netherlands (1971).

DEUTMAN, A.F. Some observations on acute maculopathies. *Trans. Amer. Acad. Ophthal. Otolaryng.* 81: *472*, May-June (1976).

DEUTMAN, A.F., PINCKERS, A. & AAN DE KERK, A.L. Cystoid macular edema, dominantly inherited. *Amer. J. Ophthal.* in press (1976).

FFYTCHE, T.J. Cystoid maculopathy in retinitis pigmentosa. *Trans. Ophth. Soc. U.K.* 92: *265-283* (1972).

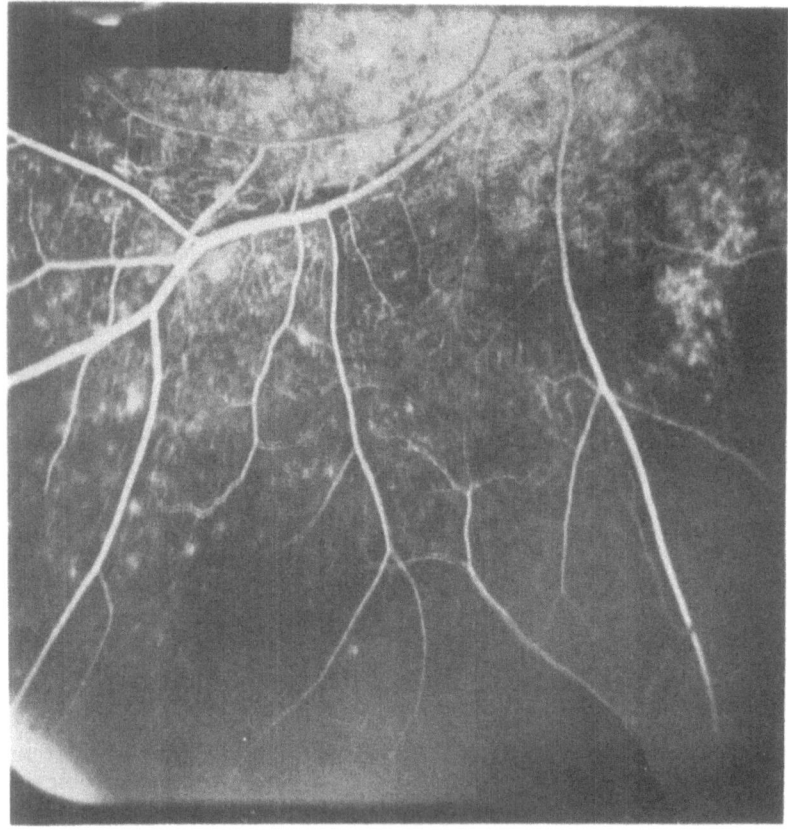

Fig. 4B.

FRANÇOIS, J., DE LAEY, J.J. & VERBRAEKEN, H. L'oedeme kystoide de la macula. *Bull. Soc. Belge d'Ophth.* 161: *708-721* (1972).

HYVÁRINEN, L., MAUMENEE, E., KELLEY, J., & CANTOLLINO, S. Fluorescein angiographic findings in retinitis pigmentosa. *Am. J. Ophthal.* 71: *17-26* (1971).

METGE, P., CHOVET, M., EBAGOSTI, A., & TASSY, A. Oedème maculaire cystoïde dans la rétinographie pigmentaire. *Bull. Soc. Ophthal. Fr.* 74: *119-123* (1974).

NOTTING, J.G.A. & PINCKERS, A. Dominant Cystoid Macular Dystrophy (D.C.M.D.) Submitted to *Am. J. Ophthal.* (1976).

PINCKERS, A., DEUTMAN, A.F. & NOTTING, J.G.A. Dominant Cystoid Macular Dystrophy (E.R.G., E.O.G., Colour Vision) Submitted to *Acta Ophthalmologica* (1976).

Keywords:
Fluorescence angiography
Hereditary retinal dystrophies
Capillary dilatation
Cystoid macular edema

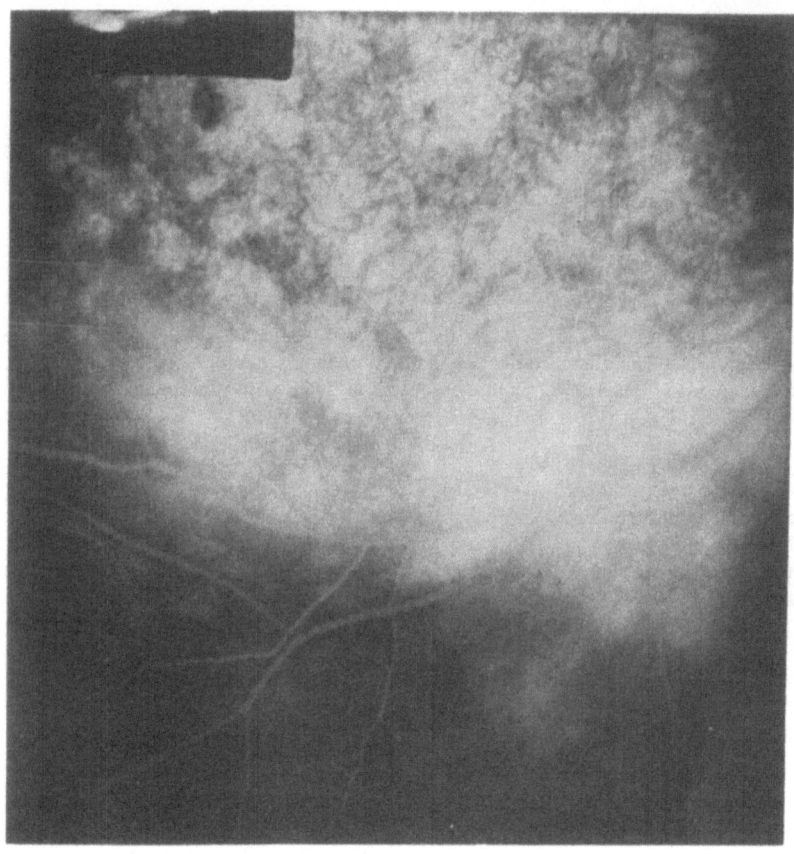

Fig. 4C.

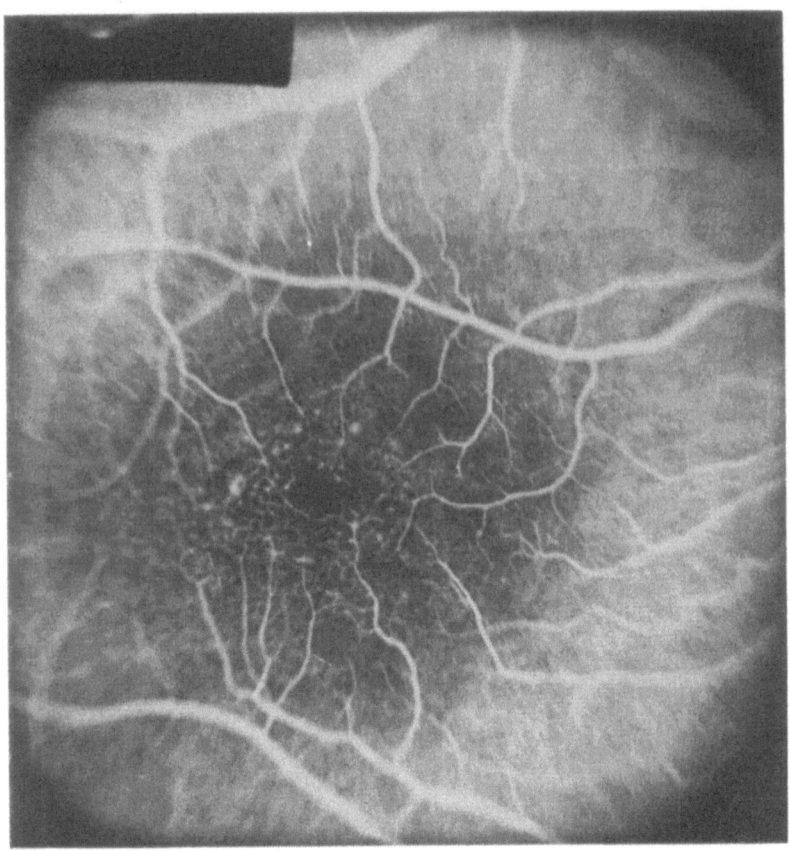

Fig. 5. Dominant cystoid macular dystrophy (D.C.M.D.). Female aged 7. Severe hypermetropia. The dilated retinal capillaries in the macular area show very clearly (a). In the late phase the classical picture of cystoid macular edema develops (b).

Authors' address:
Institute of Ophthalmology
University of Nijmegen
Philips van Leydenlaan 15
Nijmegen
The Netherlands

DISCUSSION

Dr Theodossiades: In the new entity which has been described by Dr Deutman and Dr Notting special emphasis has been given to the leakage of retinal capillaries and the disturbance of the pigment epithelium, and I would like to know if there is an effusion of the choriocapillaris as well because in some of the fluoroangiograms I think that it was evident.

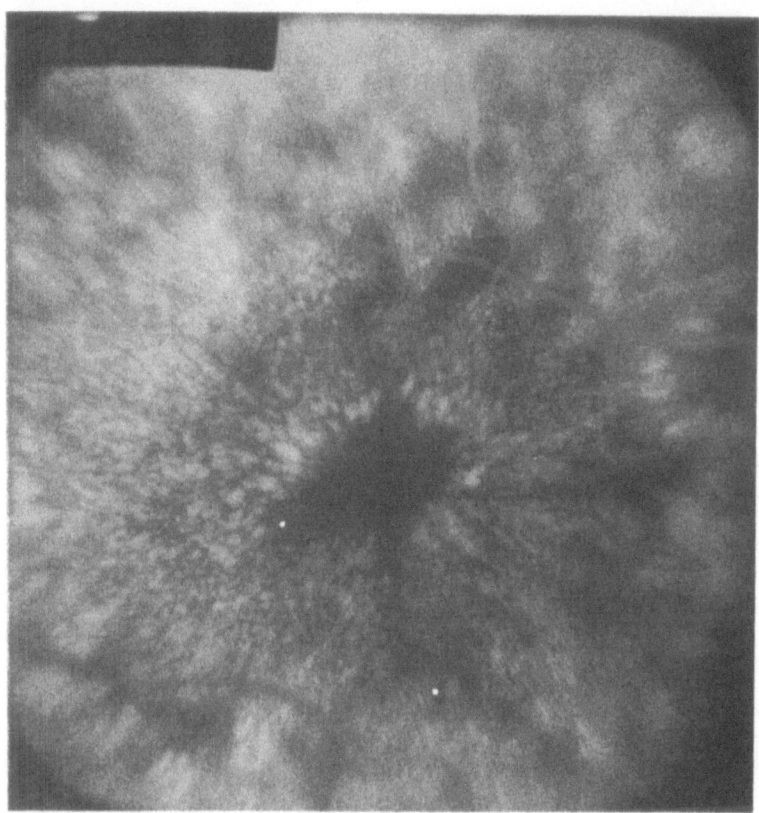

Fig. 5B.

Dr Notting: I think this is caused by the fact that these pictures were very late pictures and simulate such deep diffusion but instead it is a real late picture of cystoid macular edema coming from leakage out of the peri-macular capillaries. We could see them in the sequence very well; we could see them starting to leak and giving that very late appearance. We did not show all the stages in between.

Dr Theodossiades: You have not noted diffusion from the choriocapillaris at all?

Dr Notting: No.

EPITHELIUM PIGMENTAIRE DANS LES HEREDO-DEGENERESCENCES CHORIO-RETINIENNES A PREDOMINANCE CHOROIDIENNE

V. DRINCIC

(Belgrade, Yougoslavie)

Si l'on examine les cas publiés des dégénérescences chorio-rétiniennes à prédominance choroïdienne étudiées par l'angiographie fluorescéinique on ne peut se libérer de l'impression de ne voir, ainsi que des archéologues, que des débris de la chorio-rétine qui ont, depuis longtemps, cessé d'être une structure organisée. D'autre part, les examens histologiques, d'ailleurs parti-

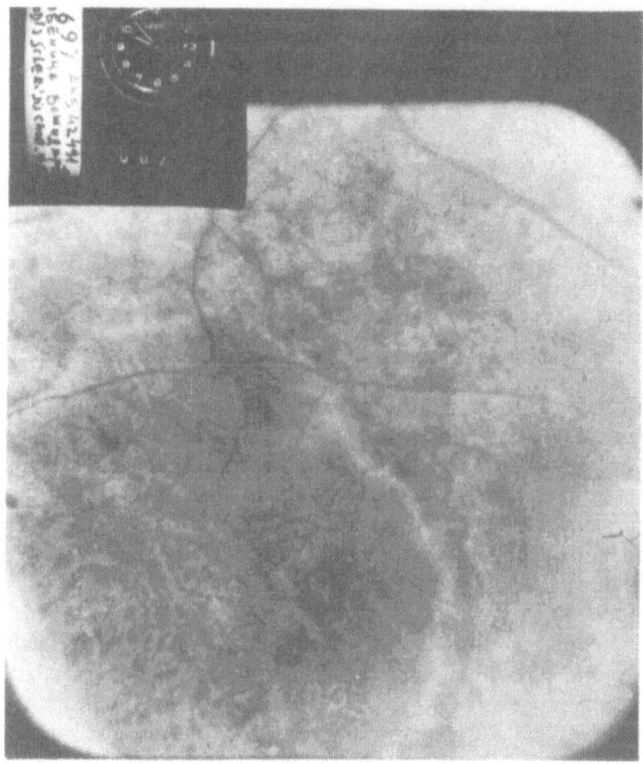

Fig. 1. *1e cas*: Atrophie choroïdienne aréolaire centrale. Phase veineuse rétinienne de l'angiographie fluorescéinique. Fuite de colorant au bord de la lésion. Autour de la lésion l'épithélium pigmentaire très dépigmenté rendant visible l'aspect tacheté de la choriocapillaire.

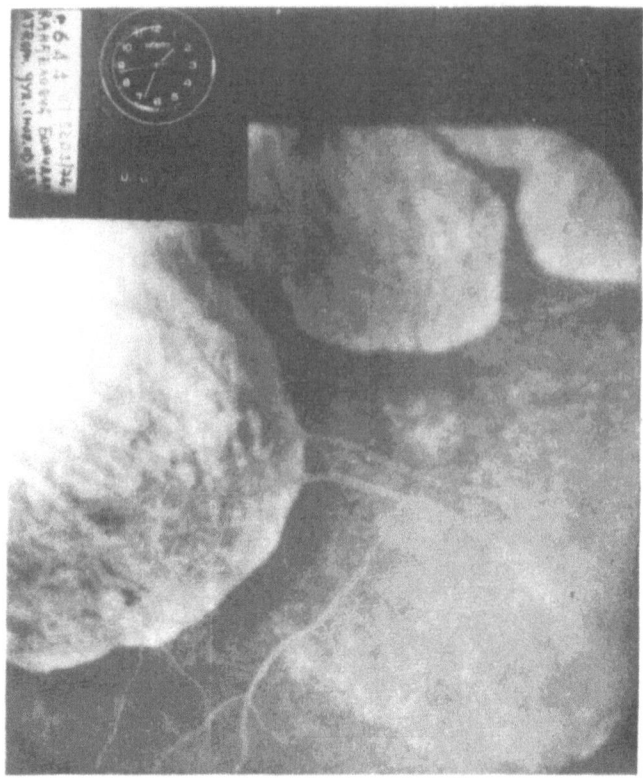

Fig. 2. *2e cas*: Atrophie gyrée de la choroïde et de la rétine. Phase artério-veineuse de l'angiographie fluorescéinique. Trois foyers d'atrophie typiques de la choroïde et dans l'angle inférieur droit de la photo un champ de l'épithélium pigmentaire dépigmenté.

culièrement rares, proviennent en général d'yeux qui n'en étaient qu'au stade terminal de l'abiotrophie.

Afin d'obtenir une image globale des différents aspects des altérations de l'épithélium pigmentaire au cours des hérédo-dégénérescences chorio-rétiniennes à prédominance choroïdienne sous le jour de l'angiographie fluorescéinique, nous avons étudié un certain nombre de malades. Les cinq cas que nous allons passer en revue illustrent ces altérations.

Premier cas: concerne un patient âgé de 46 ans, avec image ophthalmoscopique d'atrophie choroïdienne aréolaire centrale incomplète et bilatérale et baisse de vision progressive à partir de 40 ans. L'acuité visuelle est réduite à 5/60 de chaque côté. Au champ visuel périphérie normale, scotome central absolu de 10 à 20°. Courbe d'adaptation de II b (FRANÇOIS et coll., 1956). Deuteranopie acquise. L'ERG est subnormal.

L'angiographie fluorescéinique montre une dépigmentation très prononcée de l'épitélium pigmentaire ainsi qu'une prolifération poussièreuse du pigment dans la partie para-centrale du fond d'oeil. Dans la lésion atrophique centrale existent des proliférations de pigment sous forme de taches éparses. Sur le bord de la lésion atrophique on voit la fuite du colorant (Fig. 1).

Deuxième cas: Homme âgé de 25 ans, héméralope depuis l'âge de 11 ans. Il présente une cataracte compliquée polaire antérieure et postérieure bilatérale et au fond d'oeil image d'atrophie de la choroïde gyrée de 2e degré (TAKI, 1974). Acuité visuelle de l'oeil cataracté droit est à 0,5, à gauche, après la discission de la cataracte, 1,0. Le champ visuel est très rétréci concentriquement (20° à 25°). L'adaptation primaire à l'obscurité est normale, secondaire subnormale. L'ERG est bilatéralement éteint.

A l'angiographie fluorescéinique: L'épithélium pigmentaire des foyers d'atrophie choroïdienne est totalement dépigmenté et transparent au point

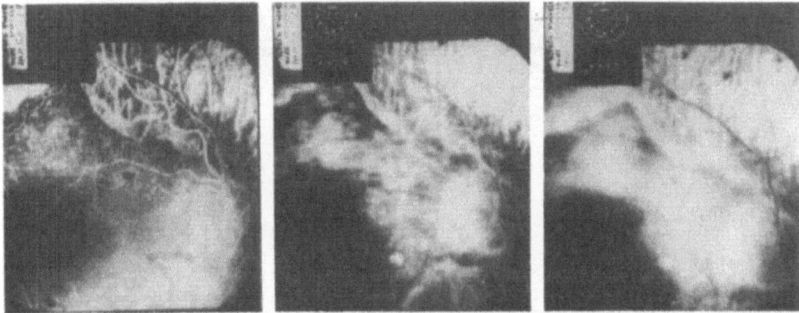

Fig. 3. *3e cas*: L'atrophie gyrée de la choroïde et de la rétine, phases artério-veineuse et tardive de l'angiographie fluorescéinique. Dépigmentation de l'épithélium pigmentaire. Fuite du colorant à travers l'épithélium pigmentaire dans la rétine.

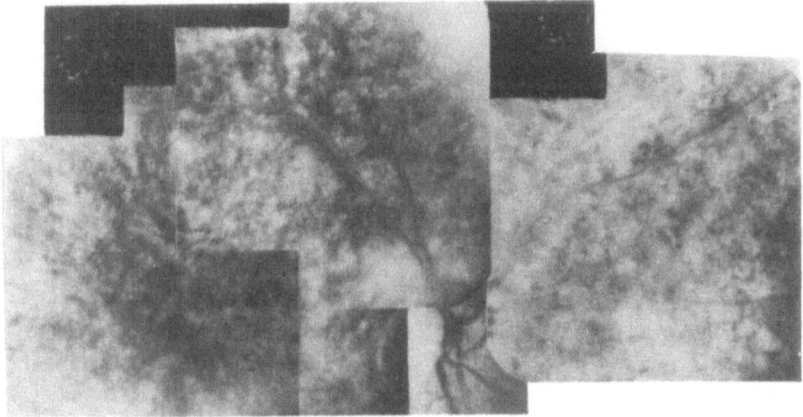

Fig. 4. *4e cas*: Conducteur de la choroïdérémie. Fond d'oeil pendant la phase veineuse de l'angiographie fluorescéinique. Dépigmentation de l'épithélium pigmentaire. Remaniement prolifératif du pigment.

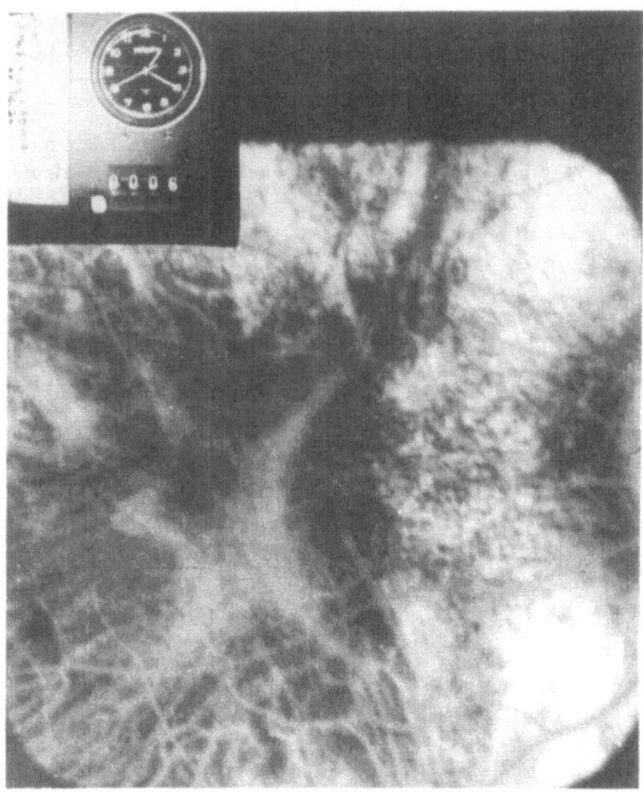

Fig. 5. *5e cas*: Choroïdérémie. Phase veineuse de l'angiographie fluorescéinique. La choriocapillaire est à reconnaître sous la forme de l'étoile hyper-fluorescente.

que le passage du colorant à travers les gros vaisseaux de la choroïde est bien visible.

A un endroit, entre la papille et le premier grand foyer d'atrophie choroïdienne, dans la periphérie, une zone arrondie d'hyper-fluorescence montre l'effet fenêtre de l'épithélium pigmentaire dépigmenté de même qu'une chorio-capillaire fonctionnelle (Fig. 2). L'aspect et le siège de cette zone laissent supposer qu'il s'agit d'un foyer d'atrophie choroïdienne en formation.

Troisième cas: Soeur du malade précédent, âgée de 34 ans. Elle est héméralope depuis l'âge de 12 ans et présente une cataracte polaire postérieure bilatérale avec image ophthalmoscopique d'atrophie gyrée de 3e stade (TAKI, 1974). Acuité visuelle de chaque oeil est de 0,2. L'adaptation à l'obscurité primaire est normale, tandis que la secondaire est nettement pathologique. Il existe un retrécissement tubulaire du champ visuel de même que la deuteranopie et la prothanomalie.

Angiographie fluorescéinique: Pendant la phase artério-veineuse on aperçoit dans les régions atrophiques à travers un épithélium pigmentaire dépourvu de pigment, la trame des gros vaisseaux choroïdiens remplis de fluorescéine. Les collections de pigments proliférés ne se retrouvent qu'en de rares endroits. En même temps apparaît une hyper-fluorescence de la région inter-papillo-maculaire ainsi qu'au dessus de la macula, avec taches de fuite du colorant à partir de la chorio-capillaire dans la rétine. La macula reste noire aussi bien dans la phase veineuse que lorsque le colorant atteint la couche des fibres optiques (Fig. 3). Cinq minutes après, l'hyper-fluorescence de la rétine imprégnée de colorant est diffuse et surtout marquée sur le bord de l'île centrale épargnée par la dégénérescence.

Quatrième cas: concerne conducteur de la choroïdérémie, agée de 70 ans, avec une acuité visuelle, champ visuel, adaptation à l'obscurité et l'ERG normal.

L'angiographie fluorescéinique: elle montre une hyper-fluorescence du fond d'oeil ainsi que les collections poussièreuses de pigment, surtout bien visibles au cours de la phase veineuse. Pas de fuite de colorant dans la rétine (Fig. 4).

Cinquième cas: est l'un des deux fils atteints du 4e malade, âgé de 33 ans. Il présente l'image de la choroïdérémie, avec un reste rougeâtre de la choroïde centrale. Héméralope depuis l'enfance. Correction de la myopie à l'âge de 24 ans et depuis l'âge de 29 ans très handicapé dans ses déplacements. Acuité visuelle avec correction myopique de chaque côté est de 1,0, achromatopsie, champ visuel tubulaire de 6 à 8°, adaptation à l'obscurité pathologique, l'ERG éteint.

L'angiographie fluorescéinique: Ce n'est que dans la phase veineuse que la fluorescéine fait son apparition dans la trame des grands vaisseaux choroïdiens de l'îlot choroïdien central. Le reste de choriocapillaires limité strictement à la région maculaire n'est rempli avec le colorant que cinq minutes après l'apparition de fluorescéine dans le réseau artériel rétinien. C'est à partir de ce moment qu'on peut distinguer la prolifération dense du pigment dans la rétine et une couche de pigments amorphes derrière la choroïde qui appartient certainement à la lamina fusca (Fig. 5).

Les conclusions portent sur trois faits importants:
— La fluorescence dans la circulation sanguine visualise dans les dégénérescences chorio-rétiniennes à prédominance choroïdienne 'depigmentatio in situ' selon le concept de Berthe Klien (Fig. 1, 2, 3, 4).
— Le pigment prolifère dans les couches internes de la rétine et il est possible de le voir au cours de l'angiographie fluorescéinique même lorsqu'il n'est pas visible par l'ophthalmoscopie. Un tel état de choses a été récemment confirmé histologiquement par Eicholz dans les rétinopathies pigmentaires sans pigment.
— Grâce à l'angiographie fluorescéinique il est possible de constater la défectuosité de la barrière hémato-rétinienne au niveau de l'épithélium pigmentaire dans les dégénérescences choroïdiennes primaires (Fig. 3).

Finalement, au stade terminal des dégénérescences chorio-rétiniennes à prédominance choroïdienne ce n'est qu'exceptionnellement qu'il est possible d'examiner avec l'angiographie fluorescéinique l'épithélium pigmentaire (Fig. 5).

REFERENCES

EICHOLZ, W. Histologie der retinopathia pigmentosa cum et sine pigmento. *Klin. Mbl. Augenheilk.* 164: *467-475* (1974).

FRANÇOIS, J., VERRIEST, G. & DE ROUCK, A. Les fonctions visuelles dans les dégénérescences tapéto-rétiniennes. *Ophthalmologica*, Suppl. 43: *1-86* (1956).

KLIEN, B. Diseases of the Macula. *Arch. Ophth.* (Chic.) 60: *175-186* (1958).

TAKI, K. Gyrate atrophy of the chroid and retina associated with hyperornitinaemia. *Brit. J. Ophthal.* 58: *3-23* (1974).

Author's address:
Hopital clinique de Belgrade
Institut Ophtalmologique
Belgrade
Yougoslavie

FLUOROGRAPHIC ASPECTS OF STARGARDT'S DISEASE
(JUVENILE FAMILIAL MACULAR DEGENERATION)

P.S. RAMALHO

(Lisbon, Portugal)

There have been several studies and reports since Stargardt's initial description in 1909 of this familial atrophic form of macular involvement of pigment epithelium. This retinal disorder of early onset (first and second decade) can be included in a wider group of diseases known as *fundus flavimaculatus*, term applied to a variety of related disorders by FRANCE-SCHETTI (1963, 1965) to describe the multiple yellow-white round or linear fishtail-like lesions affecting mainly the posterior fundus. It can occur with and without macular involvement. With the easy availability of new methods of investigation mainly the experimental studies, electron microscopy, electrophysiology, monochromatic photography and specially fluorescein angiography, there has been increasing awareness in recent years of the role of retinal pigment epithelium (RPE) in the causation of many disease formerly thought to be localized to the sensory retina. Fluorescein angiography is a good technique known to demonstrate pigment epithelial abnormalities otherwise not visible. Such studies have been carried out, both in the localized (macular) as well as in the generalized form of *fundus flavimaculatus* (ERNEST & KRILL 1966; KRILL, NEWELL & CHISTTI 1968; GASS 1970 and others).

Recently while studying juvenile macular degeneration we found in some patients with localized forms of Stargardt's disease suggestion of peripheral involvement. Similar involvement was also noticed in the non-affected close relatives of these subjects.

Because of these findings we have studied both the subjects known to have Stargardt's disease and their non-affected close relatives, with fluorescein angiography in the central and in the peripheral parts of the fundus.

MATERIAL AND METHODS

Eight (8) affected members known to have juvenile macular degeneration of Stargardt's type belonging to 4 families have been studied repeatedly at intervals (5 males and 3 females). They have been followed for 2 to 4 years. Each family had 2 affected members and their ages varied from 8 to 24 years. In 3 families they were all brothers and sisters and in one they were cousins. Their onset was during the first or second decade with more or less macular involvement in both eyes and low visual acuity (2/20-10/20).

Non-affected brothers and sisters of these 8 patients were studied and in

455

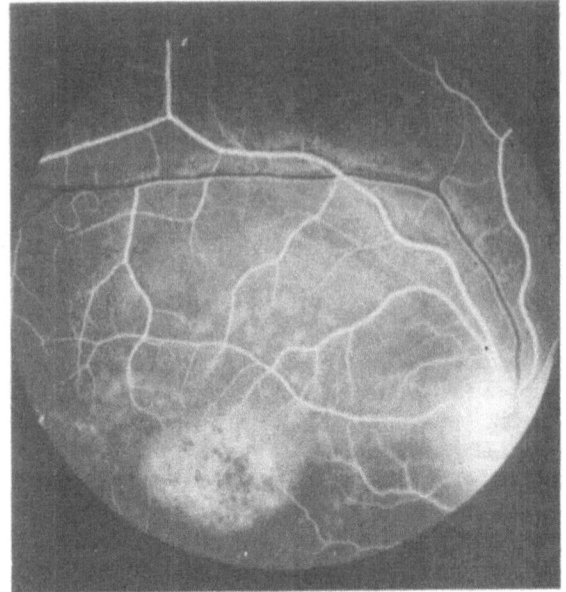

a)

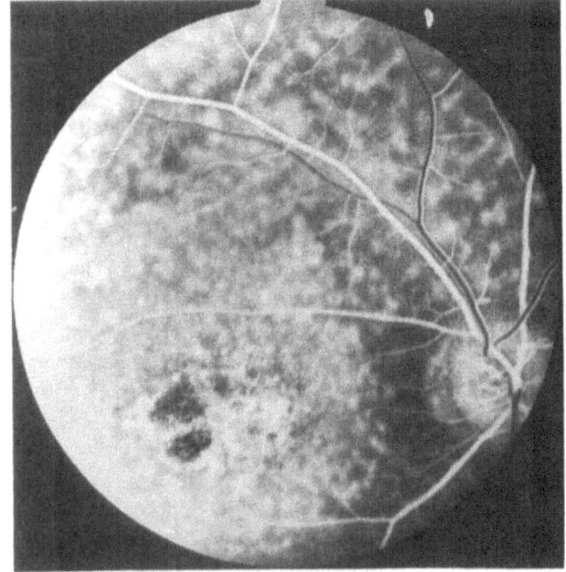

b)

Fig. 1. Right fundus angiograms of 2 young patients with Stargardt's disease (Vision = 0.4 and 0.2) showing typical pigment epithelium disturbances in the macular areas. (a) central form; (b) diffuse form. The macular fluorescence is seen in the early phases of dye transit. Some of the fluorescent spots correspond to yellow-white material (arlires-venous phase).

456

2 instances the parents, uncles, aunts and cousins also included in the investigation. Besides others routine investigation colour photography of the fundus and fluorescein angiography was performed repeatedly in all these subjects using normal technique (Kodachrome II films for colour and Kodak TRI-X-Pan for fluorescein angiography). Topcon TRC-F3 and Kowa RC2 retinal camaras were used and the films processed with standard comercial methods in the same laboratory. Central and peripheral parts of the fundus were investigated using multiple injections sometimes. Sodium fluorescein solution (3 to 5 ml of 20 or 10%) was injected into the veins of the forearm.

Colour transparencies and the negative fluorograms were studied by projection and in some cases enlarged prints were also used. The results were assessed and discussed by at least 2 members of the staff.

RESULTS AND COMMENTS

All 8 patients studied showed various degrees of macular involvement characterized by depigmentation, pigment clumping, reflex colour changes of pigment epithelium with or without deposition of yellowish material. These changes similar to reported before, were confined not only to the central macular region (central form) but also to the periphery, although not always visible (diffuse form). Some patients showed typical findings of retinitis pigmentosa including migration of pigment (bone spicules) not necessarily associated with night-blindness. The calibre of retinal vessels was in most cases reduced. The fundus was generally tessalated with pepper and salt appearance at least in some parts of the fundus. In some cases typical yellow-white fleck-like lesions could be seen in central and in peripheral parts of the retina (irregular chainlike, fishtail etc.). In one instance these lesions appeared only after 2 years of observation and coincided with lowering of visual acuity.

On careful examination of the fundus in the periphery there was always a suggestion of pigment epithelium disturbance (reflex change, tiny pigment spots, dirty, pepper and salt appearance) in localized or central forms of the disease.

On fluorescein angiography these changes of pigment epithelium were obvious. Typical filling defects alternating with hiperfluorescenceof macular area were seen both in the central and diffuse forms (Fig. 1). In the peripheral parts of the retina pigment epithelium abnormalities could also be seen in most cases of central forms of Stargardt's disease (Fig. 2).

In brothers and sisters of these patients (non-affected members) the most striking finding was that the fundus was tessalated (central and peripheral retina). The fluorescein angiography on these young subjects showed pigment epithelium defects in the mid-periphery and periphery specially in superior and temporal areas (Fig. 2a) avoiding the central region (Fig. 2b). The macula had normal appearance to fluorescein transit. These non-affected members had good visual acuity and no complaints. The parents, aunts, uncles and cousins studied did not show any particular abnormalities except tessalated fundi in some young subjects. Choroidal, capillary and circulatory changes were not seen in this study although we did not look particularly into this subject.

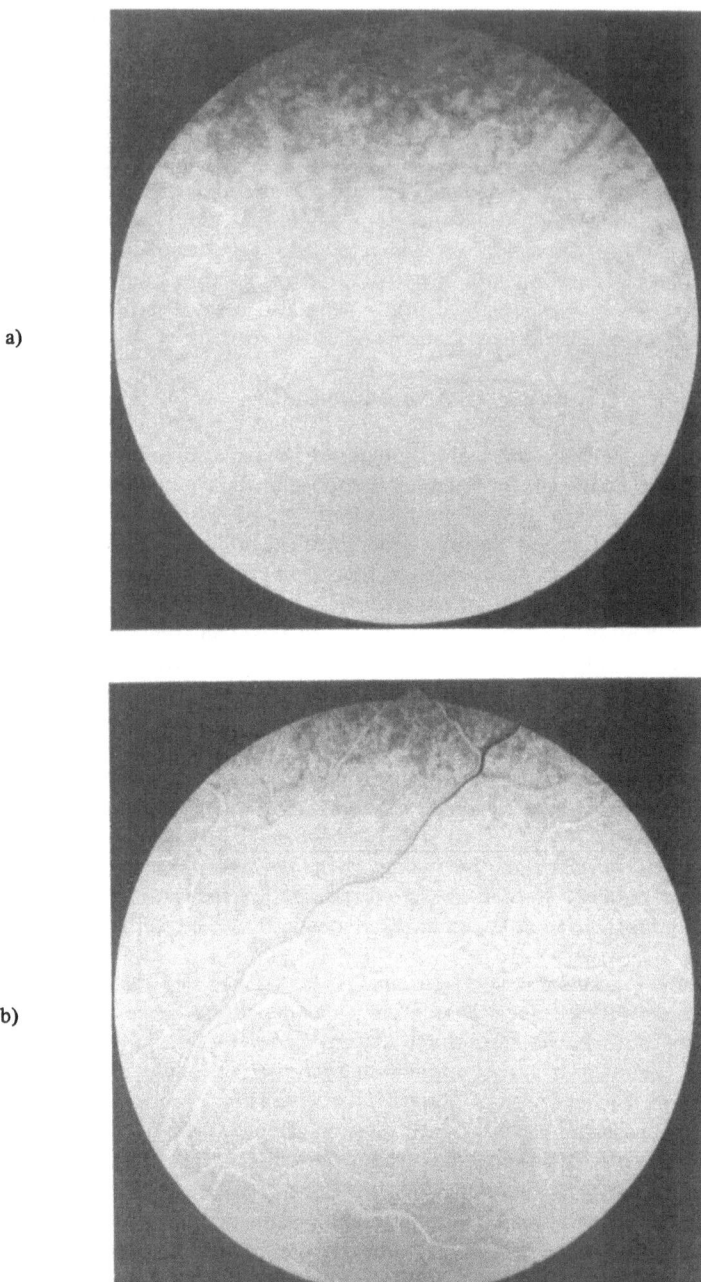

a)

b)

Fig. 2. Left fundus angiograms of superior temporal areas (late phase) showing peripheral pigment epithelium abnormalities in the central form (a). 2b — shows pigment epithelium changes in the superior temporal area. Note the macular area below is normal; Vision = 10/10 (normal 8 year old sister of the patient of figure 1a).

458

We think that this juvenile macular degeneration is a widespread pigment epithelium abnormality transmitted also to brothers and sisters of affected members in a milder form not affecting the macula and the vision.

REFERENCES

ERNEST, J. & KRILL, A.E. Fluorescein studies in fundus flavimaculatus and drusen. *Amer. J. Ophthal.* 62: *1-6* (1966).

FRANCESCHETTI, A., FRANÇOIS, J. & BABEL, J. Les hérédo-dégénérescences (dégénérescences tapéto-rétiniennes), Paris, 1963, Masson et Cie. vol. 1.

FRANCESCHETTI, A. & FRANÇOIS, J. Fundus flavimaculatus. *Arch. Ophthal.* (Paris), 6: *505-510* (1965).

GASS, J.D.M. Stereoscopic Atlas of Macular Diseases. 1970, The C.V. Mosby Company, Saint Louis.

KRILL, A.E., NEWELL, F.W., & CHISHTI, M.I. Fluorescein studies affecting the pigment epithelium. *Trans. Amer. Ophthal. Soc.* 66: *269-317* (1968).

Author's address:
Hospital de Santa Maria
Serviço de Oftalmologia
University of Lisbon
Lisbon 4
Portugal

LE SIGNE DU SILENCE CHOROÏDIEN DANS LES DÉGÉNÉRSCENCES TAPÉTO-RÉTINIENNES POSTERIEURES

P. BONNIN, M. PASSOT & M-TH. TRIOLAIRE-COTTEN

(Paris, France)

Nous appelons 'signe du silence choroïdien' un symptôme fluorographique rencontré dans les dégénérescences tapéto-rétiniennes limitées au pôle postérieur. Décrit initialement à propos de 35 cas (BONNIN, 1971), ce symptôme est caractérisé par l'absence de la visualisation normale de la choroïde par la fluorescéine. Alors que normalement la fluorescence des vaisseaux rétiniens est partiellement noyée dans la fluorescence du fond choroïdien, dans un certain nombre de cas atteints l'image des vaisseaux rétiniens est extrêmement vive et nette, au point que les moindres capillaires sont visibles, tout comme sur une préparation de rétine à plat in vitro (Fig. 1). Ceci ne correspond à aucune anomalie décelable des vaisseaux rétiniens. Ceux-ci ne sont qu'anormalement visibles du fait de la disparition de l'image choroïdiennen normale connue sous le nom de modelé choroïdien. Cette absence de visualisation de la choroïde est, fait remarquable, généralisée à l'ensemble du fond d'oeil, alors même que la maladie ne s'exprime qu'au pôle postérieur sous la forme habituelle de l'image en ocelle maculaire des dégénérescences centrales, entourée ou non des taches vivement fluorescentes des dégénérescences

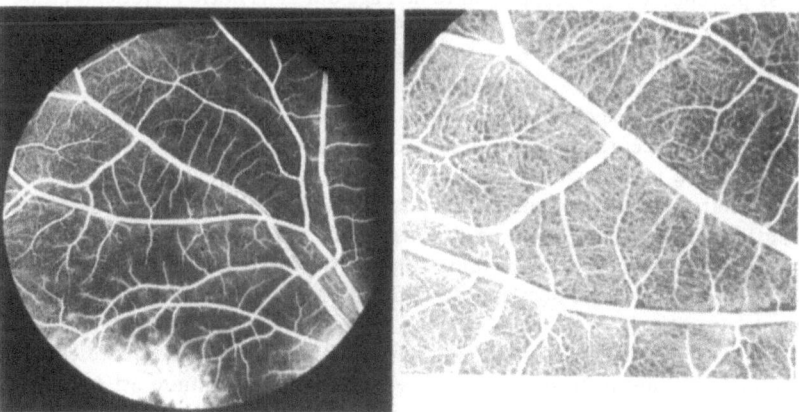

Fig. 1. Fluorographie au stade capillaire d'un oeil atteint de Fundus Flavimaculatus. Le réseau des capillaires rétiniens est anormalement visible alors que l'image habituelle du modelé choroïdien est totalement absente. A droite un agrandissement du même cliché.

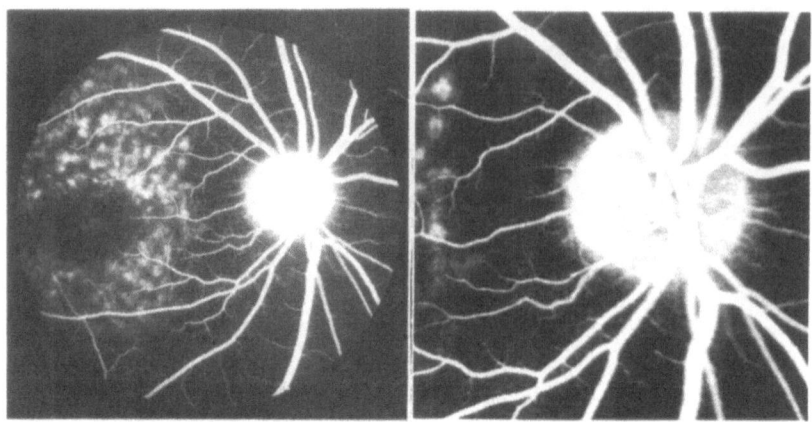

Fig. 2. Fluorographie au stade veineux d'un cas de Fundus Flavimaculatus. Le signe du silence choroïdien est évident ce qui fait que la papille parait très fluorescente par effet de contraste. A droite un agrandissement du même cliché.

péricentrales telles que le flavimaculatus (Fig. 2). Qui plus est, il nous est arrivé de rencontrer cet aspect isolément chez des sujets apparemment indemnes d'atteinte tapétorétinienne mais appartenant à des familles atteintes.

La fréquence de ce symptôme est très grande dans les dégénérescences tapéto-rétiniennes postérieures: dans 124 cas nous l'avons rencontré 104 fois, alors que 20 malades gardaient un modelé choroïdien normal. Un indice de frèquence de 83,8% ne peut être le fait du hasard. De nombreux clichés de fluorographies parus dans la littérature concernant les dégénérescences tapéto-rétiniennes du pôle postérieur mettent d'ailleurs ce signe en évidence, quoique cela ait souvent échappé à leur auteur.

Sa présence semble indépendante de l'âge qui dans notre matériel d'étude s'étend de 7 à 59 ans, avec un pic de fréquence à 18 ans qui ne fait que correspondre à l'âge oú le plus souvent le diagnostic est posé. Elle est indépendante du sexe: 60% d'hommes pour 40% de femmes dans notre série avec signe du silence choroïdien, tout comme la série sans ce symptôme.

Son existence semble liée à la présence d'une dégénérescence tapéto-rétinienne du pôle postérieur. En effet si nous l'avons noté dans 83,8% des cas de cette maladie et dans 3% de nos 32 cas d'épithéliopathie en plaques ou affections voisines, nous ne l'avons jamais rencontré dans les atteintes toxiques centrales type chloroquino-rétinopathie ni dans aucune autre affection du fond d'oeil à l'occasion de 4500 fluorographies pratiquées dans les mêmes conditions.

Bien évidemment il n'est pas retrouvé non plus dans les dégénérescences tapéto-rétiniennes diffuses où l'atteinte de l'écran pigmentaire est telle que la fluorescence choroïdienne est apparemment exagérée. Mais il ne l'est pas non plus dans les dégénérescences tapéto-rétiniennes périphériques qui respectent encore le pôle postérieur: à cet endroit le modelé choroïdien nous a toujours paru normal.

Alors qu'initialement il nous a semblé prudent de ne tenir compte de ce symptôme que chez les patients de race blanche et dont le fond d'oeil apparaissait comme normal en dehors des pôles postérieurs, l'expérience nous a montré que les sujets pigmentés non atteints présentaient, quoiqu'àun moindre degré que les européens, un modelé choroïdien décelable, alors que cinq patients mélanodermes atteints présentaient un signe du silence choroïdien net.

La pathogénie de ce symptôme nous est inconnue. A priori elle ne nous semble pas être le fait d'une augmentation de l'opacité de l'épithélium pigmentaire, qu'il faudrait très importante et homogène, que ceci soit le fait d'une plus grande densité du pigment ou que ce soit le fait d'une surcharge épithéliale; on sait que dans ce cas ce sont justement les zones surchargées qui sont anormalement fluorescentes.

Il semble bien s'agir d'un phénomène de siège choroïdien et deux faits pourraient plaider en faveur de cette hypothèse:
1. Certains auteurs (ZENATTI & ISAMBERT, 1971) ont remarqué que ces patients présentaient très fréquemment une nette diminution de l'amplitude du pouls choroïdien.
2. Les fluorographies pratiquées chez le singe après ligature de toutes les artères ciliaires courtes postérieures (HAYREH, 1971) sont tout à fait semblables à celles que nous avons observées dans nos cas, ne montrant plus, mais avec quelle finesse, que les vaisseaux rétiniens. Ne réalise-t-on pas ainsi un signe du silence choroïdien expérimental?

Par contre il faut remarquer qu'histologiquement les cas de dégénérescences centrales publiés dans la littérature ne semblent pas avoir comporté d'atteinte évidente de la choroïde, en dehors de lésions séniles banales.

Faut-il alors admettre qu'il s'agit des effets d'une anomalie de fonctionnement de la choroïde et plus particulièrement de la choriocapillaire, plus que d'une atteinte anatomique? Peut-être l'étude en microscopie électronique de la chorio-capillaire de globes atteints apporterait-elle une réponse à cette question?

Adresse de l'auteur:
C.N.O. des XV-XX
28 rue de Charenton
75012 Paris,
France

DISCUSSION

Dr Bird: We certainly noticed — particularly in the bull's eye macular dystrophies — that the choroid is very dark, which is exactly the point you are making. The film looks very thin and I suspect some additional filtering effect of the illuminating blue light or the emitting green light from the choroid in these cases. There may be some additional material at the level of pigment epithelium, perhaps a diffuse deposit of white outer segment material or something like that which blocks out the choroidal fluorescence. I am not sure that it is not a choroidal perfusion problem. It is just that you cannot see it.

IRIS ANGIOGRAPHY IN VASCULAR DISEASES
OF THE FUNDUS

M. KOTTOW, M.D.

(Bonn, W. Germany)

The present paper aims to review the effects of certain vascular diseases of the fundus on the iris vessels, as detected by iris fluorescein angiography (IFA). The technique of IFA used in these studies has been discussed elsewhere (KOTTOW & HENDRICKSON, 1975), and shall be omitted here for the sake of brevity.

RESULTS

Retinal vein occlusions

Isolated cases of IFA findings in retinal venous occlusions had been reported previously (RAITTA & VANNAS, 1960; MAPSTONE, 1970; DEODATI, BEC & LABRO, 1971), before a fairly large group of 70 venous occlusions was more systematically studied (KOTTOW & METZLER, 1976). The summarized results of these 70 patients are presented in Fig. 1. These alterations appeared more frequently in older than in younger patients, and in long-standing rather than in recent occlusions; eyes with neovascular complications of the fundus showed more iris alterations than those of the non-neovascular group (Fig. 2).

Retinal artery occlusions

Nineteen patients with retinal arterial occlusions were studied, the results being summarized in Fig. 3. These alterations did not seem to be sex or age

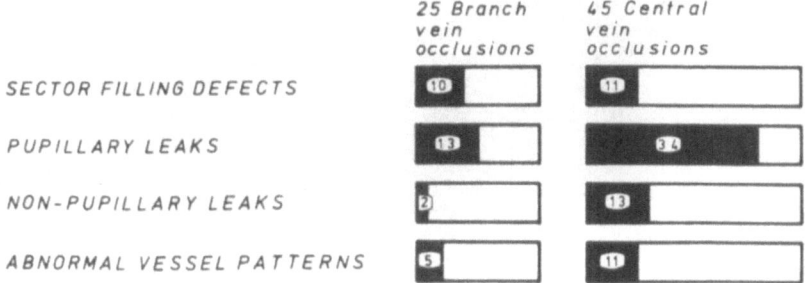

Fig. 1.   Incidence of abnormal IFA findings in 70 eyes with retinal vein occlusions.

465

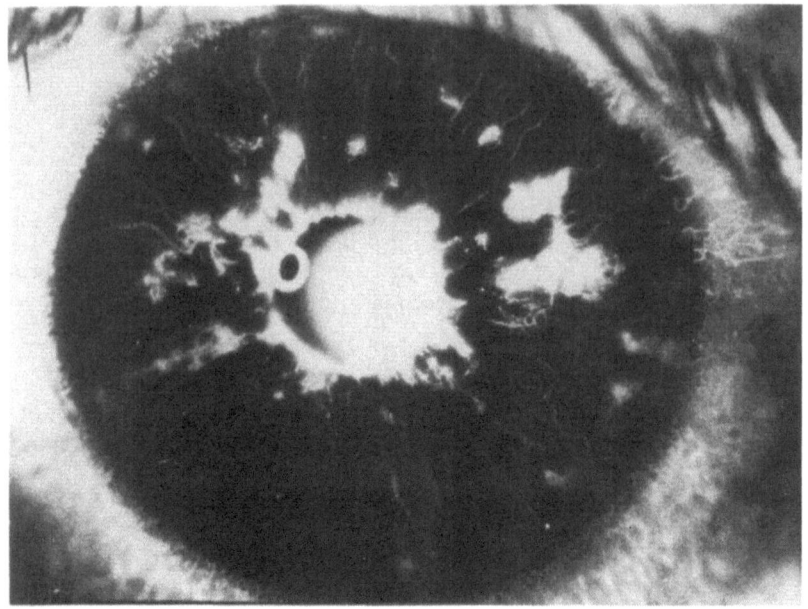

Fig. 2-A. Early phase IFA in eye with recent central retinal vein thrombosis, showing abnormal leakage of fluorescein.

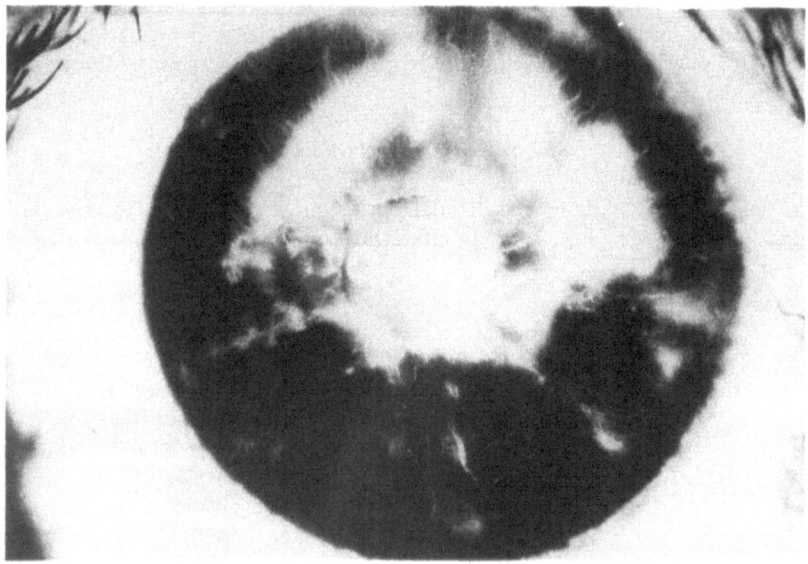

Fig. 2-B. Late phase of same eye, showing dye pools in iris stroma.

466

dependent, nor did branch artery occlusions appear to have a behaviour different from central occlusions (Fig. 4). But it could be demonstrated that the alterations were statistically significantly more frequent in eyes with abnormally high ophthalmodynamometric values, and in eyes where the occlusion was recent, i.e., less than one month old at the time of the IFA (KOTTOW & HENDRICKSON, 1974).

Stagnation thrombosis

Two patients with this type of venous thrombosis, due to a relative arterial insufficiency, have been studied (KOTTOW & METZLER, 1975). Both cases showed very heavy vessel leakages which were present 24-48 hours after the occlusive episode, and were considered to have an exaggerated arterial insufficiency type of response.

Microcystic macular edema after cataract extraction

Ten patients with this type of edema — Irvine-Gass syndrome — were studied by means of IFA. All of them consistently showed a moderate to heavy abnormal fluorescein leakage from the iris and ciliary body vessels, thus evidencing that this disease was not a localized macular derangement but some sort of massive dysfunction of the intraocular vessels (KOTTOW & HENDRICKSON, 1975).

Epinephrine maculopathy in aphakes

Twenty-five aphakic eyes were experimentally medicated with topical epinephrine, in an attempt to further understand the macular edema shown by approximately 20% of aphakes treated with this drug. A summary of the results obtained is shown in Fig. 5.

Drug-induced iris vessel leaks did not depend on the length of time elapsed since cataract extraction had been performed, nor on the type, technique or eventual complications of the surgical procedures. Intercurrent systemic diseases also seemed not to influence these results. There was an evident dose dependency, in that all the eyes that started leaking were under 2% epinephrine, none showing this reaction in the 1% epinephrine group. (Fig. 6).

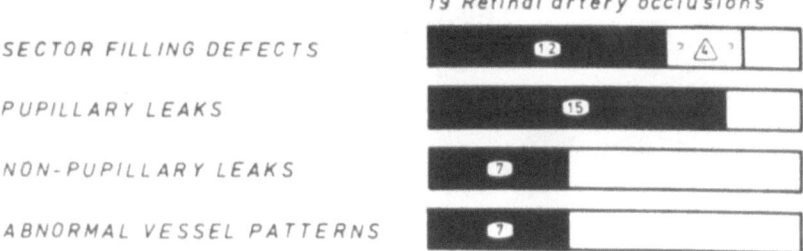

Fig. 3. Abnormal IFA findings in 19 eyes with retinal artery occlusions.

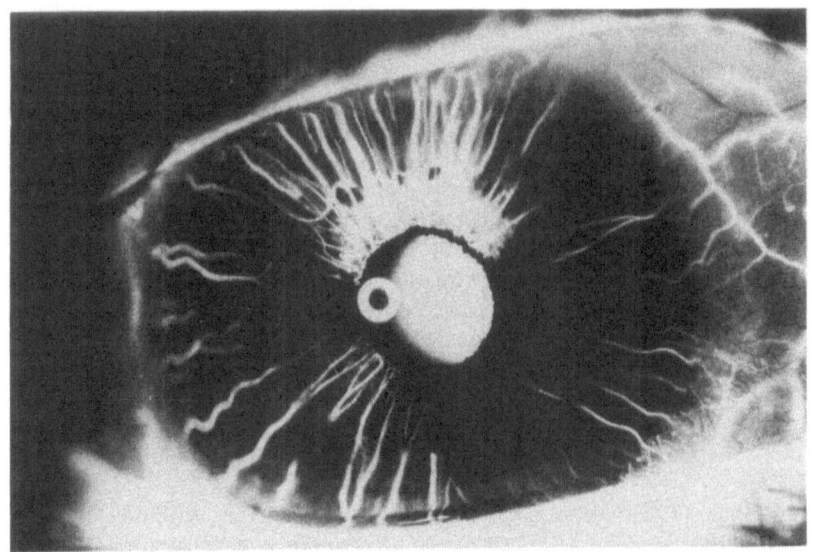

Fig. 4-A. Early phase IFA in recent central retinal artery occlusion, showing irregular arterial filling pattern.

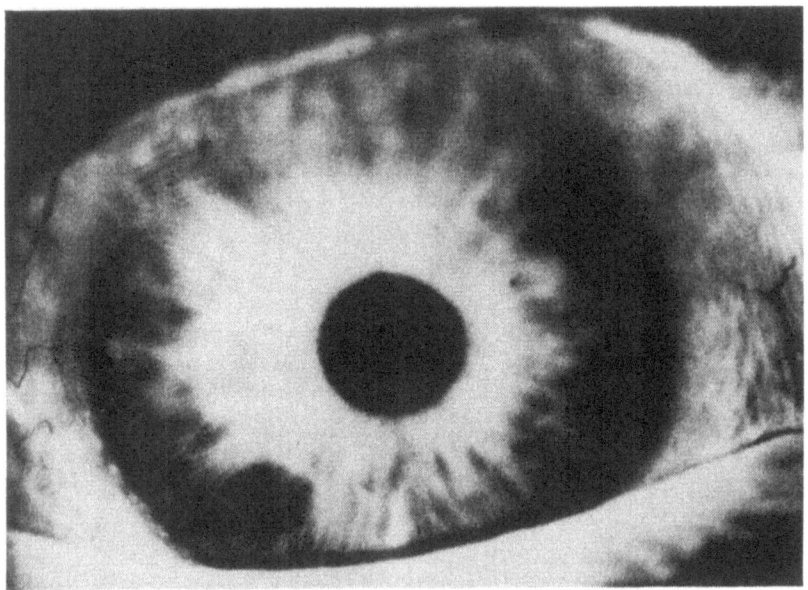

Fig. 4-B. Late phase IFA in same patient, showing marked fluorescein leakage.

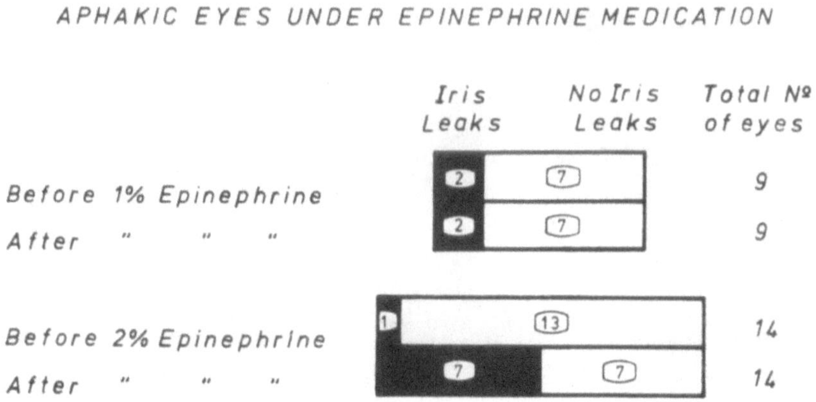

	Iris Leaks	No Iris Leaks	Total Nº of eyes
Before 1% Epinephrine	2	7	9
After " " "	2	7	9
Before 2% Epinephrine	1	13	14
After " " "	7	7	14

Fig. 5. Behaviour of 9 aphakic eyes treated with 1% epinephrine, and 14 aphakic eyes treated with 2% epinephrine.

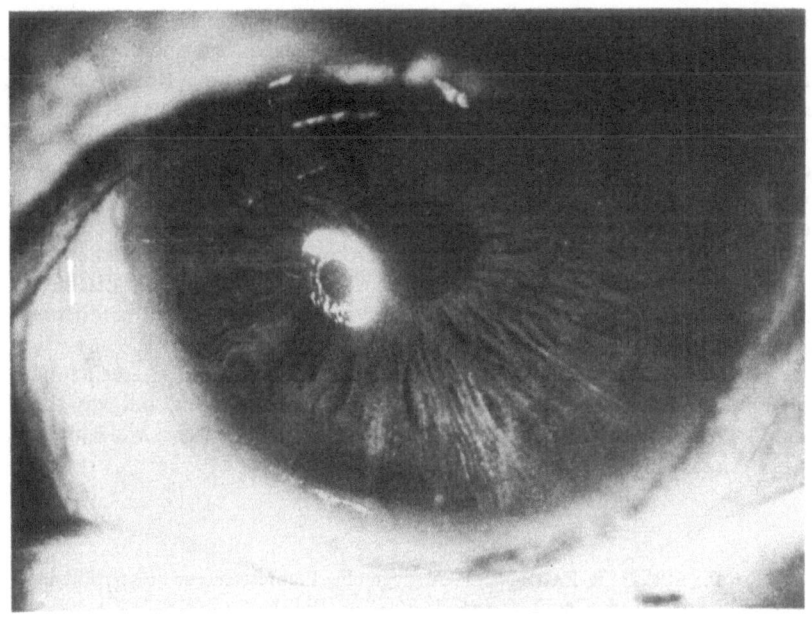

Fig. 6-A. IFA in aphakic eye before epinephrine (highly pigmented iris).

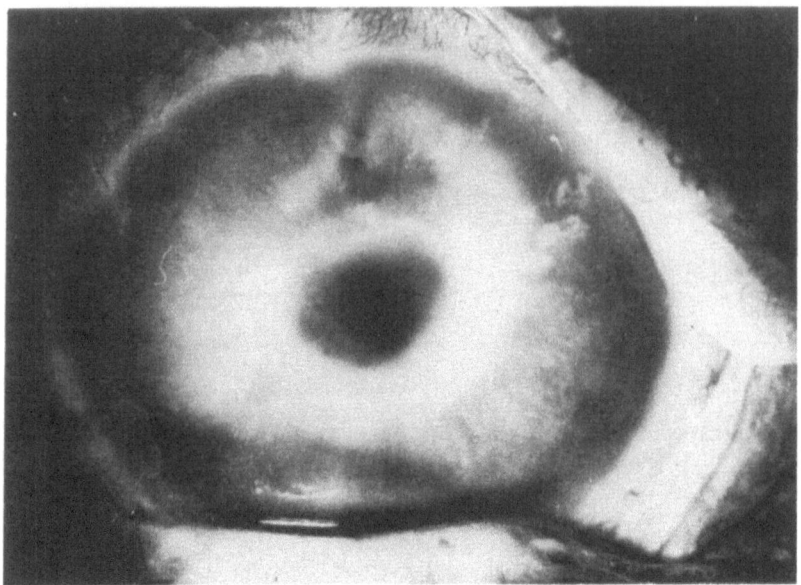

Fig. 6-B. IFA in same patient after 7 days of 2% epinephrine instillation. Note appearance of fluorescein leakage.

DISCUSSION

The results here summarized lead to at least two general conclusions:

1. Vascular occlusions of the major retinal vessels have some sort of influence over anterior segment vessels. In arterial occlusions, this influence occurs preferably early after the occlusive episode, while venous occlusions show a more delayed alteration of the iris vessels. When the occlusion affects both the arterial and the venous retinal vessels, as in stagnation thrombosis, the alteration of the iris vessels is both more immediate and more intense.

2. Macular edemata, at least of the Irvine-Gass syndrome and of the epinephrine toxicity types, are not, strictly speaking, isolated macular diseases, but should rather be considered as macular manifestations of a diffuse vascular derangement that also affects the anterior segment vessels.

It remains to be studied how such independent vascular systems as the retinal and the anterior uveal vessels can influence each other, and why the macula reacts with such peculiar intensity when involved in a widespread vascular disease of the eye.

REFERENCES

DEODATI, F., BEC, P., & LABRO, J.-P. Angiographie Fluorescéinique du segment antérieur de l'oeil. *Arch. Ophth.* (Paris) 31: *859-876* (1971).

KOTTOW, M. & HENDRICKSON, P. Iris angiography in cystoid macular edema after cataract extraction. *Arch. Ophthalmol.* 93: *487-493* (1975).

KOTTOW, M. & HENDRICKSON, P. Iris angiographic findings in retinal arterial occlusions. *Canad. J. Ophthal.* 9: *435-444* (1974).

KOTTOW, M. & METZLER, U. Stagnation thrombosis. *Ophthalmologica* 171: *192-201* (1975).

KOTTOW, M. & METZLER, U. Iris angiographic findings in retinal vein occlusions. 3rd. Mackenzie Symposium, Glasgow 1976, pp. *251-257.*

MAPSTONE, R. Ischaemia in vein occlusions. *Brit. J. Ophthal.* 54: *312-315* (1970).

RAITTA, C. & VANNAS, S. Fluoreszein angiographie der Irisgefässe nach Zentralvenenverschluss. *Graefes Arch. Ophthal.* 177: *33-38* (1969).

Author's address:
Klinisches Institut für experimentelle
Ophthalmologie
Abbestrasse 2
53 Bonn-Venusberg
West Germany

DISCUSSION

Dr Oosterhuis: Dr Kottow showed us that the iris develops more lesions in retinal artery occlusion than in retinal vein occlusion. In the first place, I would like to know if you can see more and earlier neovascularization in fluorescence angiography than when you look at the slitlamp, and second, I would like to know when you see more lesions at the iris in retinal artery occlusion than in retinal vein occlusion, why don't you see neovascular glaucoma in retinal artery occlusion?

Dr Kottow: Regarding the first part of your question. I would say that yes, you do see more. In iris angiography you can see very small vessels and this is similar to what Dr E. Norton presented a few years ago in regard to fundus angiography. He showed that after having looked at the fundus angiograms of diabetic patients, one often could then go back to the ophthalmoscope or slit-lamp and see new vessel formations that had been overlooked in the first examination. In heavily pigmented irises, the angiogram may show vessels that on slit-lamp examination had remained undetected. Regarding the second part of your question, I didn't say that arterial occlusions showed more angiographic alterations at the iris than venous occlusions, but that they appeared earlier. The only abnormal parameter which could be angiographically detected at a late stage in arterial occlusions was abnormal vessel pattern, all the other pathologic signs appeared soon after the occlusion, and that is also sooner than they appear in venous obstructions. Abnormal vessel patterns, by the way, do not necessarily mean neovascular patterns, it often means shunts or vessel arcades which are not normally seen in iris angiograms. In arterial occlusions, not all these vessel patterns are suggestive of being neovascular, and that is the reason why I specifically did not state them as neoformed vessels, but as abnormal vessel patterns. Finally, it should not be forgotten that neovascular glaucoma has been described as a complication after arterial occlusions, and that it is a fairly early complication as compared to its appearance in venous obstructions.

ALTERATION IN BLOOD FLOW IN THE PATHOGENESIS OF DIABETIC RETINOPATHY*

HUNTER L. LITTLE, M.D. & ALVIN H. SACKS, PH.D.

(Menlo Park, Calif., USA)

The pathogenesis of diabetic retinopathy is poorly understood. It is a complex series of events in which many factors contribute to the final picture. Focal retinal ischemia with hypoxia seems to be the earliest clinically detectable change and a consistent finding seen in diabetic retinopathy (KOHNER, 1974; ASHTON, 1953); focal ischemia is also a consistent finding seen in other retinal diseases mimicking it (ASHTON, 1963).

The purpose of this paper is to present evidence that abnormal red cell aggregation is responsible for causing focal retinal ischemia and hypoxia which lead to the sequence of events recognized as diabetic retinopathy. As demonstrated by Fahraeus in 1921, abnormal levels of large molecular weight plasma proteins cause pathologic red cell aggregation (FAHRAEUS, 1921). One postulates that the elevated levels of fibrinogen and alpha-2 globulin as demonstrated by Ditzel and by the authors cause pathologic aggregation of erythrocytes in diabetic patients with retinopathy (DITZEL, 1959; LITTLE et al., 1973; LITTLE et al., in press; LITTLE, in press).

METHODS AND PROCEDURES

Between November, 1972, and February, 1976, the following experimental data obtained in collaboration with Alvin Sacks, Ph.D. at the Palo Alto Medical Research Foundation through the support of N.I.H. grant No. EY 01245-01 is given as supportive evidence that abnormal red cell aggregations, resulting from increased plasma and serum macroglobulins, impair blood flow in the microcirculation and play a significant role in altering oxygen transfer to the highly metabolically active retina.

One hundred and twenty-eight diabetic patients and 43 control subjects were studied using ophthalmic and rheologic techniques to detect evidence of differences in rheologic behavior of diabetic blood and controls. Attempts have been made to determine if differences exist in rheologic behavior of blood for diabetics without retinopathy, with nonproliferative retino-

* Abstracted from Thesis by Hunter L. Little, M.D. for the American Ophthalmological Society, 1976.

Presented at the International Fluorescein Angiographic Congress, Ghent, Belgium, March 1976, the Pacific Coast-Ophthalmological Society, May 1976, and the International Course on Argon Laser Photocoagulation, Creteil, France, March 1976.

pathy, and with proliferative retinopathy. Ages of the four groups were comparable and ranged in years from 16 to 63 years with averages for the controls of 33.3, for diabetics without retinopathy of 38.4, for nonproliferative retinopathy of 43.2, and for proliferative retinopathy of 35.3.

For the purpose of the present study, the diagnosis of diabetes mellitus was made when either (1) measurements of both a plasma glucose of 140 mgm% and a two hour postprandial glucose of 160 mgm% are made or (2) daily insulin injections are required to control plasma glucose levels in order to prevent hyperglycemia and ketosis. The control group had fasting glucose measurements below 100 mgm% and no history of diabetes.

Patients seen in a retinal specialty practice, primarily concerned with diabetic retinopathy, were randomly requested to participate in the study. When practical for the patient, most accepted willingly. The studies were performed within three months and most frequently within one month of the ocular examination. Special request were made to collect controles and diabetic subjects without retinopathy since these were not routinely seen in the office practice.

Subjects were excluded because of recent surgery, complicating illnesses, transfusions, and recent innoculations. In the control group, subjects on medications or with family histories of diabetes were excluded.

RESULTS

The complete results are reported in the authors' thesis in the 1976 Transactions of the American Ophthalmological Society. For this report, only the most significant observations are reported.

All patients received a complete ophthalmological examination including refraction, external examination, slit lamp examination of the anterior segments, ocular tension, and visual fields. Visual fields were done with the Amsler grid and with the tangent screen using a two millimeter white test target at one meter.

Grading of retinopathy was carried out prior to the studies on the extent of nonperfused capillary zones and on the degree of red cell aggregation noted on rheoscopy. The grades were as follows:

0 – no retinopathy
1 – nonproliferative retinopathy
2 – proliferative retinopathy (active neovascularization)
3 – quiescent retinopathy (no active neovascularization)

BLOOD CHEMISTRY

The following chemistry determinations were made:
1. Fibrinogen versus retinopathy
2. Alpha-1 globulin versus retinopathy
3. Alpha-2 globulin versus retinopathy
4. Albumin versus retinopathy
5. Blood urea nitrogen versus retinopathy
6. Glucose versus retinopathy

The diabetic subjects were grouped according to the degree of retinopathy. Males and females were grouped separately. Graphs were made to show the relationship of each chemical measurement between the various groups. Diabetics were grouped according to no retinopathy (NR), non-proliferative retinopathy (NP), active proliferative retinopathy (PA), and quiescent proliferative retinopathy (PQ). Each point on the graph represented the average chemical measurement for each group with a plus or minus one standard deviation. The chemical measurements were plotted on the vertical axis and the patient groups on the horizontal axis.

Statistical calculation were made to test the differences between the control and the diabetic groups. For these calculations, the patients with no retinopathy and with nonproliferative retinopathy were grouped together, and the active proliferative and the quiescent proliferative patients were grouped together. These groupings were made to obtain sufficient sample sizes in statistical calculation; thus, there were six groups consisting of controls (C), nonproliferative diabetics (NP), and proliferative diabetics (PR) for both males and females. Calculations were made by listing the means of each two groups being compared and by using the standard T-test.

1. Fibrinogen

The graph illustrates a progressive rise in plasma levels of fibrinogen from twe control groups to the active proliferative group (Fig. 1). This occurred in both male and female subjects. The level for patients with quiescent proliferative disease was reduced from that of patients with active proliferative disease.

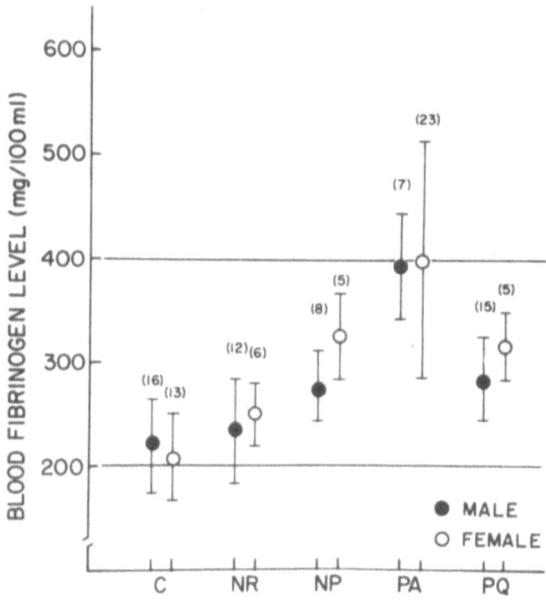

Fig. 1. Progressive rise in plasma fibrinogen levels from control group to group with active proliferative retinopathy for males and females.

Table 1 shows the significance level for each comparison of the different fibrinogen levels between the groups tested. One can see that there is statistically significant difference between the groups. The difference of highest significance is shown between female controles and female subjects with both nonproliferative and proliferative retinopathy and between male controls and males with proliferative retinopathy. These values are extremely significant as calculated by chi square indicating a significance of less then .0005.

Table I

FIBRINOGEN VS. CONTROL AND DIABETIC GROUPS

	C vs. NP	NP vs. PR	C vs. PR
Females	p∠.0005	p∠.01	p∠.0005
Males	p∠.05	p∠.01	p∠.0005

2. *Alpha-1 globulin*

The group failed to illustrate a significant rise in serum levels of alpha-one globulin (Fig. 2). Statistical calculation in Table II fail to show levels of significant difference for each comparison, with the exception of a slight significance for the difference between female controls and females with proliferative diabetic retinopathy.

Table II

ALPHA-1 GLOBULINS VS. CONTROL AND DIABETIC GROUPS

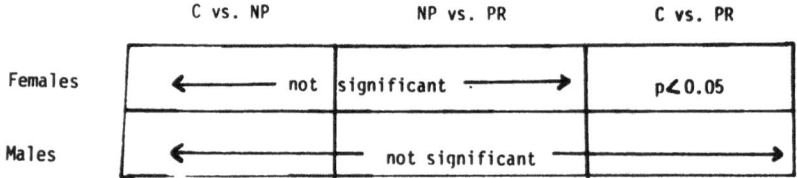

	C vs. NP	NP vs. PR	C vs. PR
Females	← not significant →		p∠0.05
Males	← not significant →		

3. *Alpha-2 globulin*

The graph (Fig. 3) illustrates a progressive rise of alpha-2 globulins as one moves from controls, to diabetics without retinopathy, then to diabetics with nonproliferative retinopathy, and finally to those with active proliferative disease. As in the fibrinogen stody, the alpha-2 globulin falls as the retinopathy undergoes regression. These observations were found in both males and females.

Table III shows the level of significance for comparison of the average alpha-2 globulin levels between the groups. Each calculation shows a signifi-

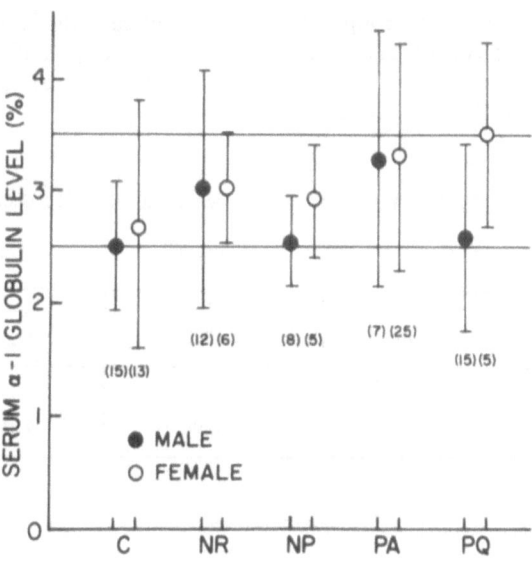

Fig. 2. Graph shows absence of significant rise of alpha-1 globulin for the different groups.

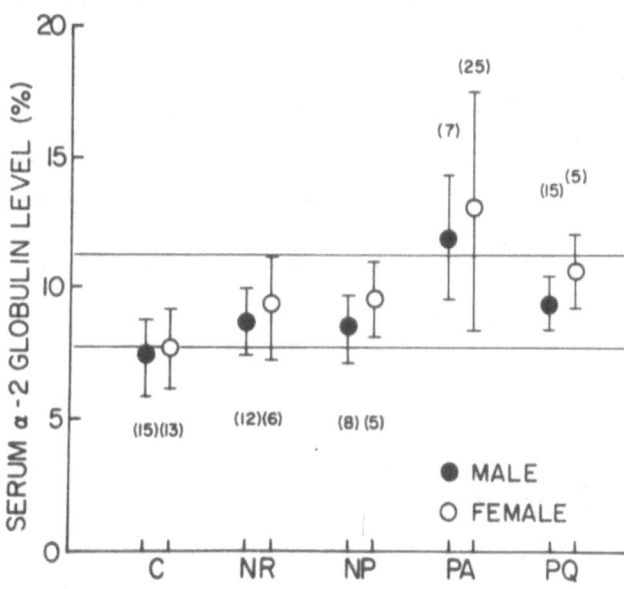

Fig. 3. Graph illustrates progressive rise of serum alpha-2 globulins from controls to diabetics without retinopathy to those with nonproliferative retinopathy to those with active proliferative retinopathy for males and females.

cant difference between groups. The most significant differences are between the female control and female proliferative group, and between the male control and the male proliferative group. These figures are extremely significant (at less than the .0005 level).

Table III

ALPHA-2 GLOBULIN VS. CONTROLS AND DIABETIC GROUPS

	C vs. NP	NP vs. PR	C vs. PR
Females	p< .025	p< .025	p << .0005
Males	p< .005	p< .005	p < .0005

5. Serum albumin

As illustrated in Figure 4, the graph depicts a progressive fall of serum albumin from controls to diabetics with proliferative disease. This drop of albumin is greater in females than in males. There is a subsequent rise in albumin for males with quiescent proliferative disease.

Table IV shows the level of statistical difference between each group when comparing levels of serum albumin. Significant differences are present between each female group listed and between male controls and males with proliferative disease.

Table IV

SERUM ALBUMIN VS. CONTROL AND DIABETIC GROUPS

	C vs. NP	NP vs. PR	C vs. PR
Females	p< .025	p< .05	p< .005
Males	not significant	not significant	p< .025

5. Blood urea nitrogen

The graph in Figure 5 depicts the sharp rise of blood urea nitrogen in females with active proliferative diabetic retinopathy.

Statistical calculations in Table V shows statistically significant differences for the three female groups and for the male control versus proliferative group. The highest significant figure is obtained when comparing blood urea nitrogen for control versus proliferative retinopathy group in females.

478

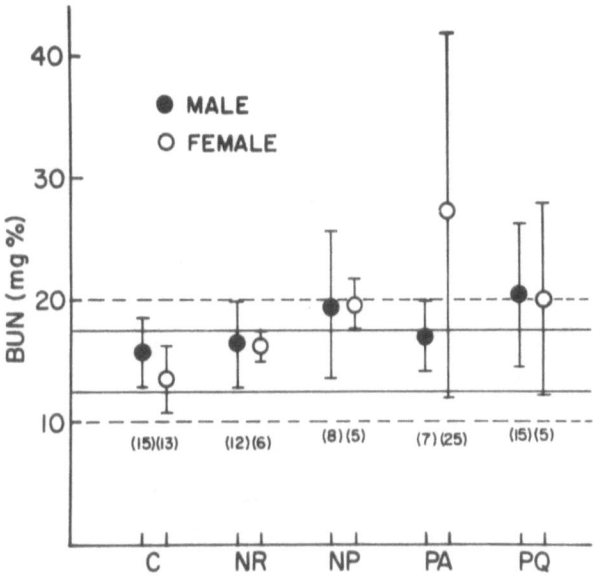

Fig. 4. Graph depicts progressive fall of serum albumin for controls to diabetics with active proliferative retinopathy.

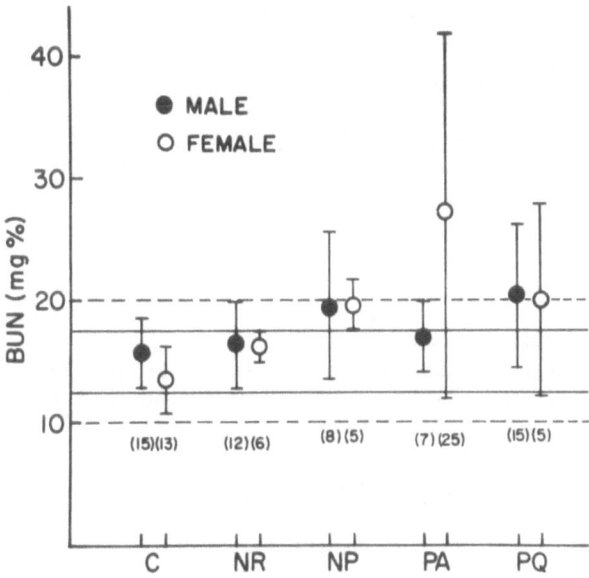

Fig. 5. Sharp rise of blood urea nitrogen in females with active proliferative diabetic retinopathy is suggestive of common factor responsible for retinopathy and nephropathy.

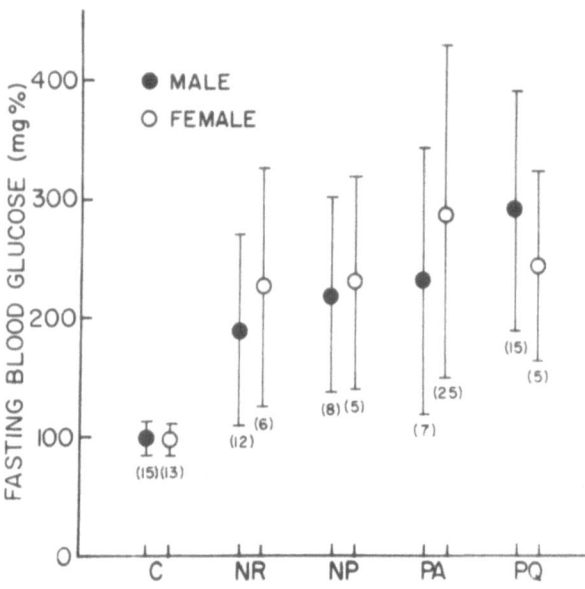

Fig. 6.   Graph shows blood glucose as a function of retinopathy for males and females.

Table V   BLOOD UREA NITROGEN VS. RETINOPATHY

	C vs. NP	NP vs. PR	C vs. PR
Females	p∠.0005	p∠.05	p∠.005
Males	not significant	not significant	p∠.01

6.   Glucose

The graph in Figure 6 shows slightly higher serum glucose levels for proliferative diabetics than for the other groups.

Table VI illustrates the statistical significance between the groups with respect to glucose levels as outlined in the other chemical studies.

RHEOSCOPY IN DIABETES

1.   Classification of red cell aggregatiok

Classification of red cell aggregation on rheoscopy is made as follows:
0 – Uniform distribution of single cells and rouleaux with essentially no indication of more than one cell thickness anywhere.

1 — Uniform background of single cells and rouleaux with a few areas of increased cell density indicating minimal aggregation.

2 — Findings identical to 1, with many areas of increased cell density but no clearly defined aggregates.

3 — The first indication of separate but loose 'lacy' aggregates. These may be interconnected but are distinguishable from the background of cells and rouleaux.

4 — Definite dense aggregates with plasma spaces replacing cellular background. Aggregates may have irregular edges or rouleaux extending from their margins.

5 — Dense, rounded, compact aggregates or clumps with essentially no single cells or rouleaux.

Table VI

GLUCOSE LEVEL VS. RETINOPATHY

	C vs. NP	NP vs. PR	C vs. PR
Females	$p < .0005$	not significant	$p < .0005$
Males	$p < .0005$	$p < .025$	$p < .0005$

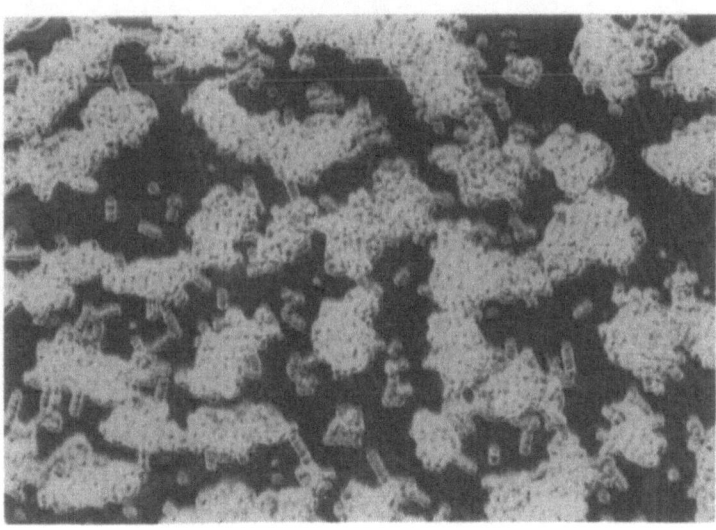

Fig. 7. Tightly clumped red cell aggregates in blood of diabetic with proliferative retinopathy.

481

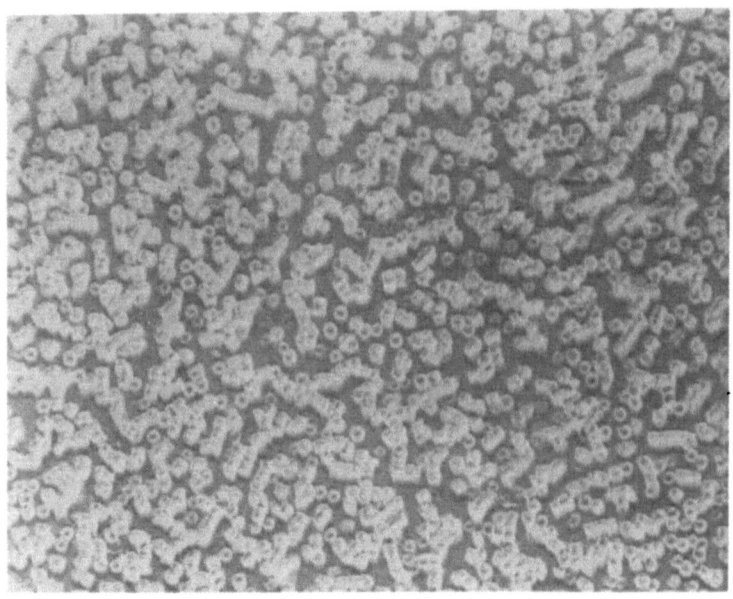

Fig. 8. Single red cells, rouleaux, and loose red cell aggregates in blood of nondiabetic control.

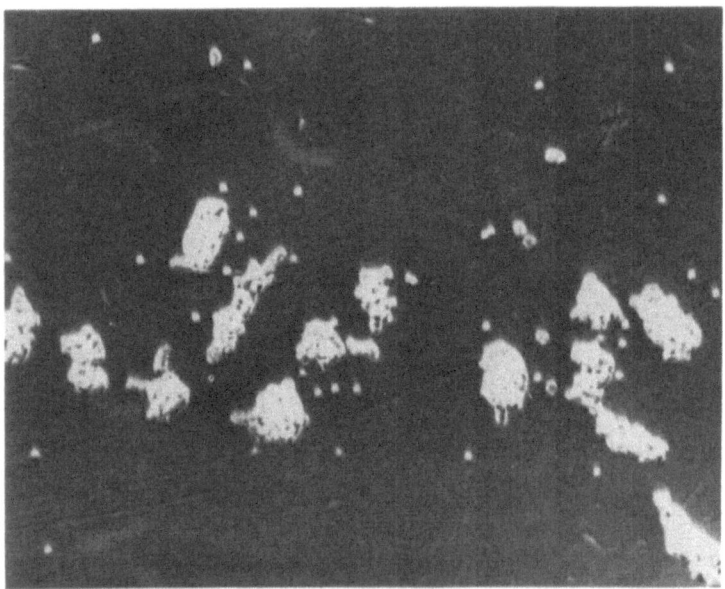

Fig. 9. Erythrocytes of the nondiabetic control when suspended in plasma of proliferative diabetic with similar blood type show pronounced aggregation.

482

2. Observations on blood of humans

a) Diabetic subjects

In diabetics with proliferative retinopathy, the following observations were made: first, at intermediate strain rates (about 22 to 45 sec^{-1}) within two minutes, blood frod diabetic patients with retinopathy developed round-to-oval, discrete, tightly clumped collections of erythrocytes exhibiting increased rigidity (Fig. 7); and second, normal rouleaux or 'stacked coin' formations were usually conspicuously absent in these specimens. With increased strain rates (90 to 225 sec^{-1}), these tight erythrocyte aggregates or clumps showed resistance to dispersion when compared to the gradual disruption of the loose aggregates and rouleaux often present in nondiabetic controls.

b) Control subjects

In the control specimens from nondiabetic subjects, no tightly bound red cell aggregates (i.e. clumps) were observed. The usual picture was one of single erythrocytes, flexible rouleaux, and loose aggregates (Fig. 8). These were easily dispersed with slight increase of strain rates (22 to 45 sec^{-1}).

3. Cross match studies

In the attempt to determine whether the clumping factor was on the surface of the red cells or in the plasma, cross match studies were performed be-

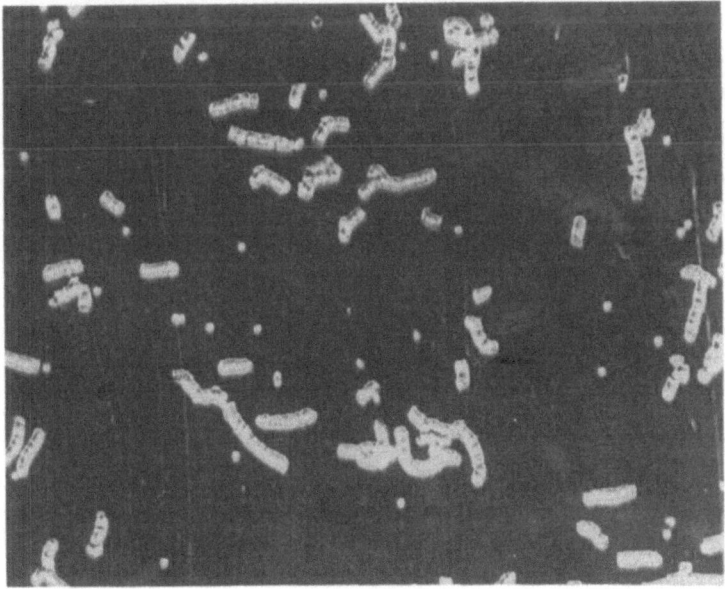

Fig. 10. Erythrocytes of the proliferative diabetic when suspended in plasma of the nondiabetic control with similar blood type show disaggregation.

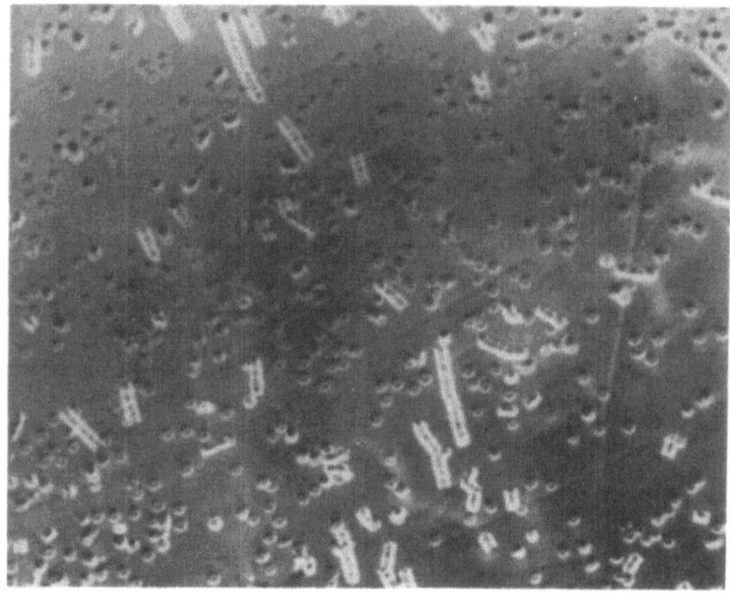

Fig. 11. Disaggregation of red cells of proliferative diabetic when suspended in auto-logous serum.

tween diabetic and nondiabetic subjects of the same blood type. One of the most significant observations in this research program occurred when erythrocytes from a nondiabetic were combined with plasma of a diabetic with proliferative retinopathy; the erythrocytes from the normal subject were markedly clumped in a manner similar to those seen in blood of the proliferative diabetic before the cross-matching (Fig. 9).

Conversely, wwen erythrocytes from the diabetic, which formerly showed marked clumping, were suspended in a plasma from a nondiabetic subject of the same blood type, the aggregates were no longer present, and erythrocytes occurred as single cells and flexible rouleaux (Fig. 10). Similar observations have with four crossmatchings using eight different subjects.

4. Red cells in serum

Red cells from the diabetic and from the nondiabetic were observed with the rheoscope when suspended in their own and in one another's serum. Aggregation occurred in neither the specimens from the diabetics nor the control subjects. In fact, erythrocytes suspended in serum were markedly disaggregated showing almost all single cells without rouleaux (Fig. 11). Thus, it was concluded that red cell aggregation in the diabetic seems to require the presence of a plasma factor.

COMPARATIVE STUDIES

Graphs and statistical evaluations were made using results from studies on 116 subject. These include 28 controls, 16 diabetics with no retinopathy or with less than five microaneurysms, 15 diabetics with nonproliferative retinopathy, and 57 diabetics with proliferative retinopathy. The latter

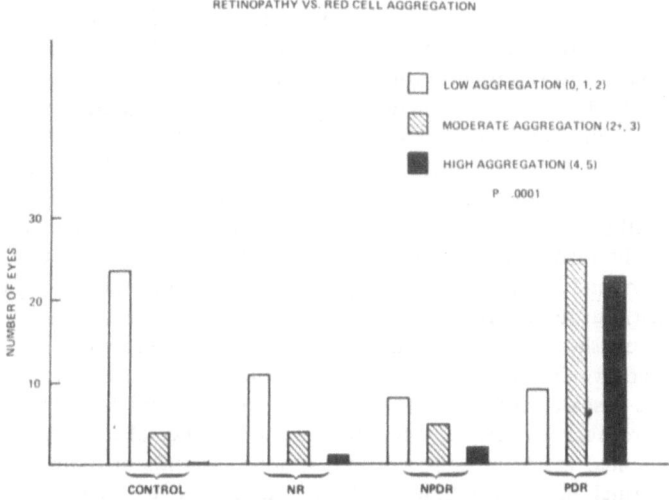

Fig. 12. Graph plotting severity of retinopathy as a function of severity of red cell aggregation.

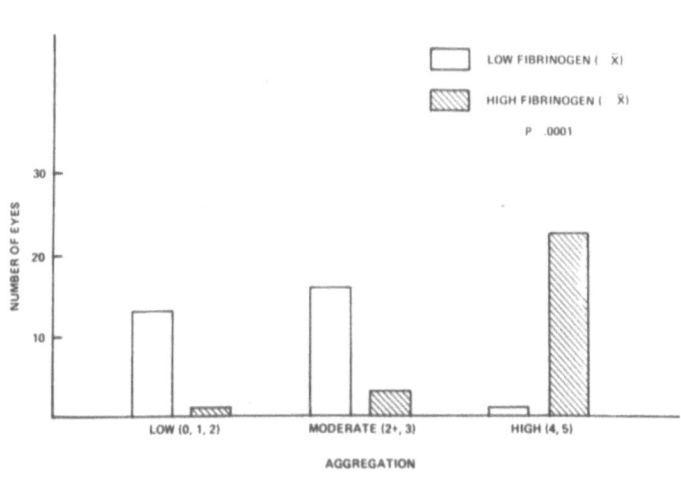

Fig. 13. Red cell aggregation as function of plasma fibrinogen level in females.

485

group with proliferative retinopathy was subdivided into 35 active and 22 inactive cases.

1. Red cell aggregation versus degree of retinopathy

The diabetic and control subjects were classified according to degree of retinopathy and degree of red cell aggregation determined by rheoscopy (Fig. 12). There was a correlation trend between severity of red cell aggregation and severity of retinopathy. Twenty-four of the 28 control subjects exhibited class 0 to 2 classification on rheoscopy. Eleven of the 16 diabetic with minimal to no retinopathy, had class 1 or 2 aggregation on rheoscopy.

Eight of the 15 subjects in the nonproliferative group exhibited class 1 or 2 aggregation and five showed class 3 aggregation. Twenty-three of 26 specimens with class 4 or 5 aggregation were from patients with proliferative retinopathy. In two cases with class 5 aggregation, retinal neovascularization occurred within six months of the rheologic studies. Of the three subjects without proliferative disease who exhibited severe aggregation, two had hypertension, and the third was a 25 year old female diabetic of four years duration without retinopathy.

Rheoscopy showed aggregation of less than class 3 in nine of 57 cases with proliferative disease; however, when one includes only cases with active proliferative disease, only four of 48 cases exhibited minimal aggregation. By active proliferative disease, one refers to the presence of multiple foci of retinal ischemia, capillary nonperfusion, venous beading, or reduplication, and intraretinal microangiography (IRMA). In such eyes, there is greater vascular than fibrous component to the proliferative disease.

In the 57 patients with proliferative retinopathy, 23 had severe aggregation of class 4 or 5; 22 of these occurred in eyes with active proliferative disease.

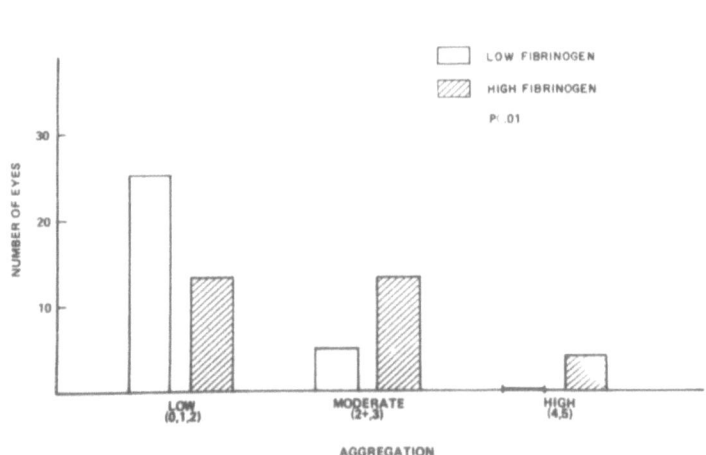

Fig. 14. Red cell aggregation as a function of plasma fibrinogen level in males.

A calculation of chi-squared for the distribution of this group of 116 patients gives a value of 45.36 which shows this to be very significant to a level of $p \ll .0001$. Thus, there is very good evidence that severity of retinopathy is related to increased degree of red cell aggregation.

2. Blood chemistry versus red cell aggregation

Diabetic and control subjects were divided into groups of either high or low levels with respect to the mean for each of the blood chemical measurements studied. Groups were then classified as to sex and degree of red cell aggregation as determined by rheoscopy. Measurements studied were plasma levels of fibrinogen, and serum levels of alpha-1 and alpha-2 globulins, albumin, blood urea nitrogen, and glucose versus red cell aggregation.

a) Fibrinogen versus red cell aggregation

The following figure summarizes data for females (Fig. 13).
A calculation of chi-squared gave a value of 43.7 indicating a statistical significance at $p \ll .0001$.
The following figure is for males (Fig. 14).
A calculation of chi-squared gave a value of 10.46 indicating a statistical significance of $p < .01$.

b) Alpha-1 globulin versus red cell aggregation

In males and females the levels of alpha-1 globulins were not statistically significantly related to red cell aggregation.

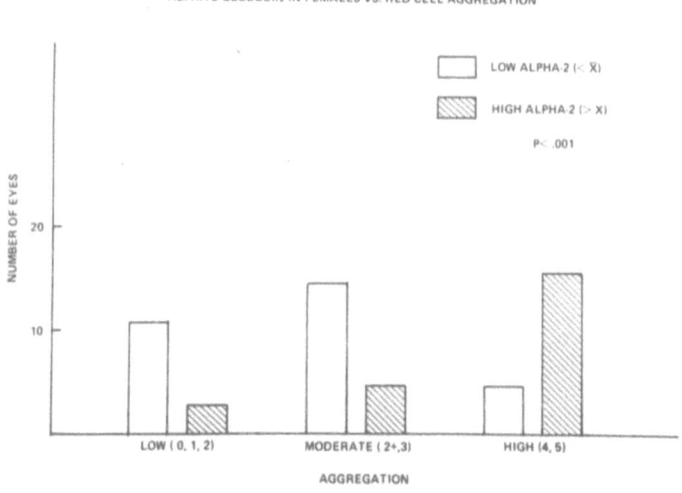

Fig. 15. Serum alpha-2 globulins in females versus red cell aggregation.

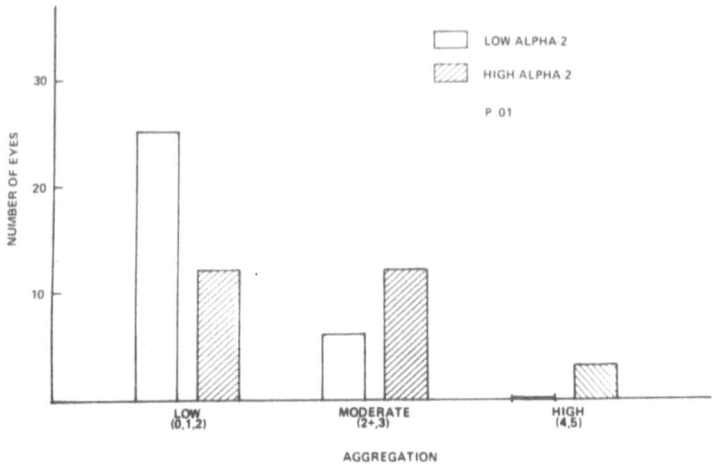

Fig. 16. Red cell aggregation as a function of serum alpha-2 globulins in males.

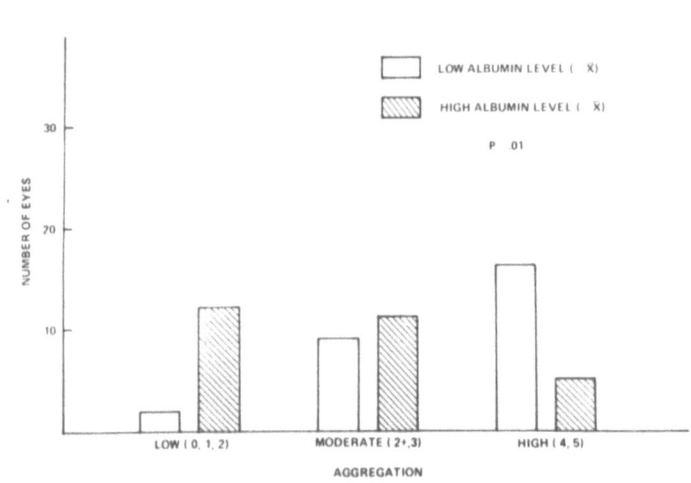

Fig. 17. Serum albumin in females versus red cell aggregation.

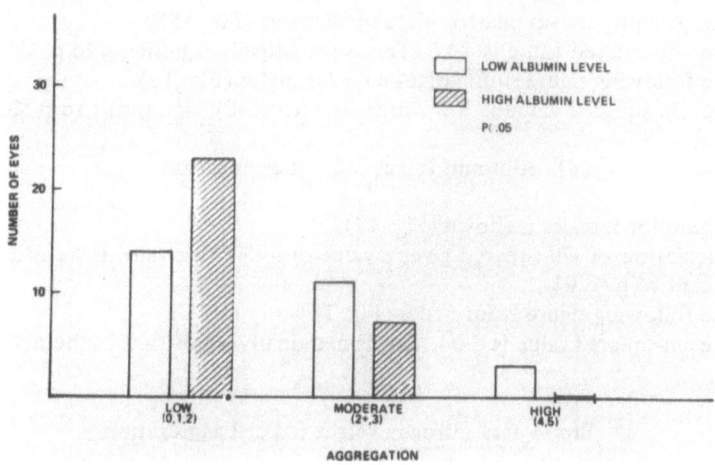

Fig. 18. Serum albumin in males versus red cell aggregation.

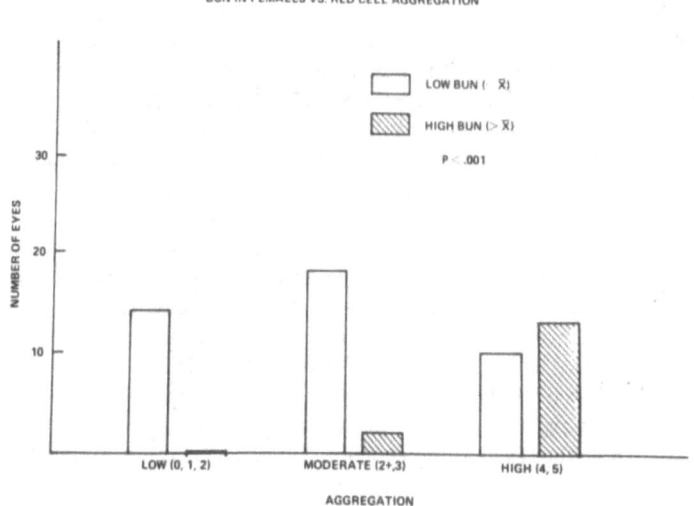

Fig. 19. Blood urea nitrogen in females versus red cell aggregation.

489

c) Alpha-2 globulins versus red cell aggregation

The followed figure summarizes data for females (Fig. 15).
The chi-squared value is 14.5. This is statistically significant to $p < .001$.
The following figure summarizes data for males (Fig. 16).
The chi-squared value is 9.2 which is statistically significant to $p < .01$.

d) Albumin versus red cell aggregation

The figure for females is shown (Fig. 17).
Calculation of chi-squared gives a value of 59.4. This value is statistically significant to $p < .01$.
The following figure is for males (Fig. 18).
The chi-squared value is 6.04. This is marginally significant at the $p < .05$ level.

e) Blood urea nitrogen versus red cell aggregation

The following figure is for females (Fig. 19).
The chi-squared value equals 18.87. This is statistically significant at the $p < .001$ level. The B.U.N. value for males was not statistically significant.

DISCUSSION

HANSEN documented that serum levels of growth hormone are a function of carbohydrate metabolism, showing high levels of growth hormone with poor metabolic control which were reversed with good metabolic control (HANSEN, 1971). Growth hormone promotes synthesis of proteins as reviewed by HALL & LUFT (1974). Thus, prolonged hyperglycemia with increased growth hormone levels in the poorly controlled diabetic could stimulate the liver to synthesize increased amounts of fibrinogen and alpha-2 globulin. Furthermore, growth hormone has a propensity to bind with plasma proteins to produce larger proteins (BALA et al., 1971) as well as a propensity to bind with plasmin (fibrinolysin) (TROUP, 1971) which would reduce the effect of plasmin on fibrinogen. This latter phenomena might account for the abnormal fibrinolytic activity in diabetics with retinopathy as reported by ALMER, MAURIZIO & NILSSON (1975).

Other evidence supporting the important role of growth hormone in the pathogenesis of diabetic retinopathy is the absence of retinopathy in human growth hormone deficient dwarfs with metabolic similarities of diabetes mellitus (MERIMEE et al., 1970) and the higher plasma levels of growth hormone in diabetics with retinopathy (KNOPF et al., 1973).

The relationship of diabetic microangiopathy to abnormal carbohydrate metabolism is reported by WILLIAMSON, VOGLER & KILO (1971). WHITE reported the higher incidence of vascular complications among poorly controlled juvenile diabetics than among well controlled subjects (PAZ-GUEVARA et al., 1975). ENGERMAN reported an increased incidence of retinopathy in poorly controlled diabetic dogs as compared to metabolically controlled diabetic dogs (ENGERMAN, in press). Thus, prolonged abnormal carbohydrate metabolism in the presence of increased levels of growth hormone seem essential in the production of retinopathy presumably by causing elevations of alpha-2 globulin and fibrinogen.

SUMMARY

This paper reports the results of a multifaceted study whose main purpose was to identify the factors that play major roles in the development of diabetic retinopathy. To this end the study consisted of a simultaneous examination of data frod three principle areas:
- direct clinical evaluation and examination of ocular states in vivo
- rheological examination of blood
- blood chemistry.

By examining and analyzing the results from these three areas, it has become evident that diabetic retinopathy is caused by abnormal red cell aggregation. This red cell aggregation has in turn been shown to be related to high levels of fibrinogen and alpha-2 globulins and low levels of serum albumin while alpha-1, beta, and gamma globulins have shown to have mini- mal changes.

The mechanism for diabetic retinopathy development may be explained as follows. Evidence indicates that diabetic retinopathy occurs as a result of impaired oxygen transfer to the retina. This tissue is most susceptible to hypoxia because of its unique vascular anatomy and its high metabolic activity. Altered hemorheodynamics in the microcirculation seems to play a major role in the production of focal ischemia and retinal hypoxia. Impaired carbohydrate metabolism with hyperglycemia stimulates release of growth hormone. This in turn activates hepatic synthesis of large plasma proteins including fibrinogen and alpha-2 globulins. These large plasma proteins bind red cells into aggregates that cause sludging in the microcirculation with increased resistance to flow. In the presence of endothelial damage, platelet adhesion to subendothelial collagen fibrils and platelet release of ADP might occur, increasing the red cell aggregate resistance to shear. Focal occlusions of the distal arterioles then occur. In areas of ischemia, there is endothelial and pericyte loss, but endothelial hyperplasia occurs in zones of hypoxia. In hypoxic zones at the margins of focal ischemia, microaneurysms and retinal neovascularization develop in association with micro and macrovascular shunts. Protein and lipid exudates from leakage of plasma and hemorrhage occur as a result of impaired capillary permeability.

The sequence of events in diabetic retinopathy can possibly be aborted with rigid control of blood sugar levels which results in decreased produc- tion of growth hormone secretion accompanied by reduced protein syn- thesis with amelioration of red cell aggregation and improved hemorheo- dynamics in the microcirculation.

REFERENCES

ALMER, L.O., MAURIZIO, P. & NILSSON, I.M. Diabetic and the fibrinolytic system. *Diabetes* 24: *529* (1975).

ASHTON, N. Arteriolar involvement in diabetic retinopathy. *Brit. J. Ophthal.* 37: *282-292* (1953).

ASHTON, N. Studies of the retinal capillaries in relation to diabetic and other retino-pathies. *Brit. J. Ophthal.* 47: *521* (1963).

BALA, R.M., FERGUSON, K.A. & BECK, J.C. Growth hormone like activity in plasma and urine, growth and growth hormone proceedings. 2nd International Symposium on Growth Hormone. Milan, May (1971).

DITZEL, J. Relationship of blood protein composition to intravascular erythrocyte aggregation (sludged blood). *Acta Med. Scand.* Suppl. 343, 164: *11* (1959).

ENGERMAN, R. Animal models of diabetic retinopathy. Trans. Amer. Acad. Ophthal. Otolaryng. (August 1976, in press).

FAHRAEUS, R. Suspension-stability of the blood. *Acta Med. Scand.* 55: *1* (1921).

HALL, K. & LUFT, R. Growth hormone and somatomedin. In: Advances in metabolic disorders. Academic Press, New York, Vol. 7 (1974).

HANSEN, A.P. Normalization of growth hormone hyper-response to exercise in juve-nile diabetics after 'normalization' of blood sugar. *J. Clin. Invest.* 50: *1806* (1971).

KNOPF, R.F., FAJANS, S.S., SUMER, P., FLOYD, J.C., JR., PRCHKOV, V.K. & CONN, J.W. Plasma levels of growth hormone and glucagon in diabetic patients and relatives of diabetic patients. *Adv. in Met. Dis.*, Suppl. 2 (7): *215* (1973).

KOHNER, E.M. Dynamic changes in the microcirculation of diabetics an related to diabetic microangiopathy. Diabetic Microangiopathy. August Krogh Memorial Symposium, p. *41* (1974).

LITTLE, H.L. The role of abnormal hemorheodynamics in the pathogenesis of diabetic retinopathy. *Trans. Amer. Ophthal. Soc.* (1976, in press).

LITTLE, H.L., SACKS, A.H., KRUPP, M., JOHNSON, P., BASSO, L., TICHNER, G., VASSILIADIS, A. & ZWENG, H.C. Abnormal hemorrheology in the pathogenesis of diabetic microangiopathy. Presented by Little, M.D. at the International Con-gress on Diabetes. Brussels (July 1973).

LITTLE, H.L., ZWENG, H.C. & SACKS, A.H. The role of altered blood rheology in pathogenesis of diabetic retinopathy. Proceedings of the XXII Congres Internatio-nal d'Ophthalmologie (1974, in press).

MERIMEE, T.J., FINEBERG, V.A., MCKUSICK & HALL, J. Diabetes mellitus and sexual ateliotic dwarfism: a comparative study. *J. Clin. Invest.* 49: *1096* (1970).

PAZ-GUEVARA, A.T., HSU, T.H. & WHITE, P. Juvenile diabetes mellitus after 40 years. *Diabetes* 25: *559* (1975).

TROUP, S.B. Fribrinolysis. In: Weed, R.I. Hematology for internist. Little-Brown, p. *218* (1971).

WILLIAMSON, J.R., VOGLER, N.J. & KILO, C. Microvascular disease in diabetes. *Med. Clin. N. Amer.* 55: *847* (1971).

Authors' address:
Palo Alto Medical Research Foundation
and Palo Alto Retinal Group
1225 Crane Street
Menlo Park, California 94025
USA

DISCUSSION

Dr Kohner: Dr Little made the important observation that it is not only the blood vessels which matter but also what is within those vessels. This also leads to the perennial problems to what comes first, the chicken or the egg? We all know that patients who have proliferative retinopathy have the most severe disease and also have the most severe platelet aggregation. We have, however, no evidence at all that either platelet or red cell aggregation is the cause of it. Indeed, there is some evidence that it may not be so. Red cell cumping, if it was in any way related aetiologically to nonperfusion in the retina, one would also expect to have an effect in other parts of the body, and of course, we know that these capillary occlusion phenomenons are to some extent specific for the retina. That is the first point. The second point is that we do not think that growth hormone alone could account for this because we know two things; one is that acromegalics do not get retinopathy and they have much higher growth hormone levels. So diabetes obviously has to be present. The second fact about growth hormone is that patients who had pituitary ablation, which is, as far as we know, complete with no growth hormone response, still have raised fibrinogen levels. Also in diabetic keto-acidosis fibrinogen levels rise before the growth hormone level rise and finally as far as the clotting's concerned, fibrinogen alone does not matter all that much. If clotting takes place, we want to know what is happening to fibrin degradation products. We looked at it in a few patients prospectively before and after pituitary ablation and so far have no significant difference. The question is have you actually measured this, if you are trying to say that it is in any way related to intravascular clotting?

Dr Little: In response to Dr Kohner's first point, capillary occlusion in diabetic microangiopathy is not specific for the retina. It occurs in the kidney, muscle, and skin; furthermore, increased red cell aggregation may play a role in the increased incidence of coronary and cerebral vascular diseases in diabetes. The retinal capillary plexus with its single end-arteriole feeder and the high metabolic activity of the retina possibly account for the increased susceptibility of the retina to microvascular occlusion and to the neovascular response.

In regard to her second point, evidence of the role of growth hormone in the production of retinopathy are as follows:
1. Merimee's study on ateliotic growth-hormone deficient dwarfs who had hyperglycemia for an average of 17 years, failed to develop any evidence of diabetic retinopathy. This was in contrast to a comparable age group of diabetics in whom retinopathy was present in 41%.
2. Campbell's study on dogs showed that diabetes occurred in dogs within three days following injection of growth hormone.
3. Johansen, Hansen, and Lundbaek have demonstrated serum growth hormone levels three to four times greater in diabetics than in normals, and Knopf, et al. showed even higher serum growth hormone levels in diabetics with retinopathy than those without retinopathy.
4. Since growth hormone stimulates synthesis of proteins, one hypothesizes that the elevated growth hormone levels in diabetes stimulate the synthesis of fibrinogen and alpha-2 globulins. Furthermore, it is possible that the growth hormone molecule may bind with plasmin, thus altering the critical fibrinogen-plasmin ratio which would further elevate fibrinogen levels.
5. The lack of a high incidence of diabetic retinopathy in acromegaly might result from the associated increase of insulin as well as growth hormone in acromegaly.

Would Dr Kohner please repeat the question concerning fibrin degradation products?

Dr Kohner: Fibrinogen degradation products which, if elevated indicate that clotting is actually taking place. But we also know that fibrinogen won't go into fibrin degradation products unless you have endothelial damage as well.

Dr Little: We have measured fibrinogen, but we have not measured fibrinogen degradation products. We have found that the degree of retinopathy is greater in patients with high fibrinogen as well as with elevated alpha-2 globulins. These findings were most pronounced in females with proliferative diabetic retinopathy.

Dr Siam: I would like to ask Dr Little about the relationship between the degree of retinopathy and the growth hormone level. We have been carrying out growth hormone essays on diabetic retinopathy of the proliferative type. We did not find any correlation between the degree of retinopathy and the growth hormone level.

Dr Little: My paper was to present evidence that plasma protein changes cause red cell aggregation and that red cell aggregation is greater in patients with retinopathy. We did not measure growth hormone. We plan to do this in collaboration with Dr Peter Forsham's, group in California. The only reason I mentioned the growth hormone change is because of its relationship to the work that has been done in Denmark, which showed elevated levels of growth hormone in diabetics. I think it ties in with our observations of changes in plasma proteins. Furthermore, the absence of retinopathy in patients who have no growth hormone but who do have abnormal carbohydrate metabolism as demonstrated by Merimee supports the essential role of growth hormone in producing retinopathy. We propose that the elevated growth hormone stimulates increased levels of alpha-2 globulin and fibrinogen which cause red cell aggregation with resulting impaired flow in the microcirculation.

The mechanism of red cell aggregation deserves a comment. Fahraeus in 1921 first emphasized the red cell agglutinating capacity of the large protein fractions in plasma and serum. Thorsen & Hint in 1950 observed aggregation of red cells by large dextran molecules. Chien & Jan in 1973 suggested that red cell aggregation results from large molecular weight molecules which prevent negative repulsive forces of red cells by forming bridges between red cells. That is, the length of the molecular bridge between the red cells is longer than the distance of the negative repulsive field. We suggest that this is the mechanism by which elevated fibrinogen and alpha-2 globulins cause red cell aggregation in diabetics with retinopathy.

Dr Peduzzi: Mr Moderator, please let me make just a little remark concerning the paper on the pathogenesis of diabetic retinopathy. The importance of the levels of fibrinogen and FDP in patients with diabetes mellitus has been pointed out by Dr Little and Dr Kohner. I feel that we should take into account the whole fibrinolytic system in these patients.

The swedish group of Malmö could in fact demonstrate that the main fibrinolytic parameters (i.e. the spontaneous fibrinolytic activity of the blood, the presence of plasminogen activator in the vessel wall, and the fibrinolytic response to venous stasis), are depressed in various degrees in diabetic patients in comparison with those of the controls.

Furthermore, the fibrinolytic activators of the vessel wall were found to be higher in patients with beginning angiopathy than in patients with more advanced retinopathy or without retinopathy.

FIRST LESIONS IN INFANTILE DIABETIC RETINOPATHY.
ANGIOFLUORESCEINIC STUDY*

D. TOUSSAINT, H. DORCHY & M. QUAETAERT

(Brussels, Belgium)

ABSTRACT

30 cases of infantile diabetic patients were studied by retinal fluorescein angiography in order to investigate the onset of the retinal angiopathy.

This study demonstrated that the appearance of microaneurysms is no necessarily subordinate to other vascular retinal modifications. It also showed the possibility of spontaneous regressions of the retinal lesions and suggested that the capillary leakage could be the first vascular retinal lesion.

INTRODUCTION

We have studied the fundus of the eye in infantile diabetic patients by fluorescein angiography in order to investigate the onset of vascular retinal lesions in cases with few or no retinal angiopathy at the moment of our first ocular investigation. Until now, there are only few angiofluoresceinic studies of infantile diabetic retinopathy (BARTA et al., 1972; BROOSER et al., 1975; KAREL et al., 1970; MARCKWORT et al., 1973).

The previous studies, mostly performed on adults, are related to retinopathies already detectable by conventional ophthalmoscopy, and where the incipient vascular lesions are obscured by numerous and intense fluoresceinic modifications. In 1974, TOUSSAINT & DORCHY have published a preliminary study of fluorescein angiography in infantile diabetes with, for the first time, a detailed description of the very first retinal lesions. We will discuss the principal data of this investigation, showing the interest of fluorescein angiography, as compared with conventional ophthalmoscopy in the diagnosis of incipient retinopathy.

MATERIAL

Our investigations were performed on 30 patients, 16 females and 14 males, varying in age from 9 to 32, where diabetes became clinically evident before or at the age of 14 (Table I). The diabetes lasted from 1 to 20 years, with our ocular investigations covering periods varying from 1 to 4 years. All patients underwent fluorographies at intervals of 6 months. Table I indicates the quality of control of diabetes and the degree of retinopathy.

---

* This investigation was supported by a grant of F.R.S.M. n° 20.512.

Table I. Roman numerals: Scott's classification of diabetic retinopathy. F: lesions only detected by fluorescein angiography. hh: punctate deep hemorrhages. HH: superficial hemorrhages.

No	Sex	Age (years)	Duration of diabetes (years)	Quality of control	Retinopathy
1	f	32	20	Good	I
2	m	28	19	Poor	IV
3	f	22	14	Poor	F
4	f	22	14	Poor	F
5	m	19	12	Insuff.	II
6	f	19	11	Insuff.	F
7	f	20	11	Insuff.	I
8	m	19	10	Insuff.	F+hh+HH
9	m	17	9	Insuff.	F
10	f	16	8	Insuff.	F
11	m	20	8	Good	F
12	f	16	8	Insuff.	0
13	f	17	8	Insuff.	0
14	m	9	8	Good	0
15	m	15	7	Good	F

No	Sex	Age (years)	Duration of diabetes (years)	Quality of control	Retinopathy
16	f	16	7	Insuff.	0
17	f	15	6	Insuff.	II–I
18	m	14	6	Insuff.	0
19	f	16	5	Good	0
20	f	15	5	Good	F+hh+HH
21	m	15	5	Insuff.	0
22	f	15	4	Insuff.	0
23	m	16	4	Good	0
24	m	16	4	Insuff.	F+hh
25	f	14	4	Insuff.	0
26	f	12	4	Good	0
27	m	13	4	Insuff.	0
28	m	13	4	Insuff.	0
29	m	15	2	Insuff.	0
30	f	12	1	Insuff.	0

For 8 (1, 2, 5, 7, 8, 17, 20, 24) of the 30 patients (26,6%) the diagnosis of diabetic retinopathy was established by conventional ophthalmoscopy with the observation of retinal microaneurysms in 5 cases (1, 2, 5, 7, 17) and retinal punctate hemorragic lesions in 3 cases (8, 20, 24). For the latter, the presence of conspicuous microaneurysms observed by angiofluoresceinic investigations confirmed the diagnosis of diabetic retinopathy.

For 7 (3, 4, 6, 9, 10, 11, 15) other patients without detectable retinal lesion by conventional ophthalmoscopy, fluorescein administration demonstrated obvious capillary leakage (Fig. 1) Therefore, the diagnosis of diabetic retinopathy was established for 15 of the 30 patients (50%). In 18 cases for

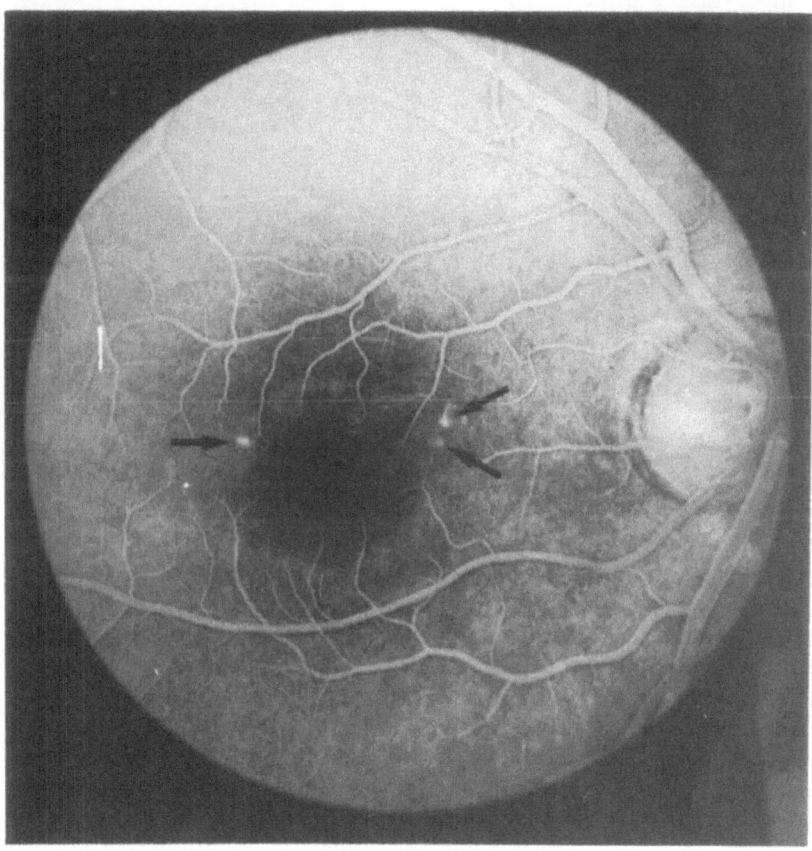

Fig. 1. O.D. Typical first lesion observed in juvenile incipient diabetic retinopathy: three small spots of fluorescein leakages (arrows).

499

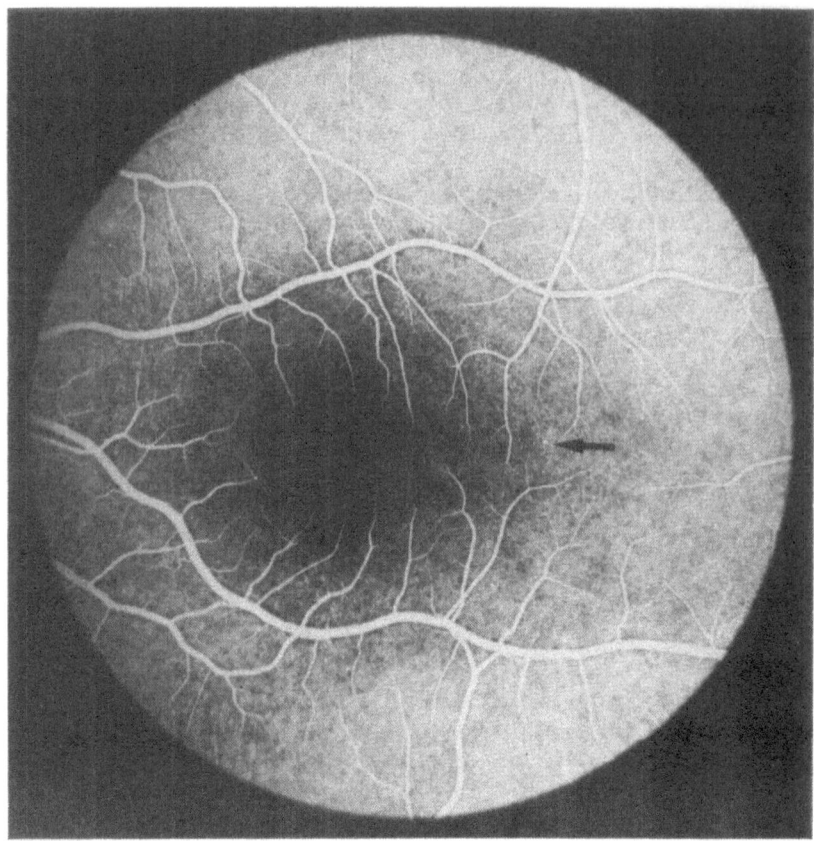

Fig. 2. O.S. Case n° 17. The arrow is pointing out a microaneurysm without any surrounding vascular modification and without any coexistent or pre-existent local leakage.

which the duration of diabetes was 6 years or more, the diagnosis of diabetic retinopathy was established by conventional ophthalmoscopy for 6 patients (33,3%) and by fluorescein angiography for 7 (38,8%). Ten of these 18 patients without any retinopathy at our first investigation developed retinal vascular lesions in the course of further examinations: fluorescein leakage for 5, fluorescein leakage and microaneurysms for 2, microaneurysms without leakage for 3. We would like to state the fact that microaneurysms have been observed appearing in capillary pattern areas entirely free from any other pre-existent of coexistent vascular lesion. No fluorescein leakage or occluded nonfunctional capillaries were observed in the vicinity of these microaneurysms (Fig. 2).

In 2 cases (15, 17) an obvious spontaneous regression of the diabetic retinal lesions was observed within the course of one year. Complete disappearance of deep round hemorrages and dotty exudates was noticed with striking restoration of capillary lumens at the level of retinal foci, formerly showing occluded nonfunctional capillaries (Fig. 3, 4, 5, 6). These spontaneous regressions of diabetic retinopathy were independent of any modification of diabetic treatment.

CONCLUSIONS

Angiofluoresceinic retinal investigation increases the possibility of diagnosis in incipient diabetic infantile retinopathy.

The appearance of microaneurysms is not necessarily subordinate to

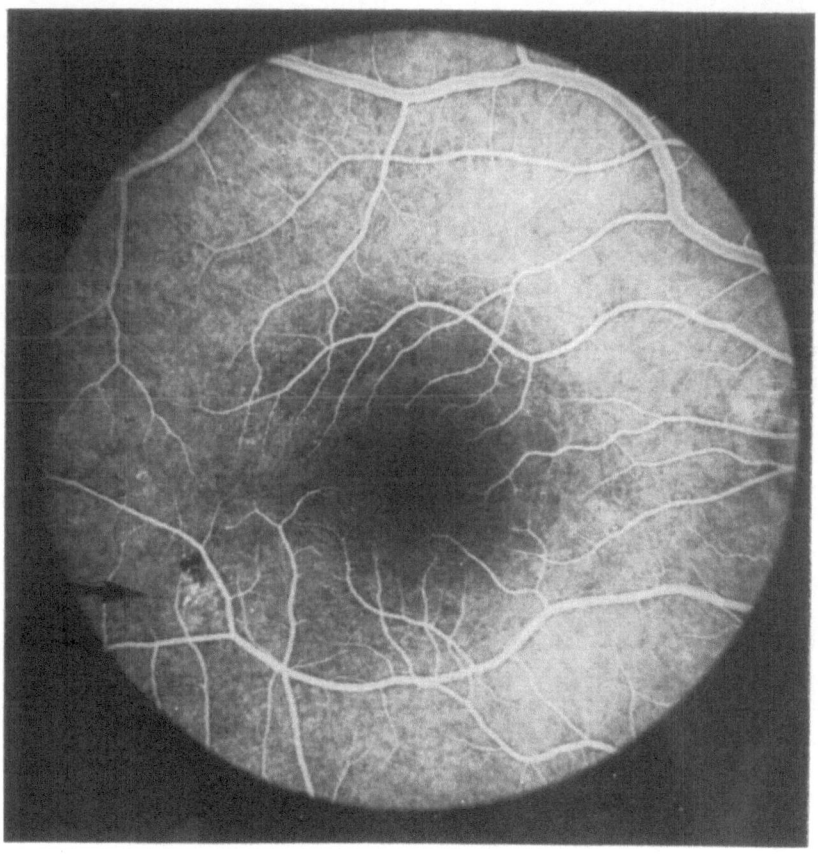

Fig. 3. O.D. Case n° 17. October 1973. Microaneurysms, deep round hemorrages and non functional occluded capillaries (arrow).

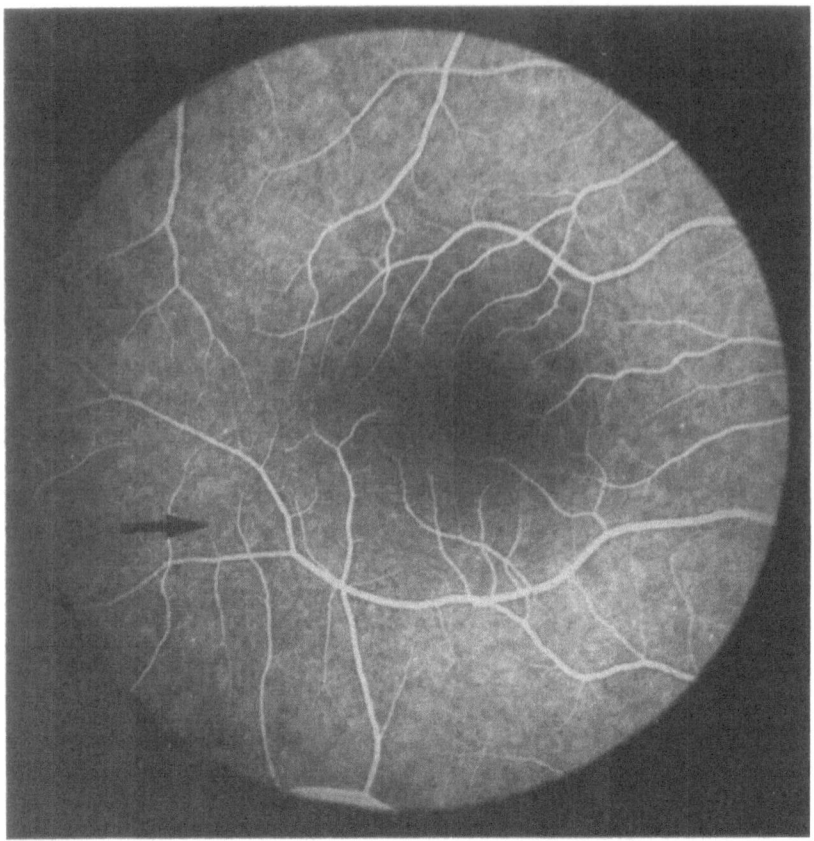

Fig. 4. O.D. Case n° 17. October 1974. Complete disappearance of all types of lesions in the same area (large arrow) as fig. 3.

other detectable clinical local or adjacent vascular modifications.

At the present time, we are not able to establish any relationship between microaneurysms and capillary leakage. Nevertheless, the high frequency of leakage in incipient diabetic angiopathy suggests that it could be the first vascular lesion in diabetic retinopathy.

Spontaneous regressions of all types of retinal lesions are not excluded in infantile diabetic retinopathies.

RESUME

L'élaboration d'angiographies rétiniennes à la fluorescéine chez 30 patients présentant un diabète infantile et pratiquées dans le but de préciser les toutes premières altérations vasculaires de l'angiopathie diabétique a démontré que l'installation des microanévrismes rétiniens n'était pas forcément conditionnée par la présence d'altérations des capillaires avoisinants; elle permet de penser que les fuites de fluorescéine existant au niveau des capillaires sont les premières lésions de l'angiopathie rétinienne diabétique et elle a démontré que dans certaines rétinopathies diabétiques infantiles on pouvait observer une régression spontanée de tous les types de lésions rétiniennes.

REFERENCES

BARTA, L., BROOSER, G. & MOLNAR, M. Diagnostic importance of fluorescein angiography in infantile diabetes. *Acta Diabet. Lat.* 9: *290-298* (1972).

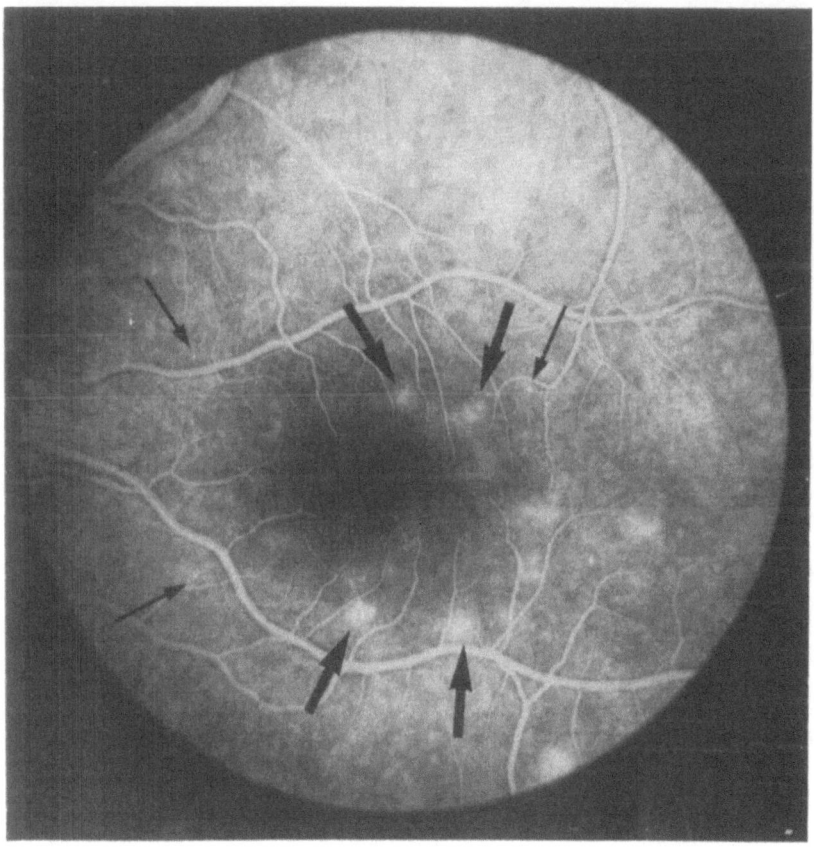

Fig. 5. O.S. Case n° 17. October 1973. Microaneurysms (small arrows). Microaneurysms and leakage of fluorescein (large arrows).

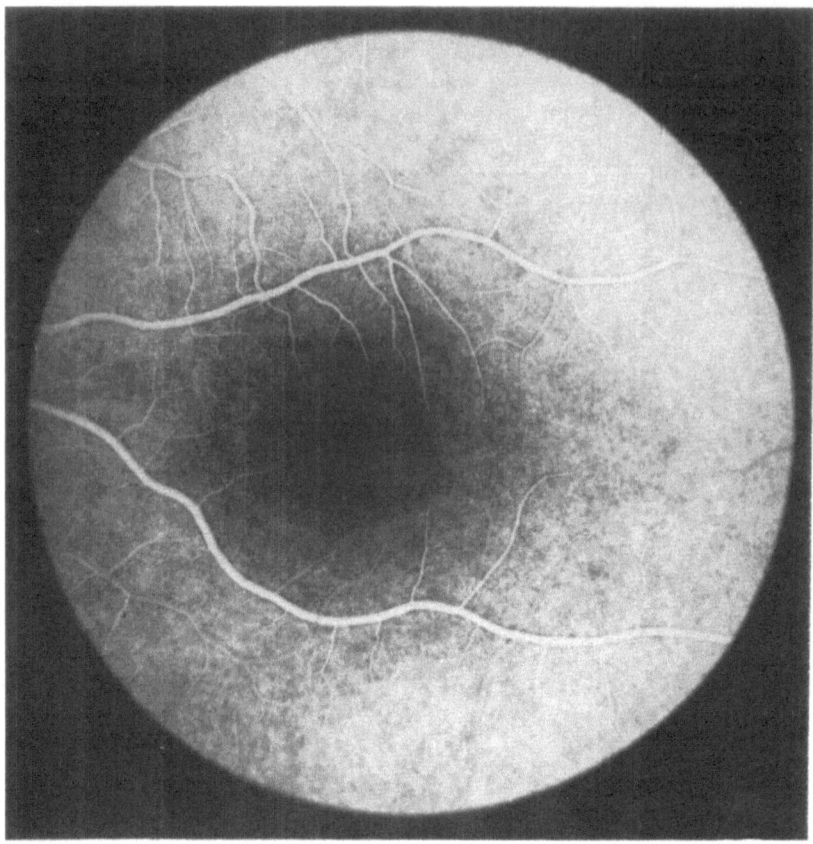

Fig. 6. O.S. Case n° 17. October 1974. Disappearance of microaneurysms. No more leakage of fluorescein.

BROOSER, G., BARTA, L., ANDA, L. & MOLNAR, M. Frühdiagnose der Mikroangiopathie bei kindlichen Diabetes. *Klin. Mbl. Augenheilk.* 166: *233-236* (1975).

KAREL, I. & PELESKA, M. Fluorescein angiography in diabetes in childhood and youth. *Cesk. Oftal.* 26: *357-362* (1970).

MARCKWORT, H.J., SCHUMACHER, R., KLUXEN, M. & SCHROEDER, U. Nachweis der diabetischen Retinopathie durch fluoreszenzangiographische Untersuchungen bei kindlichem Diabetes Mellitus. *Klin. Padiat.* 185: *408-411* (1973).

TOUSSAINT, D. & DORCHY, H. Exploration angiofluorescéinique de la rétinopathie diabétique infantile. *Bull. Soc. B. Ophtal.* 168: *783-800* (1974).

Authors' addresses:
D. Toussaint
Department of Ophthalmology
Hôpital Universitaire Brugmann
Place Van Gehuchten
B 1020 Brussels
Belgium

H. Dorchy & M. Quaetart
Diabetic Unit
Department of Pediatrics
Hôpital Universitaire St. Pierre
rue Haute
B 1000 Brussels
Belgium

DISCUSSION

Dr Brooser: We did the same investigation in 161 children and we have an even higher percentage of incipient microangiopathy as Drs Toussaint and Dorchy. We cannot explain the cause of it, but we do believe that in some cases there must be some genetic influence, some inheritance in the occurrence of the microangiopathy.

Dr Amalric: J'agrée avec les conclusions de Mr Toussaint, mais je ferai 3 réflexions.

Premièrement, en ce qui concerne l'examen. Je crois que si nous faisons des rétinographies en anérythre systématiques, avant l'angiographie, nous voyons des microanévrysmes que les clichés en couleurs ne nous révèlent pas. Ceci pour le microanévrysme seul, pour ce qui est bien entendu du leakage, c'est différent.

Deuxièmement, j'agrée avec cette évolution spontanément bénigne dans certains cas, non seulement chez l'enfant, mais également chez l'adulte jeune. J'ai vu depuis dix ans par des angiographies et des microangiographies capillaires que certains malades évoluent spontanément vers la guérison et j'ai même un cas exceptionnel de rétinopathie diabétique bilatérale, avec agrégat plaquettaire, néovascularisation et tout le tableau pathologique qui a complètement régressé; vous seriez bien incapable aujourd'hui de trouver une lésion de rétinopathie diabétique, dix ans après cette évolution aiguë.

C'est dire que sur le plan de l'évolution, troisième réflexion, une rétinopathie diabétique peut guérir spontanément. Ce qui veut dire que sur le plan de la thérapeutique j'attends avec impatience un schéma clinique parfait pour savoir le moment où il faut photocoaguler et à mon avis après dix ans d'observation angiographique le stade de la malignité d'une rétinopathie diabétique doit être à mon sens très difficile à trouver.

Dr Larsen: I would like to ask Dr Toussaint whether he found any correlation between the earliest manifestation of infantile retinopathy as compared to the duration of diabetes because during the last few years several controversial papers have been published on this.

Dr Toussaint: We have not seen any correlation between the duration of the diabetes and the mode of treatment for these young diabetics. What seems important, but it is perhaps to early to draw any conclusion, is the beginning of the puberty. To Dr Amalric I would say that in any case red free pictures have been taken. Another thing that is amazing in young diabetics is that the leakage can disappear in a few days. I have seen some cases where there is leakage on one day, and you look at them one day later and there is no more leakage.

Dr Henkind: In regard to Dr Toussaint's paper our own group, not studying diabetes but studying lupus particularly Dr Gold and Walsh's work has confirmed the work of Cruz's group in Mexico. They showed that in lupus patients where you could not see anything on the color photographs or by fundoscopy the angiogram did show microvascular abnormalities. So it is quite obvious that it is a much more sensitive test in many diseases, not only in diabetes.

CYSTOID MACULAR OEDEMA IN DIABETIC RETINOPATHY

H. FREYLER & I. EGERER

(Vienna, Austria)

INTRODUCTION

In cases of cystoid macular oedema fluorescein angiographic leakage points within the perimacular capillary bed will reveal the origin of serum spreading toward the macula. Diabetic retinopathy being associated with this type of vascular changes will not be amendable to any mode of medical therapy. By using photocoagulation the areas of capillary hyperpermeability can be eradicated, however, with the result of producing chorioretinal scars. The following study of 42 cases of diabetic retinopathy associated with cystoid macular oedema outlines characteristic fluorescein angiographic patterns, the modes of photocoagulation employed, and their final results.

METHOD OF FLUORESCEIN ANGIOGRAPHY

5 ccm of a 10% Na-fluorescein solution were injected within 3 sec. into the cubital vein. The photographs were obtained utilizing a Zeiss fundus camera, and a Robot Recorder 36 ME camera respectively, the Zeiss excitation filter 485, and barrier filter 520, using flash intensity III (480 W/sec.). The Kodak Plus X films were developed under 22° C within 8 minutes employing a Kodak HC-110 solution.

The angiograms were screened in regard to 5 different view points: density of the perimacular capillary bed, interval between the initial capillary flow of fluorescein and the first appearance of leakage, duration of presence of dye within the capillaries, and configuration of leakage patterns at the posterior pole after 3, 5, and 10 minutes respectively. Photocoagulation has been perfoimed using a Zeiss Xenon arc photocoagulator combined with the attachment of Fankhauser and Lotmar.

FLUORESCEIN ANGIOGRAPHIC CHARACTERISTICS

The time interval between the initial appearance of fluorescein within the capillary bed and the onset of extravasation averaged 8 seconds (2 to 22 sec.). 1,5 to 5 minutes (mean value 2,5 min.) had elapsed until the capillaries were completely depleted of dye, so that the pooling appeared entirely outside the vascular bed. The late (extravascular) dye patterns be classified into three different categories: Type I: a perimacular ring of dye (9 cases) (Fig. 1) Type II: same as Type I plus a concentric ring of dye just within the temporal vascular arcade (24 cases) (Fig. 2); Type III: isolated

507

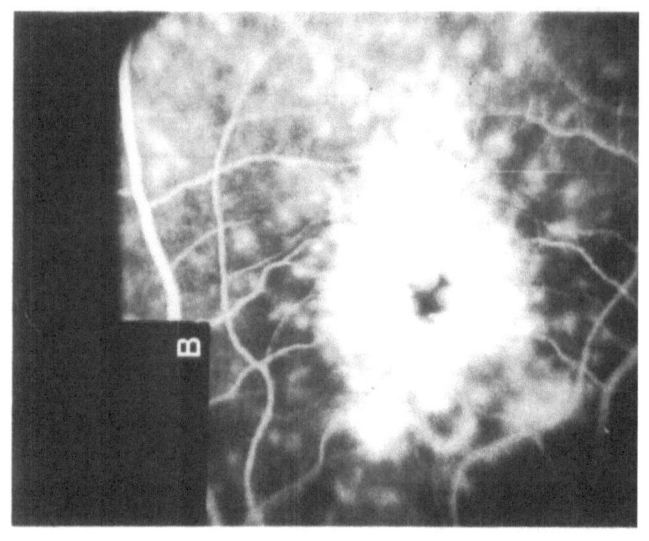

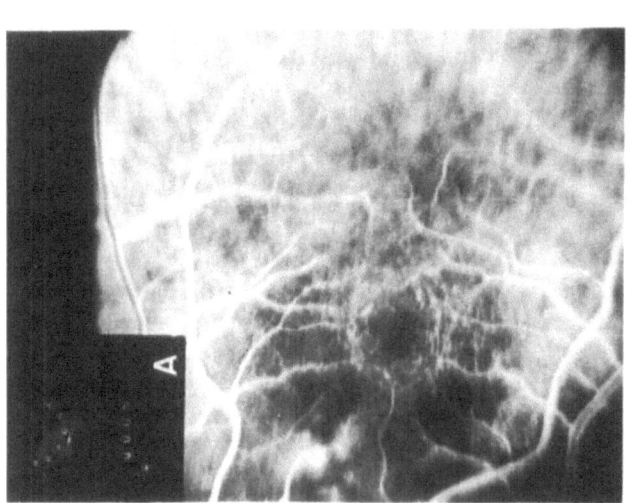

508

Fig. 1. Fluoresceinangiographic pattern of Type I: A: early venous phase; B: venous phase; from the coarsened perivascular bed the dye diffuses rapidly into the macular cysts.

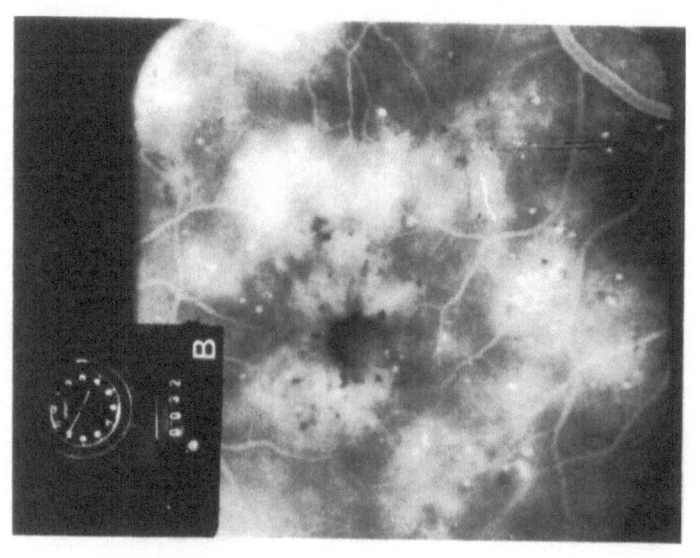

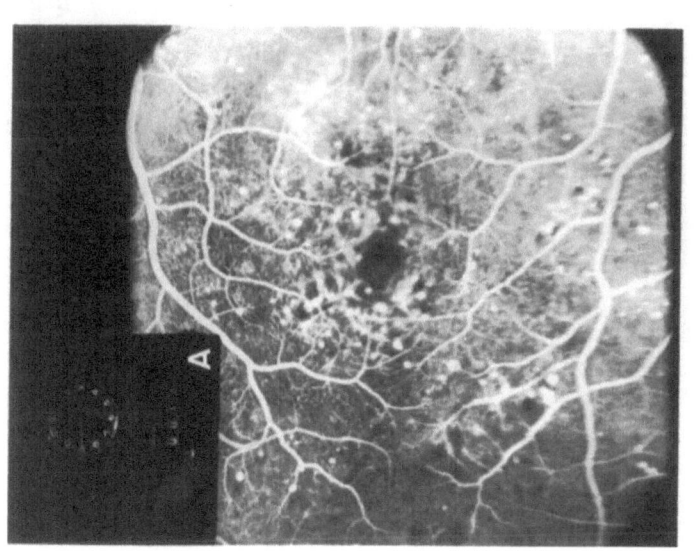

Fig. 2. Fluoresceinangiographic pattern of Type II: arteriovenous phase; B: late phase (5 min.); staining of macular area similar to Type I plus concentric ring of dye within the temporal arcade.

509

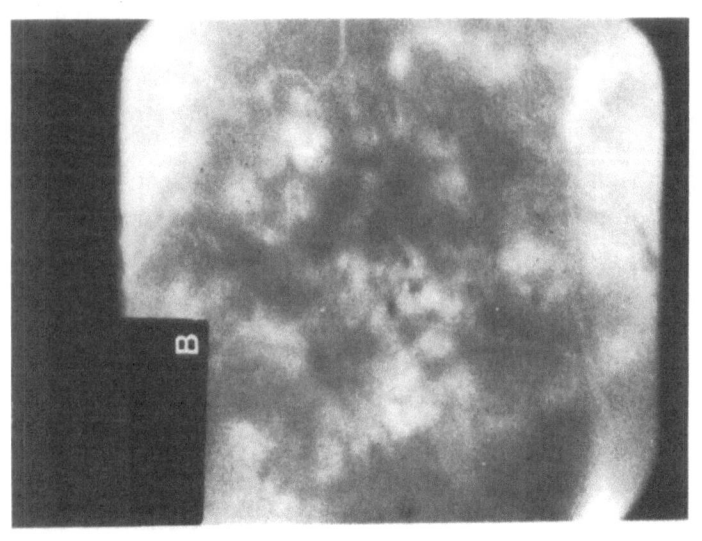

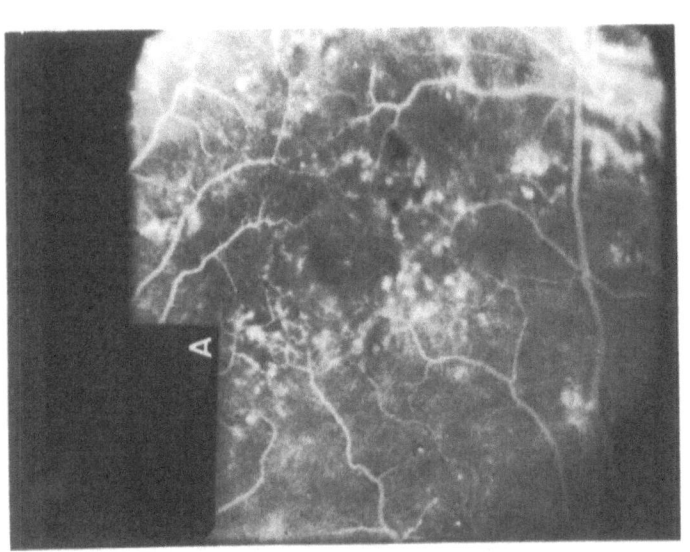

Fig. 3. Fluoresceinangiographic pattern of Type III: A: arteriovenous phase; B: late phase (5 min.); staining of the cystoid macular oedema plus concentric but non-confluent patches of dye within the temporal arcade.

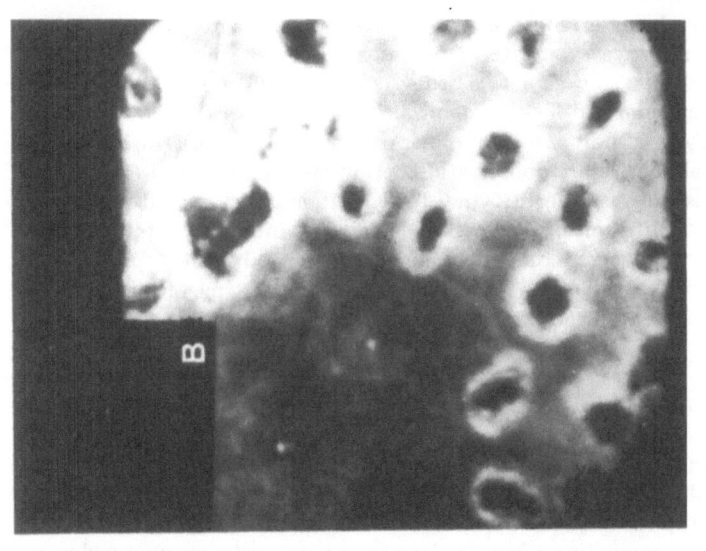

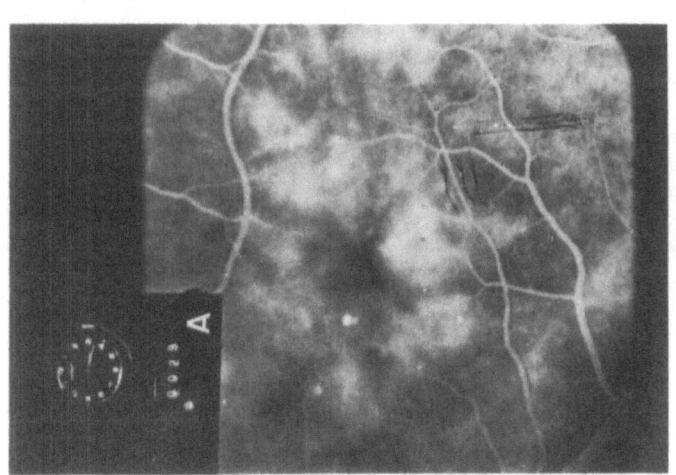

Fig. 4. Fluoresceinangiographic pattern of Type II: A: before treatment; B: 3 months after photocoagulation; the cystoid macular oedema has regressed almost completely.

511

patches of dye being arranged in a relatively circinate pattern, but without exhibiting confluence even after 10 minutes (9 cases) (Fig. 3). In cases of Type I-dye-patterns the capillary bed was fairly well preserved displaying moderate coarsening. In Type II multiple small areas of capillary dropout existed. In Type III only a small number of preserved capillaries were visible angiographically. Within an observation period of 4 years as an average (2 to 6 years), 4 cases changed from Type I to Type II, and two cases from Type I to Type III. A diffusion of dye within 10 minutes into the central macular cysts has been observed only occasionally in Type I (three times), and Type II (once), but never in Type III. In all other cases penetration of the dye into the cysts averaged 20 min. (Type I), 28 min. (Type II), and 34 min. (Type III).

Light coagulation

The first attempts of scattered light coagulation temporally to the macula using the 3° diagram and the intensity green II of the Zeiss Xenoncoagulator showed a decrease of the perimacular retinal oedema only in the nearest vicinity of the coagulations, but no decrease of the cystic macular oedema. After multiple directed coagulations of the leaking capillaries in the outer ring of dye pooling in Type II-cases using the 1° and 1,5° diagram and intensity green III, a decrease of the cystoid macular oedema was observed in about 1/3 of the patients, but an almost complete regression only in 3 cases (Fig. 4). After the coagulation of the *nonconfluent* leakage points in Type-III cases no improvement of the cystoid macular oedema was observed. It seemed that these coagulations destroyed the last still perfused capillaries in the area of the posterior pole. These cases displaying prevalence of the occlusive process of the capillaries in the fluorescein angiogram over the exudative one have the poorest prognosis. The perimacular capillary network in Type I-cases should be treated by an Argon-Laser exclusively (L'ESPERANCE, 1975). In accordance with MEYER-SCHWICKERATH (1975) a slight regression of the cystoid macular oedema was observed in some of these cases after an extensive peripheral Xenon-light-coagulation.

REFERENCES

L'ESPERANCE, F.A. JR. Ocular photocoagulation, a stereoscopic atlas. C.V. Mosby Company Saint Louis, 1975.
MEYER-SCHWICKERATH, G. Discussion to: A.E. Leuenberger, Photocoagulation of diabetic maculopathy. In: L. Guillaumat, M. Massin, L. Fison, R. Dufour, B. Daicker, New Research on the aetiology and surgery of retinal detachment. Modern Problems in Ophthalmology. Vol. 15: *333* S. Karger, Basel (1975).

Authors' address:
First University Eye-Clinic
Vienna
Austria

DISCUSSION

Dr Patz: The authors have provided a very useful classification of the pattern of dye leakage in cystoid maculopathy. We certainly found as they have more or less severe capillary non-perfusion, a loss of capillary perfusion, and that these patients responded poorly to photocoagulation. Indeed on a controlled study the treated eye faired poorer than the untreated in those patients. One other parameter that we have looked into is the patients' blood pressure. We found that no matter how good the capillary perfusion, if the patient has significant hypertension they seemed to fair poorly with photocoagulation and I like to know if the authors have looked in this particular parameter in their patients?

Dr Freyler: We did not consider hypertension; we did not include this parameter in our study.

EVALUATION OF DIABETIC RETINOPATHY

J.-H. GREITE, J.-W. HERTEL & H. MÖRCHEN

(München, W. Germany)

The evaluation of diabetic retinopathy is still an unsolved problem. The lack of useful criteria and the disadvantages of long term studies caused us to undertake a study to try to define relevant criteria for the severity of diabetic retinopathy, which would at the same time enable us to determine the progression of the disease over a shorter period. The criteria were defined on the basis of fluorescein angiography.

The study included 117 cases, 86 of which were followed over one year and the remainder over 2 to 4 years.

The population can be taken as being representative for age, sex and degree of diabetic change.

The original angiogramme negatives were used for the evaluation, as these give the best information. A grid with squareas of 1 mm² was placed over the negative under a binocular microscope, thereby dividing the angio-

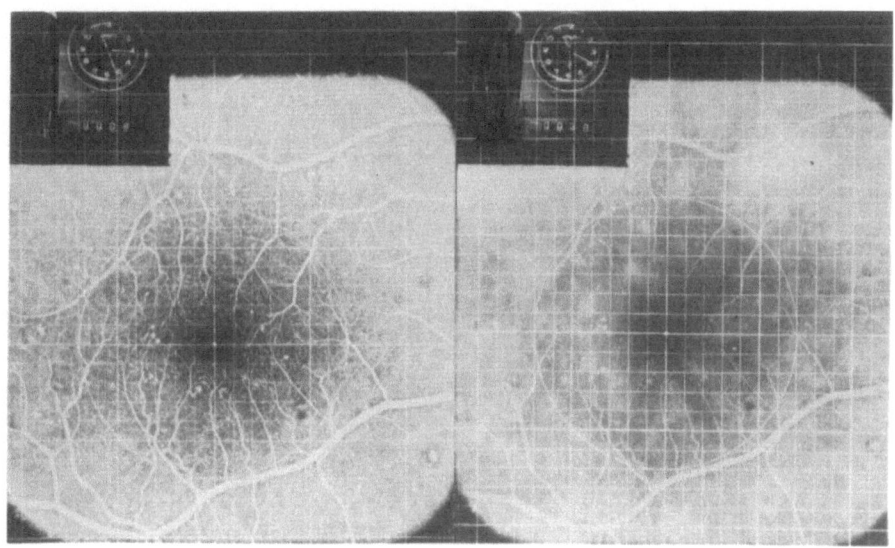

Fig. 1. Capillary and late phase of an angiogramme with overlying grid with 1 mm squares as used for counting the different parameters.

515

gramme into 520 fields. In addition, the perimacular region was examined separately within a radius of 7 mm, corresponding to 154 fields (Fig. 1). The capillary and the five-minute late phase was examined in every case. Capillary dilations, microaneurysms, intraretinal hemorrhage, hard exudates, capillary free areas, arteriolar changes, intreretinal neovascularisation, pre-retinal proliferation and leakages were counted. These data and the basic clinical data were processed by computer. It was found that capillary dilation was the best parameter for the quantitative analysis and represented the degree of severity most accurately, because the values showed the widest distribution and showed significant change over a 12 month period.

The leakages, as a functional expression of the morphological change in the capillaries, showed the very high correlation of 0.99 with capillary dilation (Fig. 2). The correlation with microaneurysms was less close (0.78). The relative distribution of the microaneurysm parameter about the linear regression line is greater than the leakage parameter and approximately constant in all regions. Microaneurysms were not noted when there were less than 10 capillary dilations present (Fig. 3). There was no statistically significant correlation between the other parameters. Intraretinal hemorrhages and lipid exudates were first noted with more than 30 capillary dilations. Capillary free areas and arteriolar changes started with more than 50 dilations, although none of these parameters were constantly present. That means that these last 4 parameters are not true indicators of the degree of the capillary change.

It was therefore logical to consider the degree of capillary dilation as the basis for a meaningful and yet practical classification. Because the frequency

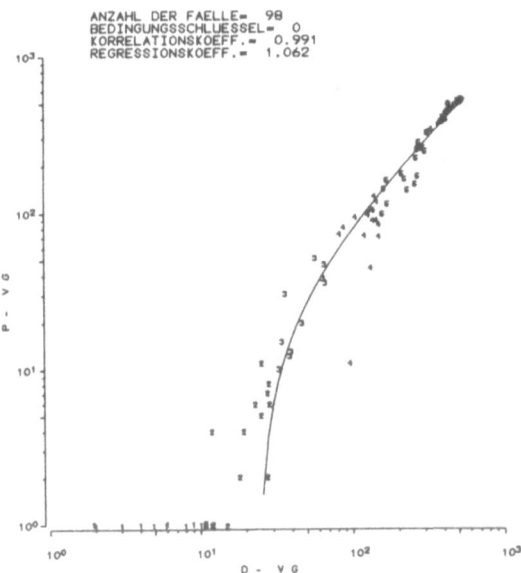

Fig. 2. Correlation bet een capillary dilatation (D) and leakages (P) in the whole angiogramme.

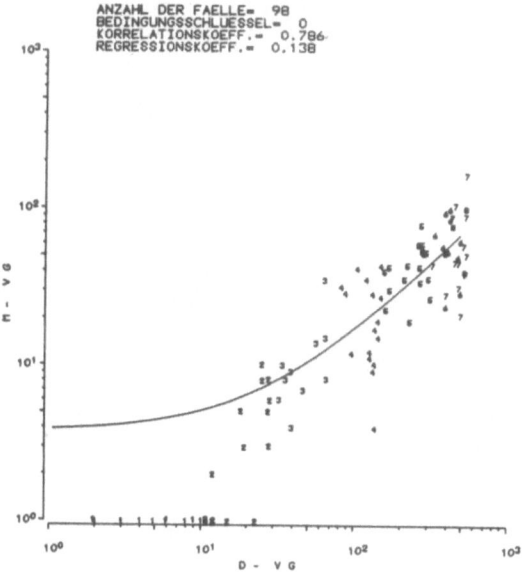

Fig. 3. Correlation between capillary dilatation (D) and microaneurysms (M) in the whole angiogramme.

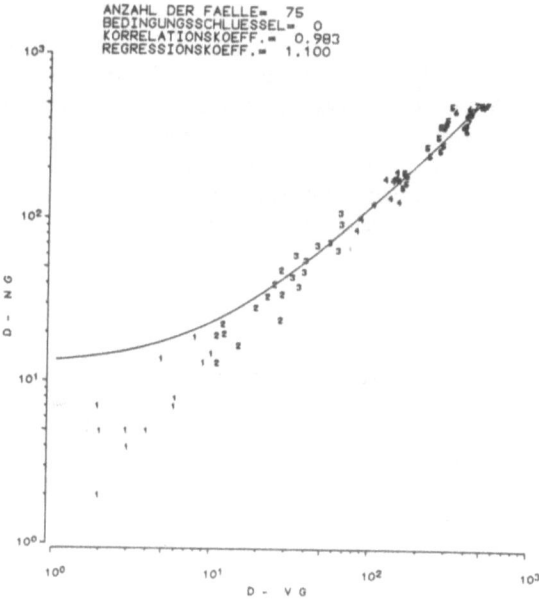

Fig. 4. Correlation between the values of capillary dilatation from the first examination (D-VG) and those after one year (D-NG) in the whole angiogramme.

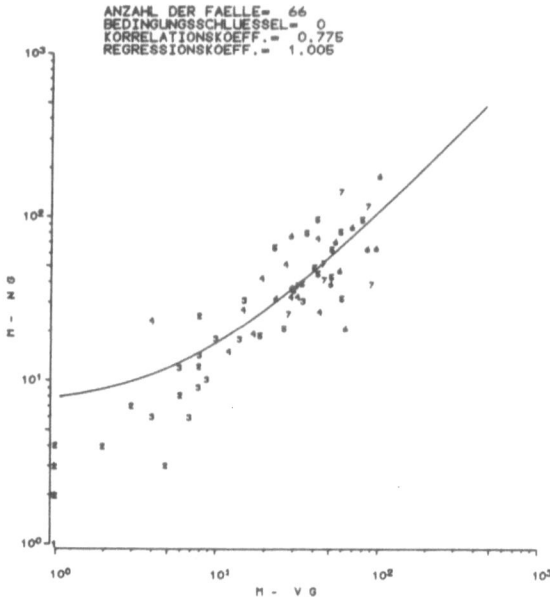

ANZAHL DER FAELLE= 66
BEDINGUNGSSCHLUESSEL= 0
KORRELATIONSKOEFF.= 0.775
REGRESSIONSKOEFF.= 1.005

Fig. 5. Correlation between the values of microaneurysms from the first examination (M-VG) and those after one year (M-NG) in the whole angiogramme.

distribution of this parameter was exponential, classification sub-groups could not be linear. Special attention was directed at the appearance of intra-retinal proliferative changes and, for a later stage, at proliferation, as these changes appeared sequentially only when approximately 2/3 of the overlooked angiogramme showed capillary dilatations.

In this way, the following nine-stage classification was defined, which served as the basis for later calculations.

stage	grids with capillary dilatation
1	1 – 10
2	11 – 30
3	31 – 70
4	71 – 150
5	151 – 310
6	over 310
7	intraretinal neovascularisation
8	preretinal vessel proliferation
9	blindness

518

Important conclusions can be drawn from the correlation analyses between the value from the first examination and those after one year. Figure 4 shows this correlation between the values of capillary dilatation. The high correlation coefficient of 0.98 and the regression coefficient of 1.10 shows that the progression is both very steady and about 10% per year. In only 4 cases was there either no progression or a slight regression. When the patient population was divided into two groups, those with good and those with poor metabolic control, it was found that those with good control had a mean progression of only 3.3%, as opposed to a mean of 15.1% for those in the poor control group. The correlation coefficients make this statement statistically highly significant. It also confirms the important influence of metabolic control on the course of diabetic retinopathy (e.g. CAIRD, 1974). Duration of diabetes, age and sex did not seem to have any significant effect on the correlation of the data. The influence of other factors such as medical treatment or photocoagulation could not yet be evaluated because of unequal distribution between the compared groups in our material.

Microaneurysms seem to have less prognostic significance. In approximately 27% of the cases, the number of microaneurysms had actually decreased after one year (Fig. 5). The transient nature of microaneurysms, which has been described in the literature (e.g. KOHNER & DOLLERY, 1970), may account for this.

The separate evaluation of the macular area showed no digression from the findings in the whole angiogram, and the findings from this area were just as significant in the early stages as those from the whole angiogram.

In order to test the validity of the experimental method, the one year changes of the relevant parameters were extrapolated over time using a special mathematical model, the principle of which is shown in the histogrammes of Figure 6. This model is based on the variation of frequency distribution over time of the capillary dilations and neovascularisation in the classification. More details will be given in the next paper. Figure 7 shows the change in the frequency distribution in stages (T_v) 1 to 9 from the first

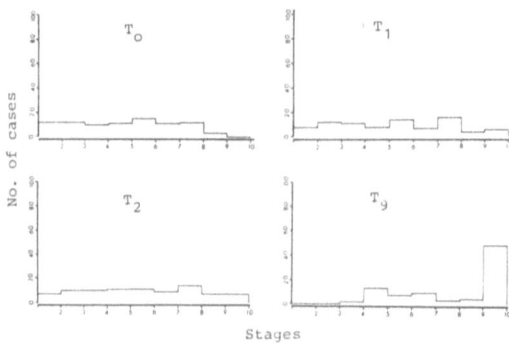

Fig. 6. Histogrammes showing the mean frequency distribution of cases in the different stages, T_0 at first examination, T_1 after one year, T_2 and T_9 calculated for two and nine years.

IV:	1	2	3	4	5	6	7	8	9	MITTELWERT	MITTL. FEHLER
T0:	12	12	10	11	15	11	12	3	0	4.6	0.00
T1:	8	12	11	8	14	7	16	4	6	5.1	0.39
T2:	7	10	10	11	11	9	14	7	7	5.5	0.57
T3:	2	10	12	12	3	13	8	16	10	6.0	0.70
T4:	1	7	11	15	4	11	5	6	26	6.4	0.79
T5:	0	7	9	15	5	3	11	8	28	6.7	0.86
T6:	0	2	10	16	6	4	2	12	34	7.0	0.93
T7:	0	1	7	14	9	5	2	11	37	7.2	0.98
T8:	0	0	5	14	9	6	2	3	47	7.5	1.03
T9:	0	0	2	13	7	9	3	4	48	7.7	1.08

Fig. 7. Extrapolated frequency of distribution of cases in the stages (IV) 1-9; from the first examination (T_0) to the ninth year (T_9). The last two columns show mean values and mean errors (Computer print out).

IV:	1	2	3	4	5	6	7	8	9	MITTELWERT	MITTL. FEHLER
T0:	0	100	0	0	0	0	0	0	0	2.5	0.00
T1:	0	70	30	0	0	0	0	0	0	2.8	0.24
T2:	0	36	64	0	0	0	0	0	0	3.2	0.34
T3:	0	0	93	7	0	0	0	0	0	3.5	0.41
T4:	0	0	62	38	0	0	0	0	0	3.9	0.47
T5:	0	0	26	74	0	0	0	0	0	4.2	0.52
T6:	0	0	0	100	0	0	0	0	0	4.5	0.56
T7:	0	0	0	86	14	0	0	0	0	4.7	0.59
T8:	0	0	0	54	46	0	0	0	0	5.0	0.65
T9:	0	0	0	17	69	14	0	0	0	5.4	0.77

Fig. 8. Extrapolated frequency of distribution of 100 cases into progressively higher stages (IV 1 to 9) who start at T_0 in stage 2.

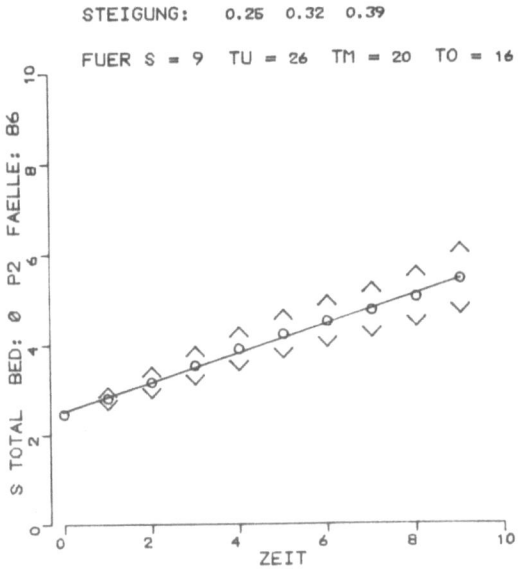

Fig. 9. Predicted progression, with deviation, of 100 cases from stage 2 against time (Zeit). (see text).

examination (T_0) to the ninth year (T_9) in matrix form. The values predicted by this model for two, three and four years were then compared with the values actually obtained from patients examined after these intervals. A very close agreement was found. In this way, it is also possible to predict the course of progression of diabetic retinopathy from any stage. Figure 9 shows a hypothetical example of expected progression of retinopathy in 100 patients, who start at stage 2 where ophthalmoscopical changes first became evident. For example, after four years (T_4), 62% would have reached stage 3 and 38% stage 4. This is shown even more clearly in the graph (Fig. 9). The average gradient of progression of 0.32 means that one grade is passed through every three years. In the next line, the time to blindness, or stage 9, is given, ranging from 16 to 26 years with a mean of 20 years (T_m). This range is of the same order as given in the literature (e.g. BERKOW, et al., 1905). For patients with good metabolic control, the predicted average time from this stage to blindness is 41 years. For those with poor control, the average is only 12 years.

In summary, the presented model proves successful and sensitive enough to differentiate between the influence of different factors on the course of diabetic retinopathy such as the state of metabolic control. It may also prove to be of value in the short term evaluation of therapeutic methods.

REFERENCES

BERKOW, J.W. et al. A retrospective study of blind diabetic patients. *J.A.M.A.* 193: *867* (1925).

CAIRD, T.I. Metabolic control. In: Lynn, J.R., Snyder, W.B. & Vaiser, A. (eds). Diabetic retinopathy: *67-70*. Grune & Stratton, New York/London (1974).

KOHNER, E.M. & DOLLERY, C.T. The rate of formation and disappearance of microaneurysms in diabetic retinopathy. *Trans. Ophthal. Soc.* U.K. 90: *369* (1970).

Authors' address:
Augenklinik der Universität München
Mathildenstrasse 8
8 Munich, West Germany

DISCUSSION

Dr Larsen: Dr Greite, with your computer technique you do not seem to be able to quantitate, for instance, vitreous hemorrhages or to include the 3-dimensions you have in new-formed vessels extending from the disc into the vitreous. I should also like to know if you have found any difference in the prognosis between cases with a periphery type retinopathy, compared to those having neovascularization extending from the disc?

Dr Greite: On the first examination we had no patients with vitreous hemorrhage and we saw only a few cases with vitreous hemorrhages at a late stage. Answering the second part of your question: we always centered the angiogram on the macula and have therefore not quantitate the changes in the periphery.

A MODEL TO QUANTITATIVELY PREDICT THE COURSE OF DIABETIC RETINOPATHY

J.W. HERTEL, J.-H. GREITE & H. MÖRCHEN

(Munich, W. Germany)

This paper contains the specifics of the paper 'Evaluation of Diabetic Retinopathy' by the same authors. All references to figures are made with respect to this paper, see pp. 515-521 of this volume.

1. EVALUATION OF THE MATERIAL OF A PATIENT ENSEMBLE WITH DIABETIC RETINOPATHY TO ALLOW STATISTICAL TREATMENT

As described in the first paper, a manual counting technique was used to extract numbers for each observable phenomenon from some 230 fluorescein angiographic photographs. Although overlapping phenomena could not be totally excluded, counting errors are small. The phenomena were labelled as parameters C, D, M, P, etc. with D for capillary dilatations. M for microaneurysms and P for permeability disturbances (leakages), for example. A computer based file was set up which allows editing and searching the data with respect to individual parameters as well as overall conditions like sex, age, blood pressure, metabolic control, and so on.

2. APPROPRIATENESS OF THE MATERIAL IN ORDER TO MAKE EXTRAPOLATIONS IN TIME, I.E. PREDICT THE COURSE OF DIABETIC RETINOPATHY

As the statistical material of 86 patients who were each examined twice with a one year time lapse in between appears sufficiently large the statistical material was investigated for its consistency and model suitability. Four major results could be established:

— The data are well mixed with respect to age, sex, blood pressure and metabolic control.

— The frequency of light cases of diabetic retinopathy versus severe cases is exponentially decreasing (as is plausible from mortality considerations).

— The parameter D displays a consistent monotonically increasing behaviour with strong correlations to P (Fig. 2) but weak correlations to M (Fig. 3).

— The parameter D from the first examination (D-VG) strongly correlates to itself (D-NG) after one year, i.e. the capillary dilatations increase consistently by 10% over the whole range of D within one year (correlation coefficient = 0.98) (Fig. 4);

These findings justify the following model validity prerequisites:

a. The taken sample is stochastic and is representative for the stationary total distribution of all cases of diabetic retinopathy.

b. The one year 'progression' of the taken sample is representative for the total distribution specified in *a*.

3. PHILOSOPHY AND FORMULATION OF A DIABETIC RETINOPATHY PROGRESSION MODEL (DRPM)

The outstanding behaviour of D resulted in its selection as 'leading parameter' in terms of classifying eight successive stages of diabetic retinopathy (plus one additional blindness stage) as shown in the previous paper. Such a classification appears necessary both for practical reasons as well as for a proper treatment of the low statistics. Thus averages of D were formed for all stages both for the first and the second examination. The DRPM then consists of a simple iterative algorithm:

– Each value of a set $\{D(t_n)\}$ is additively combined with the averages $D(t_0)$ and $D(t_1)$ of that particular stage or interval into which it falls to results in a new 'one year later' value set $\{D(t_{n+1})\}$, where t_n stands for the n-th year after the first examination.

– Each new set is depicted as a histogram (Fig. 6) showing the shift of the frequency distribution towards advanced stages.

– Averages containing error limits are calculated in a straightforward fashion showing the overall trend of diabetic retinopathy, or just the trend of a particular stage (Fig. 9).

The execution of the DRPM was done by EDP with a set of FORTRAN IV programs which were written in a generalized way such as to handle any subset of the total data allowing for differentiations with respect to conditions as metabolic control, e.g. In addition these programs allow to calculate the progression of individual stages as shown in Fig. 9. Furthermore all graphical representations are EDP produced. Particular care was taken to estimate the errors in two independant ways. Thus the error limits (Fig. 9) represent approximately a two third confidentiality range in the sense of a Gaussion error distribution.

CONCLUSION

Comparison with literature results (see the first paper) show that the DRPM is a good approximation to reality. Additional statistical material will be necessary to refine the results, but as a first approach in this area the authors are quite confident of its theoretical and practical potential.

Authors' address:
Augenklinik der Universität München
Mathildenstrasse 8
8 Munich
W. Germany

REACTIONS VASCULAIRES ET TISSULAIRES DE L'OEIL PROVOQUEES PAR LA CRYOCAUTERISATION ET PAR LA COAGULATION AU LASER. ETUDE EXPERIMENTALE A FLUORESCENCE

H. BAURMANN, K. SASAKI, L. SCHOMACHER & G. CHIORALIA

(Bonn, W. Germany)

Depuis 1973, nous étudions les effects du laser à Argon sur l'oeil (BAUR-MANN et al., 1975; 1976; SASAKI et al., 1976) que nous mettons en relation avec les résultats à fluorescence. Les détails des techniques mises au point seront publiés séparemment (CHIORALIA, sous presse). L'intérêt d'une série actuelle d'expériences est l'examen des néoformations vasculaires cornéennes d'yeux humains après le traitement au laser et la comparaison avec les effets de la cryo- et de la diathermo-cautérisation.

La provocation de la néovascularisation cornéenne, par différentes méthodes, fut étudiée chez des rats pigmentés et chez des lapins pigmentés et albinotiques. *L'argent nitrique* à un et 5% chez les rats et à 10 et 20% chez les lapins fut appliqué en contactant l'agent avec quelques lésions de la cornée provoquées artificiellement. Ce genre de provocation était efficace chez les rats; par contre chez les lapins, elle n'était pas aussi évidente qu'elle n'a était écrite par un autre auteur (LAVERGNE & COLMANT, 1964; REED et al., 1975). *La Na OH n/10ème*, 0,1 ml injectée dans la cornée du lapin a eu un bon effet (EY et al., 1968). D'autre part, nous nous sommes également intéressés aux réactions des tissus aux cryo- et diathermocoagulations et aux coagulations au laser à Argon. Les constantes pour les applications de la cryo et de la diathermie (MICHAELSON, 1952) sur la cornée paracen-

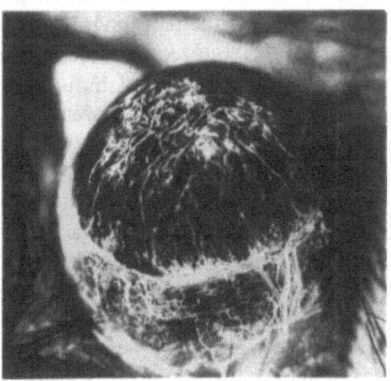

Fig. 1. Angiogramme d'un rat, 3ème seconde, 2 semaines après diathermie paracentrale. Réseau néo-vasculaire jusqu'à l'apex cornéen.

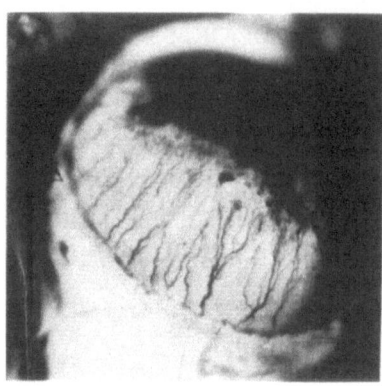

Fig. 2. Angiogramme d'un rat 60ème seconde, 1 mois après cryo paracentrale. Néo-vaisseaux avec diffusion.

trale et paralimbaire et du laser au limbe cornéo-scléral, dans les expériences de contrôle, ont été en bref les suivantes:

Cryo: 4 secondes à -30°C au maximum en une seule fois chez les rats et les lapins ou en plusieurs fois chez les lapins répété quotidiennement au maximum durant 15 jours;

Diathermie: 30 mA chez les rats 0,5 sec., chez les lapins une à 5 sec.;

Laser à Argon: chez les rats 500 mW, 50 microns, 0,02 secondes; chez les lapins 500-1000 mW, 1000 microns, une à 2 secondes.

Toutes ces provocations ont amené une néoformation vasculaire d'aspect identique chez les rats.

Le 3ème jour, les vaisseaux du limbe forment des arcades dilatées; une semaine après l'intervention, le calibre vasculaire a augmenté tandis que la croissance en longueur reste limitée; 2 semaines après l'intervention, les néoformations vasculaires ont déjà atteint le centre cornéen et un réseau capillaire s'est établi. Après un mois, il n'y a plus de modifications (fig. 1). Après l'injection intraveineuse du colorant, une diffusion en provenance des néovaisseaux est à constater (fig. 2) pendant la phase précoce et au cours des phases tardives. La microscopie à fluorescence confirme ces observations (fig. 3). Une néovascularisation cornéenne fut induite par l'injection intra-cornéenne de Na OH n/10èmem 0,1 ml, chez le lapin.

Notre activité actuelle comprend l'examen du traitement des néoformations vasculaires de la cornée avec le laser à Argon (REED et al., 1975). Les effets obtenus ressemblent à ceux décrits par d'autres auteurs (EY et al., 1968; REED et al., 1975). Les nouveaux vaisseaux démontrés semblent de taille assez mince chez le rat. L'oeil de cet animal reste tout de même un modèle favorable pour l'étude expérimentale des néovascularisations. Chez le rat, le laser à Argon a produit des néoformations vasculaires. C'est ce cercle vicieux qui nous a amené à abandonner le traitement de la cornée avec le laser (REED et al., 1975). Heureusement, jusqu'à present, nous n'avons pas dû constater, chez le lapin, une néovascularisation provoquée par le laser à Argon – même pas avec des énergies fortement elevées.

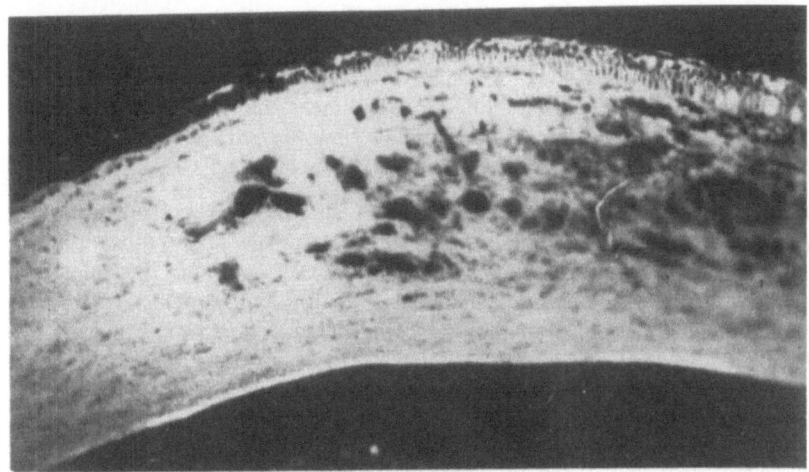

Fig. 3. Histologie à fluorescence, rat, 50 secondes après AgNO₃ 5%; néo-vaisseaux dans
la cornée superficielle et parenchymateuse.

$$\frac{10 \text{ mm}}{80 \ \mu\text{m}} \qquad 10 \text{ mm} = 80 \ \mu\text{m}$$

Nous remercions la Deutsche Forschungsgemeinschaft pour la subvention
accordée et également Monsieur Fujita et la Maison Topcon Europe N.V.

BIBLIOGRAPHIE

BAURMAN, H., SASAKI, J. & CHIORALIA, G. Altérations vasculaires du fond d'oeil
et du nerf optique après coagulation au laser. *Bull. Mém. Soc. Fr. d'Ophtal.* 87: *288-
294* (1976).

BAURMANN, H., SASAKI, K. & CHIORALIA, G. Investigations on laser coagulated
rat eyes by fluorescence angiography and microscopy. *v. Graefes Arch. klin. exp.
Ophthal.* 193: *245-252* (1975).

CHIORALIA, G. Ophthalmo-fluoreszenz-photomikroskopische Technik im Tierexperi-
ment. Dissertation, Bonn (1976).

EY, R., HUGHES, W.F., BLOOME, M.A. et al. Prevention of corneal vascularization.
Amer. J. Ophthal. 66: *1118-1131* (1968).

LAVERGNE, G. & COLMANT, J.A. Comparative study of the action of thiotepa and
triamcinolone on corneal vascularization in rabbits. *Brit. J. Ophthal.* 48: *416-422*
(1964).

MICHAELSON, I.C. Effects of cortisone upon corneal vascularization produced experimentally. *AMA Arch. Ophthal.* 47: *459-464* (1952).

REED, J.W., FROMER, C. & KLINTWORTH, G.K. Induced corneal vascularization
remission with Argon laser therapy. *AMA Arch. Ophthal.* 93: *1017-1019* (1975).

SASAKI, K., LEMMINGSON, W., BAURMANN, H. & CHIORALIA, G. Observation of
injected fluorescein diffusion after laser treatment of cat fundi. *v. Graefes Arch.
klin. exp. Ophthal.* 198: *7-16* (1976).

Adresse des auteurs:
Universitäts-Augenklinik
5300 Bonn-Venusberg
W. Germany

DISCUSSION

Dr Grayson: I would like, if I may, to address my question to both Dr Baurmann and Dr Ohtsuki, I like to compliment them on the histological preparation of the fluorescein and ask how they prevent the free fluorescein spreading when they prepare their histological specimens.

Dr Baurmann: Je remercie le Dr Grayson de ses remarques prouvant ses connaissance fondées en la matière. Notre technique est la lyophilisation des tissus après l'énucléation rapide qui, chez les rats, ne prend que quelques secondes. Chez les lapins, pour des raisons anatomiques, nous mettons 30 à 40 secondes, donc plus longtemps. Après l'énucléation, nous ouvrons le globe par une incision latérale ce qui est avantageux pour le procédé de la lyophilisation. Cette incision est effectuée en une seule seconde. Ensuite, les globes seront mis immédiatement dans le récipient contenant la carboglace (azétone). En ce qui concerne les yeux des rats, en considération de l'extrême rapidité avec laquelle ce procédé préparatif est effectué, nous pouvons dire avec une très grande certitude qu'une diffusion est évitée. Quant aux yeux de nos lapins dont les globes sont de dimensions considérablement plus importantes que celles des yeux des rats, nous ne sommes pas en mesure d'exclure avec une certitude absolue la production d'artefacts.

En vous servant du terme de 'free fluorescein spreading', vous abordez le problème très délicat des barrières. A mon avis, dans nos considérations et réflexions, il faut sélectionner minutieusement la diffusion des portions libres de la fluorescéine de celles liées aux albumines (et aux globulines à un moindre degré). Car, nos expériences nous donnent des indications que la fluorescéine libre constituant la plus petite partie, c'est vrai, est en effet capable de diffuser même sous des conditions physiologiques.

Dr Goldberg: In a study which is somewhat related to the one reported by Dr Baurmann but much more clinically oriented, colleagues of mine studied the transudative and exudative phenomena in the rabbit eye following cryocoagulations to the peripheral retina, which might simulate that performed in a human situation. We studied the amount of protein content, and the amount of fluorescein leakage into the eye following cryocoagulation, and this appeared to be prostaglandin mediated, as the leakage phenomena were largely prevented by pretreatment with aspirin and aspirin-like derivatives.

Dr Baurmann: Je remercie également beaucoup le Dr Goldberg qui a attribué de très intéressants et importants points de vue à cette discussion. Par la la littérature respective, nous avons connaissance de l'action préventive de l'aspirine. Je pense que nous saisirons votre inspiration. Il faudrait, naturellement, effectuer des séries d'expériences comparatives pour juger si l'aspirine produit un effet vérifiable sur les barrières. En principe, je n'en doute pas, mais je ne suis pas certain que nous puissions démontrer de tel effet avec notre méthode.

COMPARATIVE STUDY OF RETINAL MICROANEURYSM

K. OHTSUKI & K. MIZUNO

(Sendai, Japan)

INTRODUCTION

Pathological analysis of microaneurysm has become available in more detail with the advance of the techniques of vascular injection and retinal digestion. The development of fluorescein angiography has proved to be another benefit, likewise facilitating clinical examination of microaneurysms. However, interpretations of individual microaneurysms often encounter inconsistencies between histological and fluorescein angiographic findings. The purpose of this paper is to throw more light on microaneurysms of the human eye by step-by-step, systematic observation involving fundus photography, fluorescein angiography, incident-light- and transmitted-light fluorescence microscopy as well as routine histopathology.

MATERIALS AND METHODS

Our investigation involved 3 eyes which were surgically removed because of either glioma of the optic nerve, orbital malignant lymphoma or absolute glaucoma. Prior to enucleation, each eye was examined by fundus photography and fluorescein angiography as far as available. Thirty seconds after an injection of 7 ml of 10% sodium fluorescein, enucleation was performed, after which each eye was instantaneously placed in an acetone-dry ice bath, and its anterior segment was removed by sawing. The posterior segment was lyophilized in the same manner as described in the previous papers (MIZUNO, 1973; MIZUNO et al., 1973; MIZUNO et al., 1973, SASAKI et al., 1973). The dried posterior segments were first examined as 3-dimensional preparations suspended in xylene, then observed by incident-light fluorescence microscopy, and later dissected into 3 portions, centered about the posterior pole, equator and periphery. Each flat preparation was further examined by incident-light fluorescence microscopy and then arranged either as tissue cross-sections or as 'vascular trees'. 1. The cross sections were prepared with the flat preparation embedded in paraffin in vacuo. sectioned 10 microns in thickness and mounted on the objective glass through direct heating; these were subjected to transmitted fluorescence microscopy, and then to light microscopy after staining with PAS-hematoxylin. 2. The vascular tree was made by trypsinizing the preparation after it was treated with a graduated alcohol series to remove xylene and subsequently stained with PAS-hematoxylin. A combination of Baird-Atomic B-4 and 5 filters was regularly employed. A BV filter was used as an exciter only on occasion

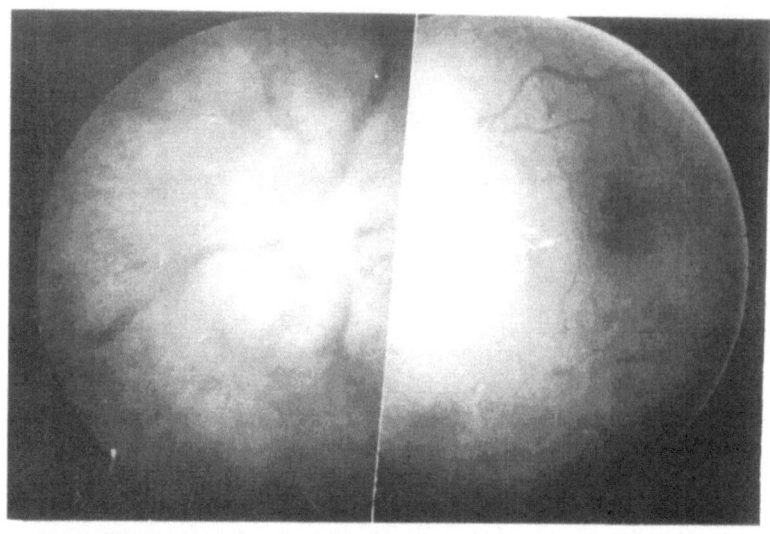

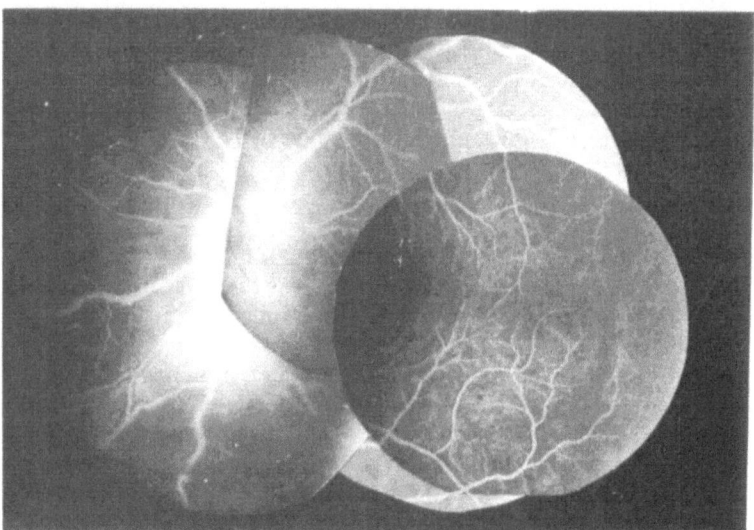

Fig. 1. *Case 1.* Papilledema due to optic glioma. Top, fundus photograph. Botton, fluorescein angiograph 30 seconds after injection.

when necessary to distinguish specific-from autofluorescence (SASAKI et al., 1973).

RESULTS

1) Microaneurysm in papilledema

A 4-year old girl had progressive exophthalmos and enlargement of the optic canal in her left eye. Funduscopy revealed extensive papilledema (Fig. 1). A fluorescein angiogram showed apparent papilledema; tortuosity of the vessels, neovascularization, microaneurysms and intensive leakage of fluorescein were seen on an around the nerve head (Fig. 1). By incident-light fluorescence microscopy, dilation and tortuosity of the capillary were found, evidently limited within the disc and in the neighboring region in either the radial peripapillary or the retinal capillaries (Fig. 2). A number of microaneurysms, varying in diameter from 20 to 90 microns and representing a variety of shapes, were observed scattered among the deformed capillaries. Microaneurysms had a surface neither smooth nor round, but rugged, bearing a rather fist-like appearance, in paraffin sections of the nerve head and its vicinity, a variety of capillary changes were identified by both transmitted-light fluorescence and light microscopy; all capillaries were seen to be distorted and dilated, delicately coiling, looping and tangled (Fig. 3). Some capillaries reunited and divided again before regaining their original forms. In the most complicated variation of changes, capillary tufts or glomeruli presented large irregular microaneurysms after fusion and eventual

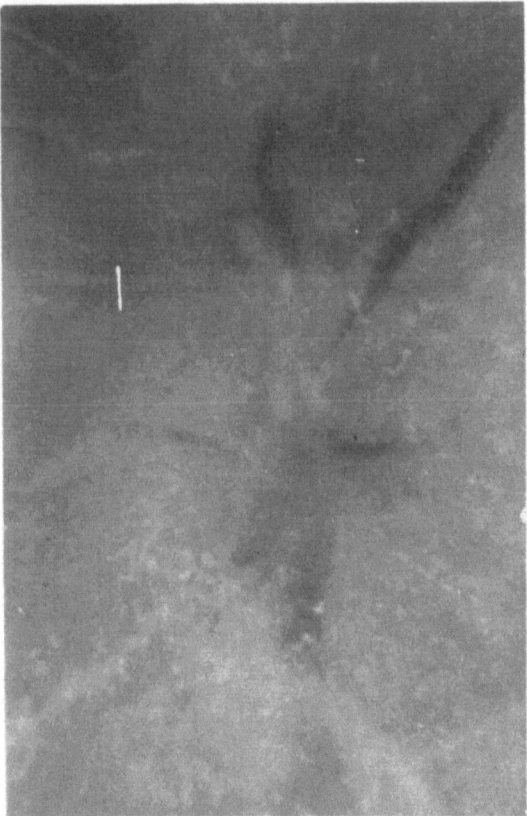

Fig. 2. Incident-light fluorescence micrograph of papilledema 30 seconds after injection in case 1. Fluorescein is leaking from the coiled capillaries and glomerular microaneurysms on and around the disc. The BV filter was used as an exciter, X 10.

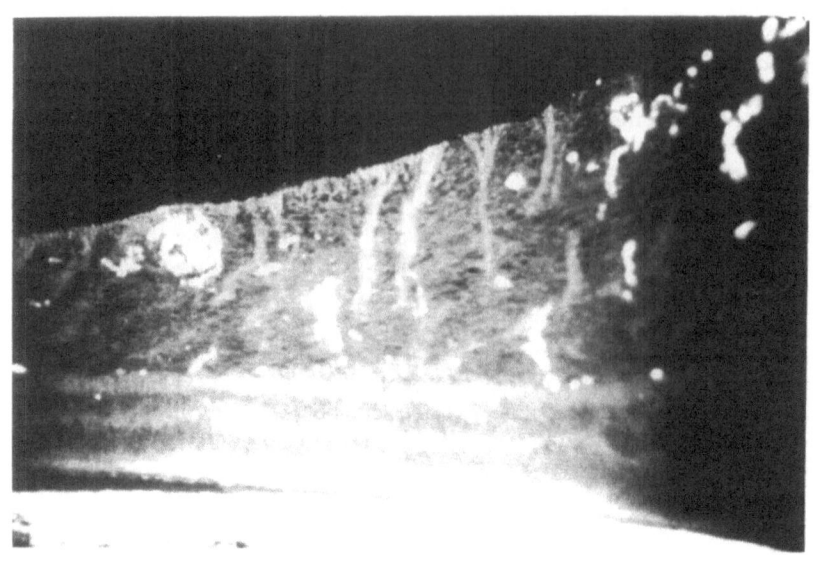

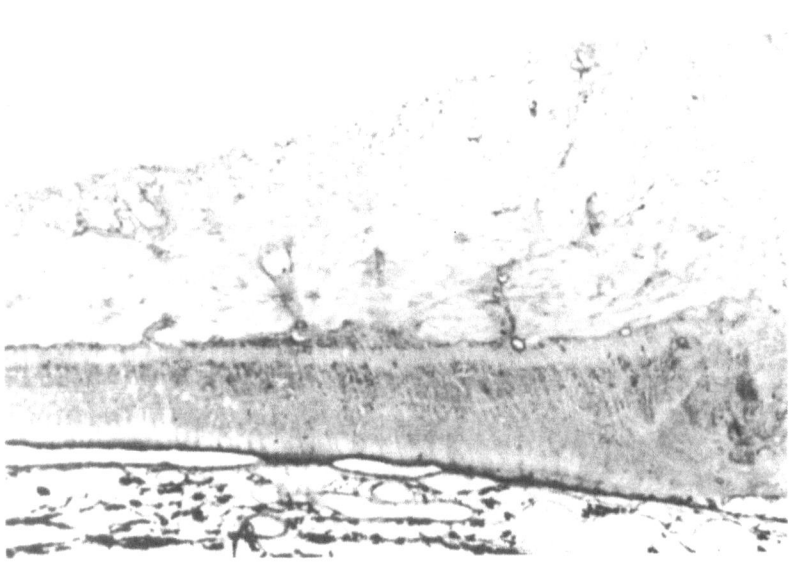

Fig. 3. Cross sections near the disc of case 1. Top, transmitted-light fluorescence micrograph after injection. Fluorescein is filling in dilated capillaries and glomerular microaneurysms. Bottom, light micrograph of the same specimen. Irregular shaped microaneurysms are seen. PAS-hematoxylin stain, X 25.

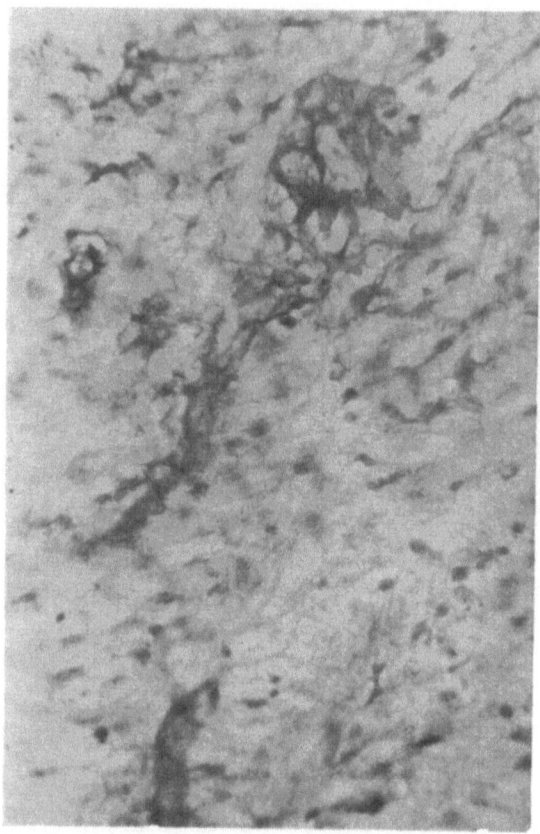

Fig. 4. High power view of one of the microaneurysms (Fig. 3, bottom). PAS-hemato-xyline stain, x 100.

necrosis of the capillary loop walls which had come in contact with each other (Fig. 4). Cells of astrocytoma (diagnosed pathologically) had invaded the optic nerve, but they were not found within the lamina cribrosa.

2) Microaneurysm in peripheral retina

In a 62-year old woman, exophthalmos slowly progressed in her left eye. At autopsy malignant lymphoma of her left orbit was confirmed. Both fundu-scopy and fluorescein angiography failed to distinguish any peripheral fea-ture of abnormality, but incident-light fluorescence microscopy could iden-tify a variety of microaneurysms in the flat preparations for the periphery. The peripheral microaneurysms were found superficially, more frequently on the venous side of the capillary bed. They appeared as bulges, saccules, elongated pouches, bizarre in form, varying in diameter from 10 to 25 mi-crons (Figs. 5, 6, 7 and 8). Microaneurysm, in several instances, apparently developed on one side of a capillary strand, with the wall associated with the intercapillary bridge (ghost vessel) (Fig. 5). In some capillary bed, a

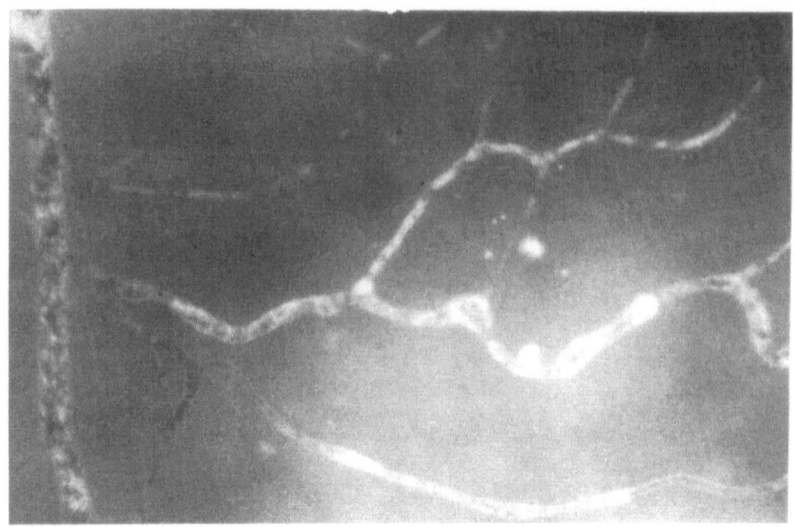

Fig. 5. *Case 2*. Peripheral microaneurysm. Incident-light fluorescence micrograph reveals that the microaneurysm connects with the ghost vessel, 30 seconds after injection, X 50.

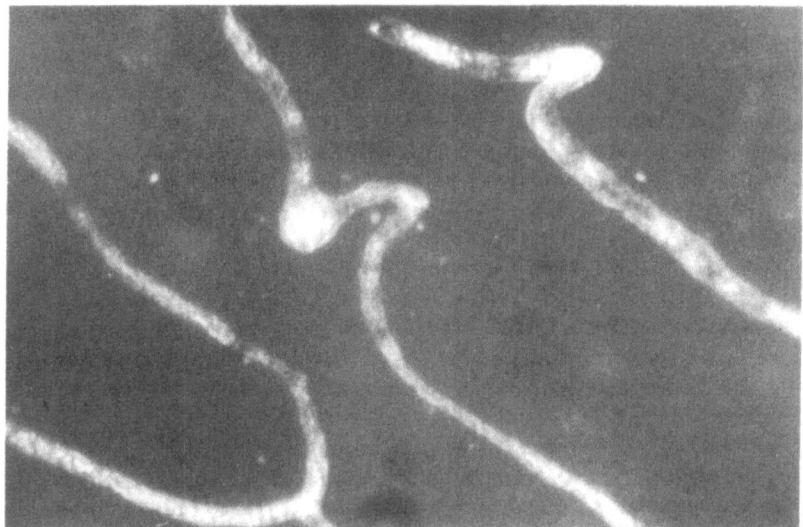

Fig. 6. Incident-light fluorescence micrograph of peripheral microaneurysm in case 2. The process of microaneurysm formation from a U-shaped kink to a saccular configulation is demonstrated in the capillary bed, X 100.

U-shaped kink was located close to a saccular configuration of microaneurysm, in which the capillary loop, with the opposing walls fusing together, made the capillary appear as a convex curve (Fig. 6). Focussing from the superficial to the deeper retinal layers showed that the convex surface is frequently directed toward the inner surface of the retina (Fig. 7). Serial paraffin sections of this part demonstrated such convex surfaces of the

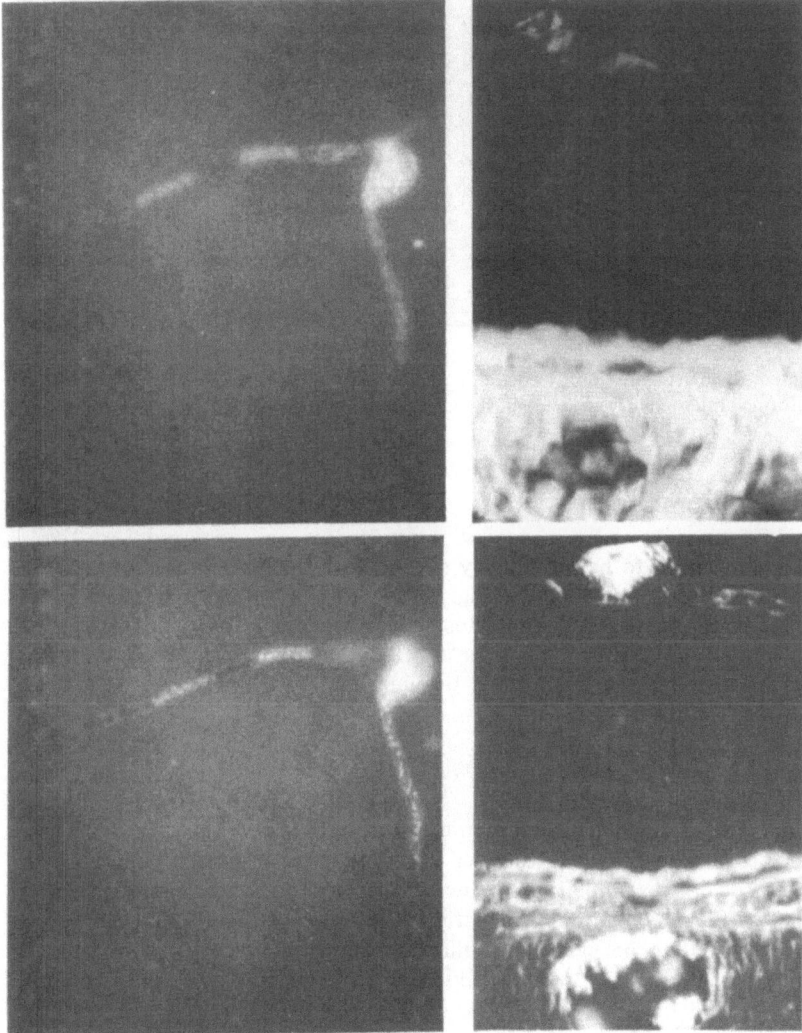

Fig. 7. Fluorescence micrographs of peripheral microaneurysm of case 2. Left, incident-light fluorescence micrographs focussed on the superficial (top) and deeper (bottom) retinal layers indicate inward outpouching of microaneurysm, X 100. Right, transmitted-light fluorescence micrographs of serial paraffin sections prepared from the same microaneurysm reveal its convex surface directs towards the inner limiting membrane, X 100.

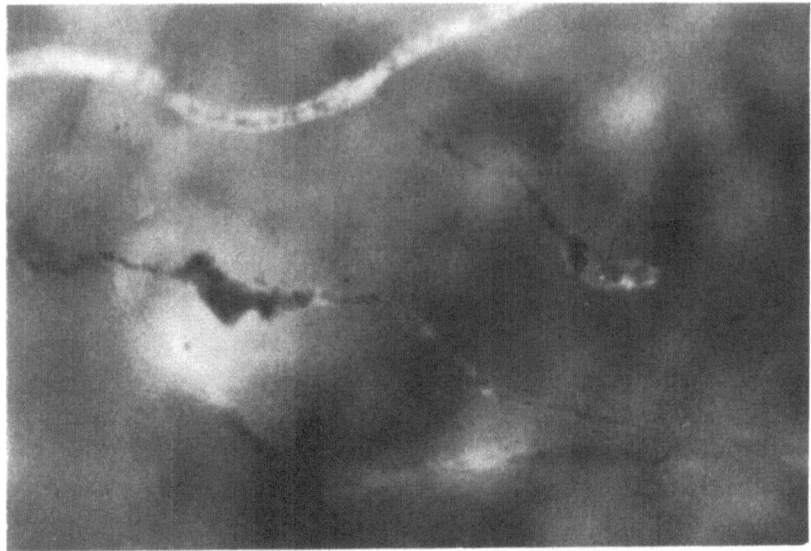

Fig. 8. Incident-light fluorescence micrograph of peripheral microaneurysm of case 2. Deformed microaneurysms and ghost vessels are barely stained with fluorescein, X 100.

microaneurysms to be moderately stained with fluorescein and adjoining to the inner limiting membrane (Fig. 7). Bizarrely deformed microaneurysms whose ends connected to the ghost vessels were also found in this part of the retina. The greater part of the cavities in microaneurysms and lumina of the ghost vessels were filled with thrombi, so that they were barely stained with fluorescein (Fig. 8).

3) Microaneurysm-like dilation in glaucoma

A 45-year old man had long-standing absolute glaucoma in his right eye. Since corneal opacity and cataract made fundus examination unavailable in this case, only examination by incident-light fluorescence microscopy was done on the whole mount preparation. The flow of fluorescein in the vessels was observed to be particularly limited within the narrow region centered around the disc. The rows of fluorescent beads on the venules and the venular capillaries indicated the presence of numerous saccular and fusiform aneurysms on these vessels (Fig. 9). They were frequently so abundant as to form rows of bead-like outpouchings out of a single venule. Their diameter ranged from 25 to 45 microns. The trypsin-digested vascular tree of this part indicated spherical bodies consisting of blood cells enclosed in a thin-walled endothelial sac (Fig. 10).This gave rise to a saccular configuration, apparently representing a focal aneurysmal dilation of the venule on both sides of the wall.

Capillary microaneurysm was previously considered to be a lesion specific to diabetic retinopathy. However, it is now generally known that all retinal capillary microaneurysms, with all possible variations in morphology or in retinopathy, are manifestations in a single pathogenic process, in other words, mainly specific, fundamental expressions of retinal capillary degenerations. However, all types of microaneurysms observed by fluorescein angiography have features in common, irrespective of their size or original disease: They are spherical or spindle shaped; fluorescent points appear to be common on them probably because of the limit of resolution in photographing the fundus. This shortcoming in photography may remain unimproved for some time. It is particular importance to perform comparative evaluation of microaneurysmal features between fluorescein angiographic evidence and the findings with the perfusion technique or those with the trypsin-digestion technique. In the present observations preliminary examinations were done as far as possible by routine fundus pictures, and by fluorescein angiography. Fluorescence microscopy by the incident light was performed on the whole mount or flat preparations. Cross sections were prepared to observe retinal features by transmitted-light fluorescence microscopy. Finally, the findings were further analyzed histopathologically. As a result, three kinds of microaneurysms were identified.

1) Microaneurysm in papilledema

Many authors have previously reported fluorescein angiographic findings in papilledema, citing the main features to be dilation and looping of the capillaries, formation of multiple microaneurysms and leakage of the dye on and around the disc. Among them, a microaneurysm found in papilledema has been briefly explained as a small spherical microaneurysm. The present findings were different from those on the ordinary angiogram: microaneurysms observed in papilledema were larger and more rugged than those in the periphery, and somewhat similar to those observed by Ashton (1951) with the infusion technique. The particularity may be due to the relatively sudden onset of venular engorgement and glomerular formation of the capillary loops. The capillary walls in the loop may then degenerate and fuse to each other to form a rugged cavity. Figure 11 represents a concept of the development of the lesions appearing in the capillaries in papilledema, from the formation of a cork-screw, in A, to the final stage of microaneurysm, in D. However, as mentioned above, this peculiarity might be present in a case with acute formation of papilledema, so that a smoothsurfaced, spherical microaneurysm might be more likely to develop in a case with slowly progressed papilledema as Ashton (1951) observed in a case with malignant hypertension.

2) Peripheral microaneurysm

Peripheral microaneurysm can be found in the extreme periphery of the senile retina with no eye disease. Ashton (1951) defined that, small in size and few in number, peripheral microaneurysms are often indistinguishable from the diabetic type of microaneurysm. A U—shaped kink and saccular configuration, demonstrated by perfusion technique were quite identical to those obtained in the present investigations. Some microaneurysms showed a particular tendency to occur at bifurcation, while others, with no such tendency, were outpouchings from one side of the capillary. It is a finding of particular interest that there is a relationship between microaneurysm and the intercapillary bridge. The bridge is generally believed to have no blood stream in its lumen and is occasionally described as a ghost vessel. However, incident-light fluorescence microscopy in this study showed the bridge to be stained, indicating that a fluid substance is sometimes exchanged between a microaneurysm and the bridge lumen. Three-dimensional observations of microaneurysm could indicate the direction of the convex surface of microaneurysm. Outpouching of the convex surface toward the inner retinal layers was confirmed in the cross sectioned preparations.

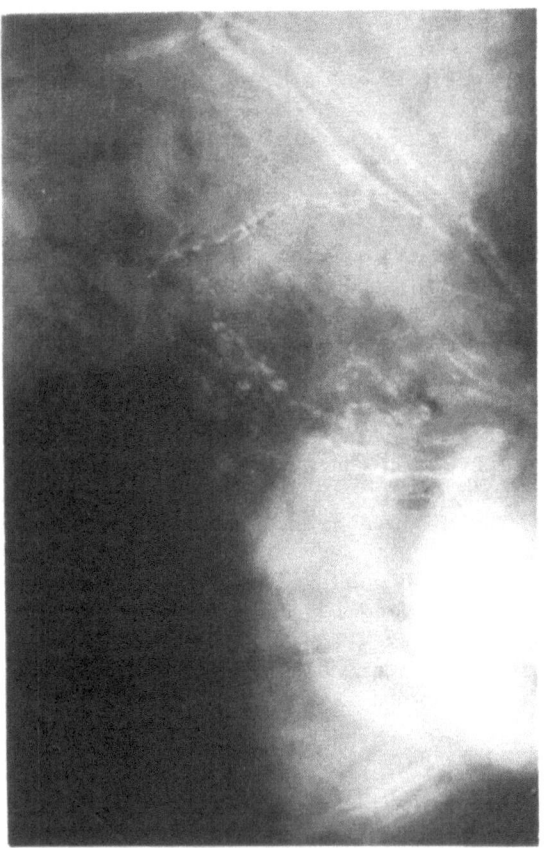

Fig. 9. *Case 3.* Aneurysmal dilation of vessels of absolute glaucoma. Incident-light fluorescence micrograph 30 seconds after injection. The rows of aneurysms are seen near the disc, X 10.

3) Aneurysm in absolute glaucoma

Fluorescein filling was limited only within a narrow region near the disc, indicating the peripheral vessels to be widely obliterated. Thus, a row of bead-like outpouchings from a single venule was confined to a small area. By the trypsin-digestion technique, Kuwabara et al. (1961) observed the presence of numerous saccular and fusiform aneurysms in cases with absolute glaucoma. It is conceivable that many more aneurysms, unfilled with fluorescein in the obliterated capillaries, may exist in other parts of the retina.

The results obtained lead us to the impression that varying features of microaneurysms, both in shape and size, are significantly related to the acuteness or chronicity of their development as well as to the severity of circulatory disturbances. A full angiographic explanation of such relationships, though unavailable at present, is expected to become possible with repeated applications of our step-by-step, systematic observation technique, which would yield pertinent data available for more detailed pathological analysis of microaneurysm.

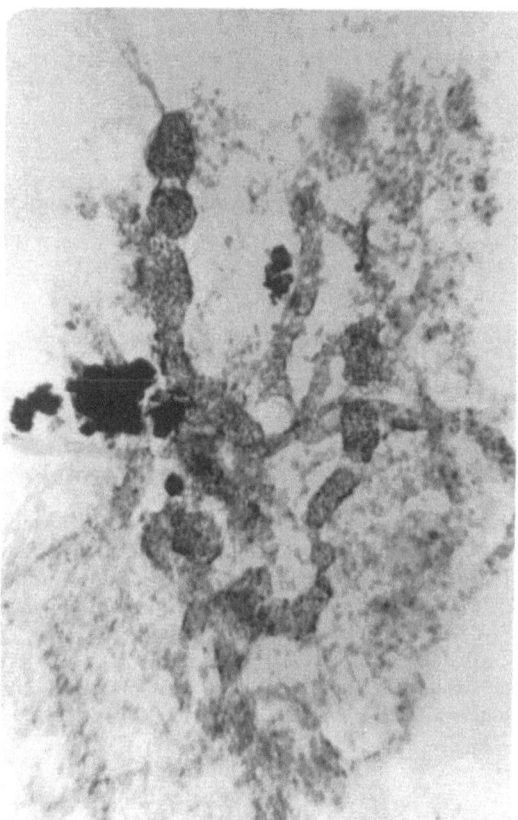

Fig. 10. The vascular tree of aneurysm prepared from the same preparation (Fig. 9). The rows of aneurysms of the venules and the venular capillaries are filled with blood cells, PAS-hematoxylin stain, x 50.

539

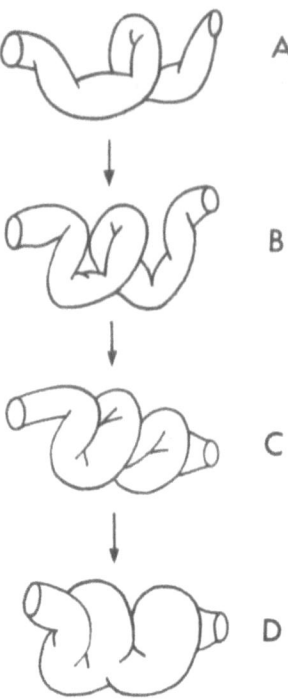

Fig. 11. Schematic representation of the development of glomerular microaneurysm in papilledema.

REFERENCES

ASHTON, N. Retinal micro-aneurysms in the non-diabetic subject. *Brit. J. Ophthalmol.* 35: *189-212* (1951).

KUWABARA T., CARROLL, J.M. & COGAN, D.G. Retinal vascular patterns, Part III. Age, hypertension, absolute glaucoma, injury. *Arch. Ophthalmol.* 65: *124-132* (1961).

MIZUNO, K. Histochemical tracing of fluorescein in retina. *EENT Monthly* 52: *15-18* (1973).

MIZUNO, K., SASAKI, K. & OHTSUKI, K. Histochemical interpretation of fluorescein angiogram. Part. 1. Technique and finding of incident-light fluorescence microscopy. *Jap. J. Ophthalmol.* 17: *202-209* (1973).

MIZUNO, K., OHTSUKI, K. & SASAKI, K. Histochemical interpretation of fluorescein angiogram. Part 2. Background fluorescence and macular dark spot. *Albrecht v. Graefes Arch. Klin. exp. Ophthalmol.* 188: *33-42* (1973).

SASAKI, K., OHTSUKI, K. & MIZUNO, K. Histochemical identification of fluorescein sodium in normal retina. *Jap. J. Ophthalmol.* 17: *323-334* (1973).

Keywords:
Microaneurysm
Fluorescein angiography
Incident-light fluorescence microscopy
Papilledema
Absolute glaucoma

Authors' address:
Department of Ophthalmology
Tohoku University School of Medicine
Sendai
Japan

540

FLUORESCEIN ANGIOGRAPHIC PATTERNS
OF RETINAL ARTERIAL ANEURYSMS*

DANIEL H. GOLD, M.D. & JOSEPH B. WALSH, M.D.

(Bronx, N.Y., USA)

INTRODUCTION

Aneurysms of the retinal arterial tree are much less common than the capillary aneurysms seen so often in diabetes, retinal venous occlusion, hyperviscosity disorders, etc. (WISE et al., 1971). They have classically been described as part of a widespread retinal vascular disorder in the spectrum of Coats' Disease/Leber's Miliary Aneurysms. ROBERTSON's report in 1973 called attention to the occurrence of retinal arterial aneurysms as a distinct entity which he termed retinal macroaneurysms (ROBERTSON, 1973). Since then several additional reports have appeared describing this disorder (SHULTS & SWAN, 1974; CLEARY et al., 1975). We wish to present the results of our study of the fluorescein angiographic characteristics of isolated retinal arterial aneurysms.

FLUORESCEIN ANGIOGRAPHIC FINDINGS

Fluorescein angiography was performed on thirteen patients with retinal arterial aneurysms. Their angiographic patterns will be described under three headings: 1) the aneurysm itself, 2) the involved artery, and 3) the adjacent retinal capillary bed.

The aneurysm

Retinal arterial aneurysms generally fill almost simultaneously with filling of the artery from which they arise. In two instances of delayed filling, there were two aneurysms adjacent to one another on the same vessel. In both cases the proximal aneurysm filled immediately while filling of the distal aneurysm was delayed (Figure 1). On occasion a retinal arterial aneurysm does not fill with fluorescein, probably indicating complete obliteration of its lumen by thrombosis or endothelial proliferation (Figure 2).

Most aneurysms filled uniformly, though some showed early filling of the proximal or peripheral portion of their lumen with delayed filling centrally or distally (i.e. distal to their site of origin from the artery) (Figure 1). This type of variation in filling is probably related to stagnant blood or thrombosis within the lumen.

* Supported in part by National Institutes of Health Grant EY00613.

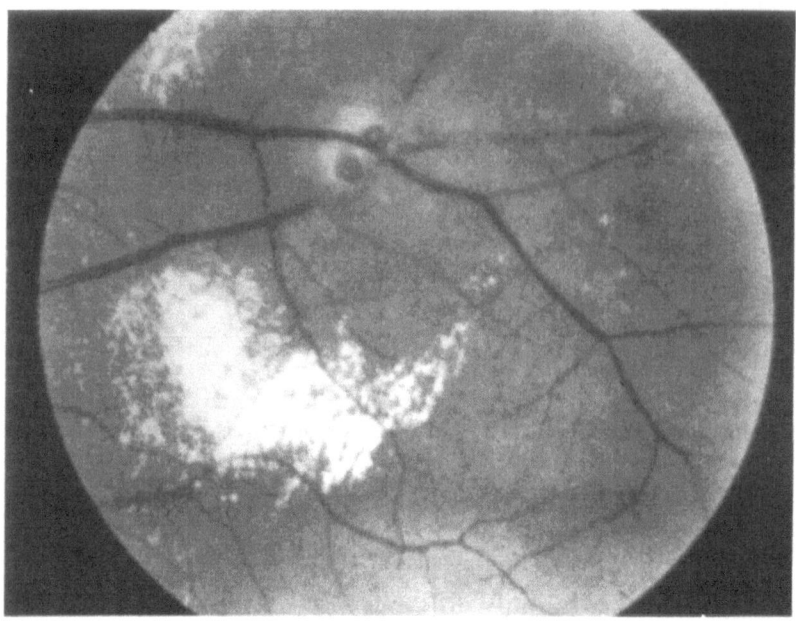

Fig. 1a. Fundus photo of two adjacent aneurysms along the superior temporal artery of a 59-year old female.

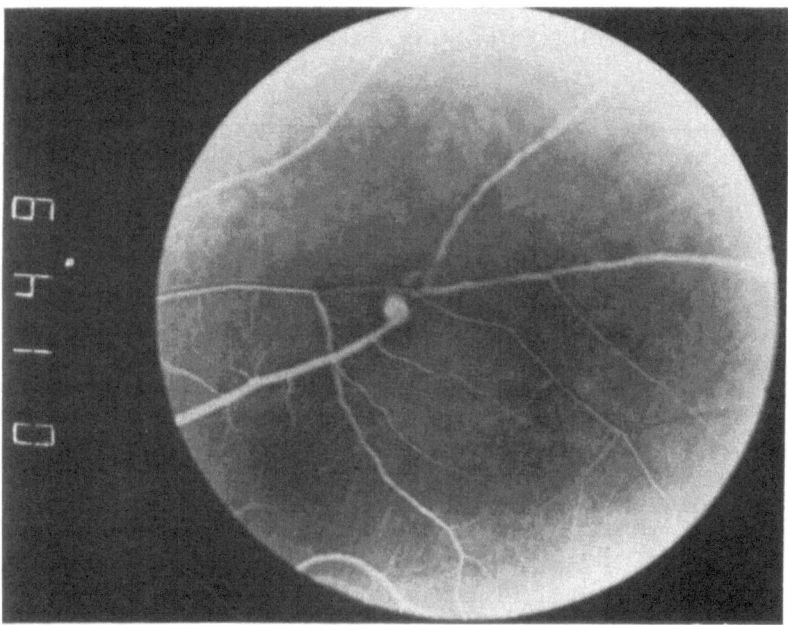

1b. Fluorescein angiography – arteriovenous phase. The proximal aneurysm is uniformly filled while a delay of the central portion of the more distal aneurysm is noted. Caliber irregularity of the involved artery is prominent.

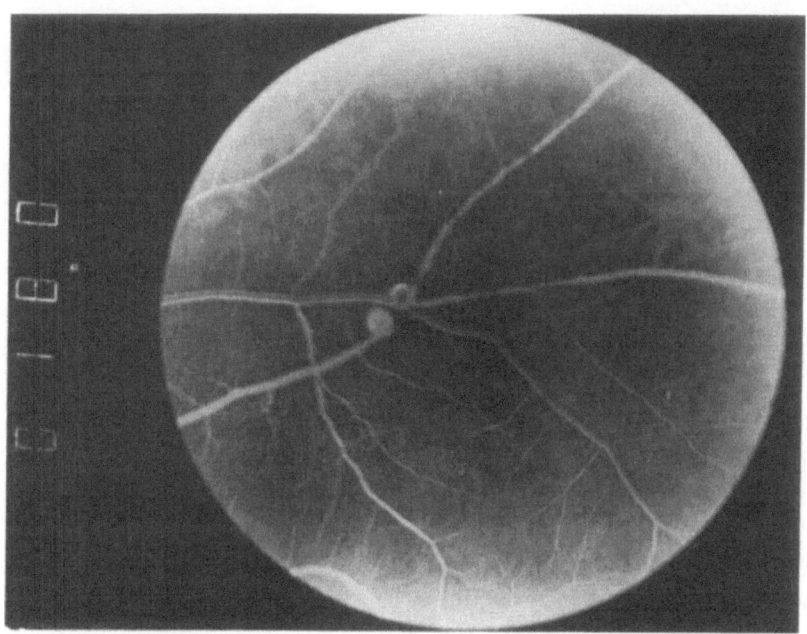

1c. Fluorescein angiography – venous phase. The distal aneurysm has filled more completely. The area surrounding the aneurysms shows blockage of background fluorescence by hyalinized tissue.

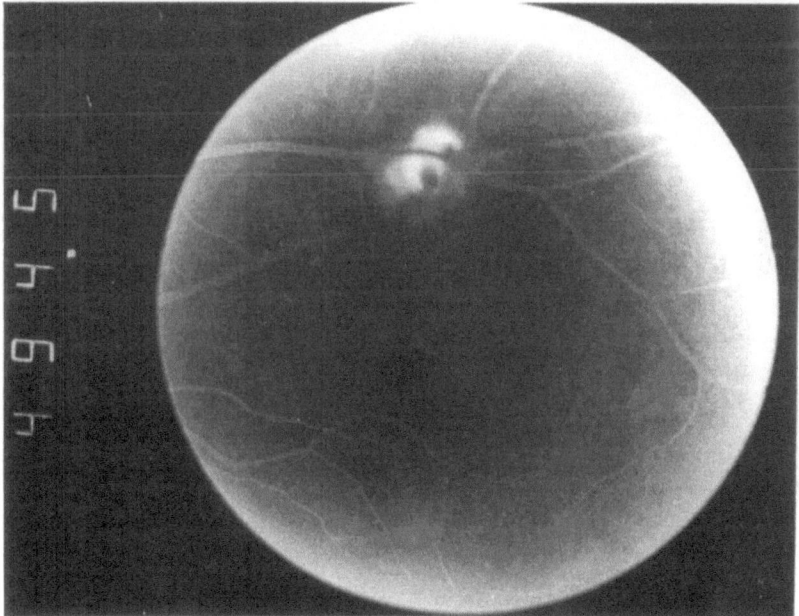

1d. Fluorescein angiography – late phase. Leakage from the aneurysms causes the highlighting of the lesions by retrofluorescence.

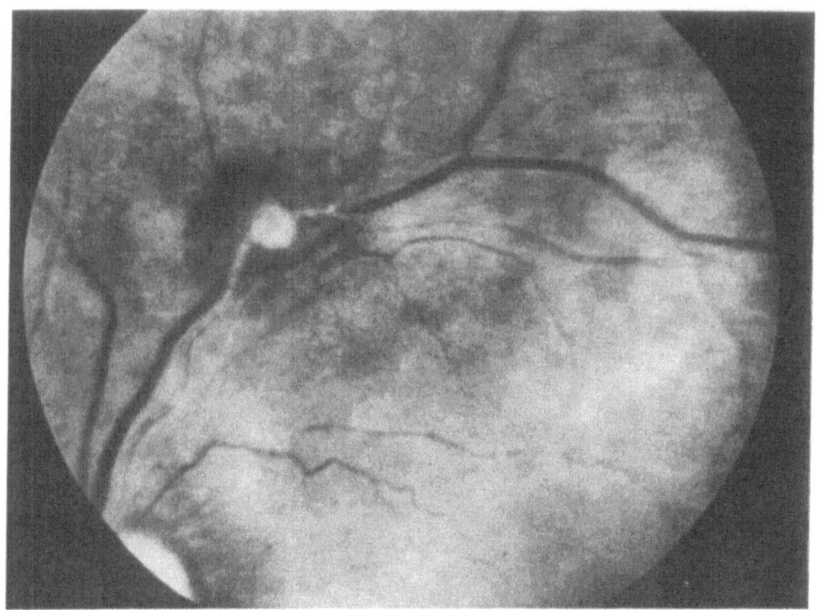

Fig. 2a. Fundus photo of a hyalinized arterial aneurysm in a 78-year old female. The involved artery is the superior temporal artery of the left eye.

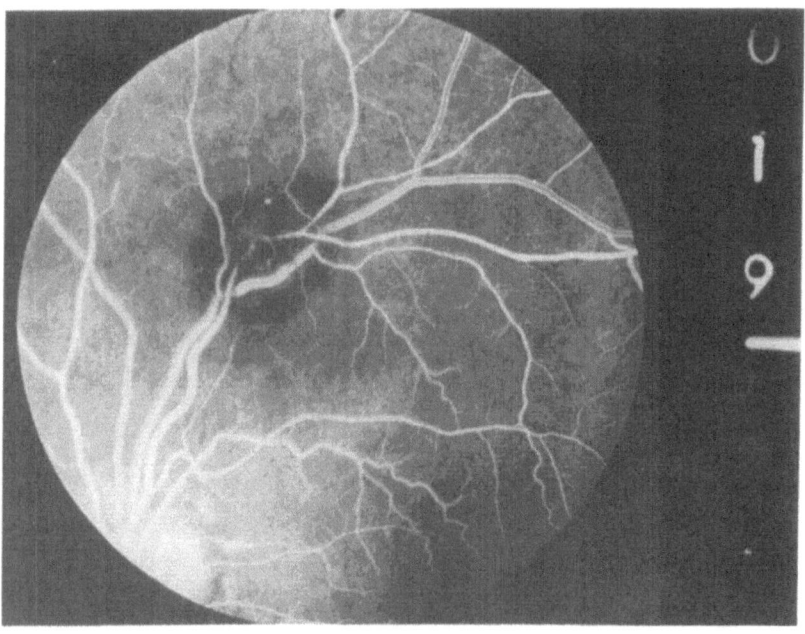

2b. Fluorescein angiogram – arteriovenous phase. No filling of the aneurysm occurs. Hemorrhage blocks the background fluorescence in the area adjacent to the aneurysm. Some dilated capillaries with a few microaneurysms are also noted adjacent to the aneurysm.

544

Leakage of fluorescein through the aneurysm wall was noted in all aneurysms which filled, though there was a good deal of variability in the extent of leakage (Figure 1). No leakage was noted in the non-filling aneurysms.

Relative or absolute blockage of the background fluorescence was commonly found surrounding the aneurysms (Figures 1, 2, 3). This varied from a small rim to one of 2-3 disc diameters in size. The blocked fluorescence was due to hemorrhage in some cases and hyalinization of the aneurysm walls in others.

Involved artery

Caliber changes consisting of narrowing or irregularity are common in both the proximal and distal segments of the involved artery (Figure 1). These changes may not be apparent when hemorrhage or exudate obscures angiographic details, but as these clear the vessel wall changes may be revealed.

In one instance, marked leakage of dye occurred through the walls of the proximal segment of the involved artery (i.e. proximal to the aneurysm) (Figure 3). The retinal artery giving rise to the aneurysm showed no fluorescein leakage in any other patient.

One patient had two 'kinks' in different branches of the distal segment of the involved artery (Figure 4). One kink leaked fluorescein while the other did not.

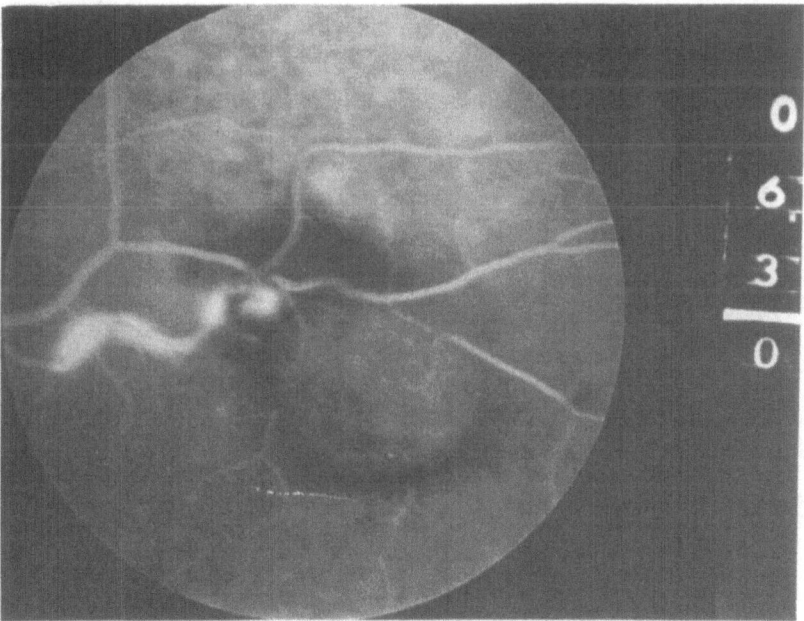

Fig. 3. Late phase fluorescein angiography of an arterial aneurysm of the left superior temporal artery in a 67-year old female. Leakage from the aneurysm and the proximal portion of the involved artery is present. An area, 2 disc diameters in size, of blocked background fluorescence is noted delineating hemorrhage.

545

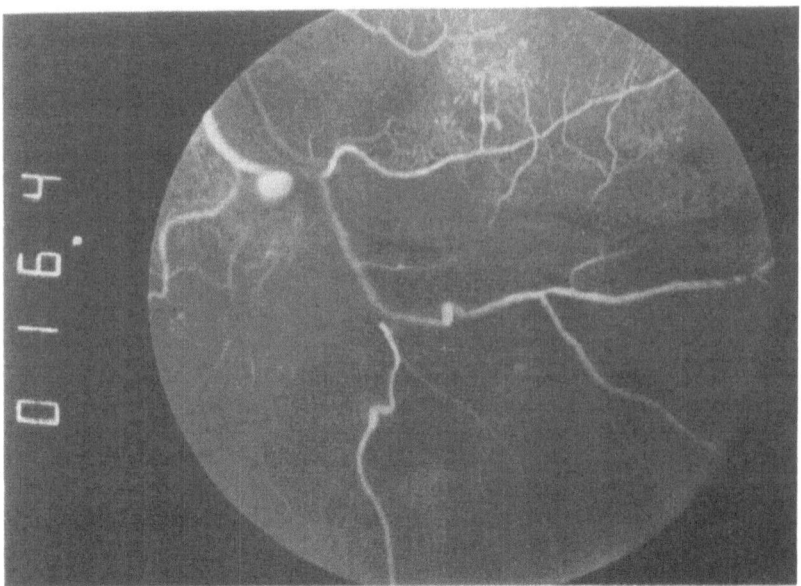

Fig. 4. Arteriovenous phase of an aneurysm in a 70-year old diabetic female involving the inferior temporal artery. Two bifurcations distal to the aneurysm two kinks are noted in the involved arterial segment. The aneurysm itself is rapidly and uniformly filled. The marked capillary bed abnormalities are likely due to diabetic retinopathy.

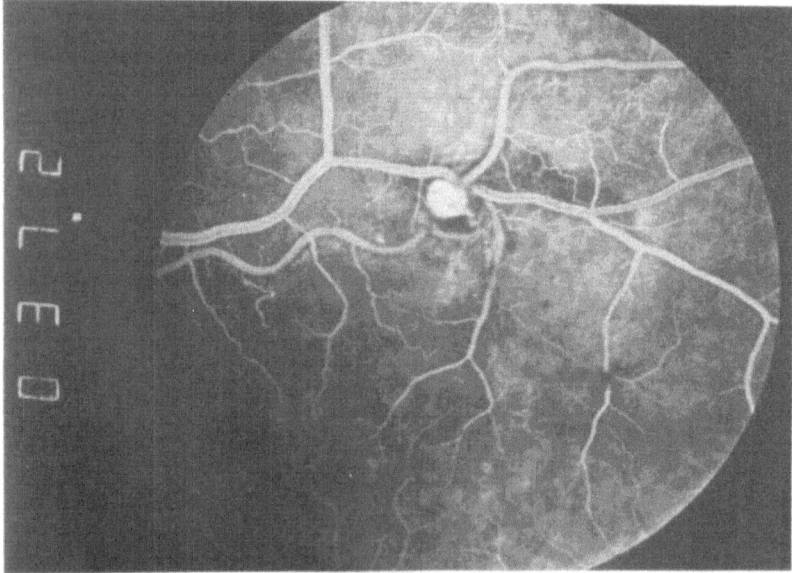

Fig. 5. Late arteriovenous phase. Same case as Figure 3 but 16 months later. The capillary bed surrounding the aneurysm exhibits areas of dilatation and micro-aneurysms as well as non-perfusion. The hypofluorescent 'cap' is present inferior to the aneurysm.

546

Detailed study of the retinal capillary bed adjacent to arterial aneurysms may be difficult due to problems such as hemorrhage and photographic resolution. Small areas of capillary dilatation and non-perfusion near the aneurysm were frequently found, as were small capillary microaneurysms (Figure 5). In these cases, late fluorescein leakage from the involved capillary bed was present.

SUMMARY

The typical fluorescein pattern of an isolated retinal arterial aneurysm is one of a uniformly filling lesion with dye entering the aneurysm as it enters the involved arterial segment. Where two contiguous aneurysms were present in the same artery, the more distal aneurysm may show delayed filling. Aneurysms which do not fill with fluorescein presumably have occluded lumens. These do not leak fluorescein, while all other aneurysms show leakage through them into the adjacent retina.

The involved artery usually has significant irregularity of its caliber, while the capillary bed surrounding the aneurysms may show dilatation, dropout, microaneurysm formation and fluorescein leakage. A frequently seen hypofluorescent 'cap' around the external aneurysms may be due to surrounding hemorrhage or hyalinization of its walls.

REFERENCES

CLEARY P.E., KOHNER, E.M., HAMILTON, A.M. & BIRD, A.C. Retinal macroaneurysms. *Br. J. Ophthalmol.* 59: *355-361* (1975).

ROBERTSON, D.M. Macroaneurysms of the retinal arteries. *Trans. Am. Acad. Ophthalmol. Otolaryngol.* 77: *OP-55-67* (1973).

SHULTS, W.T. & SWAN, K.C. Pulsatile aneurysms of the retinal arterial tree. *Am. J. Ophthalmol.* 77: *304-309* (1974).

WISE, G.N., DOLLERY, C.T. & HENKIND, P. The retinal circulation Harper & Row, Hagerstown, Maryland, pp *278-288* (1971).

Authors' address:
Department of Ophthalmology
Albert Einstein College of Medicine
Montefiore Hospital and Medical Center
Bronx, N.Y. 10467
USA

DISCUSSION

Dr Henkind: As with all things that are perhaps of interest to this group, our own group has studied a large series of monkeys and in one case, of a spontaneous hypertensive monkey with systemic hypertension, they found a retinal macroaneurysm, which fits all the criteria of human retinal macro aneurysm. So it is not limited to the human species alone. We think this particular monkey was quite old; we are now studying this by electromicroscopy. Dr Gold has not mentioned that he has two cases that he has studied clinical-pathologically in humans which will be published.

Dr Gold: We did not have time to go into the follow-up data of these patients. There were aneurysms which were patent when we first saw them and which subsequently closed off; there were other aneurysms which showed progressive hyalinization. Other aneurysms were not terribly prominent at first, but when we followed them along we found that they would get much larger. The patient who had the leaking artery and the extensive lipid in the macula had a visual acuity of about 20/400. When we saw her about a year later the artery was not leaking, the exudates had cleared up, her vision had improved to about 20/40, and the aneurysm was about twice as large.

Dr Bird: I want to ask Prof. Henkind a question. Philip Cleary certainly made the point that retinal macroaneurysms may be directly comparable to the macroaneurysms found in the central nervous system and which are probably responsible for a lot of damage in hypertensive encephalopathy or brain degeneration in hypertensive patients. I wonder whether the monkey had any cerebral aneurysms?

Dr Henkind: I am not sure. The monkey was severely hypertensive, we have the brain, we have not looked for brain macroaneurysms but we certainly will do so. I would point out that any of you who have access to large colonies of monkeys to have a survey of monkeys. We have found racemose angiomas in monkeys, macro aneurysms and also ophthalmic artery occlusion, branch artery occlusion. The only thing we have not seen is diabetic microangiopathy in a monkey.

RETINAL VASCULAR CHANGES IN TAKAYASU'S DISEASE (PULSELESS DISEASE), OCCURRENCE AND EVOLUTION OF THE LESION

MASANOBU UYAMA, M.D. & KUNIO ASAYAMA, M.D.

(Kyoto, Japan)

Takayasu's arteritis is particularly prevalent in young Japanese females, and we have encountered many patients with this disease. We wish to report our findings on 80 patients seen during the past 17 years.

In 1908, a Japanese ophthalmologist, Takayasu observed peculiar fundus changes, which have been termed 'Takayasu's retinopathy'. Absence of radial pulse was up to 1945 one of the significant findings. Since 1945, this disease has been known as 'Pulseless Disease'. Clinical and pathological investigations revealed recently that vascular disorders on the aorta develop not only at the aortic arch, but also at the thoracic and abdominal aorta.

The ocular findings we observed are summarized in Table 1. When vascular disorders on the aorta were predominant at the aortic arch, the blood flow in the upper half of the body was reduced. Thus, Takayasu's retinopathy occurred in the fundus of the eye. This is Type I, and is encountered in half the number of patients. On the other hand, when vascular disorders on the aorta were more predominant at the thoracic or abdominal aorta, the upper half of the body showed a high blood pressure. This group is Type III and here, hypertensive changes occurred in the fundus. Takayasu's arteritis included Type III also. Type II were mixtures of Type I and III.

Table I. Ocular Findings

		(80 cases)	Cases
Type I	Hypotension in upper half of the body (Takayasu's retinopathy)		38
	Stage 1 Dilatations of small vessels		20
	Stage 2 Microaneurysm formation		12
	Stage 3 Arterio-venous anastomoses		3
	Stage 4 Ocular complications		3
Type II	Mixed type		25
Type III	Hypertension in upper half of the body		16
	Fundus, not remarkable		2
	hypertensive fundus (K.W.I.)		10
	hypertensive fundus (K.W.II.)		2
	hypertensive retinopathy (K.W.III.)		2

Age and sex differences in Takayasu's arteritis are shown in Fig. 1. The disease was more prevalent in females, especially those around twenty years of age. Male patients were rather few.

The presentation here concerns Type I, namely Takayasu's retinopathy. At the mild or early stage, dilations of the small vessels of the retina were seen.

In the advanced stage, microaneurysms appeared on the entire retina, and were seen to be attached to the dilated small vessels. Retinal vessels were dilated and segmental in appearance, darker in colour, and a sludge-like blood stream was often observed in the veins.

Fluorescein angiography revealed that arm to retina time was slightly delayed, usually by 20 seconds. Intraretinal circulation was much slower. This slow arterial inflow could be observed in slow motion cine films and generally took about 30 seconds.

Microaneurysms were quite different in appearance from those seen in diabetic retinopathy. There were saccular and fusiform dilations of precapillary arterioles and postcapillary venules, and were much more numerous (Fig. 2). They most often occurred at the temporal side of the macula.

In the more advanced stages, arteriovenous communications were advanced in the periphery of the retina. According to the stage of development, arterio-venous anastmoses progressed from the periphery towards the posterior pole, and to the peripapillary region.

Fluorescein angiography revealed that retinal vessels were not perfused at the periphery to the arterio-venous anastmoses (Fig. 3). The blood pressure in the retinal artery was reduced to the extent that the blood flow could not be perfused into the peripheral vessels. Therefore, an arterio-venous by-pass or arterio-venous shunt may develop in the posterior area. Extravascular leakage through these vessels was also remarkable.

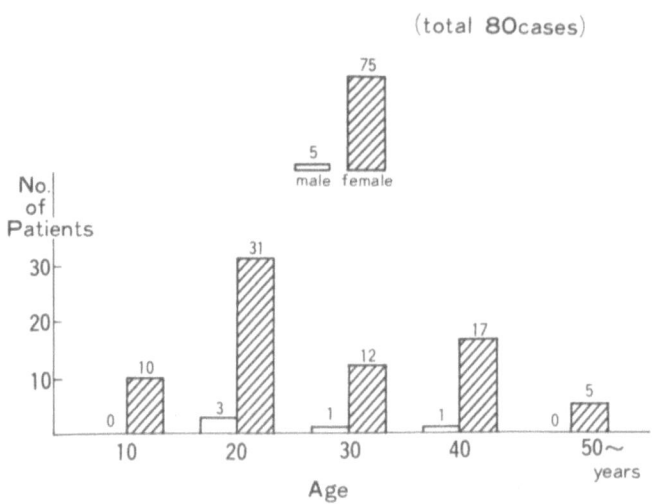

Fig. 1. Age and sex differences in Takayasu's disease.

In the final stage, vitreous haemorrhages and proliferative retinopathy occurred and vision was lost. Complications of cataract, and neovascular glaucoma may also occur.

Ophthalmodynamometry in Takayasu's retinopathy revealed 3 characteristic findings:

1. Both systolic and diastolic blood pressure in retinal arteries were quite low.

2. There was marked difference in pressure between both eyes.

3. There was considerable difference in pressure between the prone and sitting positions.

The evolution of Takayasu's retinopathy may, therefore, be divided into four stages. In the early stage, the ocular fundus shows a dilation of retinal small vessels. At the second stage, miriads of microaneurysms develop over the entire retina. Venous dilation is marked and retinal arterial pressure and

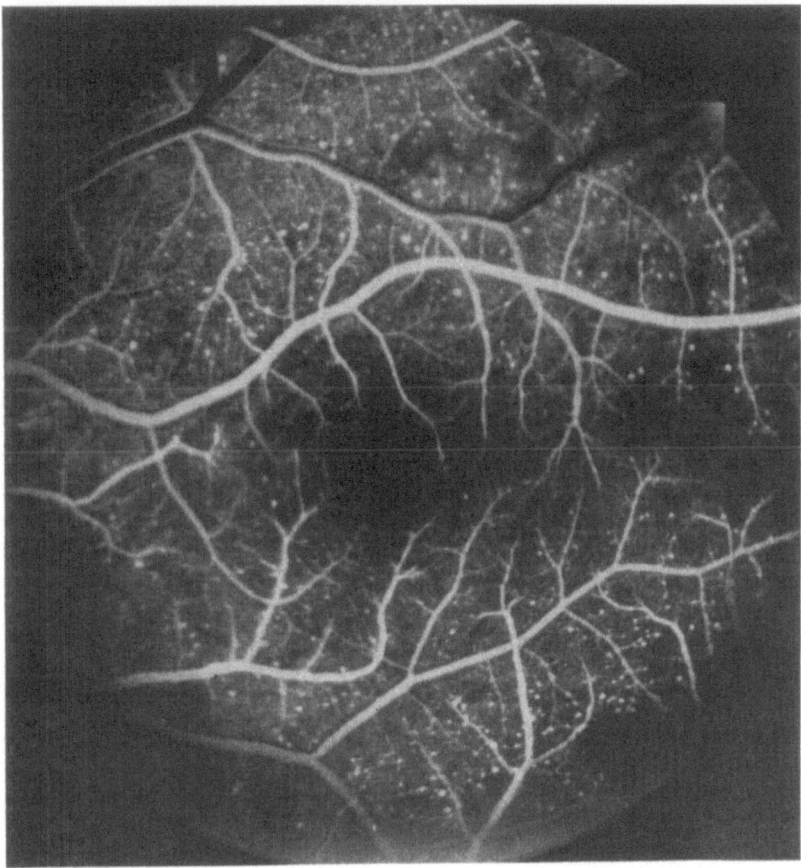

Fig. 2. Fluorescein angiogram: Takayasu's retinopathy, stage 2, Numerous microaneurysms are seen on the entire retina. Microaneurysms are fusiform or succular dilations of small vessels.

551

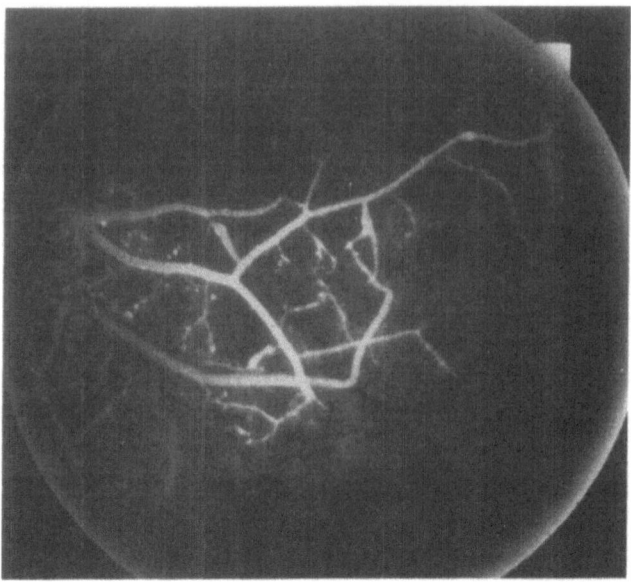

Fig. 3. Fluorescein angiogram: Takayasu's retinopathy, stage 3, Arteriovenous anastomoses are seen at the equator of the retina. Vessels at the peripheral area are not perfused.

intraocular pressure markedly decrease. In the third stage, arterio-venous communication appears. Dilations of the bulbar conjunctival vessels, and enophthalmos are seen. In the final stage, ocular complications occur.

Among the various factors affecting retinal vascular changes, decrease in blood flow is considered to be the main cause. Systolic blood pressure in the retinal artery as measured using ophthalmodynamometry is shown here at each stage of the retinopathy. Critical pressure at which microaneurysms develop on the retina was 30 mm. mercury in systolic pressure. When systolic retinal artery pressure fell below 30 mm. mercury, microaneurysms appeared. When systolic pressure was over 30 mm. mercury following medical treatment, the microaneurysms disappeared.

The critical pressure was not found for the diastolic pressure, however, retinopathy developed in proportion to the decrease in the diastolic pressure.

The intraocular pressure in Takayasu's disease was shown. With progression of the disease, intraocular pressure decreased. It is postulated that low intraocular pressures may be the result of hyposecretion of the aqueous humor, due to decrease in blood flow to the ciliary body. On the other hand, low intraocular pressure in this disease may help to maintain the intraretinal circulation, under a condition of such a low blood pressure.

In the stage of arterio-venous anastmoses, when the blood pressure level is close to the intraocular pressure, it appears that the blood flow cannot enter the blood vessels in the peripheral region.

Involvement of the main arteries arising from the aortic arch were confirmed with aortography. In the cases in which bilateral carotid and vertebral arteries were markedly stenosed or occluded, the fundi showed advanced changes over microaneurysm formation. On the contrary, in cases in which one vessel of four main trunks was patent, microaneurysms did not appear.

Therefore, microaneurysm formation on the fundus is an important sign in determining whether or not the disease is in the advanced stage.

With medical treatment, ocular lesions underwent changes. The clinical course of the retinopathy, in patients followed for at least two years was analyzed. In the fundi of the microaneurysm formation, half of the number showed no change during a two year period, and some cases advanced. In a few, however, the microaneurysms disappeared following an increase of retinal artery pressure.

In conclusion, a characteristic manifestation of Takayasu's retinopathy is the occurrence of microaneurysms in the retinal small vessels. Such a manifestation is quite evident and has a pathognomonic meaning. Retinopathy may develop with a longterm hypotension in ocular circulation. The critical systolic pressure with which microaneurysms develop is 30 mm. mercury. Arterio-venous anastomoses occur with a non-perfusion into the peripheral vessels.

REFERENCES

ASAYAMA, R. & UYAMA, M. Ophthalmodynamometric study of pulseless disease. *Jap. J. Clin. Ophthal.* 19: *397-413* (1965).

DOWLING, J.L. & SMITH, J.R. An ocular study of pulseless disease. *Arch Ophthal.* 64: *236-243* (1960).

FONT, R.L. & NAUMANN, G. Ocular histopathology in pulseless disease. *Arch. Ophthal.* 82: *784-788* (1969).

HIROSE, K. A study of fundus changes in the early stages of Takayasu-Ohnishi's (pulseless) disease. *Am. J. Ophthal.* 55: *295-1963*.

SHIKANO, S. & SHIMIZU, K. Atlas of Fluorescence Fundus Angiography, Igaku-shoin, Tokyo: *87-103*, (1968).

SHIMIZU, K. Fluorescein microangiography of the ocular fundus Igaku-shoin, Tokyo: *45-52* (1973).

UYAMA, M. Takayasu's disease (pulseless disease). *Ophthalmology* 13: *121-134* (1971).

Authors' address:
Department of Ophthalmology
Faculty of Medicine
Kyoto University
Sakyo-ku
Kyoto
Japan

DISCUSSION

Dr Goldberg: I agree that Dr Uyama's paper was a fascinating paper. I have never had the experience of dealing with such a patient, and I wonder if I might ask several questions about this disease. First, with regard to the arterio-venous communications are these high velocity shunts or, as one might expect, low-velocity shunts? Second, with regard to retinal neovascularisation, how often does this phenomenon occur, and, when it does occur, how often do these vessels bleed into the vitreous. Finally with regard to treatment do the physicians caring for these patients in Japan, direct their treatment locally against neovascularisation by means of photocoagulation or anything else, or is the approach directed to the large stenotic blood vessels in the neck or chest? If the latter is the case, and if the perfusion pressure to the eye is improved, what happens to the neovascular membranes? Do they then bleed into the vitreous as a result of increased pressure?

Dr Uyama: Arterio-venous anastomosis occurred due to the non-perfusion of peripheral retinal vessels. That is very different from arteriovenous anastomosis from venous occlusion or diabetic retinopathy. Next is the neovascularisation into the vitreous; in the final stage of the arterio-venous communication we met very few cases of neovascularisation into the vitreous, only two cases; and after that vitreous hemorrhages occurred. The third question is about the treatment: we do the treatment mainly medically, anticoagulant therapy and also steroids. At the second stage we do bypass graft of the carotid. to the aorta or 'endarteriectomy' of the aorta, but I did not do photocoagulation to the non-perfused area. However, at the stage III we also do the arterio-carotid bypass, the intraretinal arterial pressure increases so that many hemorrhages occur in the eye.

Dr Amalric: Je voudrais demander si dans cette maladie vous avez observé des oblitérations de vascularisation choroidienne? Est-ce que dans les stades tardifs on voit des oblitérations de la choriocapillaire?

Dr Uyama: Up to now I did not find any occlusion of the choriocapillaris but I would like to investigate that.

Dr Oosterhuis: I have seen your pictures with many microaneurysms and I had the impression when we consider a large number of microaneurysms that leakage was present, but was not a very prominent feature in your pictures. I have two questions. In the first place is it true that the leakage is not very marked as we see in microaneurysms in diabetic retinopathy and in retinal vein occlusion and if this is so, could it that the low perfusion pressure in the vessels influences favourably leakage?

Dr Uyama: Yes, I guess you are right. The microaneurysms in Takayasu's disease do not seem to leak at the early stage and in the later stage leakage is much more profuse from the microaneurysms.

554

RETINOPATHY DUE TO CHRONIC CARBON DISULFIDE POISONING

MASATAKA TAKAHASHI, M.D.

(Fukushima, Japan)

It is strange but true that while many cases of retinopathy due to chronic carbon disulfide poisoning have been reported in Japan, few cases have been found in other countries. As no detailed angiographic pattern of this retinopathy is known for sure, at present, the author would like to discuss it in this report.

Of 177 workers selected by random sampling, 116 were studied through fluorescein angiography. All the workers, males ranging from 33 to 56 years, have been occupationally exposed to carbon disulfide gas of very high concentration, presumably more than hundreds of ppm, since before 1961 when the gas concentration was limited below 20 ppm.

The author would like to discuss three chief findings as seen by fluorescein angiography: first, the capillary microaneurysm formation; second, the increased background fluorescence in the paramacular area indicating the defective pigment content in the pigment epithelium; and third, the abnormal retinal capillaries including dilated RPC's.

MICROANEURYSM FORMATION

Microaneurysm formation, the most typical finding, was detected in 81.03% of 116 cases. The first case (Fig. 1) is presented to demonstrate that this retinopathy, in general, can hardly be differentiated from 'diabetic retinopathy' if the patient's occupational history is not considered. Naturally, in this case there is no possibility of diabetes mellitus and other diseases, from the standpoint of familial history, past history and glucose tolerance test.

PIGMENT EPITHELIAL DISTURBANCE

Chronic carbon disulfide poisoning can affect not only the retinal capillaries, but also the pigment epithelium. Generally, the disturbance of pigment epithelium is recognized as discrete and irregular hyperfluorescent patches scattered surrounding the parafoveal area (Fig. 2) with or without detachment of the neurosensory retina. In addition, as a very interesting finding, 5 cases of central serous retinopathy were found (Fig. 3). 4.31% of 116 cases should be regarded as a relatively high incidence in comparison with 0.61% of 6450 outpatients who visited our clinic in 1974.

Moreover, localized detachment of the pigment epithelium was observed

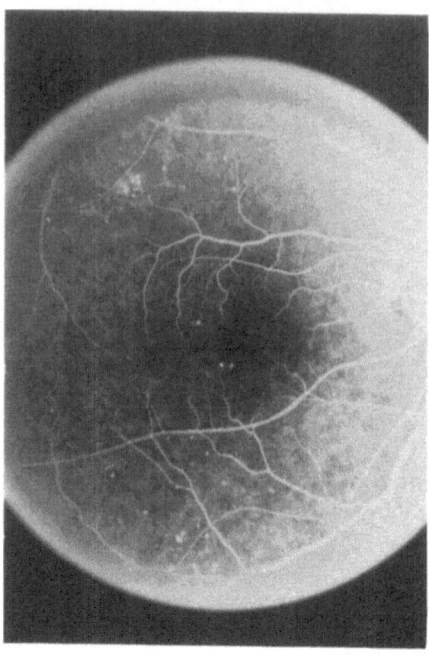

Fig. 1. A 43 year old male, exposed to carbon disulfide gas for 19 years. Microaneurysms are observed in the paramacular area.

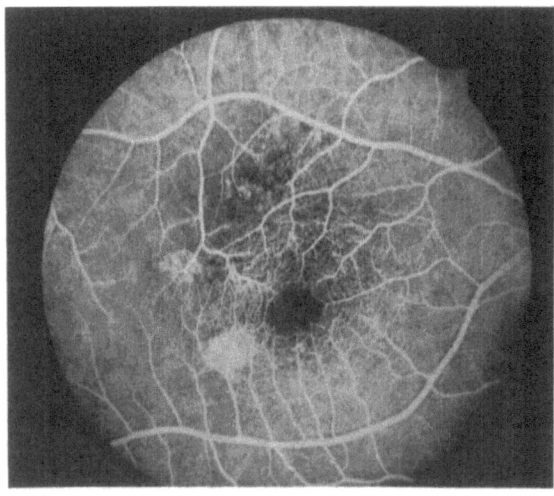

Fig. 2. A 49 year old male, exposed to carbon disulfide gas for 22 years. Hyperfluorescent patches scattered in the paramacular area.

in three cases. It is my impression that the above-mentioned involvement of the pigment epithelium is due to direct intoxication by carbon disulfide and secondary malnutrition, and, at the same time, may be regarded as the only manifestation to differentiate the disease from diabetic retinopathy because of the following statistical analysis. Namely, the pigment epithelium disturbance detected with fluorescein angiography was 47.41% of 116 chronic carbon disulfide poisoning cases, while 17.35% including no central serous retinopathy in 121 cases of clinical diabetes, ($P < 0.005$).

ABNORMAL CAPILLARY

22 of 116 cases revealed more or less abnormalities of retinal capillaries. The most characteristic change was the dilatation of RPC's (Fig. 4). Capillary obliteration without microaneurysm formation, formation of veno-venous collateral route via dilated capillaries and increased permeability of retinal capillaries were the main findings observed by fluorescein angiography.

As an additional finding, drusen were detected in relatively high prevalence, but the author wonders if this is really characteristic or/and if it is due to the poisoning. Moreover, two cases of branch vein occlusion were observed. Almost none of the cases revealed dye leakage from the capillary net of the optic disc and from RPC's.

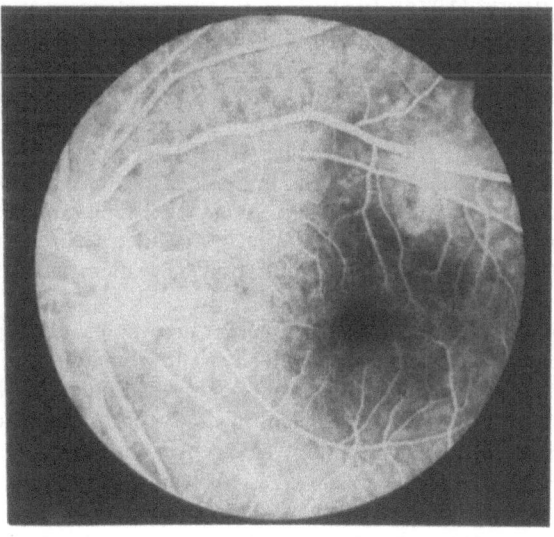

Fig. 3. A 44 year old male, exposed to carbon disulfide gas for 11 years. Central serous retinopathy was detected.

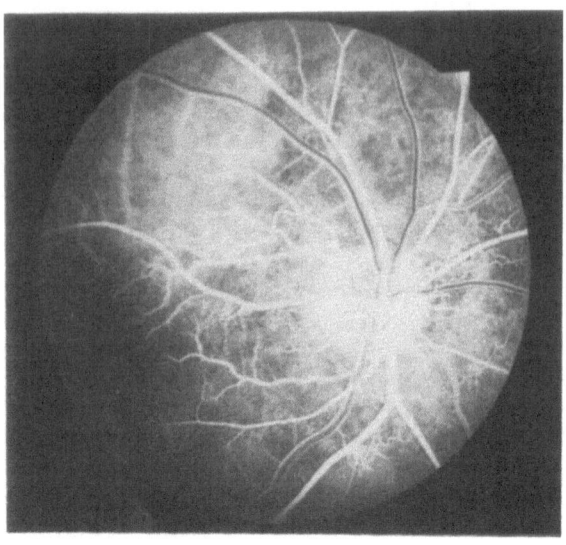

Fig. 4. A 53 year old male, exposed to carbon disulfide gas for 21 years. Remarkable capillary abnormality including RPC's.

DISCUSSION

In 1974, TOLONEN (1974) emphasized that no evidence was found for retinopathy attributable to carbon disulfide exposure and that the high prevalence of retinal microaneurysms, reported by Goto & Hotta (1970), was exaggerated by bias in selection of exposed population. According to the former, the prevalence of microaneurysm is merely 3%, almost the same rate as the controls. In contrast to this latter it revealed about 50%. As mentioned above, the author's selection reached 81.03%. Although the strict explanation of such an extreme difference between our country and Finland is impossible, one should take into consideration that the racial difference and the degree of gas concentration play important roles in the problem.

Besides capillary involvement, it is apparent that the pigment epithelium is also susceptible to carbon disulfide. The result would suggest that this retinopathy is different from diabetic retinopathy. Although the histologic changes of glomerular lesions ascertained by needle biopsies in the workers of chronic carbon disulfide poisoning are similar to those found in the Kimmelstiel-Wilson syndrome (YAMAGATA, 1966), the patients showed no clinical signs and symptoms of diabetes. Taking these two facts into consideration, we suppose that carbon disulfide poisoning is a very suggestive disease for elucidating the etiology of diabetic 'microangiopathy', although it is questionable whether it has diabetogenic effect.

REFERENCES

HOTTA, R. & GOTO, S. A fluorescein angiographic study on microangiopathia sulfo-carbonica. *Acta Soc. Ophthal. Jap.* 74: *1463-1467* (1970).

TOLONEN, M. & NURMINEN, M. Microcirculation of ocular fundus in viscose rayon workers exposed to carbon disulfide. *Alb. v. Graefes Arch. klin. exp. Ophthal.* 191: *151-164* (1974).

YAMAGATA, Y. Carbon disulfide nephrosclerosis, with special reference to the similarity to diabetic glomerulosclerosis. *Diabetes Mellitus* 9: *208-217* (1966).

Author's address:
Department of Ophthalmology
Fukushima Medical College
4-45 Sugitsuma-cho
Fukushima-shi 960
Japan

DISCUSSION

Dr Goldberg: Regarding carbon disulfide poisoning, does the agent do anything to the body that might shed some light on the pathogenesis of the retinopathy? Is there any effect on systemic blood pressure, for example? Or is there any effect on the haematological system, for example?

Dr Takahashi: The only general condition is the relative high blood pressure, over 150 mmHG.

FLUORESCEIN ANGIOGRAPHY STUDIES OF POSTERIOR POLE PRERETINAL FIBROSIS (MACULAR PUCKER)

K. PSILAS, N. STANGOS, P. TRAIANIDIS & G. GEORGIADES

(Thessaloniki, Greece)

INTRODUCTION

The syndrome of 'posterior pole preretinal fibrosis' is a form of posterior pole degeneration of diverse aetiology (WISE, 1975).

In advanced stages of this syndrome, a preretinal macular or paramacular membrane is formed. The latter contracts and causes a distortion of the retinal surface of the affected area. This results in a tortuosity of the vessels.

Numerous authors have studied this syndrome by fluorescein angiography (FAG) (BONNET, 1973; MAUMENÉE, 1967; SHIMIZU et al., 1974; SPEISER, 1975; THEODOSSIADIS et al., 1973), and were interested in the pathogenesis (BELLHORN et al., 1975; BONNET, 1973; GASS, 1970; JAFFE, 1967; REESE et al., 1970; SCHEPENS, 1955; THEODOS-SIADIS et al., 1973; WISE, 1975).

PATIENTS AND METHOD

Twenty cases with posterior pole preretinal fibrosis were studied by FAG. In 19 cases the lesion was unilateral while in one it was bilateral. They had a variety of aetiology (Table I).

In this study we made use of the Topcon Camera TRF_3 and Fluorescein 10% (8 ml).

Table I. Posterior pole preretinal fibrosis (20 cases)

Aetiology	Number of cases
1) Idoipathic	5
2) Operated retinal detachment	8
3) After peripheral xenon photocoagul.	3
4) Contusion of the eye	2
5) Peripheral retinal angiomatosis	1
6) Periphlebitis	1
Total	20

RESULTS AND DISCUSSION

From FAG studies of our cases we have made the following observations. In one case, with a very early preretinal fibrosis of the macula, asteroid in shape, the FAG studies showed no vascular or chorioretinal lesions of this area. One could see that the avascular foveal area was reduced. In more advanced cases when the newly formed membrane starts to contract, FAG shows more definitely a distorsion of the vessels in the posterior pole, already apparent by ophthalmoscopy. Personnally we had 19 such cases.

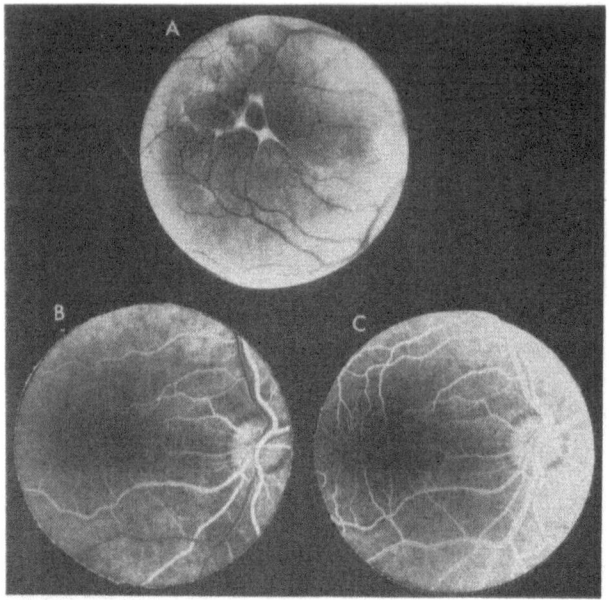

Fig. 1. A.M. ♂, age 18. A. Fundus photography. Early formation of a macular membrane.
B, C. Fluorescein angiography: no evident changes; one could perhaps see a diminution of the avascular area in the macula.

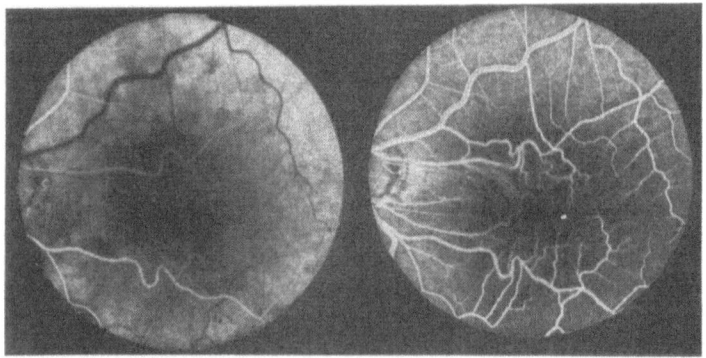

Fig. 2. B.A. ♀, age 65: Fluoroangiography. Idiopathic preretinal fibrosis.

This distorsion is more evident in small veins than arteries (BONNET, 1973; WISE, 1975) probably due to their weak walls. Among the 5 cases with idiopathic type of the syndrome, only 2 cases had 2-3 rare points of leakage in the late venous stages, arising from retinal venules and capillaries. This leakage can be explained by secondary changes in the vascular wall of the affected area. No leakage could be seen from the arteries or the pigment epithelium (Fig. 2). We found the same conditions in 3 cases of the 3rd group (Table I). By contrast in the cases of the other groups (Table I), extensive leakage was seen on the affected area. In most of these cases FAG showed further retinal or vascular lesions, due probably to the precipitating disease.

One case is of social interest and needs a more detailed description: A male patient aged 18, complaining of a recent reduction of vision of the L.E., was found to have a visual acuity 0.3. On fundus examination one could see a preretinal fibrosis of the posterior pole, also there was a retinal angiomatosis in the periphery between 11 and 2 o'clock.

FAG showed a typical picture of a preretinal fibrosis with extensive leakage in the affected area (Fig. 3 AB). The V.A. dropped to 0.1 after some days. We decided to intervene on the area of angiomatosis by photo-coagulation.

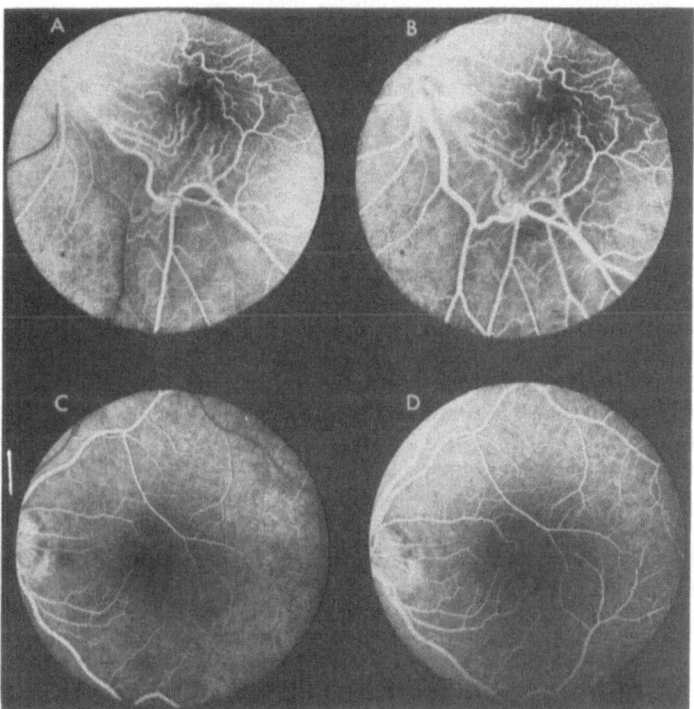

Fig. 3. Z.A. ♂, age 18: A, B. Fluorescein angiography: Preretinal Fibrosis. (In periphery these is an angiomatus formation) V.A.O,I.
C, D. The same eye one month after photocoagulation of the angiomatous formation: complete regression of the syndrome. V.A. I,O.

One month later, to our surprise, the V.A. was 1.0. Slit lamp examination showed a posterior detachment of the vitreous and an almost complete resolution of the posterior pole changes. This was also confirmed by FAG (Fig. 3 c,d). In the vitreous one could observe a floating membrane, undoubtly the same that was previously covering part of the posterior pole. In our opinion, photocoagulation precipitated the above vitreous detachment which resulted in the simultaneous removal of the preretinal membrane. GASS (1970) also reported two similar cases with spontaneous cure of this syndrome.

CONCLUSIONS

1. Fluorescein angiography in posterior pole preretinal fibrosis shows no vascular or chorioretinal changes early in the disease.
2. In a more advanced stage alterations in small vessels configuration are more evident in FAG which could be of help in the diagnosis of the syndrome in suspicious cases.
3. Fluorescein leakage is more frequently seen in secondary than in idiopathic cases, and this is more often associated with a rapidly developing lesion. Leakage is the result of secondary lesions in capillaries. The latter can regress if spontaneous cure of the syndrone takes place.
4. In differential diagnosis between idiopathic and secondary cases of the syndrome FAG is of no value, unless signs of other ocular disease exist.
5. Spontaneous cure of the syndrome is rare. We have personnally observed such a case.

SUMMARY

Fluorescein angiography was performed in 20 cases of preretinal fibrosis of the posterior pole of various aetiology (5 idiopathic and 15 secondary cases).

In the early stages of the above syndrome fluorescein angiography did not show chorioretinal or vascular changes. Fluorescein leakage is seen in more advanced cases and is more common in secondary than in idiopathic ones. Extensive leakage is frequently associated with a more rapidly developing lesion.

However, fluorescein angiography is of no differential diagnostic value between an idiopathic and a secondary case, unless other signs of ocular disease exist.

In one of our cases with a peripheral angiomatosis of the retina we observed a spontaneous cure of the syndrome one month after we treated the angiomatosis by photocoagulation.

REFERENCES

BELLHORN, M.B., FRIEDMAN, A.H., WISE, G.N. & HENKIND, P. Ultrastructure and clinicopathologic correlation of idiopathic preretinal macular fibrosis. *Amer. J. Ophthal.* 79: *366-373* (1975).
BONNET, M. Le syndrome de Jaffe. *Arch. Opht.* (Paris) 33: *209-224* (1973).

GASS, J.D. Macula dysfunction caused by preretinal vitreous membrane contraction. Stereoscopic atlas of macular diseases 200 (Mosby édit., Saint Louis) *208-214* (1970).

JAFFE, N.S. Macular retinopathy after separation of vitreoretinal adherence. *Arch. Ophthal.* (Chicago) 78: *585-591* (1967).

MAUMENÉE, A. Further advances in the study of the macula. *Arch. Ophthal.* (Chicago) 78: *151-165* (1967).

REESE, A., JONES, I. & COOPER, W.C. Vitreo macular traction syndrome confirmed histologically. *Amer. J. Ophthal.* 69: *975-977* (1970).

SCHEPPENS, C.L. Fundus changes caused by alterations of the vitreous body. *Amer. J. Ophthal.* 39: *631* (1955).

SHIMIZU, K., YOKOCHI, K. & OHMI, E. Pre-retinal macular fibrosis: a clinical and fluorescein angiographic presentation. *Jap. Ophthal. J.* 18: *381-393* (1974). In: Ophthal. Lit. vol. 28, No 5 (3513).

SPEISER, P. Spontane epiretinale Fibroplasie. *Ophthalmologica* (Basel) 170: *217-222* (1975).

THEODOSSIADIS, G., KOLIOPOULOS, J., KARANTINOS, D. & VELISSAROPOULOS, P. Traction idiopathique maculaire. Existe-t-elle comme entité clinique? *Bul. mem. Soc. Fr. opht.* 86: *341-344* (1973).

WISE, G.N. Clinical features of idiopathic preretinal macular fibrosis. *Amer. J. ophthal.* 79: *349-357* (1975).

Authors' address:
30 rue Ste Sophie
Thessaloniki
Greece

ANGIOGRAPHIC CONSIDERATIONS ABOUT
THE PRERETINAL MEMBRANE

JORGE MOSQUERA & ALEJANDRO GONELLA

(Buenos Aires, Argentina)

At the retino-vitreous plane is a virtual space limited on one side by the vitreous hyaloid condensation and on the other by the internal limit of the retina, which can become real under pathological circumstances.

In some patients, due to causes which are not, as yet, too well defined, a membranous neoformation develops and occupies that space, receiving the name of pre-retinal membrane.

Many authors have described the different types of pre-retinal membrane in the posterior pole, and the same have been adequately studied from the ophthalmologic, biomicroscopic, histopathologic and clinical point of view.

Several angiographic appearances have been described in connection with these structures, which appear to originate from vitreous hyalocytes in

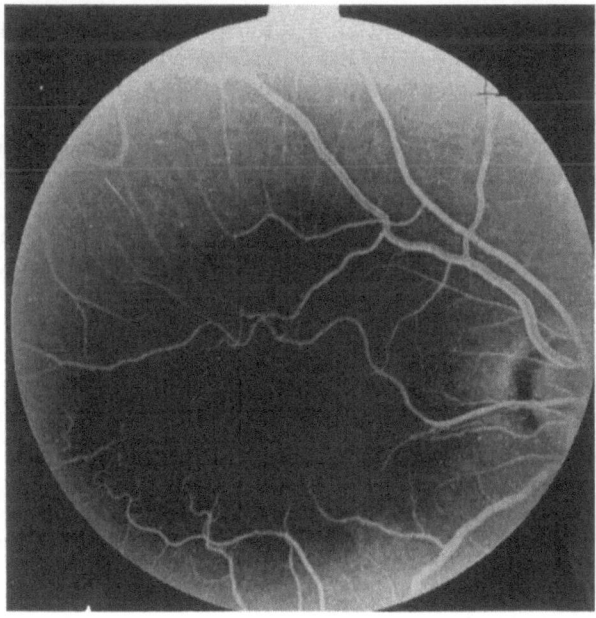

Fig. 1. Preretinal membrane without pathological fluorescence. Only the distortion of the vessels of the macular area is visible.

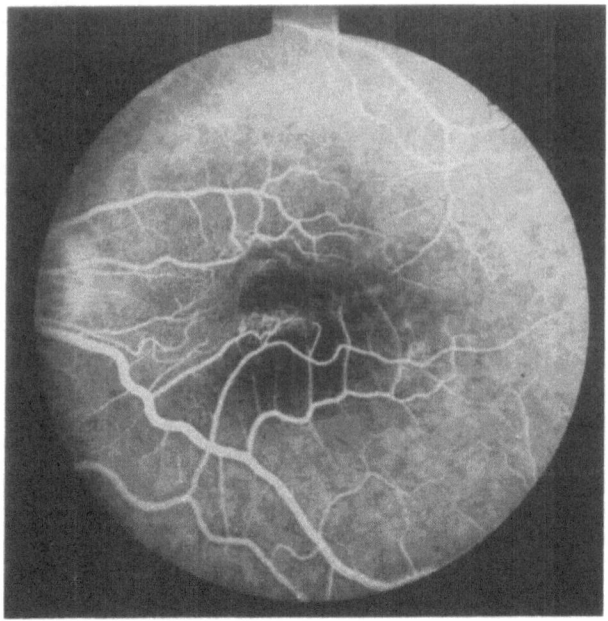

Fig. 2. Preretinal membrane with pathological fluorescence and with neovascularization. The newly formed vessels are visible in the macular area.

the posterior hyaloid, bearing in mind that the hyaloid are specially numerous in the macular zone, though there is no conclusive evidence of his.

The presence of an anomalous membrane in the retino-vitreous plane produces the following changes in that area:

a. Changes in the retina: radial folds arising from the new formed tissue.

b. Alterations in the perimacular vessels: they become irregular and sinuous, and may eventually change in calibre.

c. Abnormal vascular permeability: in some patients, the retinal vascular walls become permeable, allowing exudation into the interstitial space.

d. Neovascularisation of the affected area: it is signified by the appearance of microaneurysms, newly formed vessels, shunts in veins and arteries, invariably accompanied by a pathological permeability.

e. Micro- and macrocystic oedema of the macula.

f. Macular hole: it appears in some cases and seems to be related to the vitreous strength. However, the difficulties in finding an operculum in many cases would indicate there are other causes which may be the origin.

Bearing in mind the afore-mentioned points and from a strictly angiographic point of view, we suggest the following classification for the appearance of the pre-retinal membranes of the posterior pole:

I. Without pathological fluorescence;

II. With pathological fluorescence:

(A) Without neovascularisation

(B) With neovascularisation

(C) With false macular hole
(D) With cystic oedema of the macula
(E) With macular hole.

TYPE I: WITHOUT PATHOLOGICAL FLUORESCENCE

It is characterised by the modification in the perimacular vessels and sometimes by variations in their calibre. There is no neovascularisation or exudation into the interstice. The picture may range between mild, in which case
a comparison with the contralateral will be necessary, to severe, which can
be readily recognised by an experienced specialist.

TYPE II: WITH PATHOLOGICAL FLUORESCENCE

(A) Without neovascularisation

The pathological fluorescence seems to originate in the retinal capillaries
and may belong to one of two types. It can be diffuse, along one or more
vessels, or be localised, more or less pointed. Occasionally, hyperfluorescence appears due to alteration of the pigmentary epithelium, with transmission defect.

(B) With neovascularisation

These unmistakable cases present all the range of the vascular pathology,
with newly formed vessels, microaneurysms, arteriovenous shunts and
pathological permeability.

(C) With false macular hole

In some pre-retinal membranes there is a circular condensation through
which the red underlying retina can be seen. This is the cause of error in
diagnosis, as it is not a true macular foramen. Generally, it does not occupy
the central zone, and this helps to diagnose them correctly.

(D) With cystic oedema of the macula

It presents the typical picture of a late retention of dye as microcysts and
macrocysts.

(E) With macular hole

In these patients, the shape of the foramen is usually irregular or oval, in
contrast with the perfect roundness of idiopathic forms. No operculum can
be found, and there is an elevation of the retinal edges and fundus fluorescence of variable magnitude.

According to our experience, this classification has proved useful and
makes it possible to classify patients rapidly. Also it is possible to follow the
influence of some therapeutic methods which are under study, in the evolution of this disease.

REFERENCES

BONNET, M. Le syndrome de Jaffe. *Arch. Ophthal.* (Paris) 33: *209* (1973).

CORREA MEYER, R. & CORREA MEYER, P. & BARSANTE, C. Angio Fluoresceino-grafía: *37-54.* Bahía (1973).

JAFFE, N.S. Vitreous traction at the posterior pole of the fundus due to alteration in the vitreous posterior. *Trans. Amer. Acad. Ophthal. Otolaryng.* 71: *642-652* (1967).

LINDER, B. Acute posterior vitreous detachment and its retinal complications. *Acta Ophthalm.* Suppl. 87 (1966).

WISE, G. Clinical features of idiopathic preretinal macular fibrosis. *Am. J. Ophthalmol.* 79: *349-373* (1975).

Authors' address:
Puerredon 442, 3° piso Dto 14
Buenos Aires
Argentina

DISCUSSION

Dr Theodossiadis: I would like the follow-up of the patients who were presented. In our experience it is very difficult to divide this syndrome into separate categories. Macular puckering is frequently a progressive disease and one category goes on to the other very often.

Dr Gonella: This is true and we want also to remark that from a strictly angiographic point of view you can find separate stages. This was surprising to us and that is why we presented this classification. We believe that they present evolution.

Dr Theodossiadis: But in cases in which you have not noticed neovascularization, if you see the same case one or two years later, you may have new vessel formation and leakage from the vessels.

Dr Gonella: Yes, I agree. I only said that with fluoroangiography we can say that the patient is in that stage of the evolution.

Mr Blach: Dr Henkind, before you ask your question, I wonder if you do not have any pathology of this condition?

Dr Henkind: I suspect that this is a very common condition, because we personally have over 250 cases. As you know the late George Wise reported on 150 in his Schoenburg lecture. I do not agree with the classification and I do not think it should be split. I think there is an idiopathic variety of preretinal macular fibrosis, which must vie with senile macular degeneration as the commonest non-diabetic manifestation of the posterior pole; perhaps drusen are more common. Never does a week go by when we do not see this condition in the clinic. I ask my colleagues Dr Gold and Dr Walsh: of the approximately 250 cases of the idiopathic variety we have seen perhaps one case had neovascularization. I do not believe that neovascularization plays a role in this disease.

To answer the question posed by professor Blach, yes indeed we have histopathology. The correct term for this condition is preretinal macular gliosis. Without question, this membrane arises from glial cells in the retina, presumably Müller cells; they could, however, be other glial elements. It is surprising how common we find this on routine autopsy eyes. We have done two cases with clinical-pathological correlation.

Furthermore an entity that I will share with you now, because it is astounding to us. We have studied 10 consecutive eyes of patients with retinitis pigmentosa. This was done by Dr Friedman of our group. Everyone of those where a tapetal sheen was said to be present, it turns out that the tapetal sheen is a preretinal membrane, identical to preretinal macular fibrosis; that is a membrane on the surface composed of glial elements. I personally feel that vitreous has nothing to do with this entity. This entity can be seen after posterior vitreous detachment that has occured years before.

Dr Norton: I agree with Paul that it is a very common entity. However, I do think there is something gained by at least dividing them into those that really do not affect vision and those that significantly affect vision. Paul, I think that almost every day I see this entity; clinically I think, I can recognize them: membranes growing over the surface of the retina. In general the type you are talking about, the type George Wise described, is a non-progressive disease. We saw back a 100 cases of which we have photographs taken 5-7 years before and only one of the 100 had progressed. So the type we are talking about is not a really progressive disease. The other type, after retinal detachment surgery, is a very much more severe type as it involves the entire thickness of the retina. This is the type that leaks, this is the type that may get neovascularization. They are the serious problems. They come on, as you know, more or less six weeks after surgery and they then stabilize. I have followed them for 5-10 years and they never seem to change after that period of time. I shall comment later this afternoon on the treatment of these cases.

Dr Henkind: We have not taken these cases, we have split them off. From your own group, Machemer claims that some or many of those membranes are epithelial membranes coming from the pigment epithelium and that may be true. Our cases never have shown a break that would be through and through. I agree that you must classify them; there is a primary group which is a common entity, which occurs as far as I know in any race, whereas, for example, senile macular degeneration is rare in the black population. But the detachment type is an entirely different entity, which is much more severe. I do not think it is the same disease at all.

Dr Goldberg: Since the late Dr Wise thought that at least some cases of preretinal fibrosis are related to incipient or total retinal vein thrombosis, I wonder if we can ask any participants in the discussion whether or not they have clinical, angiographic or histopathologic evidence of central vein thrombosis in any of their patients.

Dr Henkind: I can answer that when George Wise first described that clinically in the fifties, he had noted several cases of this entity occurring generally in branch vein obstruction. Since he only had a few cases at that time, he thought that was the common etiology. But prior to his death he stated

571

that that was an uncommon cause. There is no question that 5 or 10% or more of branch vein or central vein occlusions will have this entity, but if you split those cases up, you still end with a substantial number of idiopathic cases for which there is no antecedent ocular history at all. I do not know what triggers it off but would bet we are going to find on routine autopsy eyes somewhere between a 10 or 20% incidence in patients over the age of 60. It is just a matter of looking for these things.

Dr Hayreh: Coming back to the premacular fibrosis, it occurs quite often in eyes with occlusion of the central vein when the associated macular edema lasts for a considerable length of time.

FLUOROGRAPHY OF THE FUNDUS PERIPHERY WITH RHEGMATOGENOUS RETINAL DETACHMENT

KENSEI MINODA & SADAO KANAGAMI

(Tokyo, Japan)

There are a few reports on the fluorescein angiography of peripheral fundus with retinal detachment (ROSEN, 1969; SATO et al., 1971; SHIMIZU, 1972). SATO (1971) and SHIMIZU (1972) described that the areas of equatorial degeneration in the detached retina are characterized by the presence of vasoobliteration, formation of arteriovenous shunts proximal to the degenerative zone, hyperpermeability of the retinal vessels and capillary dilatation.

It remains, however, unsolved whether or not these vascular changes in the peripheral retina may exist before the onset of retinal detachment. In other words, it must be clarified that these abnormalities in the retinal vessels are primary or secondary changes in the retinal detachment.

Comparison of fluorographic findings in detached eyes with those in their undetached fellow eyes may give us some information to analyze significance of the vascular changes described above. The present study reports fluorographic findings in peripheral retina of 100 detached eyes and 11 undetached fellow eyes.

MATERIALS

During Oct., 1974 to Feb., 1976, 171 cases of rhegmatogenous retinal detachment were operated in our clinic. Fluorographic data of sufficient

Table I. Age distribution and shape and location of retinal breaks in 100 detached patients

Breaks \ Age	0-9	10-19	20-29	30-39	40-49	50-59	60-
Equatorial Hole	1	10	12	10	6	2	
Equatorial Tear			2	4	12	15	11
Intermediate Tear				2		4	3
Macular Hole				1	1	4	
Oral Disinsertion		1	3				
not found				1	2	1	
	1	11	17	18	21	26	14

573

Table II. Fluorographic findings in peripheral retina of 100 detached eyes

Findings Age group	Vaso- obliteration	Vascular Arcade	Vaso- dilatation	Leakage
< 40	35	28	31	31
40 ⩾	29	14	29	30
Total	64	42	60	61

Table III. Peripheral retina with vasoobliteration (64 eyes)

Age Breaks	< 40	40 ⩽
Equatorial Hole	27	7
Equatorial Tear	3	13
Intermediate Tear	2	4
Macular Hole	1	3
Oral Disinsertion	1	0
not found	1	2
	35	29

quality have been obtained in 100 detached eyes and 11 undetached fellow eyes. Age distribution and the shape and location of the retinal breaks in the patients are shown in Table 1. These cases were apparently well representative of rhegmatogenous retinal detachment as a whole, in terms of age distribution and the shape and location of the retinal breaks. Our cases were classified into 6 groups, 1) detachments with equatorial holes mostly in the juveniles, 2) arrow-head or horseshoe tears at the equator which were common in the older age group, 3) tears at the intermediate zone between the equator and posterior pole, 4) macular hole, 5) oral disinsertion and 6) the group in which retinal breaks were not found.

RESULTS

The principal findings of the fluorography in the peripheral retina of the detached eyes was extensive vasoobliteration at and distal to the equatorial degenerative area. This avascularity of the peripheral retina was most frequently observed in the juveniles with equatorial holes (Table 2, 3). At the borderline of the peripheral avascular area, retinal terminal vessels frequently formed vascular arcade consisting of complex arterio-venous shunts. In some cases, this vascular arcade was distributed in almost straight line (Fig. 1), whereas in other cases the arcade showed a zig-zag course (Fig. 2). Filling of fluorescein dye into the vascular arcade was always slow and the

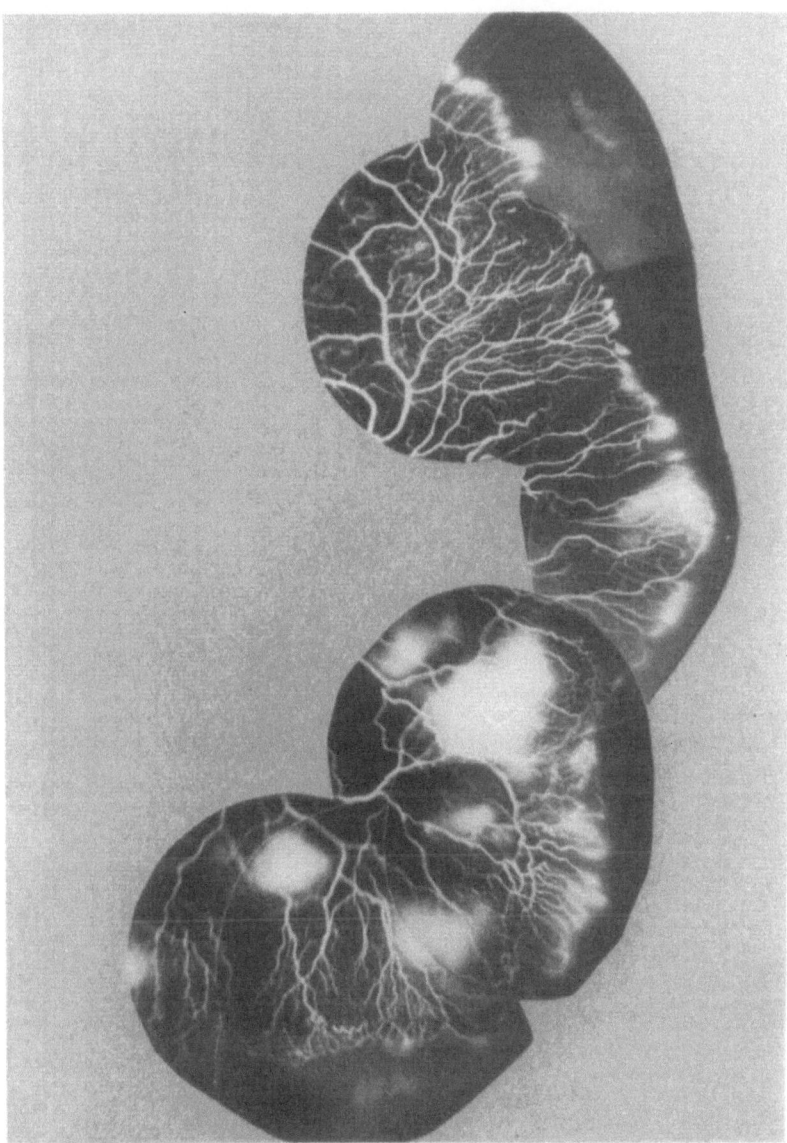

Fig. 1. Fluorography of left detached eye of 14 year old girl, showing extensive vaso-obliteration at the temporal periphery of the retina and conspicuous vascular arcade at the borderline of the avascular area. Extravasation of the dye is observed at the arcade and its neighborhood. Round holes were found at the upper-temporal and the lower-temporal portions of the avascular area.

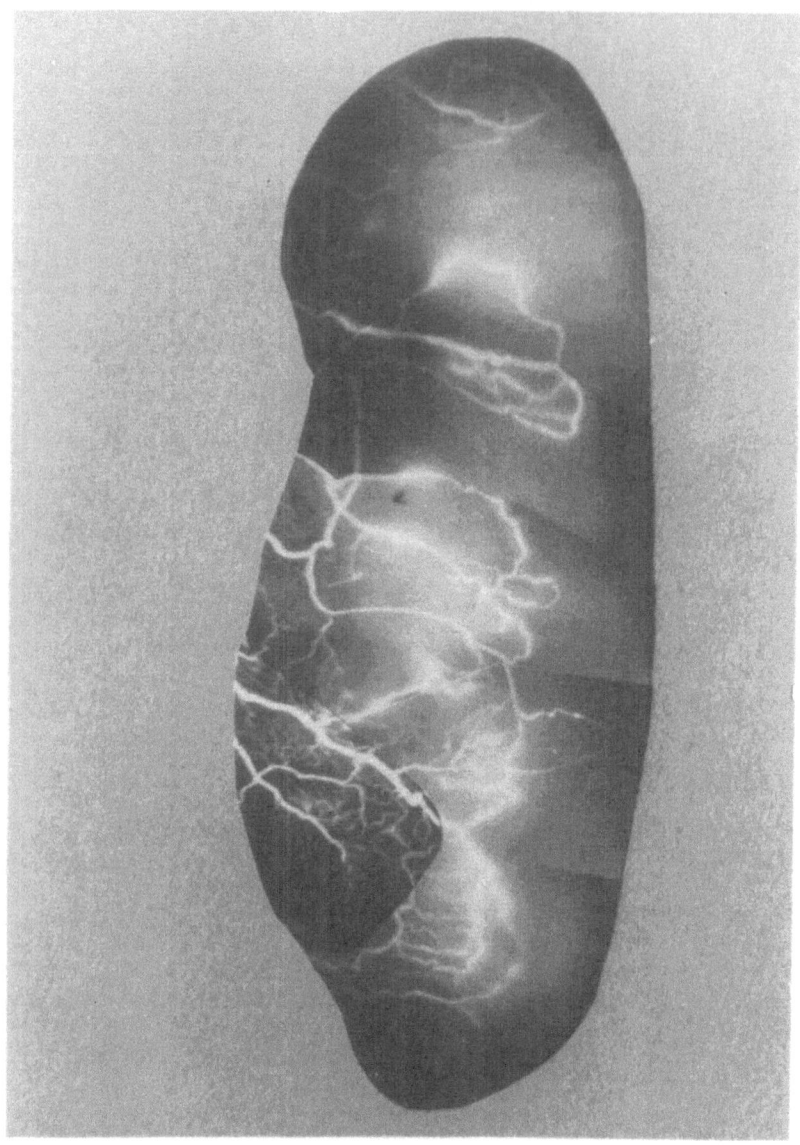

Fig. 2. Temporal equator of left detached eye of 20 year old girl. The vascular arcade adjacent to the vasoobliterated area is irregularly distributed as compared with Fig. 1, and terminal vessels sometimes show microaneurysm-like enlargement. Absence of capillary network is obvious at the area proximal to the arcade, where round hole was located.

capillaries at this area showed extensive dilatation (Fig. 1, 2). Some capillaries at the arcade area demonstrated microaneurysm-like distension and capillary network near the arcade often disappeared (Fig. 2). At the borderline of avascular area, terminal vessels sometimes demonstrated club-like enlargements or terminal buds (Fig. 5). At the late venous phase, extravasation of the dye was frequently observed at and proximal to the vascular arcade (Fig. 1-2). The frequency of these vascular changes and their relation to the configuration of retinal breaks and the age of the patients are shown in Table 2-4. It was obvious that the vascular change described above were characteristic of the group of equatorial holes in the juveniles. On the other hand, the group of equatorial tear in the older age frequently showed almost normal vascular pattern in the peripheral retina, except at the restricted portion of the tear.

Fluorographic findings in 11 undetached fellow eyes were essentially same as those in the detached eyes, except that in the former, leakage of the dye at the vascular arcade was less frequently observed than in the latter (Fig. 3-6). Vasoobliteration, vascular arcade and capillary dilatation at the peripheral retina were frequently observed in the undetached fellow eyes as much as in the detached eyes (Table 5).

DISCUSSION

It should be noted that extensive vasoobliteration at the peripheral retina, the vascular arcade and the capillary dilatation at the borderline facing to

Table IV. Peripheral retina without vasoobliteration (36 eyes)

Breaks	Age < 40	40 ≤
Equatorial Hole	1	1
Equatorial Tear	3	24
Intermediate Tear	0	1
Macular Hole	0	2
Oral Disinsertion	3	0
not found	0	1
	7	29

Table V. Fluorographic findings in 11 detached eyes and their fellow eyes

Eyes	Findings Vaso-obliteration	Vascular Arcade	Vascular Dilatation	Leakage
Detached	9	9	8	7
Fellow	10	9	8	2

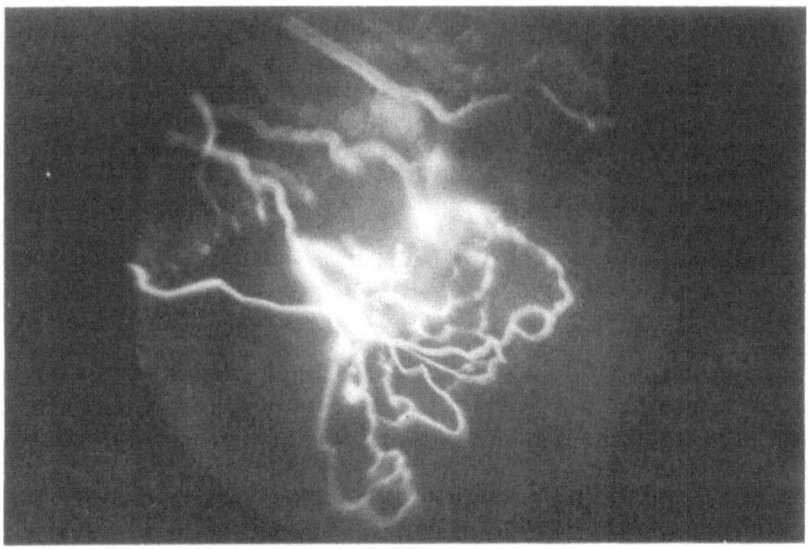

Fig. 3. Vascular arcade projecting into the avascular area in left detached retina of 32 year old female. At least three venules and one arteriole construct the arcade and they demonstrate distinct dilatation and hyperpermeability and form microaneurysm at several portions.

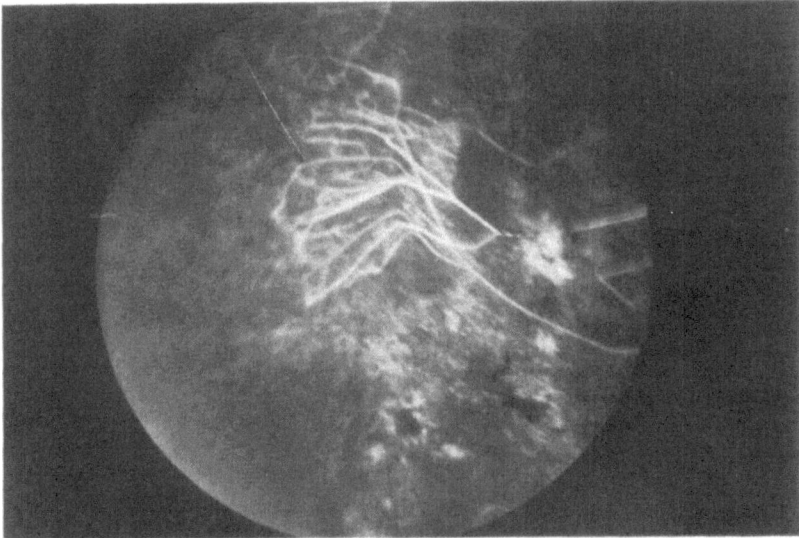

Fig. 4 Temporal equator in the undetached fellow eye of the same patient, showing vascular arcade facing to the vasoobliterated area. The extent of the avascular area and the shape of the vascular arcade resemble those in the detached eye, though dilatations of the vessels and extravasation of the dye at the arcade of the fellow eye is not distinct as compared with in the detached eye.

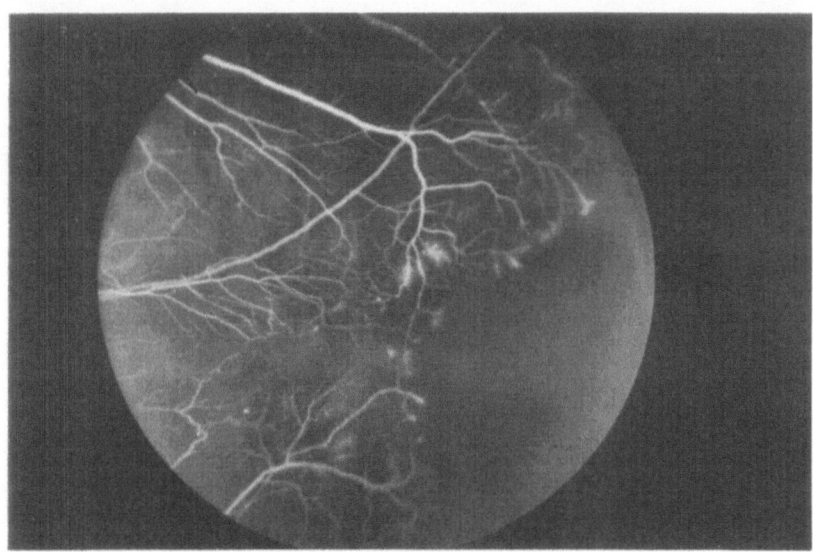

Fig. 5. Infero-temporal equator in left detached eye of 22 year old male, showing terminal enlargements of the vessels, or terminal buds at the border-line of the avascular area.

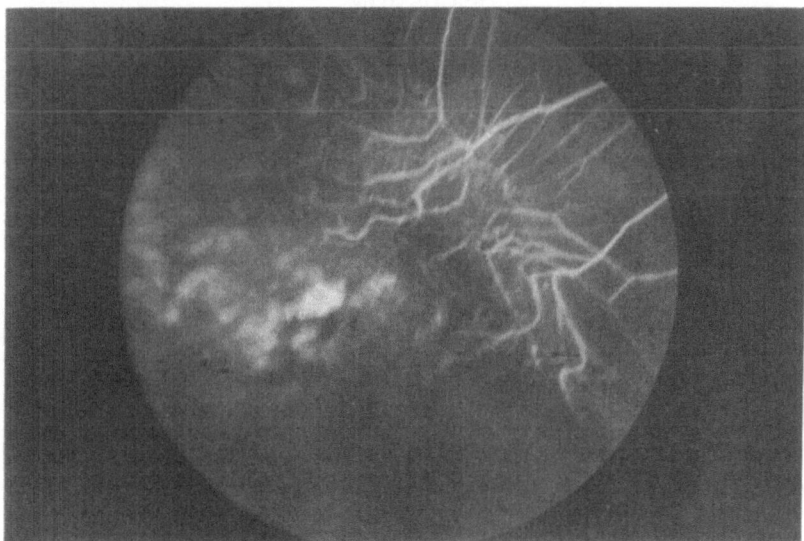

Fig. 6. Infero-temporal equator in the undetached fellow eye, showing avascular area so extensive as in the detached eye. Hyperfluorescence at the degenerated pigment epithelium is shown in the avascular area.

the avascular area were frequently observed in the undetached fellow eyes as well as in the detached eyes. In addition, these vascular changes were most frequently encountered in the group of equatorial hole in the younger age. It seems reasonable, therefore, to assume that the vascular abnormality at the peripheral retina is not a secondary change in the retinal detachment but that this change may play a principal role to produce equatorial holes in the juveniles.

On the other hand, the group of equatorial tears at the older age frequently showed almost normal vascular pattern at the peripheral retina, thus suggesting that formation of arrow-head or horseshoe tears may be associated mainly with vitreous traction but not with retinal vascular change.

REFERENCES

ROSEN, E.S. Fluorescence Photography of the Eye, Butterworths, 1969.
SATO, K. et al. Fluorescein angiography on retinal detachment and lattice degeneration. Part I. Equatorial degeneration with idiopathic retinal detachment. *Acta Soc. Ophthal.Jap. 75:635-642* (1971).
SHIMIZU, K. Fluorescein Microangiography of the Ocular Fundus, Igaku Shoin, LTD. Tokyo, 1972.

Authors' address
Department of Ophthalmology
Tokyo Kosei Nenkin Hospital
Tokyo, Japan

DISCUSSION

Dr Patz: I like to congratulate Dr Minoda on his excellent presentation. In the first case the vascular pattern suggested to me the possibility of arrested retrolental fibroplasia. I wonder if the birthweight of the child is known?

Dr Minoda: Yes, you point it out very exactly. This first case was prematurily born and presented the onset of retinal detachment when 13 years old. We recently found the late onset of rhegmatogeneous retinal detachment in patients prematurily born and this occurs rather frequently. We do not know exactly the frequency but we have to be very careful if we find juvenile patients with a rhegmatogenous retinal detachment. The second case, however, which I showed was not premature. He was 9 years old. This case demonstrates extensive vasoobliteration at the temporal periphery.

Dr Siam: There are two comments on this paper. The first concerns the number of macular holes: 6 out of 100 which I think is too high. I am convinced that there is a high incidence, but never up to 6%. What changes did you find around the macular holes in these cases? The second question is what changes did you find all over the detached retina, not only in the area of the periphery. Our experience is that they leak more than normal vessels and this is also in the undetached retina and on the optic disc with edema of the disc in the area of the detachment.

Dr Minoda: The relatively high incidence of macular holes can be explained by the fact that the surgery of macular holes is a difficult surgery. Patients with retinal detachment and macular holes are thus referred more rapidly to our clinic. That might be the reason why we have a rather high incidence of macular holes. In the cases of macular holes you can see the leakage of dye through the macular hole region; however, the interesting thing that I like to point out is that in cases of macular hole we sometimes found similar changes at the peripheral fundus. This may seem peculiar, but if we follow the macular hole region for rather a prolonged period, we sometimes find holes or tears in the peripheral region. This might be the reason why we have this type of changes in the periphery.

PERIPHERAL VASCULAR DISEASES

M. SPITZNAS

(Essen, W. Germany)

Because of the limited speaking time I have to confine my discussion on the vascular diseases of the retinal periphery to a brief description of the two most important disorders of this region, which are Eales' disease and Coats' disease.

The term Eales' disease is often used synonymously with idiopathic periphlebitis. This is wrong. Eales' disease has to be understood as a separate, most probably non-inflammatory entity. In contrast to idiopathic periphlebitis, Eales' disease shows a 3:1 predominance of male patients, a marked tendency toward bilateral disease in males, a different appearance of vascular sheathing, an absence of inflammatory cells in the vitreous and no response to steroid treatment. The etiology of Eales' disease is unknown, but from our long-term observations on close to 400 eyes with Eales' disease the following pathogenetic conclusions can be drawn:

Primarily, Eales' disease seems to be disorder to the walls of the peripheral shunt vessels, which are so characteristic for the circulation of the peripheral retina. The wall structure of these vessels differs from other retinal vessels and their lumen is wider than that of the retinal capillaries. It is conceivable that, in the normal state, the majority of blood cells reach the retinal veins via these shunt vessels, since the retinal capillaries measure only 3.5 to 6 μm and are therefore poorly perfused with particulate blood components. The first and most delicate finding in Eales' disease is a focal occlusion of these shunt vessels. In cases with well dilated pupils the occlusion can be demonstrated by fundus photography which reveals avascular areas in the peripheral retina. Fluorescein angiography shows the corresponding lack of perfusion.

In many cases, the veins coming from such avascular areas show delicate white lines limiting the blood column on both sides over variable distances. This is probably due to a loss of transparency of the vascular wall so that it becomes visible as a pale line along both borders of the blood column. This phenomenon is usually produced by a change in the vessel wall such as hyalinization or intramural deposition of material of any kind. It is conceivable that this is the beginning of a process that finally leads to an occlusion of the vessel. This is confirmed by the observation that increased sheathing leads to narrowing of the blood column and not to widening of the total diameter of the vessel. The occlusion of peripheral vessels causes considerable hemodynamic disturbance, leading to congestion on the arterial side with widening and tortuosity of the feeling vessels which often assume a corkscrew appearance. As the disease progresses, the peripheral avascular areas become more extended. As a compensation for the missing peripheral shunt vessels, there is a dilation of the more posterior capillary channels which often assume the pattern of rungs of a rope-ladder. A further finding are microaneurysms on the patent capillaries in the vicinity of unperfused areas.

At this point the primary process specific for Eales' disease seems to terminate. The changes described result in more or less extended areas suffering from malnutrition or hypoxia. What follows now is the stereotypical proliferative response of the retinal vascular system, similar to that seen in other disorders associated with retinal hypoxia, such as sickle-cell disease, retrolental fibroplasia, branch vein occlusion and diabetic retinopathy. In the early stages, the new-formed vessels spread at the level of the retina. In many cases, however, they also invade the vitreous cavity. The new vessels show a marked impairment of permeability, which leads to massive dye leakage in fluorescein angiography. Fibrous tissue is frequently observed to accompany the vessel proliferations.

The connective tissue strands tend to attach to the retina, creating tears and retinal detachment when they shrink. As in diabetic retinopathy, the newformed vessels tend to rupture, thus giving rise to recurrent, more or less extended vitreous hemorrhages, which are the leading symptom of Eales' disease. The treatment of choice in Eales' disease is photocoagulation which, in our series at Essen, was able to bring the disease to a morphological standstill in 91% of the cases.

In contrast to Eales' disease, which seems to be primarily a disease of the non-cellular components of the vessel wall, Coats' disease seems to be primarily a disorder of endothelial cells and of intramural pericytes. Light and electron microscopic studies revealed a loss of both these cell types together with a progressive thickening of the basement membrane.

The clinical picture of Coats' disease probably depends on the degree of involvement of endothelial and/or mural cells. The loss of endothelial cells causes a breakdown of the blood-tissue barrier. This process leads to a visible leakage of dye in angiography. Such dye leakage remains confined to the circumscribed areas of endothelial damage and is therefore fundamentally different from the profuse extravasations seen in neovascular disorders, where the entire new-formed vessels are penetrated by dye. Clinically the break-down of the blood-tissue barrier is manifested by the appearance of lipoid deposits adjacent to the diseased vessels. In contrast to a decrement of endothelial cells, the loss of mural cells causes a mechanic weakening of the vessel walls. As a second step, the intravascular pressure leads to dilation of the vessels and to formation of aneurysmatic outpouchings. The role of blood pressure is confirmed by the observation that the aneurysmatic changes are located mainly in the arterial portion of the vascular system. It is interesting to note, that dye leakage is more pronounced on small aneurysms than on large aneurysms.

In spite of the fact that the changes described are usually observed together, there are cases where the changes consist almost exclusively of massive vessel dilation and aneurysm formation, while others show nothing but extensive accumulation of exudates. These exceptions are probably due to a selectively higher involvement of either mural cells in the first or endothelial cells in the latter case. The thickening of the endothelial basement membrane finally leads to a collapse and an occlusion of the vessel. Fluorescein angiography shows such regions of vessel occlusion as dark areas. Where these changes are little pronounced, there is a rarefaction of the capillary bed and a coarsening of the normal capillary pattern. In more pronounced cases the avascular areas are bordered by dilated shunt vessels. In the vicinity of such areas of impaired circulation lipoidal exudates, dilated vessels and aneurysms are very pronounced.

Also in Coats' disease the treatment of choice is the destruction of the diseased vessels by photocoagulation. In our series, the progression of the disease could be stopped in 90% of the cases. In 71% the destruction of the diseased vessels was followed by a spontaneous regression of exudates.

Author's address
Universitäts-Augenklinik
Hufelandstrasse 55
4300 Essen
W. Germany

DISCUSSION

XXXX: In 1973 we conducted a study of 31 cases of Coats' disease at the Wills Eye Institute in Philadelphia together with Dr Tasman. I tend to disagree with Dr Spitznas on two points. We found that the large aneurysms the so-called light-bulbs, in Coats' disease did indeed leak profusely. Secondly, we also found microaneurysms and coarsening of the capillaries in areas away from the exudation.

Dr Spitznas: I think we are not in disagreement. Coats' disease is a vascular disorder so you can find vessel changes in areas where you do not find exudates. They are even cases where there are no exudates at all, and still it is a Coats' disease. As to the leakage: on the slide with the many angiograms I wanted to show that the largest aneurysms are the ones that leak least, so they hardly lose any dye. Am I misunderstanding you?

XXXX: I wanted to state that the large aneurysms do leak profusely and we found that the large aneurysms did leak profusely. We definitely established that there were two types of Coats' disease, namely the one were you found aneurysms and coarsening of the capillary bed in areas with exudates and others were you found coarsening of the capillaries and microaneurysms without any exudates at all.

Dr Spitznas: Yes, agree: I showed pictures of that.

XXXX: I just wanted to state about the microaneurysms that did leak profusely, because we found this in many instances.

Dr Spitznas: Well, on the larger aneurysms we have made a different observation.

THE VALUE OF FLUORESCEIN ANGIOGRAPHY IN
SICKLE CELL RETINOPATHY*

MORTON F. GOLDBERG M.D.

(Chicago, Ill, USA)

INTRODUCTION

Sickle cell retinopathy comprises a constellation of abnormal signs in the retinas of patients who inherit hemoglobinopathy genes. Proliferative changes (neovascularization) and visual disability are most characteristic of the doubly heterozygous hemoglobinopathies, sickle cell-hemoglobin C disease (SC) and sickle cell beta-thalassemia (S-thal), although patients with the homozygous form, sickle cell anemia (SS), are also affected (GOLDBERG, in press). Most retinal changes occur in the fundus periphery, although the posterior pole may also show abnormalities. Beginning with erythrocytic occlusion of retinal arterioles, sickle cell retinopathy proceeds naturally through the stages of arteriolar-venular anastomosis, neovascularization (sea fan formation), vitreous hemorrhage, and retinal detachment.

Fluorescein angiography is invaluable in the study of sickle cell retinopathy, particularly with respect to understanding the following: retinal vascular flow dynamics; remodeling of microvascular beds in the retina; macular ischemia; central retinal artery occlusion; and detection and evaluation of retinal neovascularizations (sea fans), both before and after obliterative therapy.

RETINAL VASCULAR FLOW DYNAMICS

As a result of arteriolar closure, blood from obstructed vessels runs off through pre-existing capillaries into adjacent vessels. The involved capillaries enlarge and become prominent as arteriolar-venular anastomoses or shunts (Fig. 1). Fluorescein angiography clearly shows that these channels represent *low* velocity, rather than high velocity, shunts (GOLDBERG, in press) (Fig. 2). The transit time within the normal retinal vascular tree is usually less than 3 seconds, but increases, sometimes to over 40 seconds, in the partially occluded peripheral retinal vasculature of the sickle cell patient. This duration exceeds that required for the deoxygenation of a normal erythrocyte and its conversion to a sickle-shaped cell. Sickle cells, being considerably more rigid than normal pliable erythrocytes, act as micro-

* Supported in part by contract 72-2956B and grant IP18HL 15168 from the National Heart and Lung Institute, National Institutes of Health, Bethesda, Md., U.S.A., and by an unrestricted grant from Research to Prevent Blindness, Inc., New York, N.Y., U.S.A.

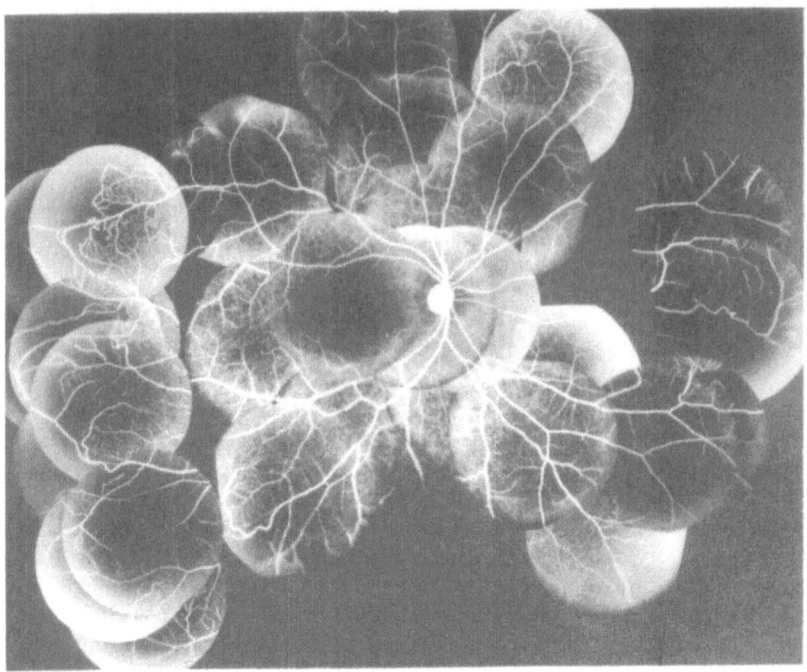

Fig. 1. Angiographic montage of young man with SS hemoglobin. Note loss of macular and perimacular vessels. In temporal periphery (at the equator and posterior to the equator) are a series of long arteriolar-venular anastomoses (stage II of proliferative sickle retinopathy). The fundus peripheral to these A-V loops is totally avascular.

emboli and propagate the vaso-occlusive process, thereby contributing to the vicious cycle, namely, arteriolar closure →slow flow →hypoxia →conversion of erythrocytes to sickled forms →further arteriolar and capillary closure, and so on.

REMODELING OF THE VASCULATURE

Fluorescein angiography every three to four months has demonstrated that peripheral retinal arterioles (and their dependent capillaries and venules) close, open, reclose, and reopen repetitively (GALINOS et al., 1975). Since closures tend to outweigh openings, the net effect is a gradual, intermittent centripetal movement of the peripheral vascular arcades away from the ora serrata toward the posterior pole. This process takes several years to evolve completely, but rarely is it severe enough to spread contiguously into the macula. On the other hand, angiography reveals that the macular vessels themselves may be primarily involved in the occlusive process (STEVENS et al., 1974). It is theoretically and clinically important to realize that macular function may persist despite loss of one or more perifoveal arterioles and despite occlusion of one or more of the innermost capillary arcades surrounding the foveal avascular zone. Progressive occlusion of several peri-

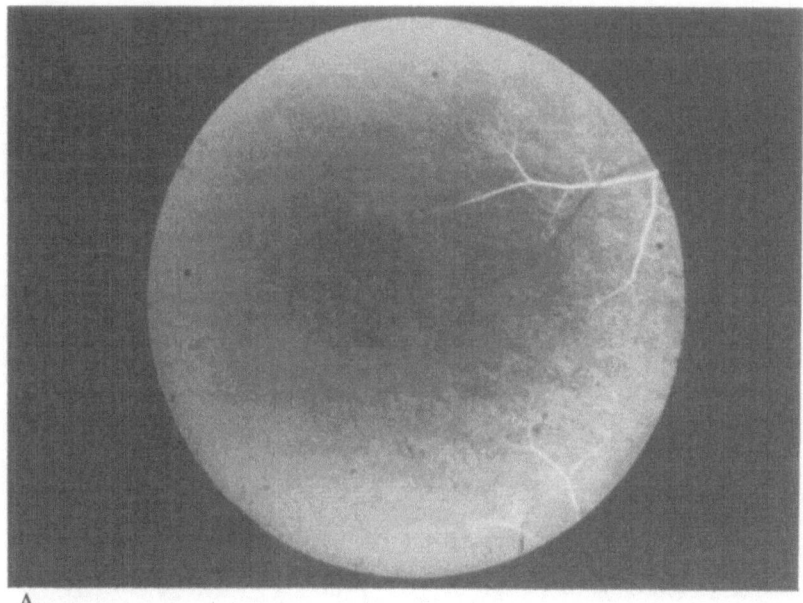

A.

B.

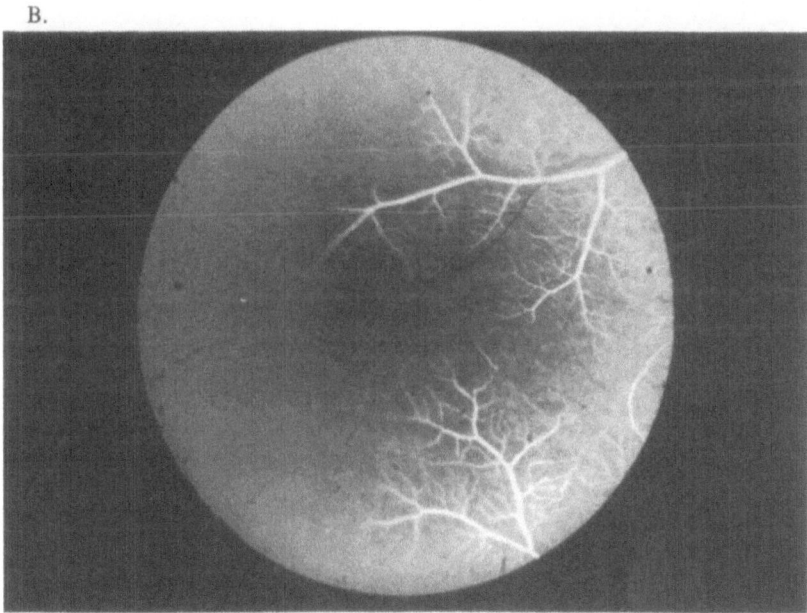

Fig. 2 (A-F). The 10-o'clock position of the angiographic montage shown in Fig. 1. Note extremely slow transit time (over 20 seconds). This is sufficiently prolonged to allow deoxygenation and intraocular sickling within a single transit. The A-V anastomosis represents a *low* velocity shunt.

589

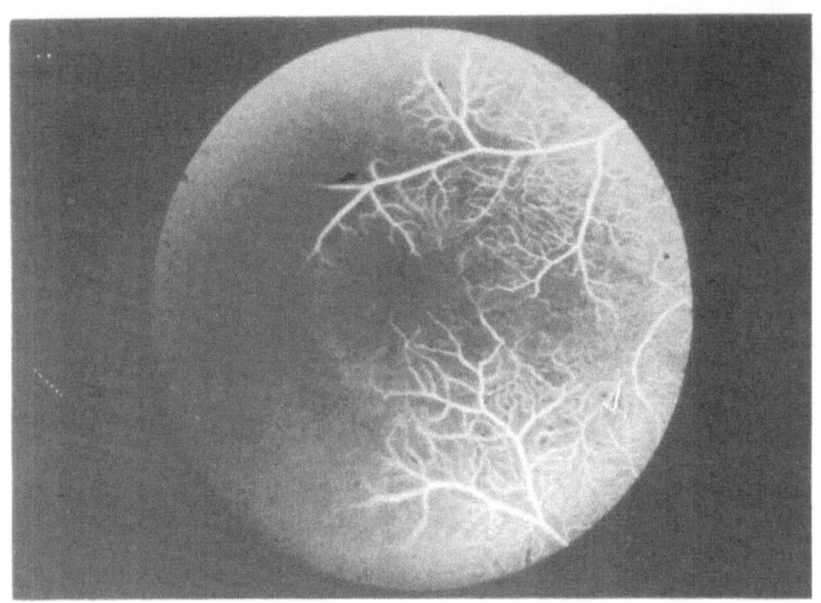

2C

2E

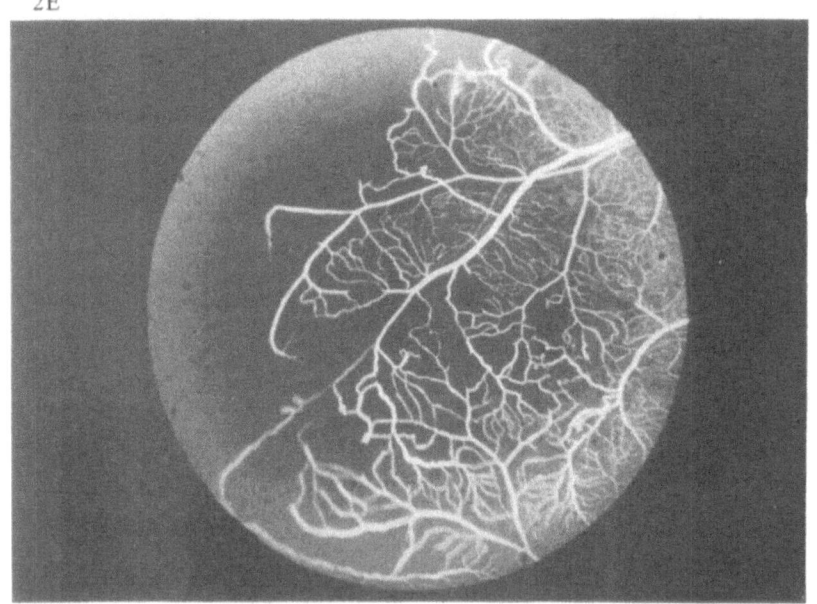

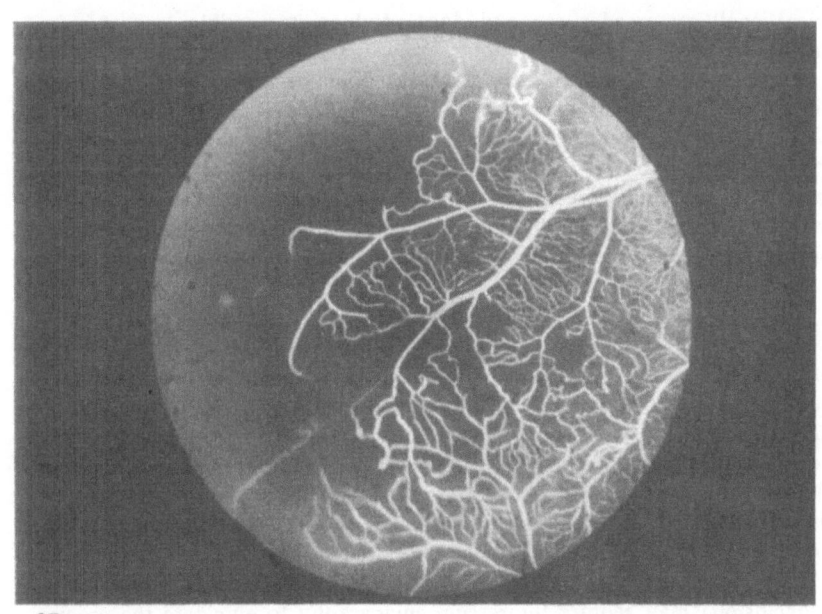

2D

2F

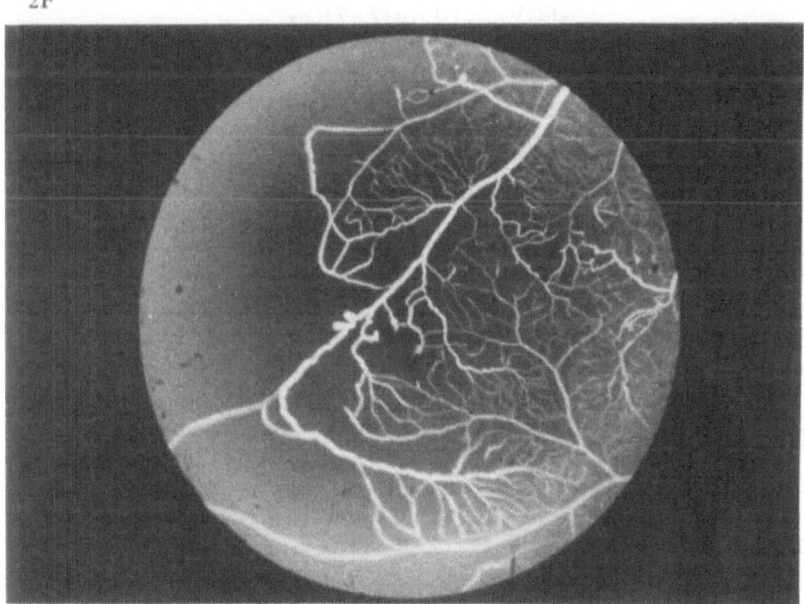

foveal capillary arcades can and does produce irreversible loss of some macular function.

Because visual symptoms are not caused by peripheral occlusions and remodeling, and because visual symptoms are not necessarily induced even by macular vessel occlusions, fluorescein angiography is essential for detection of these abnormal and potentially deleterious vascular insults. Occlusions are a necessary precondition for development of neovascularization (with its consequences of vitreous hemorrhage and retinal detachment) and for loss of central vision (if macular ischemia is profound enough).

CENTRAL RETINAL ARTERY OCCLUSION

The presence and importance of vascular occlusions on the *arterial* side of the vascular tree in sickle cell retinopathy is nowhere better shown than in central retinal artery occlusion. Because this blinding event occurs in children and other young persons with sickle cell disease, in whom vascular sclerosis and induced thrombosis are virtually nonexistent, the role of embolic sickled erythrocytes in the pathogenesis of arteriolar vascular occlusion is emphasized. Clinically unexplained partial or total loss of vision in children (presumably due to macular vessel occlusion or central retinal artery occlusion) may require fluorescein angiography to elucidate the precise course of events. The same may be true in patients who have poorly understood strabismus or amblyopia.

NEOVASCULARIZATION

Neovascular patches in the equatorial fundus arise after the foregoing stages of vascular occlusions and anastomoses. Until the neovascular stage in the evolution of sickle cell retinopathy has been reached, there is little likelihood that the peripheral retinopathy can, by itself, interfere with vision. Neovascular patches (sea fans), however, continually transude copious amounts of plasma into the vitreous. This violation of the vitreous can cause syneresis, and the induced traction can add to that caused by the fibrous and glial tissue that accumulates at the neovascular patch. Vitreous hemorrhage, retinal tears, and retinal detachment are the logical sequelae. Accordingly, successful prophylaxis against vitreous hemorrhage and retinal detachment requires detection of sea fans, preferably before visual symptoms arise. Early sea fans can be difficult to detect, because their tiny naked neovascular channels are close to the surface of the retina and blend into the red fundus background. Occasionally, they are obscured by small glial or fibrous plaques. Angiography is diagnostic of their presence, due to the telltale, enlarging cloud of intravitreal fluorescein that is readily detected by ophthalmoscopy (with an appropriate blue filter in the ophthalmoscope) or by photography. Once detected, sea fans are easily obliterated by photocoagulation (GOLDBERG, 1971; GOLDBERG & ACACIO, 1973; GOLDBAUM et al., in press). In some patients, vitreous blood is dense enough to obscure the location of the responsible sea fans. Under these circumstances, the fluorescent cloud (though not the actual vessels) is often still detectable with an indirect ophthalmoscope, allowing trans-scleral cryocoagulation of

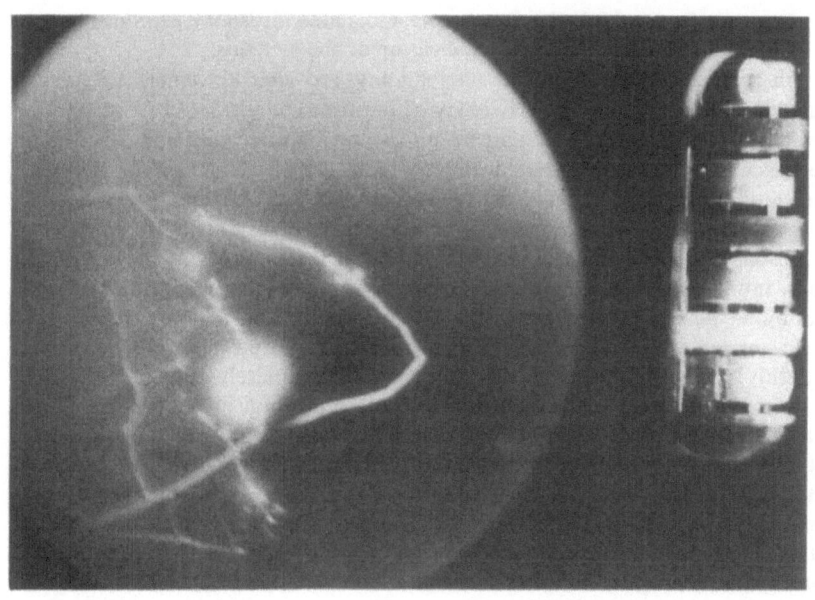

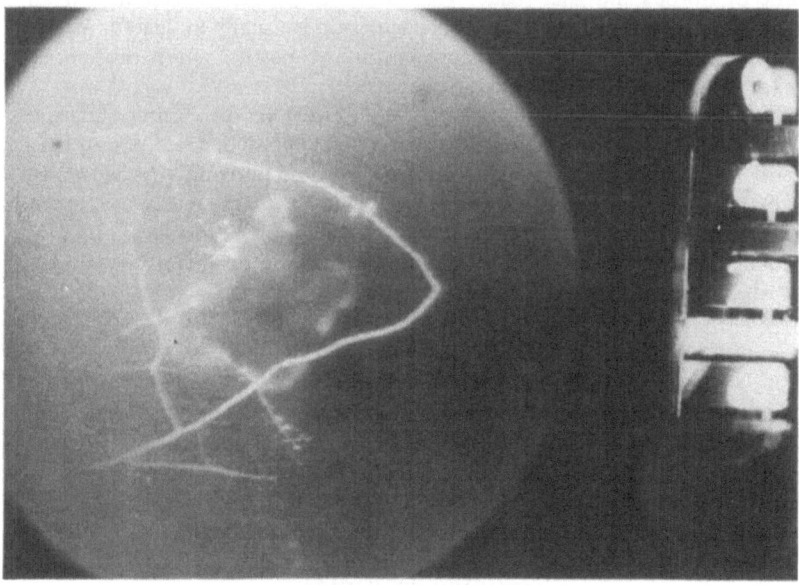

Fig. 3 (A-B). Photocoagulation of perfused sea fans results in permanent infarction of neovascular tissue, as shown angiographically by subsequent nonperfusion.

the location from which the fluorescein emanates. This may prevent repetitive hemorrhages and allow gradual clearing of the vitreous.

Fluorescein angioscopy and angiography are also extremely useful in determining the extent and efficiency of photocoagulation. In our currently preferred technique of xenon arc or argon laser photocoagulation, small flat neovascular beds are coagulated directly (focally), and larger or elevated sea fans are infarcted by closing their feeding arterioles. Following placement of coagulations to as many sea fans or feeding arterioles as possible, fluorescein angioscopy is performed (Fig. 3). If dye still leaks from any neovascular beds, immediate retreatment is carried out. One day later, fluorescein angiography is performed for purposes of documentation, and retreatment is again carried out if necessary. The process is repeated at intervals (daily, monthly, quarterly, etc.) until the retina is completely free of perfused neovascular areas. The persistence of visible red blood in photocoagulated sea fans does not necessarily represent active perfusion; permanently isolated, trapped columns of erythrocytes can retain their red color for up to one year despite total infarction of the sea fan. Thus, only angiography or angioscopy can indicate whether or not retreatment of red neovascular channels is necessary. Ultimately, infarcted sea fans lose their red color, shrink, and turn white.

Sea fans may appear white, fibrous, and nonperfused even without coagulation treatment. In some cases, autoinfarction (spontaneous remission) has occurred (NAGPAL et al., 1975). In others, an actively perfused neovascular bed is camouflaged by fibroglial reaction to previous local transudation and hemorrhage. Some of these more nature fans may have less propensity for further spontaneous hemorrhage than those without a supporting mantle of fibrous and glial tissue. This cannot be predicted accurately in an individual case, and as a result, photocoagulation is usually indicated. Angiography confirms which of these fans continue to perfuse and is thus necessary for the clinical decision-making process.

Unusual, and sometimes dangerous, complications of photocoagulation can only be deciphered with an angiographic approach. Choroido-retinal-vitreous neovascularizations have occurred in some patients after excessive photocoagulation (GALINOS et al., 1975). Only the availability of sequential, rapid-phase angiography has allowed the detection of the uveal origin of blood in these choroido-retinal vitreous anastomotic proliferations (GALINOS et al., 1975).

SUMMARY

In sickle cell retinopathy, fluorescein angioscopy and angiography are invaluable diagnostically and therapeutically. Peripheral and macular vascular occlusions are often undetectable without the intravascular contrast agent. Decisions for initial and repetitive prophylactic and therapeutic coagulations of neovascularizations require the performance of these techniques.

ACKNOWLEDGMENT

Angiographic montage prepared by Michael Woolf, M.D., and Bruce Busse.

REFERENCES

GALINOS, S.O., ASDOURIAN, G.K., WOOLF, M.B., GOLDBERG, M.F. & BUS-SE, B.J. Choroido-vitreal neovascularization after argon laser photocoagulation. *Arch. Ophthalmol.* 93: *524-530* (1975).

GALINOS, S.O., ASDOURIAN, G.K., WOOLF, M.B., STEVENS, T.S., LEE, C.B., GOLDBERG, M.F., CHOW, J.C.F. & BUSSE, B.J. Spontaneous remodeling of the peripheral retinal vasculature in sickling disorders. *Am. J. Ophthalmol.* 79: *853-870* (1975).

GOLDBERG, M.F. Treatment of proliferative sickle retinopathy. *Trans. Am. Acad. Ophthalmol. Otolaryngol.* 75: *532-556* (1971).

GOLDBERG, M.F. Retinal vaso-occlusion in sickling hemoglobinopathies. In: Bergsma, D., Cotlier, E. & Bron, A. (eds.): The eye and metabolic disease: birth defects original article series. National Foundation/March of Dimes, in press.

GOLDBERG, M.F. & ACACIO, I. Argon laser photocoagulation of proliferative sickle retinopathy. *Arch. Ophthalmol.* 90: *35-44* (1973).

GOLDBAUM, M.H., GOLDBERG, M.F., NAGPAL, K., ASDOURIAN, G.K. & GALINO, S.O. Quantitative photocoagulation and the treatment of proliferative sickle retinopathy. In: L'Esperiance, F. (ed.): Current diagnosis and management of chorioretinal disease. St. Louis, C.V. Mosby Co., in press.

NAGPAL, K., PATRIANAKOS, D., ASDOURIAN, G.K., GOLDBERG, M.F., RABB, M. & JAMPOL, L.M. Spontaneous regression (autoinfarction) of proliferative retinopathy. *Am. J. Ophthalmol.* 80: *885-892* (1975).

STEVENS, T.S., BUSSE, B.J., LEE, C.B., WOOLF, M.B., GALINOS, S. & GOLD-BERG, M.F. Sickling hemoglobinopathies: Macular and perimacular vascular abnormalities. *Arch. Ophthalmol.* 92: *455-463* (1974).

Author's address:
University of Illinois
Eye and Ear Infirmary
1855 West Taylor Street
Chicago, Ill. 60612
USA

DISCUSSION

Dr Baurmann: It is a question for both Dr Spitznas and Dr Goldberg. In both cases in many of your pictures we could not see any background fluorescence. What about the perfusion of the choroid in these regions? Did you do any investigation with the method of Amalric and Bonnin, with red light?

Dr Spitznas: No.

Dr Goldberg: There is at least one major reason that background fluorescence is not obvious in many of our patients, since virtually 100% are negro patients with extremely dense retinal pigment epithelium. We have studied many of these patients with indocyanin green and have tried to visualize choroidal vascularization. Neo-vascularization in the choroid is very uncommon. There are one or two cases in the literature (one from Condon & Serjeant in Jamaica in the West Indies, where major infarct of the choroid occurred in a young patient with a variant of sickle cell disease). As you might expect, there was widespread pigmentmottling corresponding to the damage of the retinal pigment epithelium. This is a very unusual event in sickle cell retinopathy.

Dr Deutman: This is a question regarding treatment to both Dr Spitznas and Dr Goldberg. I saw a slide of Dr Goldberg where he just treated the vascular malformation. I know that some people have advocated that you should treat the peripheral avascular area. I should like your comments on this.

Dr Goldberg: I suspect that one can accomplish the job by many techniques. One can directly obliterate neovascular tissue in a very effective way, particularly when the neovascular tissue is flat against the retina and there the complication rate is acceptable. In our experience, however, when the neovascular tissue is pulled into the middle of the vitreous chamber, by detached vitreous, direct obliteration of the neovascular bed is dangerous and is frequently complicated by immediate vitreous hemorrhages or vitreous hemorrhages within 24 hours. For those situations we prefer to infarct the neovascular bed by closing its anteriolar supply and we will repeat fluorescein angioscopy, without the film, on a daily basis until we obliterate the feeding arteriole. I would guess, although we have not yet done it, that one could get an indirect involutional effect on the neovascular tissue by treating the peripheral ischaemic zone. It may well be that this will have the lowest rate of complication of all, but it may take a rather prolonged time for the neovascular tissue to involute, and we feel, largely on subjective grounds, that one should eliminate perfusion of the neovascular bed as quickly and as permanently as possible.

Dr Spitznas: I have nothing to add to this, this question was also directed to me. I would like to add something. Dr Goldberg, as far as I understand you, sickle cell retinopathy comes to a stand-still in many of the cases after peripheral photocoagulation. Do you have any explanation for that effect? The same thing holds true for Eales' disease, I would have an explanation for Eales, but is there any explanation that you could offer for sickle cell?

Dr Goldberg: I do not have an adequate explanation. It is true that, if one obliterates these neovascular beds by infarcting them, or by direct photocoagulation if the patches are flat against the inner surface of the retina, recurrent growth of neovascular tissue does not occur in that specific meridian. But that does not prevent onset of neo-vascular growth at the clockwise or the counterclockwise site around the previously treated area. That particular meridian having undergone treatment, is safe for all practical purposes for years, and we are following such patients for over 10 years.

Dr Henkind: I would like to ask Dr Goldberg a question. It has been my feeling that in areas where you develop collaterals, and if one sticks to the definition of collaterals, neovascularization generally does not occur. I have yet personally to see neovascularization occurring from a collateral vessel, even in diabetes or any other process. From what I heard, you are suggesting that there were instances were neovascularization did develop from collaterals. It seems to me that the mechanisms are so different for producing the two different kind of lesions that when you do develop collaterals it must be exceptionally rare for neovascularization to develop in that identical geographic area. I would like your comments on that.

Dr Goldberg: I agree that neovascularization from true collaterals is unusual, if you mean by collaterals an arteriolar-arteriole connection or a venule-venular connection. On the other hand, neovascularization appears to be extremely common when direct arteriolarvenular connections occur, and this is what we observe in patients with sickle cell disease. There may, in fact be true collaterals, either at the arterial side of the vascular tree or at the venular side of the tree, but they are very uncommon, and in those uncommon circumstances I have not seen neovascularization either.

Dr Henkind: Did you say: you do see from A-V collaterals, if that is so, it must be peculiar because the diabetic situation were A-V shunting is common there has never been a single example of neovascularization that I know of.

Dr Goldberg: We may be defining collaterals differently. I was referring to collaterals as connecting vessels that remain either on the arteriolar side of the vascular tree or exclusively on the venous side of the tree. And while such connections can occur in sickling I have not seen neovascularization under these circumstances. On the other hand direct A-V connections, which for purposes of terminology, we prefer to call A-V anastomoses or A-V connection and we avoid the term collateral; under such circumstances neovascularization as you could see in at least 4 circumstances in the same area of the retina followed sequentially every 3 months, neovascularization was extremely common. In our own series of selected patients, up to 60% with sickle cell hemoglobin C disease have neovascularization. In Patrick Condon's unselected series from Jamaica 40% or thereabouts have neovascularization. So this is a common problem following the onset of A-V communication.

Dr Henkind: There is a paper in the literature which describes the difference between collaterals, shunts and neovascularization. As a matter of fact that is the title of the paper. The strict definition of these entities really, I would suggest the people in the audience who have not read it, to read it, because it really defines clinically as well as experimentally this type of lesion. One of the authors was Dr Wise, I think, I was the other one. My personal feeling about these things, I think I heard Ed. Norton say a few days ago, and I think he is absolutely correct, that there are only a few potential responses of, for example, the pigment epithelium and there are only a few potential responses of retinal vascular disease. We will make progress when we will get accurate definitions. I fully agree with you, Morton, but I am not sure what we agree on until we get the definition down.

Dr Ryan: I was very interested, Dr Goldberg, to hear your report on sickle and sarcoid cases that developed neovascularization in the vitreous coming from the choroid. Davis has observed this in diabetes, and I wonder if you would care to comment or to speculate on the pathogenesis; i.e., the role of ischemia and the role of the vitreous, in addition to the rupture of Bruch's membrane? How do you explain this relatively uncommon complication of photocoagulation?

Dr Goldberg: This is an extremely serious complication of photocoagulation, but it might be not that uncommon. We have been able to collect 6 such patients now, all having had excessive, intense photocoagulation in the peripheral fundus. They represent a von Hippel haemangioma, sickle cell disease, and sarcoidosis. But other individuals have observed the same thing in Eales' disease and in diabetic retinopathy. In our own cases we can go back to the immediate posttreatment color photographs in every single case and it is quite clear that our overtreatment was due to using a laserbeam with too small a beam diameter and too high a power setting. In every single case there was a rupture of Bruch's membrane with pigment churning and a small amount of blood coming from the choroid through Bruch's membrane into the retina and in some cases into the vitreous. Clearly this was excessive treatment and in every case the common denominator, which was subsequently followed by choroidal-vitreous neovascularization was rupture of Bruch's membrane. In the experimental lab my colleagues Drs Michael Goldbaum, Daniel Wolpe, and I have tried to reproduce this in primate eyes by using both argon and xenon energy sources and were unable to break Bruch's membrane unless the power had been raised extremely high which with the laser generally means a small beam diameter and high watt setting. In the Xenon cases it generally means a very prolonged burn and a high power setting. Our own experience is limited, but we have not yet seen this complication in a human after Xenon treatment, although such cases have been reported in the literature.

Dr Ryan: In the therapy of subretinal neovascularization in certain macular cases, there can be recurrence of the subretinal neovascularization and hemorrhage. Bruch's membrane and the pigment epithelium can be ruptured, yet you do not get intravitreal neovascularization. What is the role of the retina, what is the role of ischemia, and possibly the role of vitreous in those disorders that aid to the development of intravitreal neovascularization? It is interesting to me that the cases in which neovascularization develops from the choroid to the vitreous were cases of proliferative retinopathy, rather than cases of subretinal neovascularization.

Are you aware of any such cases that do not have other potential factors for proliferative retinopathy that can develop neovascularization extending from the choroid to the vitreous?

Dr Goldberg: In this situation, in the macula there are frequently breaks in Bruch's membrane and drusen, many of which contain capillaries. I think this situation is related to the progressive growth of granulation tissue, representing a healing or reparative response to the tissue injury created by the photocoagulator. Such a situation is potentially very dangerous, and for that reason I prefer not to treat such patients.

FLUORESCEIN ANGIOGRAPHY IN RETROLENTAL FIBROPLASIA

ARNALL PATZ, M.D., DANIEL FINKELSTEIN, M.D. & JOHN PAYNE, M.D.

(Baltimore, Md, USA)

FLYNN and co-workers (1971, 1975) at the Bascom Palmer Institute in Miami, were the first investigators to utilize fluorescein angiography in the diagnosis of acute proliferative retrolental fibroplasia. Their studies have contributed significantly to the understanding of the active stages of RLF. Our findings confirm those of FLYNN and co-workers, and attest to the usefulness of this technique in not only the diagnosis, but the clinical management of the cases. Utilizing the technique in older patients with arrested RLF, some of whom may have shown only high myopia as a residual, we have noted that the retinal vessels, in some cases, never regained complete competence and show considerable fluorescein leakage from the peripheral vasculature (PAYNE & PATZ, in press; PATZ, 1975).

FLYNN and co-workers described a mesenchymal shunt at the area of vascularized and avascularized retina. Just posterior to the shunt vessels the

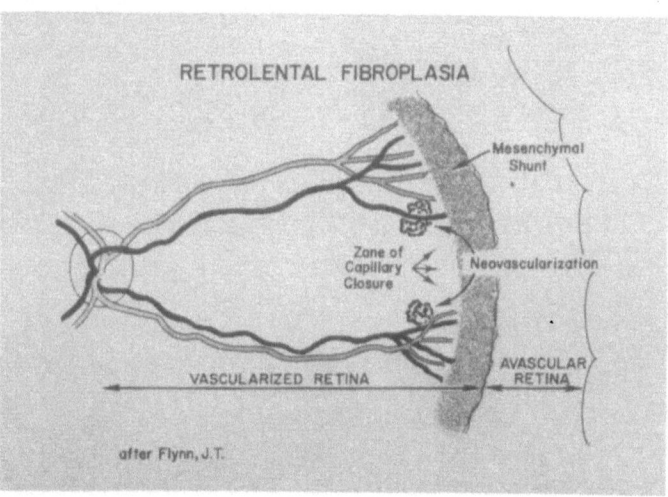

Fig. 1. Schematic diagram of pattern of active proliferative retrolental fibroplasia, modified from FLYNN and co-workers. Note the temporal straightening of the major retinal vessels instead of the normal arching over the macula. At the junction of the vascularized and avascular retina, shunting between the arterioles and venules occurs. Just posterior to the 'mesenchymal' shunt, areas of neovascularization develop.

surface or intravitreal proliferation of vessels is noted. These investigators have found that when the retinal vascularization proceeded past the junction area of new vessel formation, that spontaneous regression was starting. We have confirmed this observation in our own cases.

Some practical aspects of fluorescein angiography for the small premature infant:

1. The dose of fluorescein should be on an approximate per kilo basis and the average premature infant of 5 lbs. weight is given a dose of 0.3 cc. of 10% solution. If the fluorescein is injected through an intravenous infusion set, care should be taken that the dye be injected as near to the entrance needle site as feasible. Furthermore, a small flush of saline (1/4 to 1/2 cc) should follow to push the bolus of dye through the I.V. tubing and into the circulation. When giving the injection through the I.V. tubing, the photographer should be alerted that the appearance time in the retinal circulation may be delayed several seconds past that normally anticipated.

2. The chin-rest attachment must be removed from the standard fundus camera.

3. The patient who will be recumbent should either be sedated or under anesthesia.

To appreciate the fluorescein angiography findings in acute proliferative retrolental fibroplasia it is appropriate to review briefly the basic patho-

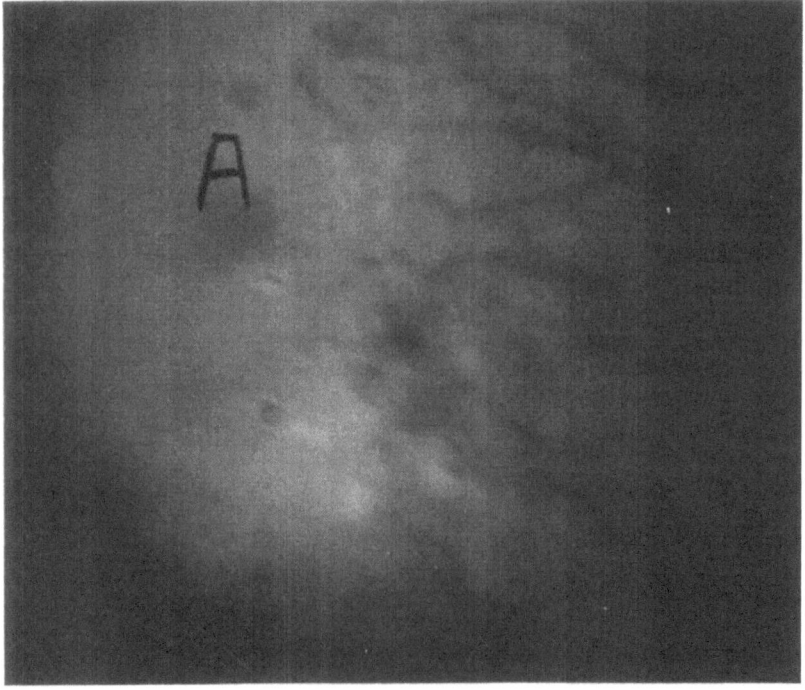

Fig. 2A. Red-free photograph of temporal periphery at junction of vascularized and avascular retina.

600

genesis and mechanism of oxygen action on the immature retina (ASHTON et al., 1954; PATZ, 1957).

The effects of oxygen on the infant or experimental animal, with an incompletely vascularized retina, can be conveniently divided into the *initial* response to oxygen and a *secondary* one after removal to room air. In the initial or primary response there is a severe vasoconstriction. During the exposure to oxygen, direct injury to the vessel endothelium occurs and ultimate obliteration of the more immature vessel complexes results. After removal to air, new vessel formation occurs at the area of retinal capillary damage and obliteration. These new vessels erupt through the surface of the retina to grow into the vitreous in the classical manner of proliferative retinopathy very similar to that seen in diabetes and sickle cell disease. The changes after the intravitreal proliferation of new vessels are relatively non-specific. These vessels almost invariably leak proteinaceous material and in more advanced cases hemorrhages occur from these intra-vitreal new vessel formations. Traction produced by vitreo-retinal adhesions detaches the retina. Active RLF may regress at any stage of the proliferative disease. Vitreo-retinal traction in the temporal periphery frequently produces a dragging of the retinal vessels across the disc and a displacement temporally (heterotopia) of the macula may occur.

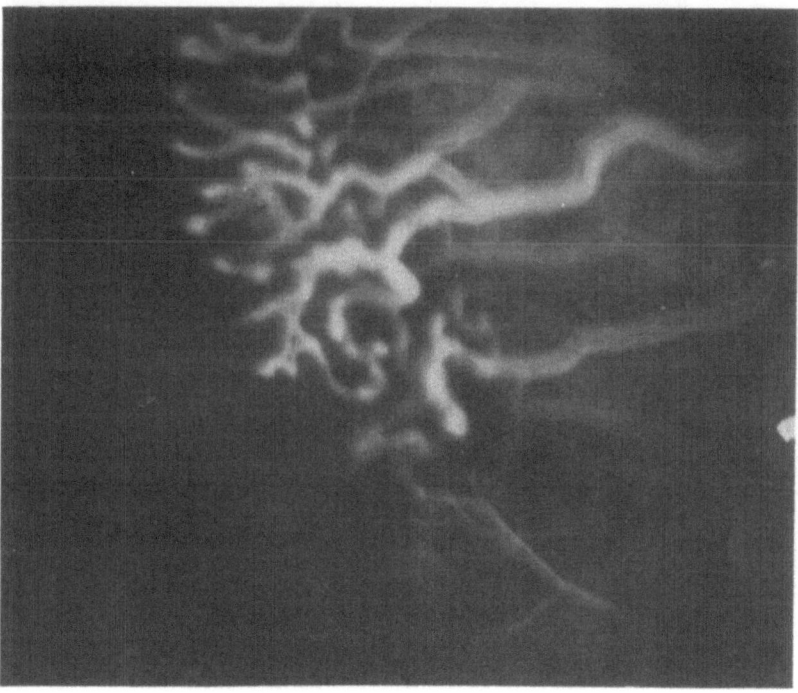

Fig. 2B. Early fluorescein transit of area in Figure 2A, showing telangiectatic vessels classical of arrested retrolental fibroplasia.

CASE HISTORY

The patient is a nine and a half year old white female, who gives a history of having been born one month prematurely with a birthweight of 4 lbs., 6 oz. The patient received no supplemental oxygen after birth. She was noted to have a deviating left eye at three months of age.

Examination showed visual acuity corrected in the right eye to 20/200 and the left eye hand motion. Refraction showed a high degree (11 diopters) of myopia in the right eye. The patient experienced a recent hemorrhage in the left eye. The hemorrhage obscured all details of the left fundus. Intraocular pressure measured 11 mm in each eye. Ophthalmoscopic on the right eye showed a myopic conus. The retinal vessels emerged from the optic disc in a normal arcuate pattern over the macula area. There was no dragging of the vessels across the disc and no heterotopia of the macula. In the temporal periphery there were areas where the retinal vasculature stopped just posterior to the equator. Fluorescein angiography showed at the junction of retinal vascular-avascular zone, the classical telangiectatic appearance of the vessels as demonstrated on fluorescein angiography.

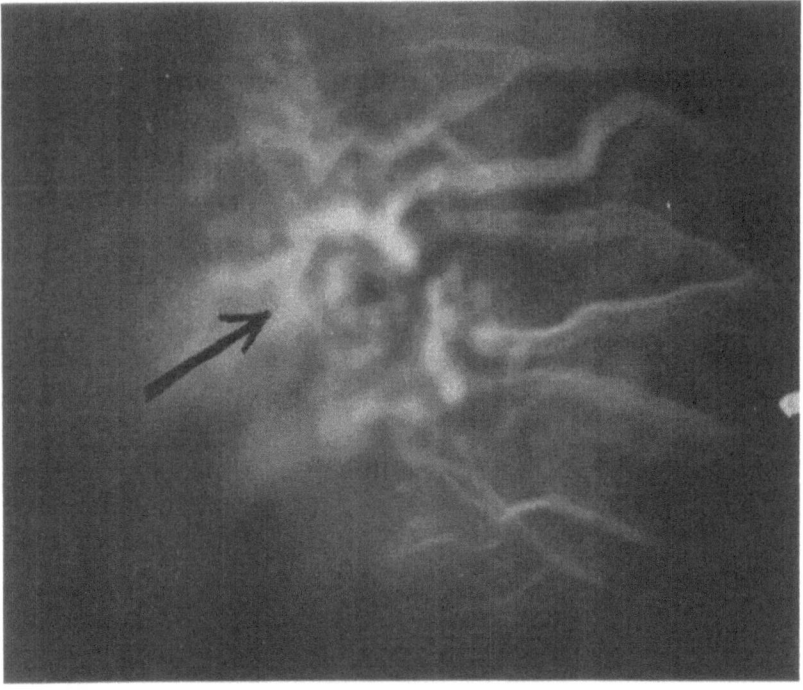

Fig. 2C. Fifteen seconds later in dye transit. Note early leakage of dye around telangiectatic vessels (arrow).

REFERENCES

ASHTON, N., WARD, B. & SERPELL, G. Effect of oxygen on developing retinal vessels with particular reference to the problem of retrolental fibroplasia. *Brit. J. Ophthal.* 38: *397* (1954).

CANTOLINO, S.J., O'GRADY, G.E., HERRERA, J.A. & FLYNN, J.T. Ophthalmoscopic monitoring of oxygen therapy in premature infants: fluorescein angiography in acute retrolental fibroplasia. *Am. J. Ophthal.* 72: *322* (1971).

FLYNN, J.T. Acute proliferative retrolental fibroplasia: Evolution of the lesion. *Graefe's Arch. Klin. exp. Ophthal.* 195: *101* (1975).

PATZ, A. The role of oxygen in retrolental fibroplasia. E. Mead Johnson Award Address. *Pediatrics* 19: *504* (1957).

PATZ, A. The role of oxygen in retrolental fibroplasia. *Graefe's Arch. Klin. exp. Ophthal.* 195: *77* (1975).

PAYNE, J. & PATZ, A. Fluorescein angiography in retrolental fibroplasia. Int. Ophth. Clinic, Little, Brown & Co, Boston (in press).

Authors' address:
Wilmer Ophthalmological Institute
Johns Hopkins Hospital and University
601 North Broadway
Baltimore, Maryland 21205
USA

DISCUSSION

Dr Fonda: I want to put three questions to Dr Patz. We know, as also Dr Hill in the first day of this symposium has pointed out, that the velocity distribution in a vessel follows a parabolic curve so in the vessels you can find zero velocity and maximum velocity, and you can compute a mean velocity. Did you compute the mean velocity or the maximum one? This I think may be important because vasoconstriction is involved. The second question is: was the velocity measured in arteries or in veins? The third: how long was the tract of the vessel for velocity measurements? This is very important because, for a precise measurement of the velocity, there must be no collateral branch between the two measurement points on the vessel.

Dr Patz: In reference to whether it was a mean or maximum velocity, this I do not recall specifically. Dr Collin Dollery who had been utilizing this technique, was visiting us and Bob Flower worked out a calculation which, to the best of my recollection, was a measure of the maximum velocity. The measurement was made in the retinal arterioles and was made over a distance of approximately 4 disc diameters, which was the widest field that we can get, using the lowest magnification of our photographic system. Utilizing the reference point of one disc diameter in the young kitten as one mm the time lapse in term of the wavefront passing that distance was used to calculate the velocity.

Dr Fonda: Did the vessel tract have some branches?

Dr Patz: Yes, this was recognized but the comparison was made in terms of controlled and treated and whatever the influence of the branching was, it was assumed to have reasonable effect in both. I am sure that this would have an action on true velocity. We were not specifically interested whether there was a 20-fold or a 40-fold change. This was just a way for us to compare the effect of arterial P 02. We were interested to find the critical level in the kitten at which changes of any type could be measured indicating, a response of the vessels to oxygen. Our data were qualitative as far as looking at the eye itself; our quantitative measurements were primarily the arterial P 02 level to try to get some estimate in terms of the comparison to the critical situation in the nursery, to see if we might get some guideline as far as safe oxygen levels.

ALTERATION OF RETINAL HEMODYNAMICS IN RETROLENTAL FIBROPLASIA*

W. LEMMINGSON

(Karlsruhe, W. Germany)

INTRODUCTION

When newborn animals with an immature retina are exposed to highly concentrated oxygen for a period of at least 24 hours a well-marked vasoobliteration appears in the retinal periphery. In previous experiments (LEMMINGSON, 1972, 1974) we were able to demonstrate that prior to the onset of the oxygen induced vasoobliteration some important alterations of retinal hemodynamics take place. The purpose of this paper is to give a brief summary of those hemodynamic alterations in the retina in order to get a hypothesis for better understanding of the pathomechanism of the vasoobliteration in experimental retrolental fibroplasia.

MATERIALS AND METHODS

Vitalmicroscopical observations have been performed in kittens aged 2 to 8 days during the artificial oxygenation in a concentration of 40 to 50 per cent. The vitalmicroscopic technique for the observation of the microcirculation with magnifications up to 130 times have been described in details elsewhere by LEMMINGSON (1972). In order to make both components of the intravasal flow, the marginal plasma layer and the axial red cells column visible, the vitalmicroscopic technique was combined with a low dosed fluoresceine-angiography.

RESULTS

The initial alteration of retinal hemodynamics becomes visible about 10 minutes after the oxygenation was started. Using low magnifications it looks prima vista like a generalized vasoconstriction being accompanied by a disappearance of terminal vascular bed in peripheral areas. If this initial effect is a true vasoconstriction as interpreted by ASHTON et al. (1954) some additional criteria of vasoconstriction must be present like a proportional narrowing of both the intravasal axial red cells column and the marginal plasma layer as well as an incomplete perfusion of terminal vascular bed. In spite of this we have to remember that under normal conditions, which means before the artificial oxygenation has started, there is a relation

---

* Supported by Deutsche Forschungsgemeinschaft

of about 1 to 4 between the width of the marginal plasma layer and the axial red cells column in a medium sized artery as seen in Fig. 1a and b. It is a wellknown fact that in retinal vessels by means of incident light microscopy the marginal plasma layer cannot be optically separated from the axial red cells column. Only in exceptional cases the retinal vessels wall is visible and allows to determine both components that means the width of the marginal plasma layer and the diameter of the axial red cells column (Fig. 2). Using sodium-fluoresceine in low concentrations to dye the marginal plasma layer so that the axial red cells column remains visible, we are able to measure and calculate the value of both components in each phase of our experiments. As seen in Fig. 3 there is during the artificial oxygenation a significant decrease of the axial red cells column diameter and a simultaneous increase of the width of marginal plasma layer. Making calculations on this basis we see that the cross section of the axial red cells column in an arterial branch is diminished about 4 times compared with the value before the oxygenation (Fig. 4). It has been pointed out in the same experiment

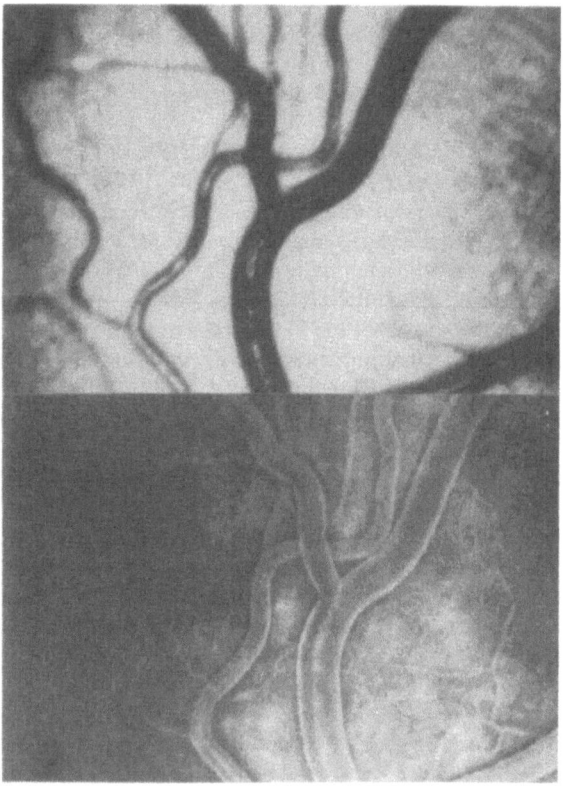

Fig. 1 a and b. The width of the marginal plasma layer in retinal vessels demonstrated by fluoresceine-angiography. a. The visible diameter of the vessels before and b. during the routine fluoresceine-angiography.

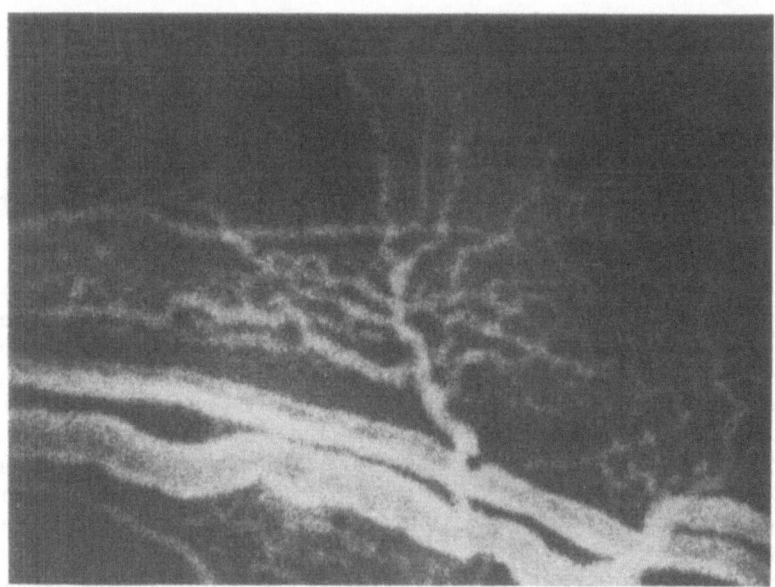

Fig. 2. Demonstration of the marginal plasma layer and of the axial red cells column in a medium sized artery by means of low dosed fluoresceine-angiography.

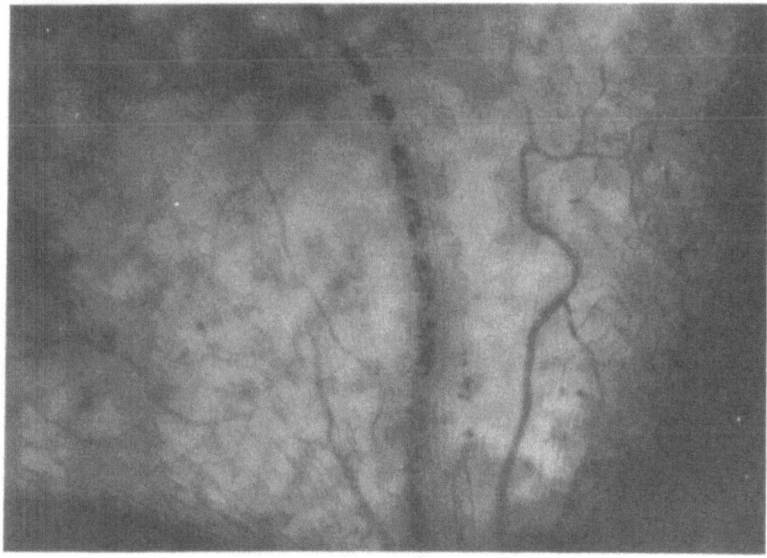

Fig. 3. An exceptional observation of vessels wall and the marginal plasma layer by means of incident light vitalmicroscopy. Magnifications 65 times.

that during the artificial oxygenation there is a significant decrease of the axial red cells column accompanied simultaneously by an increase of the marginal plasma zone so that the vessels calibre still remains unchanged.

During this phase of the alteration we observed that the narrowed red cells column is no longer situated exactly in the axis of the vessels lumen, but fulfils oscillating movements just like having lost the conduct by the vessels wall. This will be demonstrated in the short film following this paper. paper.

All these findings indicate that the phenomenon described here is a plasma skimming and not a vasoconstriction. If this conclusion is correct, we must be able to find some other criteria of plasma skimming specially in the perfusion of capillary bed during the oxygenation. In Fig. 5a the diminished red cells flow in the main arterial branches is accompanied by a disappearance of the visible capillary network. We have now to find out whether this finding represents a circumscript vasoobliteration or only a hemodynamic alteration of the same area. As demonstrated in Fig. 5b the lack of visible capillary network is not always identical with real obliteration. When sodium-fluoresceine is injected some of the formerly disappeared capillary areas become visible again because of their perfusion by plasma only. In connection with the oxygen induced plasma skimming in the perfusion of capillary bed another phenomenon takes place. The flow of erythrocytes which runs under normal conditions continuously through

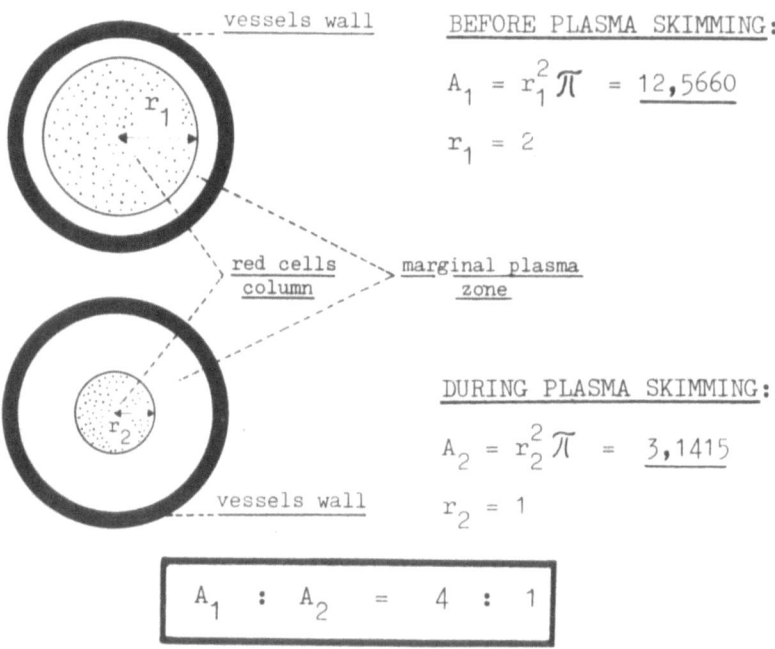

vessels wall

red cells column

marginal plasma zone

vessels wall

BEFORE PLASMA SKIMMING:

$$A_1 = r_1^2 \pi = 12,5660$$

$$r_1 = 2$$

DURING PLASMA SKIMMING:

$$A_2 = r_2^2 \pi = 3,1415$$

$$r_2 = 1$$

$$A_1 : A_2 = 4 : 1$$

Fig. 4. Schematic drawing of the calculated reduction of the cross section of red cells column by plasma skimming.

608

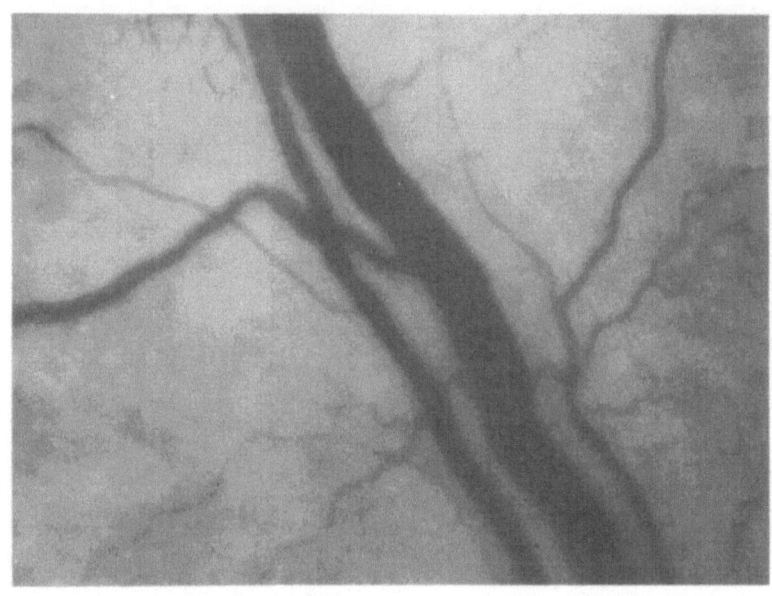

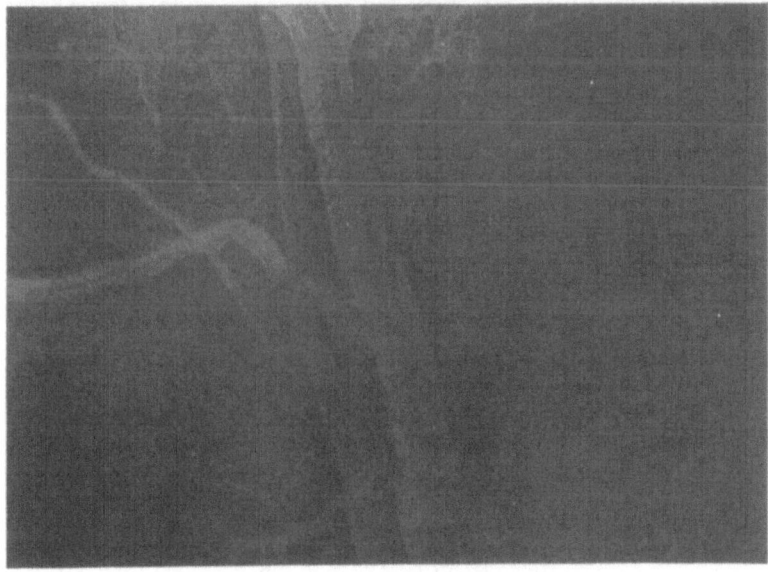

Fig. 5 a and b.   a. Disappeared areas of capillary network due to plasma skimming.
b. The same area during the fluoresceine-passage. There is no capillary obliteration.

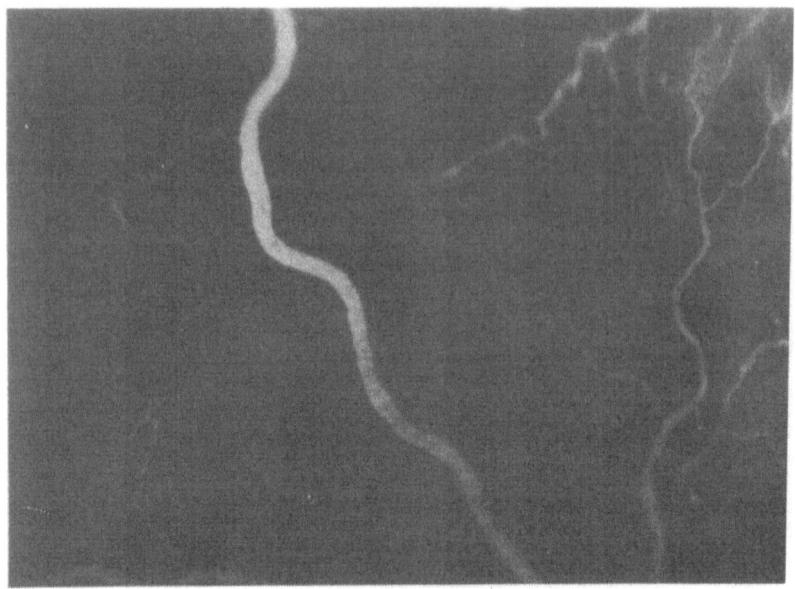

Fig. 6. True capillary obliteration situated at both sides of shunting circuits demonstrated by fluoresceine-angiography. Magnifications 90 times.

each single capillary loop, gets restricted more and more to a few circuits functioning like preferential channels connecting the arterial side of the vascular bed directly with the venous one. In this hemodynamic situation the net capillaries placed at both sides of such shunting circuits are not passed by erythrocytes any more. They thus lost their oxygen supply and undergo unoxemic damage which leads to a progressive obliteration. This is demonstrated in Fig. 6. The plasma skimming is still running on until the retinal vascular bed is completely obliterized. Based on the plasma skimming the pathomechanism of the oxygen induced vasoobliteration in the experimental retrolental fibroplasia can be explained more easily than by other hypotheses.

REFERENCES

ASHTON, N. & C. COOK. Direct observation of the effect of oxygen on developing vessels. Preliminary report. *Brit. J. Ophthal.* 38: *433-440* (1954).

KROGH, A. Anatomie und Physiologie der Capillaren. Springer, Berlin (1929).

LEMMINGSON, W. Änderungen im Durchblutungsmuster der Retina durch Plasma-Skimming. *Klin. Mbl. Augenheilk.* 159: *790-793* (1971).

LEMMINGSON, W. Vitalmikroskopische Untersuchungen zur Morphologie und Pathogenese der experimentellen O_2-Schädigungen der Retina. *Adv. Ophthal.* 25: *240-322* (1972).

LEMMINGSON, W. Hemorheological changes in experimental retrolental fibroplasia. Sec. Intern. Congress of Biorheology, Rehovot 29.12.74-7.1.75.

Author's address:
Augenklinik Diakonissen-Hospital
Diakonissenstrasse 28
7500 Karlsruhe
W. Germany

DISCUSSION

Prof. Hill: Could I express my appreciation of Dr Lemmingson's paper, and put two questions. First, I should like to know whether he was able to estimate the flow rate or the change in relative flow rate when the skimming that he reported, occurred? And second, I should like to ask; did any change occur in an animal studied by the same technique and under the same conditions but not subjected to a raise in oxygen tension?

Dr Lemmingson: The measurement of the diameter of the axial red cells column is a relative one only, we used for this purpose a low dose of fluorescein less than 1/3rd of the normal concentration in order to separate the marginal plasma layer from the axial red cell column. As to the second question, we do not know of any other condition where we can cause the same phenomenon I demonstrated here than by using oxygen in the newborn animals.

EQUATORIAL DEGENERATIONS WITH ATYPICAL VESSELS

A. WESSING & B. SCHLICKE

(Tübingen, West Germany)

Equatorial or lattice degeneration shows a very typical angiographic pattern. The symptoms can be summarized as follows:

In close vicinity to an equatorial or lattice degeneration a peculiar lack of vessels can be noticed. The vessels cease already at a certain distance centrally; by way of small collaterals the flow of dye is drained off into the corresponding vein. In this way rightangled kinking of the vessels and rope-ladder formations develop.

As SATO has already pointed out in Tokyo in 1972 even the normal peripheral fundus shows a relatively poor vascularisation. However, it seems that together with the appearance of equatorial degenerations the whole peripheral margin of the vascular network is shifted centrally. New arterio-venous shunts, which correspond to the original peripheral shunt-capillaries, are developing at a more central site.

These facts are of some importance for the prophylactic treatment of degenerations. Prophylactic coagulations at the site of the dystrophic retina may produce retinal tears. Therefore it is recommended to coagulate a relatively large safety-zone. Using photocoagulation the degeneration should be surrounded by the coagulations in a certain distance as defined by the keep-off-technique.

The angiographic picture changes with the incidence of retinal tears. By exceeding the margins of the degeneration and of the nonperfused retina the tears extend into areas with an intact vascular system, where they produce a heavy vascular reaction.

As long as the retina is still in place we only see a focal capillary dilatation. However, with the onset of retinal detachment all vessels in the vicinity of the tear are considerably dilated. The capillaries are forming a large widemeshed network. Arterioles and venoles are crossing among them like wide channels and their shunting function is getting obvious.

Fluorescein leakage may occur from the ruptured capillaries at the edge of the tear. It may originate also from the bigger vessels. The disturbance of permeability seems to be a rather complex process. Damage of the vessel wall is not only confined to the site of the tear, but occurs also in the more distant vicinity of a retinal break, even though the tear may be rather small. Thereby the outer vessel arcades near the ora are most heavily involved. In

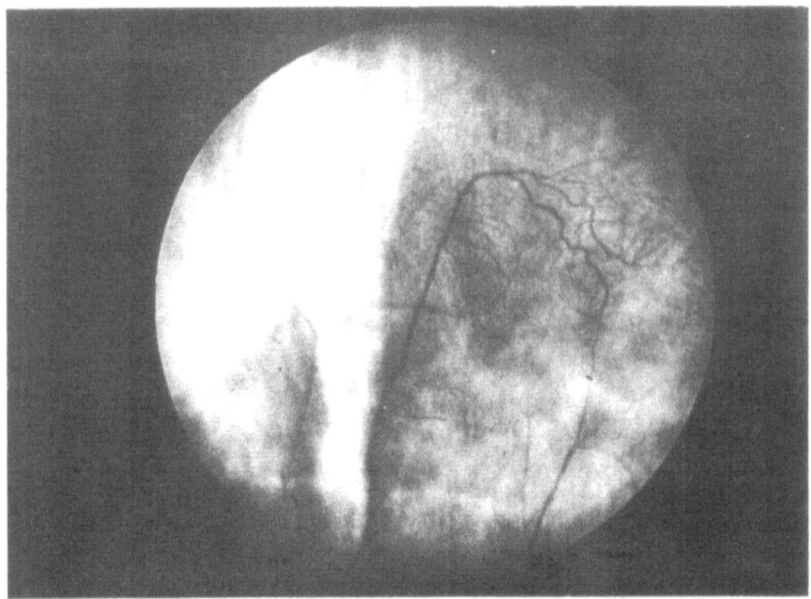

Fig. 1.   Atypical vessels in lattice degeneration.

these cases the retinal tear seems to be merely a local event within a much more extensive disease-mechanism.

Also a centrally located retinal break shows this peculiar vasodilatation, always provided the retina being detached. In the undetached retina the vessels remain intact.

After the onset of such a vascular reaction, normalization seems to proceed very slowly. Pretty often after buckling or encircling procedures one can observe persisting vascular dilations occasionally even microaneurysms, which again confirms the observations of ROSEN (1968) and SATO (1972).

With this let us return to equatorial degenerations. Occasionally we find equatorial degenerations, which contrarily to the above-mentioned, show an increase of vessels (Fig. 1). There are thin, long stretched vessels, which reach into the area of degeneration. Their thick packing gives the impression of an augmentation of vessels. The peripheral ending is formed by large vesselarcades running parallel to the ora. In the angiogram they are wide calibred and they often carry microaneurysms; however leakage almost never occurs.

Among the great number of patients with lattice degeneration cases with this type of vessel formation are rare. Within 10 years we have seen 14 such cases in the Essen Eye Hospital. Younger patients between 15 and 30 years of age were involved. The eyes were moderately myopic to a degree of 7 to 9 diopters.

614

Undoubtedly there is a striking contrast between these cases and the typical pattern of vascularisation in equatorial degenerations. Similarities with Eales' disease are called to mind. However, there is a fundamental difference since dye-leakage does not occur. AMALRIC (1969) has published similar pictures in juvenile retinoschisis. However, our own cases did not show any sign of retinoschisis. We have had the impression, that the atypical vessels presented here fit much more into the picture of the retinopathy of prematurity. They may represent nothing else than a form fruste of this peculiar disease. In regard to this one should keep in mind that eyes with retrolental fibroplasia are often myopic (FOOS 1975, TASMAN 1975) and furthermore that retrolental fibroplasia may occur even in children who have been carried to term and who have never been living in an oxygenatmosphere (BROCKHURST & CHISHTI 1975).

IN CONCLUSION

The question of a correlation between vessel malformations in the periphery of the fundus and formation of equatorial degenerations cannot be answered sufficiently. The purpose of this paper was to point out that atypical findings do occur and that they are probably occupying a key-position in the pathogenesis of peripheral retinal degenerations.

REFERENCES

AMALRIC, P. Angiographie fluorescéinique dans le dédollement juvénile. *Mod. Probl. Ophthal.* 8: *394-406* (1969).

BROCKHURST, R.J. & M.I. CHISHTI. Cicatricial retrolental fibroplasia, its occurrence without oxygen administration and in full term infants. *Graefes Arch. Ophthal.* 195: *113-128* (1975).

FOOS, R.Y. Acute retrolental fibroplasia. *Graefes Arch. Ophthal.* 195: *87-100* (1975).

ROSEN, E.S. A photographic investigation of simple retinal detachment. *Trans. Ophthal. Soc. U.K.* 88: *331-342* (1968).

SATO, K. Shunt formation in lattice degeneration and retinal detachment. A fluorescein angiographic study. *Mod. Probl. Ophthal.* 10: *133-134* (1972).

SATO, K. Fluorography of the peripheral retina in normal ocular fundus. In: Fluorescein-Angiography herausg. von K. Shimizu. Igaku Shoin Tokyo 1974: *153-154*.

TASMAN, W. Retinal detachment in retrolental fibroplasia. *Graefes Arch. Ophthal.* 195: *129-139* (1975).

WESSING, A. Fluoreszenzangiographie bei Netzhautablösung und ihren Vorstadien. In: Die Prophylaxe der idiopatischen Netzhautablösung. Herausg. von H. Fanta und W. Jaeger. Bergmann, München 1971: *92-101*.

WESSING, A. New aspects of angiographic studies in retinal detachment. *Mod. Probl. Ophthal.* 12: *202-206* (1974).

Authors' address:
Universitäts-Augenklinik
Schleichstrasse 12
D-7400 TÜBINGEN
W. Germany

DISCUSSION

Dr Amalric: Sur le travail de Mr Wessing, j'agrée avec les images qu'il nous a montrées concernant l'angiographie fluorescéinique autour des déchirures rétiniennes mais je voudrais apporter quelques commentaires. Si on parle toujours dans ces cas là de la rétine, on n'a pas évoqué le problème de la choroïde périphérique. Je ne veux pas en parler pour discuter la pathogénie de son atteinte mais simplement pour parler des images que nous constatons. Car si la rétine a sa circulation très diminuée à la périphérie, il doit en être de même pour la choroïde. J'ai réalisé dans certains cas des angiographies de la périphérie choroïdienne jusqu'à l'ora serrata chez des aphaques et on voit qu'il y a un arrêt circulatoire très important jusqu'à la zone avoisinant le corps ciliaire où une bande fluorescente apparait. Il en résulte que lorsque nous voyons des images avec des hyperpigmentations avec des hyperfluorescences dans la périphérie, je pense qu'elles ne sont pas physiologiques; et lorsque nous voyons des modifications dans la zone qui correspond sur le plan rétinien à des déchirures, je me demande s'il n'y a pas un processus mixte à la fois choroïdien et rétinien. Ceci pour permettre d'ajouter que dans certaines maladies que nous considérons comme typiquement rétiniennes comme le rétinoschisis héréditaire lié au sexe, on s'aperçoit qu'il y a des lésions choroïdiennes dans les régions qui correspondent au rétinoschisis. J'ai eu la bonne fortune d'angiographier récemment deux familles avec plusieurs enfants atteints de rétinoschisis héréditaire par les différentes méthodes d'exploration de la choroïde, infra-rouge, technique en lumière anérythre, angiographie fluorescéinique. C'est uniquement dans ce sens là que je voulais ajouter ces quelques mots: dans la périphérie rétinienne pensons aux vaisseaux rétiniens, mais n'oublions pas les vaisseaux choroïdiens.

Dr Wessing: I have only one comment to add. I am sure that they are choroidal lesions in these cases. We try to do angiograms of the choroid in cases of giant tears but especially in these cases we did not find any lesion in the choroid. We found it very surprising but maybe the reason is that it is difficult to reach the far periphery on angiogram.

ANGIOMATOSIS RETINAE

S.L. FINE

(Baltimore, USA)

The subject of angiomatosis retinae continues to receive much attention in the medical literature. WELCH (1970) has reviewed in detail the history of von Hippel-Lindau disease including advances in diagnosis and therapy. HAINING & ZWEIFACH (1967) have described some of the fluorescein angiographic features of retinal tumors (HAINING, 1967). This report will emphasize the prominent role of fluorescein fundus photography in: (1) understanding the pathogenesis of retinal angiomas; (2) illustrating the pathological circulatory dynamics through the angiomas and surrounding retina; (3) demonstrating peculiar anatomic features of some lesions, such as surface neovascularization; and (4) as an adjunct in evaluating the response to light coagulation or cryotherapy. Finally, the limits of fluorescein angiography for determining adequacy of therapy will be discussed in view of previously published cases of clinical-histopathologic correlation showing

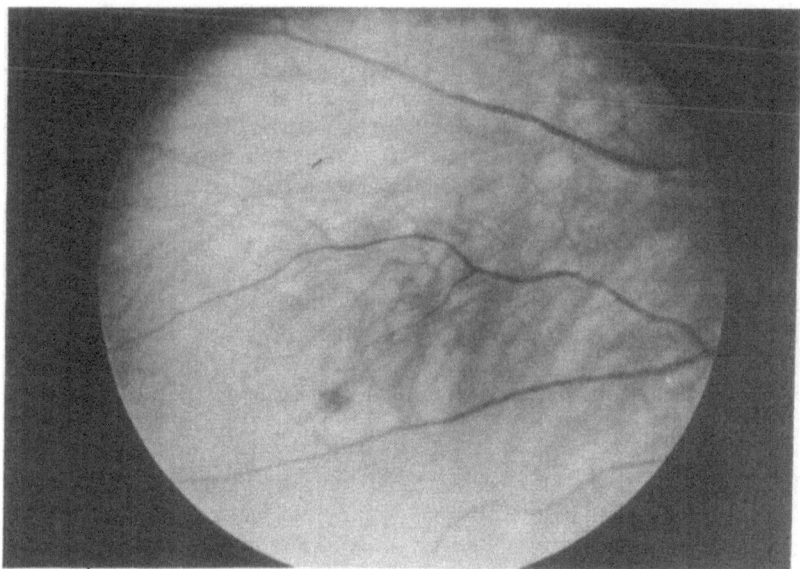

Fig. 1. Small tumor nodule without dilated feeder vessel (Patient of Dr. Robert B. Welch, Baltimore).

617

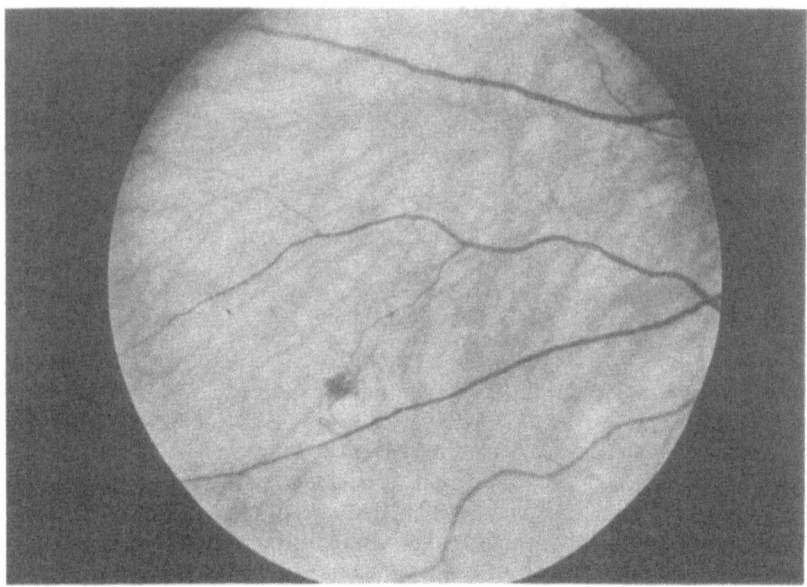

Fig. 2A. Same as Figure 1, fourteen months later, with tumor nodule slightly enlarged and draining venule more prominent.

viable tumor cells in areas thought to have been destroyed by clinical and fluorographic examination.

The early or stage 1 lesion is described by DUKE-ELDER (1967) as an angioma with vascular dilatation. Previous investigators speculated that the basic lesion was a malformation of an entire vascular unit (arterioles, capillaries, and venules), all three of which enlarged as the tumor grew (GOLDBERG & DUKE, 1968). Subsequently, JESBURG and others (JESBURG et al., 1968) demonstrated that angiomatous lesions could develop from retina considered normal by clinical examination without evidence of accompanying dilated feeding and draining vessels, thus raising the possibility that angiomas may develop de novo in an individual with the appropriate genotype. This latter thesis received additional support when WELCH showed a small red nodule in normal retina (Figure 1) without a dilated feeder vessel. Fourteen months later, the nodule had enlarged slightly with a visible draining venule (Figure 2A), and the tumor now filled fluorescein (Figure 2B) which it had not done appreciably at the time of the initial examination.

The bright red color of many tumor nodules has long been thought to reflect the relatively high PO_2 in the tumor caused by arteriovenous shunting through the lesion. Fluorescein angiography substantiates the validity of this theory by demonstrating unequivocally the rapid flow and shunting through the tumor. The draining venule characteristically fills with dye several seconds before the arterioles and capillary bed distal to the tumor (Figure 3). Retinal tumors which do not exhibit the fire-engine red color

618

may be deeper in the retina or may be covered by exudate and/or glial tissue which imparts a yellowish to grayish cast to the lesion.

Another feature which may enhance the bright red color or some tumors is the presence of fine new vessels on the surface. Neovascularization can be appreciated readily with fundus biomicroscopic exam or by inspection of stereo-color photographs (Figure 4A). Fluorescein angiography demon-

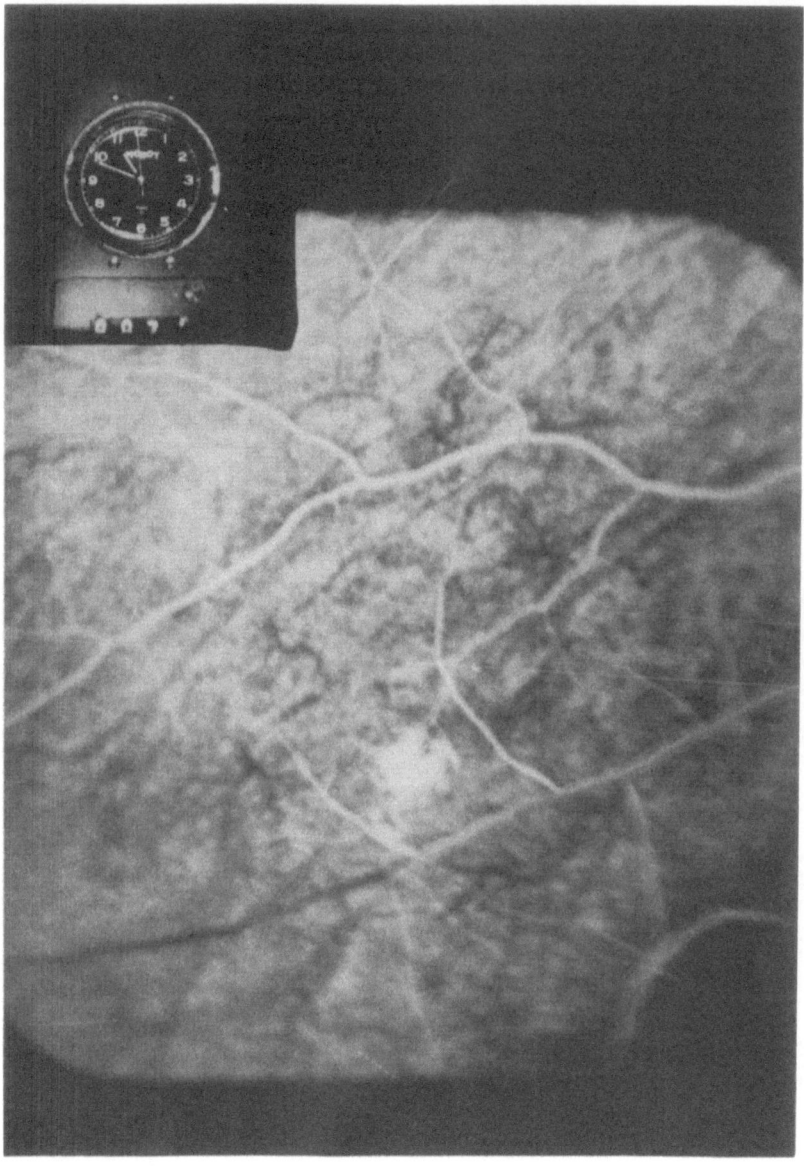

Fig. 2B.   Tumor nodule fills with dye.

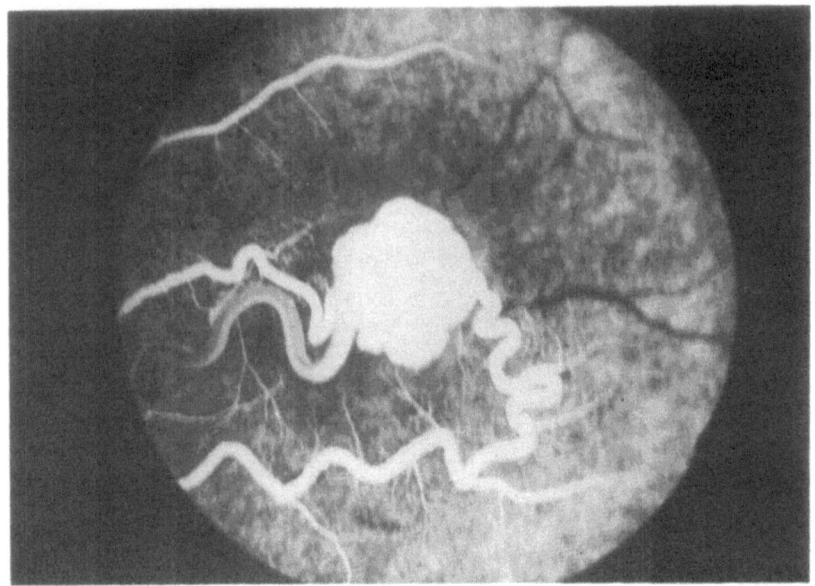

Fig. 3. Venule draining tumor fills with dye before arteriole or capillary bed distal to tumor, demonstrating arteriovenous shunting through tumor.

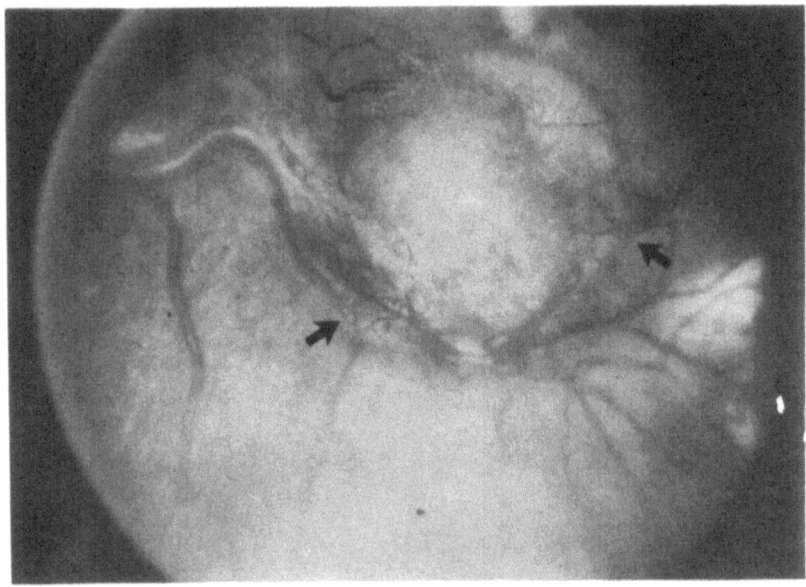

Fig. 4 A. Surface neovascularization over tumor contributes to bright red appearance.

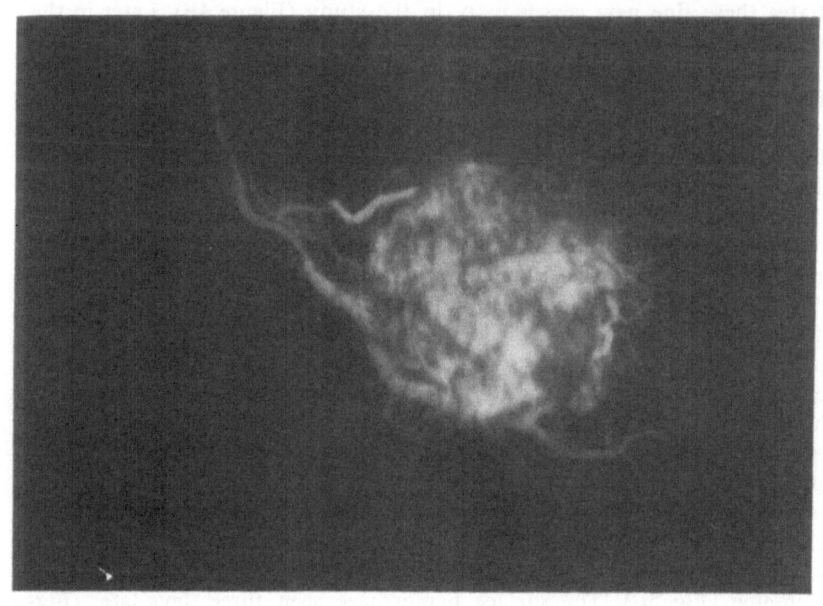

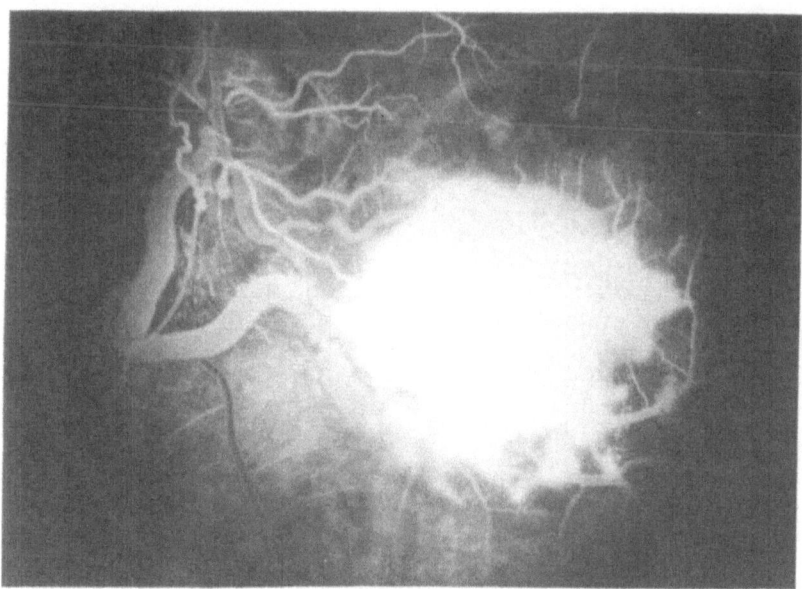

Fig. 4B, 4C. Surface neovascularization leaks dye and causes blurred edges to tumor nodule.

strates these fine new vessels early in the study (Figure 4B). Later in the angiogram, one sees blurred margins at the tumor edge (Figure 4C) in contrast to the smooth margins in tumors without surface neovascularization (Figure 3).

Consideration of treatment is important since most investigators believe that untreated tumors eventuate in loss of vision first by causing lipid accumulation in the macula and later by retinal detachment and absolute glaucoma. VAIL cited a success rate of 70 percent with diathermy (VAIL, 1958), but WELCH outlined certain advantages of light coagulation and cryotherapy which have resulted in their acceptance as the preferred modes of therapy today. The value of fluorescein photography in evaluating the effectiveness of therapy and in determining the need for additional treatment is illustrated in the following case. The patient is a 21-year old black female whose right eye has 1/200 vision due to an exudative detachment of the temporal retina including the macula and twelve retinal angiomas of varying dimensions. The left eye has 20/15 vision with a single angioma, approximately one disc diameter in size, superotemporal to the posterior pole (Figure 5A). Note the dilated feeding and draining vessels on both the red-free photograph and the fluorescein angiogram (Figure 5B). Immediately after xenon arc photocoagulation, note the intense pigment epithelial whitening (Fig. 5C). The surface hemorrhage seen three days later (Figure 5D) is not an uncommon finding. Four months later, visual acuity remained 20/15, and the lesion appeared to be replaced by scar (Figure 5E). Note attenuation of feeding and draining vessels compared to pre-treatment photograph. Despite the ophthalmoscopic appearance, fluorescein angiography showed persistent filling and leakage in the inferonasal part of the

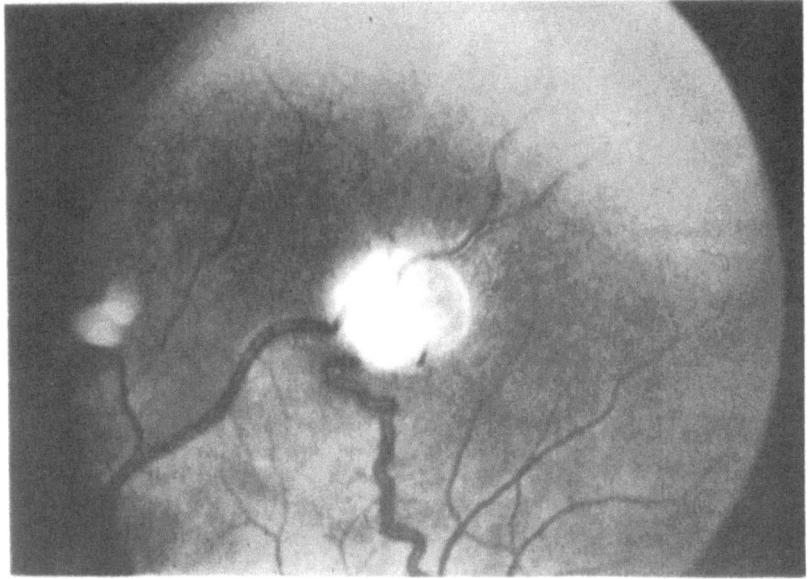

Fig. 5A. Tumor superotemporal to left macula, pre-treatment.

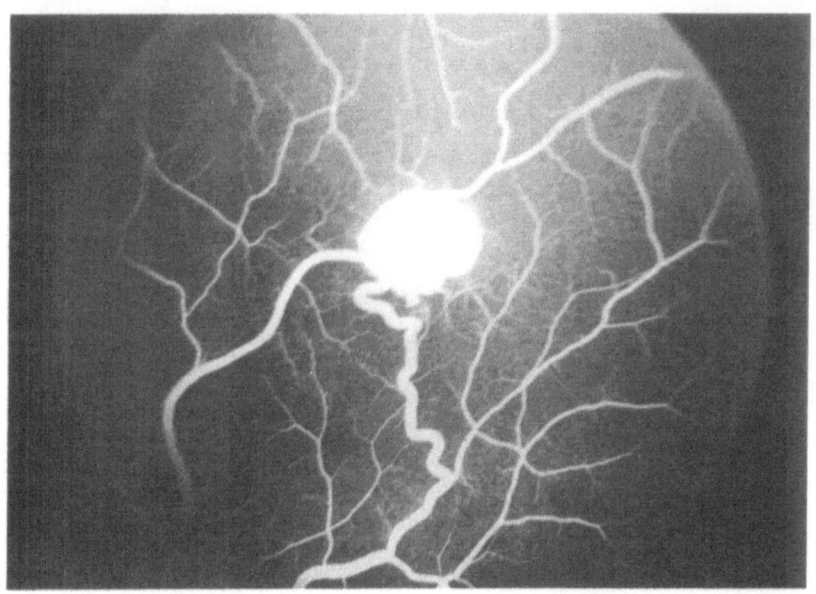

Fig. 5B. Fluorescein angiogram pre-treatment.

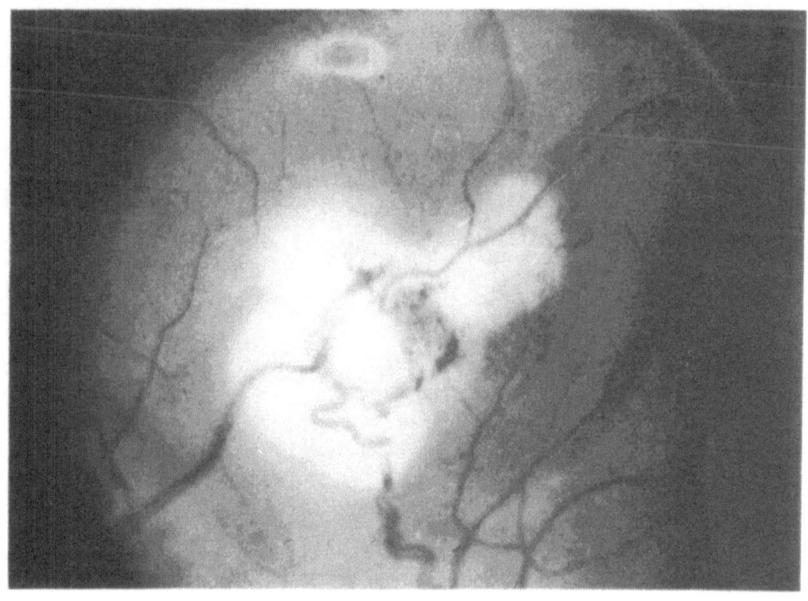

Fig. 5C. Immediately post-xenon arc photocoagulation.

623

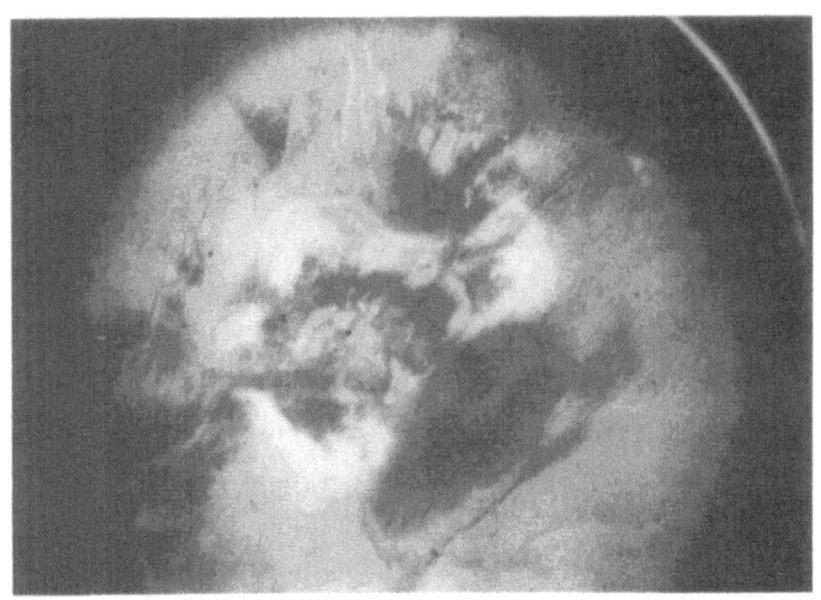

Fig. 5D.   Surface hemorrhage four days after xenon arc treatment.

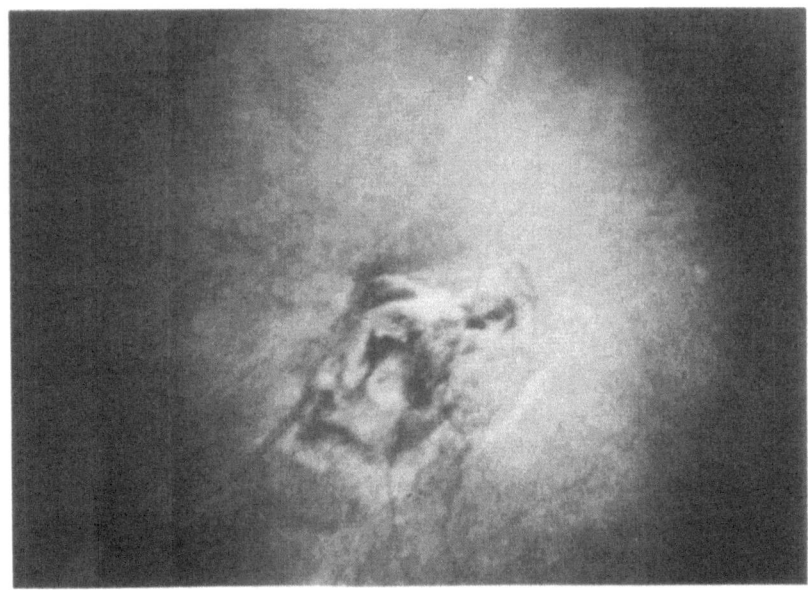

Fig. 5E.   Scar four months after xenon treatment.

624

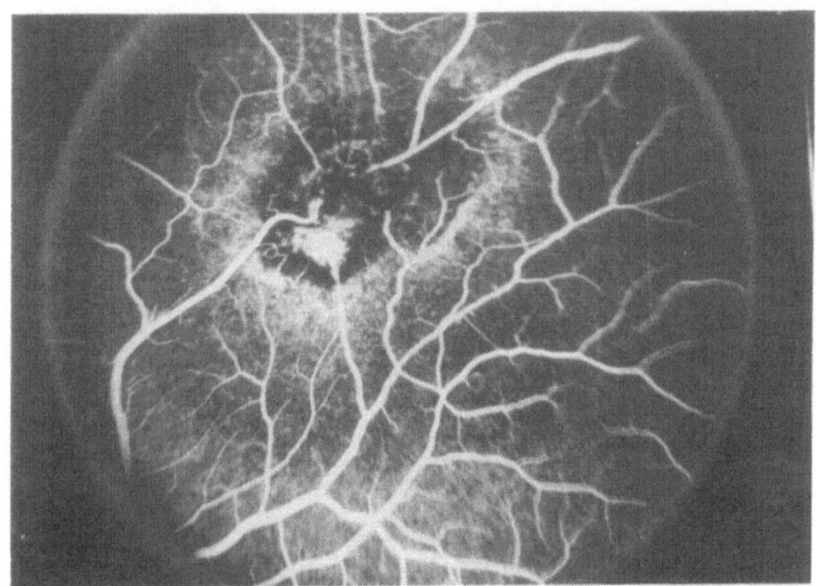

Fig. 5F. Fluorescein angiogram four months after xenon treatment shows persistent vascular channels in tumor.

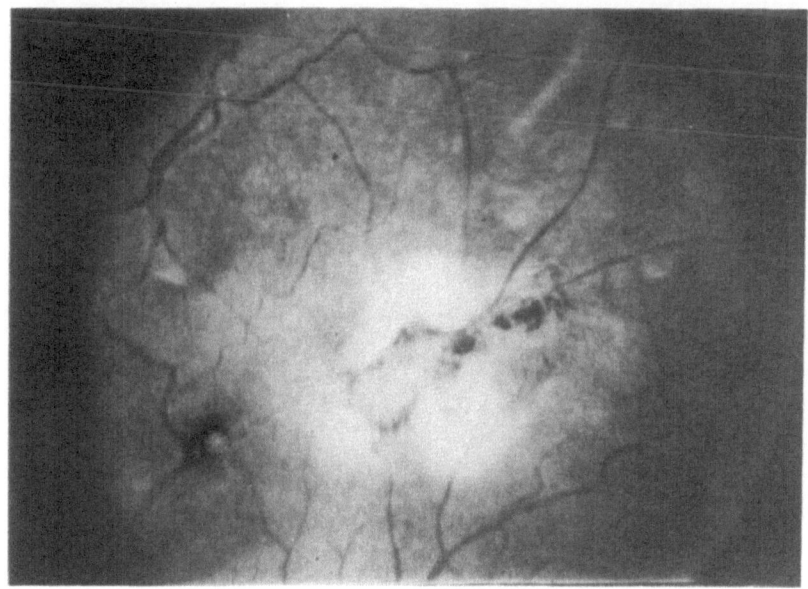

Fig. 5G. Immediately after second photocoagulation treatment.

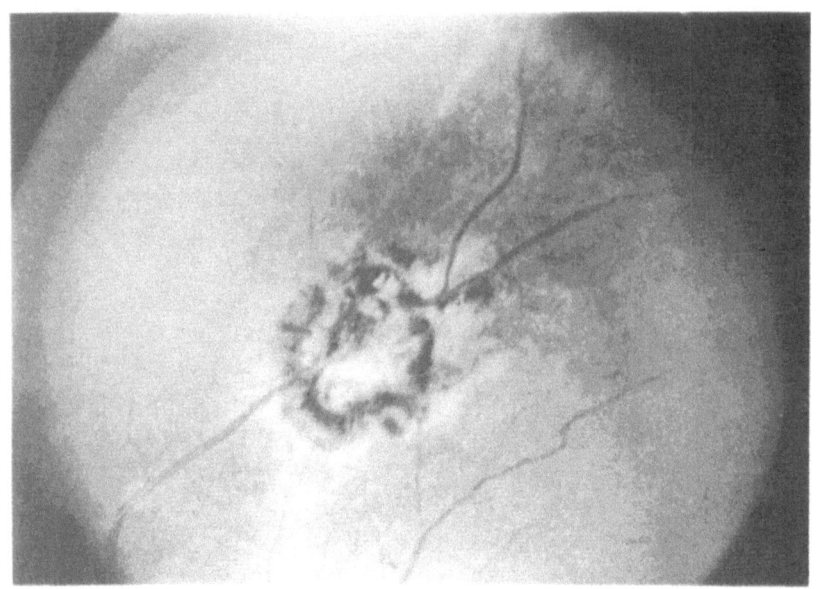

Fig. 5H. Six months after second treatment.

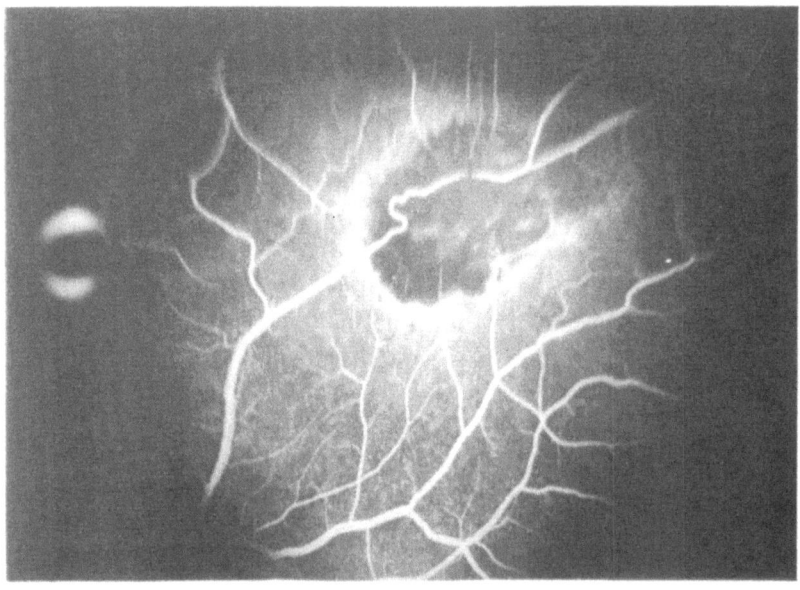

Fig. 5I. Fluorescein angiography six months after second treatment showing no patent channels in tumor.

626

lesion (Figure 5F), thus necessitating additional photocoagulation (Figure 5G). Six months after the second treatment episode, a black scar is noted (Figure 5H), and no fluorescein filling or leakage is seen (Figure 5I). Although it might have been reasonable to postpone the second treatment until the remaining tumor elements became ophthalmoscopically visible in addition to angiographically apparent, this case illustrates the advantages of contrast photography over ophthalmoscopy alone. It is important to note, however, that GOLDBERG and others have shown histologically viable tumor elements in cases where tumor was thought to have been completely destroyed after both xenon arc (GOLDBERG & DUKE, 1968) and argon laser treatment (APPLE, GOLDBERG & WYHINNY, 1974). On the other hand, WATZKE reported one case showing complete histologic destruction after cryotherapy to the tumor (WATZKE, 1974). Most investigators believe that argon laser, xenon arc, cryotherapy, and diathermy all have a role to play in the management of retinal angiomas depending upon the size of the tumor and its location in the fundus. Thus, the ophthalmic surgeon managing the patient with von Hippel's disease should be skilled in each of these therapeutic modalities. Although the detailed features of a particular retinal lesion which would cause one to consider one form of therapy over another are beyond the scope of this report, the importance of fluorescein angiography in demonstrating the pathogenesis, documenting the appearance, and following the lesions after treatment is indisputable.

REFERENCES

APPLE, D.J., GOLDBERG, M.F. & WYHINNY, G.J. Argon laser treatment of von Hippel-Lindau retinal angiomas. II. Histopathology of treated lesions. *Arch. Ophthalmol.* 92: *126-130* (1974).

DUKE-ELDER, S. System of Ophthalmology. Vol. X. *Diseases of the retina.* St. Louis, C.V. Mosby, Co., p. *738* (1967).

GOLDBERG, M.F. & DUKE, J.R. Von Hippel-Lindau disease: histopathologic findings in a treated and an untreated eye. *Am. J. Ophthal.* 66: *693-705* (1968).

HAINING, W.F. & ZWEIFACH, O.H. Fluorescein angiography in von Hippel-Lindau disease. *Arch. Ophthalmol.* 78: *475-479* (1967).

JESBURG, D.O., SPENCER, W.H. & HOYT, W.F. Incipient lesions of von Hippel-Lindau disease. *Arch. Ophthal.* 80: *632-640* (1968).

VAIL, D. Angiomatosis retinae, eleven years after diathermy coagulation. *Am. J. Ophth.* 46: *525-534*, (1958).

WATZKE, R.C. Cryotherapy for retinal angiomatosis. A clinicopathologic report. *Arch. Ophthal.* 92: *399-401* (1974).

WELCH, R.B. Von Hippel-Lindau disease; the recognition and treatment of early angiomatosis retinae and the use of cryosurgery as an adjunct to therapy. *Trans. Amer. Ophthalmol. Soc.* 68: *367-424* (1970).

Author's address:
Wilmer Institute
Johns Hopkins Hospital
601 N. Broadway
Baltimore, Maryland 21205
USA

627

DISCUSSION ON COMPLICATIONS

Dr Gass: Dr Schafroth from Bern spoke to me about a recent catastrophe they had as a result of fluorescein angiography. I thought it worthwhile for him to just mention this case in the hope that other people who have any problems with fluorescein angiography will bring them to our attention.

Dr Schafroth: Two weeks ago we performed a regular angiography with a rather old patient and after five minutes this patient fell into a shock. We brought him at once to the department of reanimation where he had adequate care. Despite of all that, after 2 hours he died. The autopsy was done but the final results are not yet known. It seems that there were no signs of acute anaphylactic shock. It is our general impression that this was perhaps an unhappy coincidence. But all the same once such a thing happens to you, you look differently at angiography. Before we always thought that such complications are very rare and we had our preparation for emergency cases but no more. We feel that there are moral and ethical implications especially if you know that in several places in Europe, such mortal complications have occurred. Several years back a paper have been published in the American Journal of Ophthalmology collecting the complications but in the meantime fluorescence angiography has become so much more used all over the world that such a review should be done again. The main points we should be able to get are first the incidence of severe complication, bad shocks or mortal cases and second to know the reason if possible, if there were any signs of allergy or perhaps if we can make out a group of high-risk patients. All the patients we heard of were rather old and most of them had diabetes. This knowledge would help us first to select high-risk people where angiography should be performed only with a strong indication and with great care, and second to prepare adequate measures if any group of reactions can be expected. This survey should be carried out by means of a questionary sent by one of the well established centers for angiography.

Dr Gass: I would urge that any one who had a serious complication let Dr Schafroth know about it, or sent the information to one of the authors who have written about this matter before, so that it can regularly be brought up to date.

Dr Gold: I would like to make a comment about the question of serious complications after fluorescein angiography. Most of the attention given to this topic in the past has been related to complications of an allergic nature. We have found, unfortunately, that it is not uncommon for patients to have episodes in which they feel somewhat faint shortly after the injection of fluorescein. In patients with borderline cardiac or cerebral perfusion, a drop in blood pressure may be enough to precipitate frank infarction. Fluorescein angiography may be associated with such a drop in blood pressure, and this may actually be the most common potentially serious side-effect of the procedure. I know of several cardiac deaths and a stroke following fluorescein angiography.

Dr Siam: Talking about these serious events I like to make two remarks on two patients. One of them was a diabetic with a blood pressure of 190/110

629

and after the fluorescein injection his blood pressure dropped to 40. I was lucky because I happened to have the anaesthetist beside me. It took us several hours to bring the blood pressure up and to save the patient. The other incidence was in a young man of 23 who had a severe renal retinopathy on both eyes. One hour after the fluorescein angiography had been done this young man went into a state of hypertensive encephalopathy and severe coma. He stayed in the hospital for about one week. We do not know if this had something to do with it, but he seemed to be perfectly fit before the angiography was done.

Mr Rubinstein: I myself, obviously, as I hope, all of you, have a kit for this kind of resuscitation in my fluorescence angiography outfit, but all the reactions apart from one that I ever had in these many years with these many patients where really things that one would call vaso-vagal attacks. Obviously in somebody with some cardiac problem or somebody old you might have trouble. How can one prevent that? I do not think we should really try to limit fluorescein angiography because we will not be able to wheat I think ever those people that are going to do it or not and they often do it before you inject. It is not fluorescein that hurts them, it is the surgical procedure or the intention of the surgical procedure that hurts them.

Dr Schafroth: I did not want to go into details about our case. But since this possibility was mentioned I want to say that our patient had signs of chronic intracranial pressure with a questionable papilledema, which was the reason why he was sent. He was an out-patient. He had also signs of a rather peculiar chronic stroke and probably had a bad intracranial circulation. Our idea at the moment is exactly what you said. Probably by the procedure the blood pressure sunk for a certain time and this was sufficient to reduce the intracerebral circulation so much that an apoplexy could develop. If we know that these patients are especially prone for that reaction, we know already much and we can abstain from angiography in them, unless there is a very strong reason.

Dr Amalric: Je crois avoir publié il y a quelques années un travail sur les accidents et incidents par l'angiographie fluorescéinique* et j'ai eu à l'époque une malade, jeune, qui a failli mourir à la suite d'une angiographie. Ayant fait la bibliographie à cette époque, il y avait déjà trois cas de décès par angiographie. Il ne s'agissait pas d'une malade âgée, il s'agissait d'une malade jeune qui avait une tumeur de la choroïde bilatérale pour laquelle j'avais fait une angiographie un mois auparavant dans de très bonnes conditions sans aucun accident. Un mois plus tard, après radiothérapie locale sur les deux yeux et une récupération visuelle partielle, j'ai voulu faire une nouvelle angiographie. Ce n'est pas 5 minutes après que s'est produit l'accident, c'est pendant l'angiographie au temps veineux. La patiente est tombée dans le coma avec une hémiparésie et une hypotension catastrophique. Nous avons fait, avec le médecin qui était avec moi, une injection intraveineuse de cortisone et nous l'avons mise en perfusion. La tension est restée très basse

* Incidents et accidents au cours de l'angiographie fluorescéinique. *Bul. Soc. Ophtal. de France* 12: 968-972 (1968).

pendant plusieurs minutes puis elle a récupéré progressivement. Nous l'avons portée à la clinique en ambulance car l'angiographie se déroulait dans mon cabinet. Le soir tout est rentré dans l'ordre et elle est repartie chez elle le lendemain. Ceci étant, comme elle avait une tumeur métastatique, nous avons pensé qu'il était possible que cet accident était sous la dépendance d'une métastase cérébrale mais cela était faux car j'ai revu la malade deux mois plus tard et il n'y avait aucun signe de complication cérébrale. Elle est morte deux ans plus tard. Lorsque j'avais fait la bibliographie de la question à cette époque, je vous parle de 1969, même avant 1969, j'avais remarqué dans 3 cas où il y avait eu décès, il y avait certainement des problèmes comme ceux qu'a évoqué Siam

Le tableau d'une hypotension brutale réclame une thérapeutique d'urgence. Ce tableau est réellement dramatique et dans de tels cas, je crois qu'il faut avoir sous la main non seulement les injections classiques mais tout l'ensemble de réanimation que nous connaissons.

GENERAL REVIEW

E. NORTON

(Miami, USA)

To summarize a four day symposium in a few minutes is impossible. I will be only able to give my evaluation of the important discussions that have been presented. I will have to omit some papers which either have less significance or were so clear they were complete in themselves. Please forgive my human failing or biases.

The first thing to discuss are the changes in instrumentation and technique. At the last symposium in Tokyo we were all excited about the wide angle fundus camera that was going to be developed. It is apparent at this meeting, that they are readily available. We have a beautiful exhibit by Lee Allen and his group from Iowa. If you look at that exhibit, I think you will realize this technique has limited usefulness. It is going to be good for some diseases where you want a panoramic view, but you cannot help but be impressed, as you go through the exhibit, that whenever you have a beautiful picture it is always the one taken with the Zeiss that we conventionally use. Wide angle photography is going to be a supplement to what we have , but I do not think it is going to replace it. I do not know obviously what is going to happen with the Canon fundus camera because I have not even seen it.

Another advance in photography is the simultaneous stereo photography on a single 35 mm frame. As you may know Dr Donaldson in Boston has developed a simultaneous stereo fundus camera which he has had for many years. It is a beautiful camera but each eye has a different frame. The pictures have to be specially mounted and specially filed so that if you have a big department it makes filing complicated, especially the time in mounting and filing them. However, it is a beautiful camera but it is not in mass production and probably never will be. With respect to the one which is on exhibit here by Topcon, I think the pictures they have (it is the first time I have seen them) are excellent. I have felt for a long time that a simultaneous stereophotograph even if the field be small is worth it, because we definitely need to quantitate some of our observations and we know that even Lee Allen's prism does not give absolutely reproducible results in stereophotography. The big question is will this give reproducible results and while I expect it will, it has not been put to that test yet.

We have had TV fluorescein angiography for a long time. Since the first meeting, it has been discussed. Progress is slow but I do think that with the addition of the image intensifier and the subsequent use of computers, this will be in use much more frequently, maybe not for the next meeting but maybe a later meeting.

At the first meeting in Albi we had quite a bit of time spent on filters. It is interesting to me that this time we basically had only one paper on filters. At that first meeting, Lee Allen gave a very beautiful presentation of what

633

the ideal filter would be. I do not think that this new filter meets his specifications. I am impressed that Dr Missotten's statements regarding the transmission of pigment epithelium were very important for this new filter. That is that more light is going to come out and that is what they all are noting about it. Mr Justice just told me, he loves it because he can see the fundus so well while he is taking the picture. But more light is coming out because more light is going through the pigment epithelium to excite the choroid and more fluorescence is coming back to be recorded and for you to see. Apparently, it is a good filter; I am impressed that it is going to be more valuable to study the choroid and it might be less valuable to study the retina, because the background fluorescence seems to overpower the retinal vasculature. I may be wrong in this observation.

I do not think we can leave this part of the discussion without mentioning the complications. Complications should be a subject at the next symposium. We ought to get together and get some of the data on reactions to dye. Any time you are going to put a needle into a person you must expect a significant number of people to react, even if you just inject saline. Just coming at them with a needle, may cause a drop in blood pressure and you can expect that if they have marginal blood supply either to their cerebrum or to their myocardium, there may be trouble. This is not necessarily due to the dye.

About the paper on light damage; it is something we all want to keep in mind, as we develop new cameras and change different illumination systems we can damage the eye with light.

At the risk of hurting the feelings of some people and displaying my own ignorance with respect to flow, it is still in an experimental state. We have not gotten it to a point that it is helping us clinically. That may be our fault. Basically, we have with the standard technique we use today a qualitative method of evaluating flow at one or three frames a second and that seems to be sufficient for the diseases we recognize today as having impaired flow. Obviously if we had an easy way to measure flow we might learn that a lot more diseases are influenced by flow, but for the present I think it is still an experimental technique.

On vein occlusion, I did ask Eva Kohner to put in her slide and I want to show that one slide because it gives a very nice summary of the pathophysiology. It is a very straightforward situation and I think that it fits in with all the papers that were presented on vein occlusion, and particularly the importance of capillary non-perfusion areas and their influence on prognosis. The classification of branch vein occlusion presented by Desmond Archer is straightforward and is in your abstract. The classification that was mentioned in the discussion of central retinal vein occlusion by Sohan Hayreh is important. We have reached the point now, with this understanding of branch vein occlusion, that we are ready for a clinical trial to evaluate the influence of photocoagulation on the end-result of this disease. There are several papers which would suggest that it is very valuable. We all know that there are other people who have reported that it is no better than the natural course of the disease. We need the classifications if we want to be able to establish a good clinical trial, randomized and so on. I think we are ready for that in branch vein occlusion. We will get rid of the conflicting data and we will find out whether we are doing good to the patients or not.

Choroidal circulation: As you know, I was sitting next to Pierre, so I would not dare to omit it. In this meeting there is increased interest in the choroid and I have noticed this in each succeeding meeting. Our interest is still not enough because our friends from Tokyo have not studied the choroid as well as they might in their paper on Takayasu's disease, but they will I am sure. We have a lot of conflicting data. Conflicting because we had the morphologic presentations by Dr Heimann and Dr Koichi Shimizu and the acute experimental studies by Sohan. I have little doubt that this is a very important subject. Somehow as I listen to them I do not think they are quite as far apart as it seems. The primary difference appears to me to be whether there is a blood supply that is primarily to the macula as Dr Amalric has said for some time or not, and Dr Hayreh obviously has not been able to demonstrate this. That might be important in senile macular degeneration for example. We have to settle that point and at the moment I do not think we can. I have the feeling after listening to all the papers on choroidal circulation, even the introduction of ICG, which gives very nice photographs of the flow in the choroid, that we still do not know much more on the choroid than what Pierre Amalric described clinically more than a decade ago. I am sure it is important and that this study of choroidal disease will be one of the major breakthroughs of the next decade.

As far as choroidal tumors, obviously we had a striking contrast in opinions. The real controversy that exists today is: whether to observe melanomas when you see them or whether to take them out? When the patient has 20/20 vision it is a difficult decision. If the patient does not have good vision and has a normal eye on the other side it is not a very difficult decision. You may not feel it is important but I might just tell an anecdotal case of a patient who had a melanoma in the fundus with a very strongly positive P 32 uptake of 190%. She was advised to have the eye removed. We happened to see the patient and advised that it be observed and naturally the patient would follow someone who is giving a recommendation like that rather than having her eye removed. We continue to follow the patient and are now in the 7th year and during this time she has lost the use of her other eye. The lesion has yet to change, we get photographs of it twice a year. I just urge you to be careful in taking out small tumors. I do not think the pathologists know what a malignant melanoma is. I talked to Zimmerman and I am convinced that he does not even know what a malignant melanoma really is. If you think historically, when I was a resident anyone having an iris melanoma had the eye removed if you could not excise it. Today, seldom does anyone take the eye out for an iris melanoma, because we know that people do not die from an iris melanoma so we follow them as long as the eye is good. You have to think a little bit about it. I am not saying we are right in following them; we may prove to be wrong and it might be a costly mistake but I do think we need some very good studies on following these pigmented lesions of the fundus and finding out what their natural course is. I am not going into the P 32 test. Don Gass pretty well covered it; it is a good test, but I just cannot see taking an eye, which you think clinically has a choroidal haemangioma and taking that patient up to the operating room, under general or retrobulbar anesthesia, expose the eye, place an instrument over the lesion and push it against the eye to try to prove that you are right. I just think that it is not the thing to do.

I was pleased to see the paper from New York on the lesions simulating melanomas in sarcoid. I have not seen such lesions. We have seen several patients that simulated those lesions presenting with scleritis, with reticular cell sarcoma, but I have not seen it with sarcoid. Retinitis has been more often seen with sarcoid.

The problem of senile disciform degeneration is still with us and I don't think we have learned much new. The precursor signs were outlined but really add little to our knowledge. Maybe the perimetric profiles, the mesopic profiles, might be helpful if someone is embarking on a clinical trial.

The problem of drusen of the disc had a lot of discussion. The big advance is the recognition that these things can give rise to vascular membranes and can give hemorrhages.

I do not want to get into the controversy of Dr Cope's paper whether or not the patient had retinitis pigmentosa and drusen of the optic nerve, the audience can make up their own minds. I would like to say, however, since I have seen it so often, when you have a patient who has obvious ocular disease and has no neurological signs (and I am an ex-neurologist), do not subject him to the 2,000 dollar neuro-surgical massage. At least wait a while. They do not need double barrel arteriography, they do not need pneumoencephalography, unless you clearly have clinical signs other than the eye that would make you follow that course.

One of the most exciting aspects of this meeting is the continuous contribution which, while slow in coming, is probably as important as anything; the histopathologic correlation of lesions with the photographs, the fluorescein angiograms and then getting the eye and studying it. I think just one case like that is invaluable. Dr Ryan, Donald Gass, Paul Henkind's group and several others are to be congratulated. This is what we must look for and try to get the patients to sign up with an eye bank so if anything happens we get the eyes.

Coming to the pigment epithelium it is interesting that, as Paul said a while ago, the pigment epithelium can only respond in a few ways to an insult, and one of them is to turn a little creamy white; it does not matter what the insult is, an infarct, or a direct infection of the cells. We saw the cases with Harada's and S.O. with very similar appearance. We had central serous cases that looked very much like Harada. It is interesting that when these diseases all heal, (and I did not mention placoid) they all heal with more or less the same picture: a diffuse disturbance in the pigment epithelium; it reminds me of congenital rubella as you look at their fundus. I do not know what that means. Obviously there is great emphasis on auto-immune processes. This is the fashion today, at least in the United States, when an internist does not know what to call a disease it is auto-immune. While that is something to think about, we have not ruled out infection, whether it be viral or something else in many of these conditions.

One thing that struck me though as I listened to the papers and thought about it; we had a butterfly dystrophy presented by August Deutman with heavy pigment under the macula, we all know that Best's vitelliform can be yellow and we think that it is in the pigment epithelium, we had these patients with uveal effusions, with Harada's disease, with central serous; they have a serious loss of visual function and then when they recover they have these diffuse changes in the pigment epithelium and yet the vision can return to 20/20; they see very well. There is no correlation between what we see with the ophthalmoscope or what we record in the fundus and the visual acuity. That means that there is pigment epithelium probably there, it is just that the pigment is not necessarily important in each individual cell to give us normal function, or at least reasonably normal function.

The subject of genetics was discussed by Dr Deutman and you all know his contributions, you only have to read his book and to follow his papers. The most interesting thing to me was the report of a new entity of hereditary cystoid macular edema, which he has described as a dominant case that goes on to atrophy of the posterior polar area in the late stage or in the older group.

I might digress just for a moment about the paper of Dr Kottow on iris angiography and the correlation of the vascular changes in the iris and cystoid macular changes (CME). It was interesting and the fact that he could produce it with 2% Epinephrin was also interesting. Since we do not know the etiology of CME it does suggest that it is a more diffuse disease than just the macula.

Diabetic retinopathy has been a plague to us for a long time and will continue to be. The pathogenesis remains unknown despite Hunter Little's paper. But I do think that Hunter Little made at least a contribution to our understanding; this aggregation of cells could be a factor, obviously I do not think it is going to be one factor, but it could be a factor in producing the areas of capillary closure and infarcts in the retina. After all, we see capillary closure in sickle cell disease; it is not exactly the same, there the red cells have trouble, because of flow and change in shape, getting through the capillaries. Maybe, there is something with aggregation of red cells in the production of retinopathy.

From the first time we had fluorescein angiography and studied diabetics, most of us immediately went to juvenile diabetics and did studies on them to try to find out which came first; what you could see with the ophthalmoscope or was there a change in function that we could not recognize. Dr Toussaint answered that question first and I admit it is contrary to what I have observed but I have not observed it as well as he has, so I accept it. He had 7 cases in which he could not see anything in the fundus but could show changes in the permeability of the retinal vessels. It is a very important observation. The variability of this permeability is an important observation; the fact that it could come and go. I do not know what to make of it but it is very important.

I am going to skip Dr Hertel's model. I think it is interesting but I am not quite sure how it will predict the course of diabetic retinopathy because it does not take into account the major cause of blindness in diabetic retinopathy and that is the proliferative phase. It does not take into account the new vessels on the disc or the new vessels elsewhere, but there may be a correlation that we don't know yet. If you keep studying, it may be you can demonstrate that there is a correlation between what goes on in the macula and what goes on at the disc and in the periphery, but unless you do I do not think it is going to predict the course of diabetic retinopathy.

I might just digress at the moment. You know there has been a study in the United States for the past ..., my goodness I do not know for how long, a collaborative study on diabetic retinopathy. Since it has been released to the newspapers this week I believe I can comment on it. This study involves a little less than 1,800 patients. To get in the study they had to meet certain criteria which were photographically controlled by a reading centre. The treatment was a standard type of treatment and basically was the type of treatment advocated by Hunter Little in ablative treatment of diabetic retinopathy. The patients had to agree to be in the study obviously. It is experimental work on humans as all clinical trials have to be and they had to agree to be followed. There had to be a certain degree of retinopathy. While there was one exception basically the patient had to have proliferative retinopathy in at least one eye. We have analyzed the results on a regular basis and the statisticians, at least, are absolutely convinced that the eyes that had neovascularization on the disc and were subjected to pan-ablation photocoagulation have had a significant decrease in the incidence of blindness when compared to the control eyes. If they had new vessels on the retina elsewhere with vitreous hemorrhage the statisticians are convinced that it is also significant. All other types of diabetic retinopathy have not shown significant variation. At the present moment we are treating the second eye of all patients who fall into either of these categories, i.e., neovascularization on the disc or neovascularization elsewhere with vitreous hemorrhage.

Obviously some eyes have gone blind and cannot be treated. This is a very important study. It will be published in the April issue of the American Journal of Ophthalmology; those of you who get the AJO by air-mail will probably get it today.

The Japanese retinopathies are most interesting. One could not present a better paper than the paper on Takayasu disease. The paper on carbon disulfide was provocative in that it gave a fundus picture similar to that of diabetic retinopathy. As I was writing the note I decided this could be a perfect thing to try to initiate in an animal model. I met Arnall Patz and he had already started animal experiments on carbon disulfide so I guess next time we shall have some reports on that, Arnall.

The problem of preretinal fibrosis versus macular pucker was a little confusing. The entity that Paul Henkind was talking about of preretinal fibrosis, definitely should be separated from the severe macular puckers. Donald Gass does not agree with me; he thinks that it is a spectrum and they all ought to be considered the same; they are just variations within that spectrum. But I agree with Paul, I think they are two quite distinct entities and they ought to be separated. The general feeling at this moment at least in our institution, based on Paul's work plus some of our own work is that preretinal fibrosis, which is a relatively benign condition for visual function, is a proliferation of glial cells through breaks of the inner limiting membrane in the retina, whereas macular pucker and what has been called massive vitreous retraction or massive periretinal proliferation may well have its origin from the pigment epithelial cells growing on the surface to the retina. I might just tell you, that I personally never have seen a patient improve more than a line or so who had a severe pucker after retinal detachment operation. I have seen some membranes peel off just like what was presented here on preretinal fibrosis, but I have never seen a pucker after detachment operation improve more than a few lines. We recently, 3 weeks ago, had a patient come in with a vision of 5/200, six weeks after a retinal detachment operation. Dr Machemer took this patient to the operating room, did a pars plana vitrectomy and went in with a needle and peeled off the membrane, I do not have the photographs, but the pucker has gone away and the patient is 20/50, which I think is fantastic. So a whole new field is opening up involving operating right on the surface of the retina.

Peripheral vascular diseases: I do not have very much to say other than the fact that I am very impressed by the quality of the peripheral fundus photography. It is improving at each meeting, beautiful! It is interesting that we have basically two types of changes occurring in the periphery; one in which they apparently start out with normal peripheral retina and then ablate the peripheral vessels. Usually you can see little ghost vessels going out. The other happens in infants when the child fails to develop the peripheral vessels and that is why I think Arnall immediately asked about the birthweight of this patient with the avascular peripheral zone. I also think that some day we may find a correlation between the development of the retinal vasculature in the infant and equatorial degeneration. You certainly see it in patients with retrolental disease, it is different but it may well be just a forme fruste of some sort of related equatorial degeneration to whatever retrolental fibroplasia is. It is important that you all realize that retrolental fibroplasia is not a disease of the past; primarily because the pediatricians are not content to let the cerebrum be damaged just to save the vision. It is a delicate balance to have to walk. We must all be alert to retrolental disease.

The scientific aspects of this meeting as all meetings had some high points and some low points but I personally leave with a feeling that this has been a good to excellent symposium. There has been some new knowledge especially from people from countries that are diverse from my own background. There has been enough controversy without blood shed so we can go home and try to come up with some new experiments to answer the unresolved questions. There have been some excellent basic review papers from the younger participants.

On behalf of the committee, accept our sincerest appreciation for your participation – Bon Voyage.